T0201241

Current Therapy in Endodontics

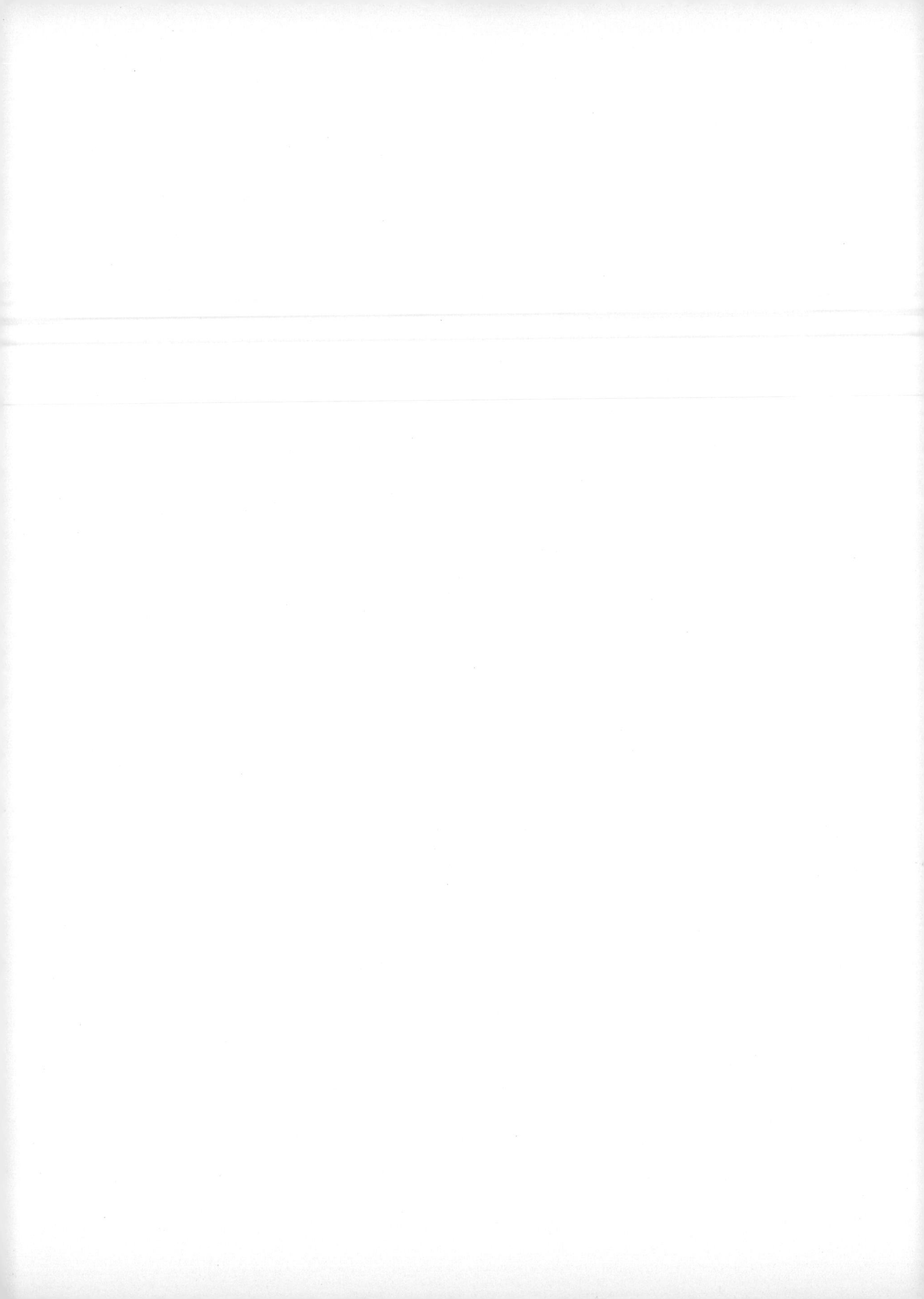

Current Therapy in Endodontics

EDITED BY

Priyanka Jain MSC, MDS, BDS

Specialist Endodontist
Dubai, UAE

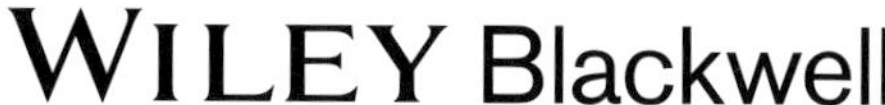

This edition first published 2016 © 2016 by John Wiley & Sons Inc.

Editorial offices: 1606 Golden Aspen Drive, Suites 103 and 104, Ames, Iowa 50010, USA
The Atrium, Southern Gate, Chichester, West Sussex, PO19 8SQ, UK
9600 Garsington Road, Oxford, OX4 2DQ, UK

For details of our global editorial offices, for customer services and for information about how to apply for permission to reuse the copyright material in this book please see our website at www.wiley.com/wiley-blackwell.

Authorization to photocopy items for internal or personal use, or the internal or personal use of specific clients, is granted by Blackwell Publishing, provided that the base fee is paid directly to the Copyright Clearance Center, 222 Rosewood Drive, Danvers, MA 01923. For those organizations that have been granted a photocopy license by CCC, a separate system of payments has been arranged. The fee codes for users of the Transactional Reporting Service are ISBN-13: 978-1-1190-6755-/ 2016.

Designations used by companies to distinguish their products are often claimed as trademarks. All brand names and product names used in this book are trade names, service marks, trademarks or registered trademarks of their respective owners. The publisher is not associated with any product or vendor mentioned in this book.

The contents of this work are intended to further general scientific research, understanding, and discussion only and are not intended and should not be relied upon as recommending or promoting a specific method, diagnosis, or treatment by health science practitioners for any particular patient. The publisher and the author make no representations or warranties with respect to the accuracy or completeness of the contents of this work and specifically disclaim all warranties, including without limitation any implied warranties of fitness for a particular purpose. In view of ongoing research, equipment modifications, changes in governmental regulations, and the constant flow of information relating to the use of medicines, equipment, and devices, the reader is urged to review and evaluate the information provided in the package insert or instructions for each medicine, equipment, or device for, among other things, any changes in the instructions or indication of usage and for added warnings and precautions. Readers should consult with a specialist where appropriate. The fact that an organization or Website is referred to in this work as a citation and/or a potential source of further information does not mean that the author or the publisher endorses the information the organization or Website may provide or recommendations it may make. Further, readers should be aware that Internet Websites listed in this work may have changed or disappeared between when this work was written and when it is read. No warranty may be created or extended by any promotional statements for this work. Neither the publisher nor the author shall be liable for any damages arising herefrom.

Library of Congress Cataloging-in-Publication Data

Names: Jain, Priyanka, 1976- editor.
Title: Current therapy in endodontics / [edited by] Dr. Priyanka Jain.
Description: Ames, Iowa : John Wiley & Sons, Inc., 2017. | Includes bibliographical references and index.
Identifiers: LCCN 2016024814 (print) | LCCN 2016026084 (ebook) | ISBN 9781119067559 (cloth) | ISBN 9781119067733 (pdf) | ISBN 9781119067740 (epub)
Subjects: | MESH: Root Canal Therapy–methods
Classification: LCC RK351 (print) | LCC RK351 (ebook) | NLM WU 230 | DDC 617.6/342059–dc23
LC record available at https://lccn.loc.gov/2016024814

A catalogue record for this book is available from the British Library.

Wiley also publishes its books in a variety of electronic formats. Some content that appears in print may not be available in electronic books.

Set in 8.5/12pt, MeridienLTStd by SPi Global, Chennai, India.
Printed and bound in Singapore by Markono Print Media Pte Ltd.

1 2016

I would like to dedicate this book to my parents, who have always encouraged and supported the pursuit of knowledge and for making me who I am. Thank you Mom and Dad.

Contents

List of figures

List of tables

Contributors

Angelo Barbosa de Resende, BDS
Endodontic specialist, Professor of a Specialization in Endodontic at
ABO PE - Associação Brasileira de Odontologia - Seção Pernambuco- Brazil

Brian Beebe, DDS, PC
Private Practice,
Bozeman, Montana, USA

Edward Besner, BS, DDS, FICD, FACD
Formerly Associate Clinical Professor, Department of Endodontics, Georgetown University School of Dentistry, Washington DC.
Lecturer in Endodontics, Institute for Graduate Endodontists, New York.
Consultant in Endodontics, Veterans Administration Training Center, Washington DC.
Founder and Past President, Virginia State Academy of Endodontics.
Diplomate of the American Board of Endodontics

Sami M. Chogle, MSD, BDS
Associate professor and Program Director,
Post- Doctoral Endodontics
Boston University, Henry M. Goldman School of Dental Medicine,
Boston, Massachusetts USA

Carla Cabral dos Santos Accioly Lins, PhD, MSc, BDS
Endodontic Specialist of Federal University of Pernambuco-Brazil.
Professor Adjunct, Department of Anatomy, Federal University of Pernambuco-Brazil

Kakul Dhingra, MDS, BDS
Private Practice,
Mumbai, India

Reza Farshey, DMD, CAGS
Private practice, Chevy Chase, Maryland, USA
Clinical Assistant Professor, University of Maryland School of Dentistry

Diógenes Ferreira Alves, PhD, MSc, BDS
Professor of a Specialization in Endodontic at ABO-PE/FOR (Associação Brasileira de Odontologia - Seção Pernambuco), Department of Endodontics, Federal University of Pernambuco, Recife, Brazil

Mansi Jain, AAID, MDS, BDS
Senior Lecturer, Inderprastha Dental College and Hospital, Uttar Pradesh, India.
Private Practice, Delhi, India

Priyanka Jain, MSc, MDS, BDS
Specialist Endodontist, Dubai, UAE
Clinic Tutor (Part time), Department of Endodontics, University Dental Hospital, Sharjah, UAE

James D. Johnson, DDS, MS
Chair and Clinical Professor
Program Director, Advanced Education Program in Endodontics
Department of Endodontics, School of Dentistry
University of Washington
Seattle, Washington, USA

Zuhair Al Khatib, BDS, MS
Formerly, Head of Endodontic Department, Dental Center, Dubai Health Authority, Dubai, UAE
Private Practice, Dubai.

Sahng G. Kim, DDS, MS
Associate Professor of Dental Medicine at Columbia University
Director, Post- Doctoral Endodontics, Department of Endodontics,
Columbia University College of Dental Medicine, New York, USA

Kathleen McNally, DDS
Advanced Education Program in Endodontics
Endodontics Department
Naval Postgraduate Dental School
Bethesda, Maryland

Scott B. McClanahan, DDS, MS
Chair and Professor,
Program Director, Advanced Education Program in Endodontics
Division of Endodontics, School of Dentistry
University of Minnesota,
Minneapolis, Minnesota, USA

Stephen P. Niemczyk, DMD
Director (Endodontic Microsurgery), Advanced Education Program in Endodontics Harvard School of Dental Medicine, Boston, Massachusetts.
Director (Director Endodontic Microsurgery), Advanced Education Program in Endodontics, Dental Division, Albert Einstein Medical Center, Philadelphia, Pennsylvania.
Private Practice in Endodontics, Drexel Hill, Pennsylvania, USA.

Mohammed AlShahrani, BDS, DScD, CAGS, FRCDC
Endodontist
Riyadh, Saudi Arabia

Faysal Succaria, DDS, MSD
Diplomate of the American Board of Prosthodontics,
Private Practice, Dubai, UAE

Mahantesh Yeli, MDS, BDS
Chair and Program Director, Graduate Endodontics,
Department of Endodontics,
SDM College of Dental Sciences and Hospital, Dharwad, India

Foreword

The clinical practice guidelines for endodontic therapy are changing at an accelerating rate due primarily to the abundance of impressive investigations published in peer-reviewed endodontic journals. The advances we are making in accurate pulpal and periapical diagnosis, treatment planning, new technologies enabling even higher quality endodontic therapy, pain prevention, and early detection of vertical root fractures are all due to the dedicated dental scientists who have expanded our body of knowledge.

One of the goals of this textbook is to distill the plethora of scientific investigations and reframe the findings to help dentists incorporate the latest developments and discoveries into clinical endodontic practice. Back in the 20th century, the studious dentist could become conversant with all the important endodontic literature. Those days are over! Thus, to gain the most current knowledge about every aspect of endodontics, Dr Priyanka Jain invited prominent professors and lecturers from around the world to contribute to this new textbook. Another goal of this textbook is to enable the curious clinician who wants to drill down into the literature to cite (or reference) the clinically relevant consort studies, meta-analyses of the literature, and/or systematic reviews of the latest investigations that enable the doctor to provide the best endodontic treatment available today.

Readers will meet some of the contributors, and Dr. Jain as well, along the way. When these moments occur, take the time to thank these men and women for their dedication to advancing endodontic science and generously sharing their knowledge with their colleagues.

Stephen Cohen, M.A., DDS, FICD, FACD
Diplomate, American Board of Endodontics
San Francisco, CA, USA

Preface

The discipline of endodontics has evolved rapidly over the years, both in terms of our understanding of the pathobiology of the disease process and in the evolution of new materials and technology, especially since the turn of the millennium. Developments, scientific studies, and research have contributed significantly to improved understanding, including possibilities and limitations. This new knowledge offers tremendous potential for endodontic success.

Although new materials and devices are important, the theoretical background and understanding of their clinical application is of even more significance. Keeping this as the main objective, I have endeavored to bring about work that incorporates the recent and current advances in the field of endodontics into one single textbook, to provide an up-to-date orientation in the daily endodontic practice while at the same time not losing sight of the basics. This book discusses the current advances in endodontics in the fields of materiality, technology, and the techniques that connect innovative science and materials with biological and evidence-based understanding.

The book starts with a brief discussion of diagnosis of endodontic problems, which can be a challenging part of the treatment. Prior to performing any endodontic procedure, it is crucial to establish pulpal and periradicular diagnosis. The chapter discusses the most currently used and introduced pulpal tests.

Radiology is an indispensable tool in endodontic practice. It is also an expanding science driven by constant changes in technology. The introduction of two-dimensional digital imaging allows us to attain accurate and clear instant images. The chapter on radiology talks about the recent advancement in this field in the form of cone beam computed tomography (CBCT), as well as improved understanding in radiographic interpretation as applied to endodontic practice. CBCT provides three-dimensional images that can be constructed by computer software to view tooth anatomy at any angle or direction. This provides a new level of information that improves our ability to diagnose and treat.

New and improved devices available for the endodontist today include battery-driven or electric motors with gear-reduction handpieces using nickel–titanium (NiTi) rotary file systems and new-generation electronic apex locators (EALs). Rotary NiTi files are an engineering wonder that continues to evolve. The new rotary instruments in NiTi are widely and universally accepted and have simplified the most complex part of the root canal treatment. The latest advancement comes in the form of the concept of reciprocation. The newer NiTi files that employ reciprocation are driven in a specifically designed motor and handpiece to rotate the file in different directions during instrumentation. The reciprocating motion is thought to minimize the risk of file separation. This has been discussed in great detail under rotary instruments.

A new resinous obturating material called Resilon has been introduced as a substitute for gutta-percha It has all the physical characteristics of gutta-percha (it is thermoplastic and soluble) and it also guarantees adhesion to the dentinal wall. This is used with resin-based cements and is becoming increasingly popular.

The introduction of surgical microscope, in combination with ultrasonic devices, makes it possible to conduct therapeutic endeavors and deliver treatment successes with great ease and clarity that were virtually unattainable previously. Today, in many specialist dental schools all over the world, endodontics is taught and carried out using the microscope. The operating microscope has transformed surgical endodontics into a microsurgical procedure. All the surgical phases – the incision, the root end preparation, and filling, as well as the suturing – can all be carried out using the microscope. This has definitively increased the predictability of the results, improved the prognosis, and raised the quality of success.

Lasers have also become an increasingly useful tool in endodontics. Their precision and less-invasive quality make them an attractive technology in our specialty.

Regenerative endodontics is also a very exciting area of endodontic treatment today. First introduced as a protocol in 2004, the concept of revascularizing a previously necrotic canal has become reality and is an area where we can expect significant development over the coming years.

Another area in its infancy but gaining popularity with tremendous scope is the field of teledentistry. Its use in endodontics has been briefly discussed to give the reader an insight into the opportunities this offers.

Many eminent national and international specialists, who excel in the art and science of endodontics, have made their contributions to this book. The authors recognize the fact that books alone cannot enhance our clinical skills, however well the information is presented. Theory must be incorporated into working knowledge through practice.

Every attempt has been made to incorporate all of the more widely used materials, but the list is exhaustive and it is beyond the scope of this book to cover each and every material and device on the market. The more common ones have been discussed. The text presents the material in a reader-friendly manner, with many clinical pictures and illustrations. Each chapter is accompanied by an extensive bibliography, allowing readers to explore in greater depth. We hope that this is just the beginning for the reader toward development in this exciting and fascinating field.

Enjoy the book, and we welcome your feedback at any time.

Acknowledgements

It has always been my desire to write a book, which would serve as a medium of information to learn and practice the art and science of endodontics. It took close to 2 years in conceiving and executing this project to completion. A book of this magnitude and scope can never be accomplished by a single person, and it is the outcome of the tremendous efforts and dedication of numerous individuals. This book is a true team effort. I would like to acknowledge and thank each one of my coauthors for their commitment and academic excellence toward this project. They are the true heart and spirit of this textbook.

Therefore, my sincere gratitude to:

Dr. Reza Farshey, author of the chapters on diagnosis and imaging technologies, Dr. Mahantesh Yeli and Dr. Kakul Dhingra, authors of the chapter on root canal filling, Dr. Sami Chogle and Dr. Faysal Succaria, authors of the chapters on restoration of endodontically treated teeth, Dr. Zuhair Al-Khatib, author of the chapter on traumatic injuries, and Dr. Edward Besner for his contribution on root resorption. Dr. Carla Cabral, Dr. Diogenes Ferreira Aves, and Dr. Resende, authors of the chapter on visualization in endodontics, Dr. James D. Johnson, Dr. (Capt.) Scott McClanahan, Dr. Kathleen McNally (Col. US Army) and Dr. Niemczyk, for their work on the chapter on microsurgery. Dr. Sahng G. Kim, for his expertise on pulp regeneration, Dr. Sami Chogle and Dr. Mohammed Al-Shahrani for their contribution and research on the chapter on lasers, and Dr. Mansi Jain for contributing to teledentistry.

I would also like to thank Dr. Isha Manon and Dr. Vikram Sharma for their constant moral support and help during the course of this project. Sincere thanks to Mr. Kumar Krishna Mohan, 3D graphics artist, for his help for the images and illustrations.

Sincere thanks to Dr. Stephen Cohen for providing the foreword for this book. He has always been my inspiration and I was very honored when he agreed to write the foreword.

I would like to thank my husband and children for their patience and support. It was not easy for them, especially towards the last stage when I went into hibernation.

Last but not least, I would like to thank Wiley and their team for their professional expertise in making this book a reality. Many thanks to Rick Blanchett, Teri Jensen, and Catriona Cooper for believing in this project and their professionalism and constant support ever since.

CHAPTER 1
Diagnosis

Reza Farshey[1,2]
[1] *Private practice, Chevy Chase, Maryland, USA*
[2] *Clinical Assistant Professor, University of Maryland School of Dentistry*

Dentistry has always been a fusion of science and art. Science provides the foundation for dentists to deliver optimal care. Evidence-based practice has successfully worked its way from medicine into dentistry. Every treatment decision that is made is at least partly influenced by the scientific support for its rationale. However, the science behind diagnosis relies on advancements in diagnostic equipment and armamentaria. The most consistent marker for an accurate diagnosis remains the clinician's ability to correctly process the diagnostic findings.

When patients are asked to grade the level of pain in an inflamed tooth after a painful stimulus is applied, it is foolish to assume a uniform and consistent response will be obtained from all patients. The International Association for the Study of Pain defines pain as an unpleasant sensory and/or emotional experience associated with actual or potential tissue damage [1]. Obviously, the physiologic condition of the tooth plays a major factor in pain perception, but the emotional aspect of this experience can modulate the pain levels among different patients. Factors such as past experiences, temperament, culture, gender, age, and overall pain tolerance can affect the responses. Recognizing this nuance is the trait of a good diagnostician. This is the *art* of diagnosis.

This chapter explores the various components that make up the examination process. A systematic approach to diagnosis is presented in order to gather the information thoroughly. A few clinical tips are offered to help clinicians with some of the confusing scenarios encountered during an examination.

Chief complaint

The chief complaint (CC) identifies the reason for the patient's visit. The information used to construct the CC is derived during the interview portion of the examination. This represents the very first interaction between the patient and the clinician. It is best to use the patient's own words when constructing the CC, rather than writing down a factual, objective sentence based on the initial interaction with a patient. For example, a chief complaint that reads *I have pain in my lower right back tooth after I bit down on an olive pit* is more complete than one that states *pain in the lower right tooth* or *evaluate lower right tooth*. Documenting the patient's own words often provides valuable information that can help steer the clinician toward an accurate diagnosis. It also allows the clinician to become familiar with the patient. Does the patient's demeanor suggest a high level of anxiety? Does the patient possess clarity of communication, or is the patient very vague and ambiguous when describing the purpose of his or her visit? Clinicians often overlook the significance of this last point. A patient lacking clarity of communication can make diagnosis more challenging for the clinician. Lastly, a well-documented CC allows the clinician to separate a coincidental finding or a coincidental diagnosis from the diagnosis that addresses the patient's CC.

Current Therapy in Endodontics, First Edition. Edited by Priyanka Jain.
© 2016 John Wiley & Sons, Inc. Published 2016 by John Wiley & Sons, Inc.

Medical history

Every patient who presents for evaluation or treatment should complete a thorough medical history form. The patient, or guardian if the patient is a minor, should sign and date the form. Prior to examining the patient, the clinician is responsible for reviewing the medical history with the patient, highlighting any medical conditions, a list of current medications, and any drug allergies. The clinician should initial the form to indicate that a review of the medical history has been completed. The medical history forms should be reviewed with the patient at every subsequent appointment and should be updated once a year to reflect any changes to the patient's medical history.

Many medical conditions require the clinician to modify a proposed dental treatment. Modifications to treatment can include shortening the appointment time, postponing elective treatment to a later date, or prescribing a course of antibiotics, just to name a few. Having a basic understanding of various medical conditions is paramount to providing appropriate care to patients with intricate medical conditions. The list of the medical conditions requiring a modification in dental treatment is vast. However, many textbooks and references are available to guide the clinician on how best to provide dental care for patients with medical conditions [2]. The clinician should also consult with the patient's primary health care provider if any aspect of the patient's medical history is not clear.

Recording the patient's blood pressure and pulse at the initial visit is an important step that provides the clinician with a broad snapshot of the patient's health status. Elevated blood pressure is associated with increased cardiovascular health problems. Even though hypertension is the most commonly diagnosed disease worldwide, undiagnosed hypertension is still prevalent in various patient populations. The findings of one study concluded that 20% of the sample patient population examined had undiagnosed hypertension [3]. Therefore, the clinician has an important role in screening for hypertension. Because the initial blood pressure readings can be elevated due to *white coat hypertension*, it is prudent for the clinician to obtain blood pressure readings at subsequent dental visits and compare the values.

If a patient presents with swelling or any other signs or symptoms of a dental infection, the patient's temperature should also be obtained and recorded. A febrile state justifies the use of antibiotics as part of a comprehensive dental treatment. The clinician should exercise caution when prescribing medications that may be contraindicated by the patient's medical history. Awareness of various drug–drug interactions that can adversely affect the patient's overall health is equally important. Online portals such as *HYPERLINK "http://www.pdr.net" www.pdr.net or lexicomp at HYPERLINK "http://www.wolterskluwercdi.com" www.wolterskluwercdi.com* are useful tools to aid clinicians in prescribing the appropriate pharmacological regimens for patients.

Relevant dental history

Clinicians often underestimate the importance of gathering an accurate account of the relevant dental history. Most clinicians transcribe the patient's description of the chronology of events as the dental history. Even though that is an important component, it is not the complete scope of the dental history. This chronology of events is better known as *history of present symptoms*. The other component of the dental history involves documenting any recent dental treatment in the offending area. If the patient is a new patient, the clinician should ask the patient about recent dental treatment. The information obtained can sometimes provide clues to guide the clinician toward an accurate diagnosis. For example, recent crown placement [4] or prior pulp capping [5] are positive findings that can lead to breakdown of pulp, even if the patient did not present with symptoms immediately after treatment was rendered.

Extraoral examination

Extraoral examination is the first opportunity for the clinician to examine the patient. This examination consists of a visual and a physical component. The clinician should look for any facial asymmetry. Asymmetry in the infraorbital, zygomatic, buccal, mandibular, or nasolabial regions may be an indication of facial swelling that has emerged from an intraoral source (Figure 1.1). If asymmetry is evident, the clinician should palpate the area to determine whether the swelling is firm or fluctuant, localized or diffuse.

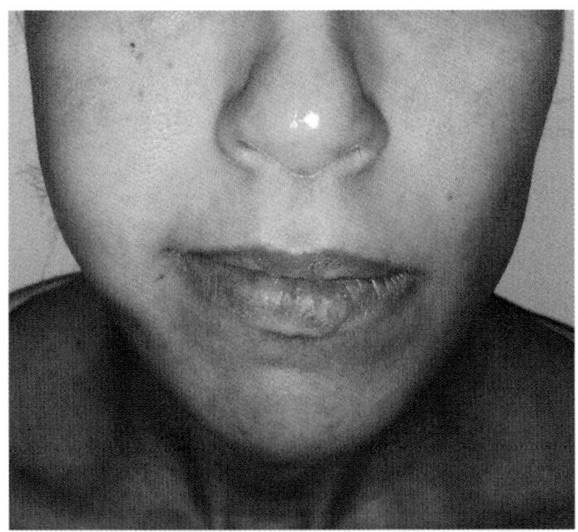

Figure 1.1 Extraoral examination includes a visual assessment of facial asymmetry.

Swelling from an infection often includes localized lymphadenopathy as a concomitant finding. Therefore, palpation of the cervical and submandibular lymph nodes is an important part of every examination sequence, and a firm or tender lymph node should be recorded in the patient's chart.

Intraoral examination

The information obtained from the patient's chief complaint, the relevant dental history, and extraoral examination should direct the clinician to a more-specific area of the mouth for further examination. The intraoral examination is a focused examination of the internal structures in the suspected region of the mouth. For this examination to be thorough, it is prudent to implement a systematic approach to the examination process. A good examination sequence follows a pattern of *broad to narrow*.

The soft tissues are examined first. The tongue and the uvula should be positioned at the midline. The gingiva, mucosa, cheek, and tongue are dried using a dry gauze pad, and inspected for any abnormalities. The abnormality can be in color or texture. The presence of ulcerations is also an abnormality that must be noted. When recording an abnormality, a description of its color, texture, size, and location should be noted. The general rule is to reexamine the site in two weeks. If the abnormality is still present, the patient should be referred to an oral pathologist for further evaluation.

The clinician should then move to the quadrant of interest, to further examine the soft tissues. Intraoral swelling or the presence of a sinus tract should be noted. Swelling should also be palpated to determine if it is diffuse or localized and whether it is firm or fluctuant. This is an important point to emphasize, because a fluctuant swelling indicates whether a treatment of incision and drainage may be appropriate.

A sinus tract is defined as a pathway from an enclosed area of infection to an epithelial surface [6]. A sinus tract develops when a chronic infection drains to the surface and forms a nodule, known as a *parulis* (Figure 1.2). A sinus tract should be traced, when possible, because the location of the parulis may be distant to the source of the infection [7]. To trace a sinus tract, a thin gutta-percha point is placed through the tract until resistance is felt (Figure 1.3). A radiograph is exposed, allowing the clinician to see the path of infection to the source.

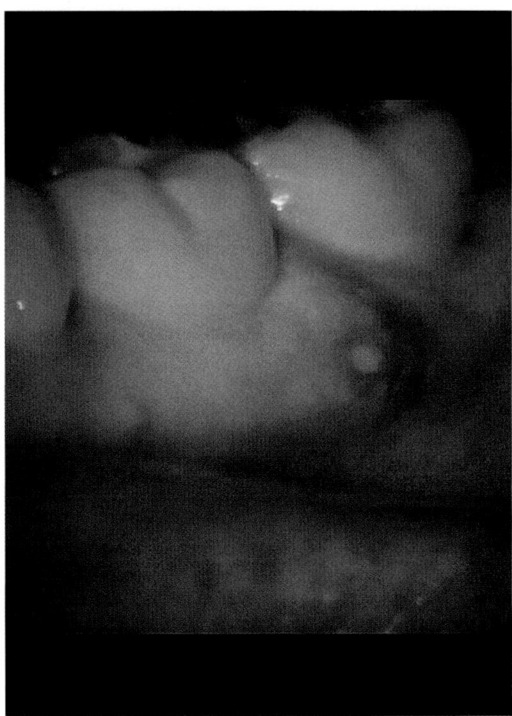

Figure 1.2 The presence of a sinus tract must be noted in the examination report.

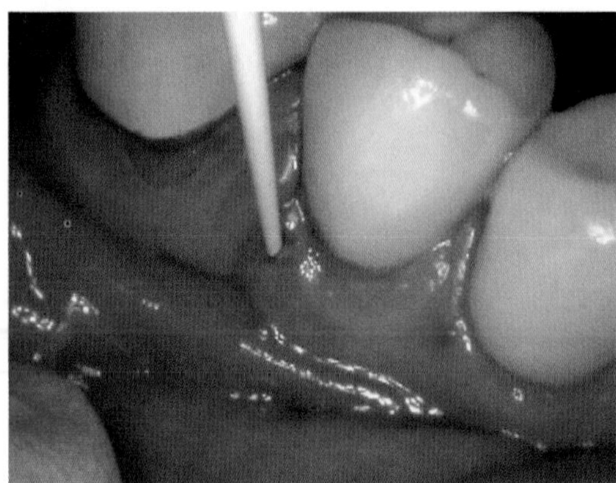

Figure 1.3 A gutta-percha point is placed through the opening of the sinus tract until resistance is felt. A radiograph is obtained to identify the path of the sinus tract.

Palpation

The purpose of palpation is to assess the texture, rigidity, and tenderness of the tissues around the teeth. Palpation is performed using an index finger. This helps identify any areas of swelling that were not previously identified. Any tenderness to palpation, as compared to the contralateral side, should be recorded in the patient's chart.

Percussion

Percussion testing helps identify inflammation in the periodontal ligaments of a given tooth, termed *periradicular periodontitis*. If the patient's chief complaint includes pain when chewing or sensitivity to pressure, it can most likely be duplicated by performing a percussion test. The test is performed by gently tapping the occlusal surface using a blunt instrument, such as the back end of the mirror handle (Figure 1.4). It is prudent to test the contralateral side first so the patient can get accustomed to what a *normal* response feels like. The clinician should employ a simple system to record the values during percussion testing. Using one of three possible values of *normal, slight,* or + are sufficient to provide the necessary information for diagnostic purposes. Many clinicians assign multiple + values, such as +++, to emphasize the degree of sensitivity in a given tooth. This approach rarely adds any clinical significance, and it serves to complicate the diagnostic process by introducing an arbitrary component to the test. Having a simple value of *normal, slight, or* + is more than sufficient to underscore its importance.

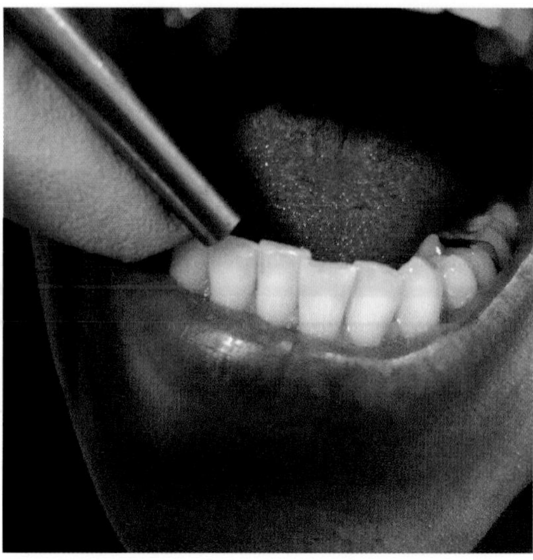

Figure 1.4 Percussion testing is best performed by tapping a tooth using the back end of a mirror handle. The tapping force should be consistent when testing multiple teeth.

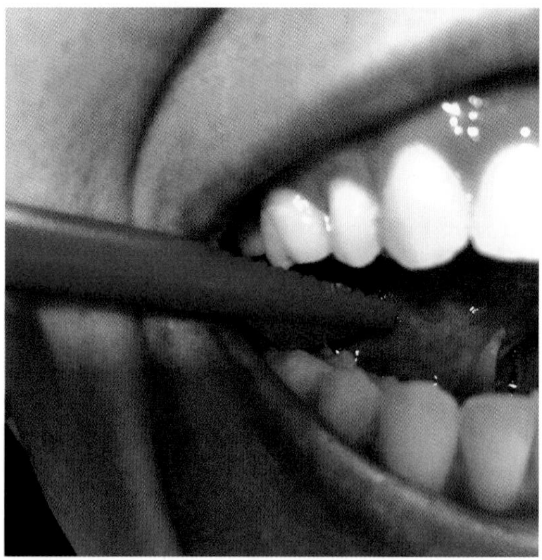

Figure 1.5 The Tooth Slooth is used to test for biting sensitivity in a given tooth.

The Tooth Slooth (Professional Results, Laguna Niguel, CA) can also be used to determine whether periradicular periodontitis is present. The plastic device is placed on the occlusal aspect of a given tooth, and the patient is asked to bite down on the stick (Figure 1.5). A painful response to biting down confirms inflammation in the periodontal ligaments of the tooth. Additionally, when the patient reports pain on release, this is usually an indication of a cracked tooth. Refer to page 10 for more information on crack classifications.

Periodontal examination

The periodontal examination includes recording the probing depths of a given tooth, and mobility, if present. Grading the degree of mobility is rather arbitrary and ranges in increasing degree from +1 mobility to +3 mobility.

Probing depths should be measured in six areas of a tooth. The mesial, mid-root, and distal areas of the buccal and lingual aspects are measured. A probing depth greater than 4 mm signifies a possible periodontal attachment loss and may be a significant factor in the overall diagnosis.

Pulp testing

The patient's responses to pulp tests provide the requisite information that allows the clinician to formulate a pulpal diagnosis. Therefore, it is easy to see why pulp testing is one of the most important components of the diagnostic process. When diagnostic mistakes occur, they commonly result from misinterpretation of pulp test data, which can lead to an inconclusive diagnosis or misdiagnosis. Two common methods for pulp testing are electrical and thermal stimulations.

Electrical stimulation

Electrical stimulation is performed using a commercially available device, commonly referred to as the electrical pulp tester (EPT) (Figure 1.6). The tooth should be dried adequately and the probe from the device must be coated with toothpaste, which helps in the transfer of the current. Care must be taken to ensure the probe is placed over an area of natural tooth surface. Small probes are available that are suitable for placement under a crown margin, where tooth structure may be exposed. The patient needs to hold the probe in place to activate the current. Current is transferred to the tooth in increasing intensity until the patient feels a tingling sensation. The results of the EPT are usually interpreted as positive or negative (if no sensation is felt). The numerical reading is not usually of diagnostic importance, unless the value for one tooth is demonstrably higher than that for the other teeth. Even so, no definitive conclusions can be drawn from the disparity in values, only that test results may be questionable and further testing should be performed.

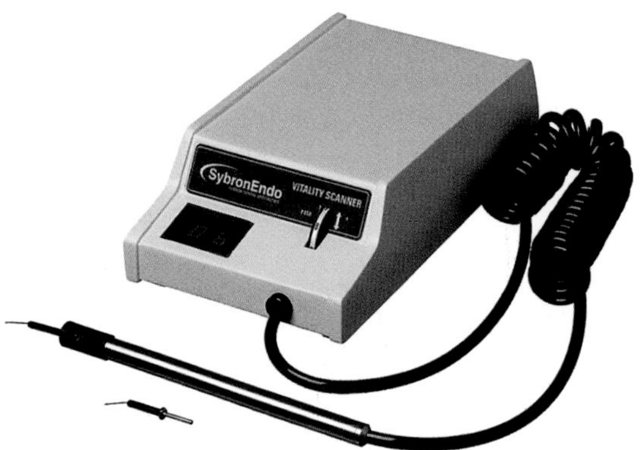

Figure 1.6 The Vitality Scanner 2006 from Kerr is a common electrical pulp testing device used in endodontic diagnosis. (Image courtesy of Kerr Endodontics.)

Thermal testing

Thermal testing is best performed using a refrigerant spray. The most effective refrigerant spray contains 1,1,1,2-tetrafluoroethane as its active ingredient and is commercially available as Endo-Ice (Hygenic Corp., Akron, Ohio) (Figure 1.7). Endo-Ice is easy to handle, easy to store, and environmentally safe. Endo-Ice has a low liquid temperature of −26.2 °C, which can decrease the intrapulpal temperature of a tooth effectively, thus making it useful for diagnostic testing [8].

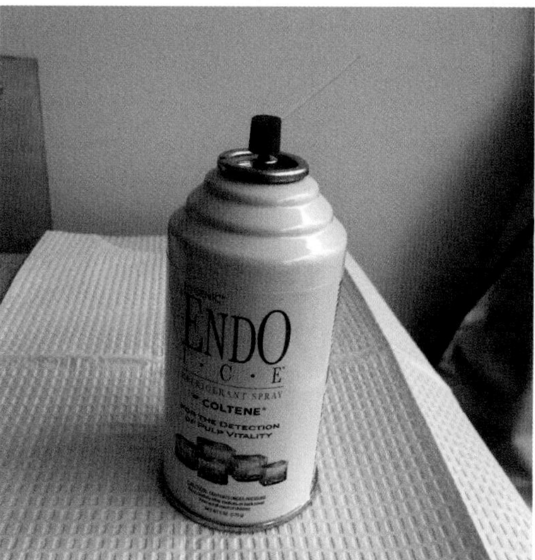

Figure 1.7 Endo Ice has an effective working temperature to make it an ideal refrigerant for thermal testing.

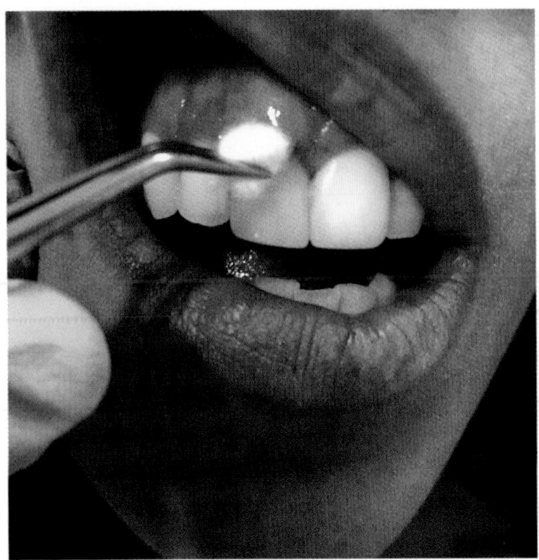

Figure 1.8 Placing the pellet on the cervical third of the tooth ensures an accurate patient response.

Thermal testing should first be performed on a contralateral tooth to identify the *baseline* response for a given patient. The baseline response is the typical response of a normal tooth to thermal testing. This helps the clinician to identify a suspect tooth during testing, by identifying when a response deviates markedly from the baseline response. Endo-Ice, or any other suitable refrigerant, is sprayed liberally on a size #2 cotton pellet, and the pellet is placed immediately on the cervical third area of the tooth (Figure 1.8). The pellet is removed when the patient experiences a sensitive response. The patient is then asked about the onset, intensity, and duration of the sensitivity. The patient's response allows the clinician to formulate a pulpal diagnosis. For example, an immediate sensitive response that disappears rapidly on removal is generally accepted as a *normal* response. A hypersensitive response to thermal testing that disappears rapidly on removal is associated with *reversible pulpitis*. If the hypersensitive response is prolonged, or if sensitivity lingers after the stimulus is removed, then the pulp is in a state of *irreversible pulpitis*. Finally, a lack of response to the cold stimulus indicates *pulpal necrosis*.

Comparison of methods

A number of studies that conclude cold testing is more reliable than electrical testing [9] [10], and conventional wisdom supports this conclusion. For example, cold testing can enable the clinician to distinguish among the different stages of a vital pulp (normal, reversible pulpitis, and irreversible pulpitis), whereas EPT is usually interpreted as all or none (vital or necrotic).

The future

Laser Doppler flowmetry (LDF) is based on a technology that objectively measures the vitality of the pulp by way of assessing the blood supply rather than the sensory function. An infrared light beam is projected through the crown of the tooth. Based on the Doppler principle, if the frequency or the wave of the light beam is shifted, then there are moving red blood cells in the pulp. If the light remains unshifted, the pulp tissue is deemed necrotic. Many studies have found LDF to be accurate, reliable, and reproducible in assessing the pulp status [11]. However, the technology has not yet reached a point where the testing mechanisms or the equipment are practical and cost effective for everyday clinical use [11–13].

Pulse oximetry is an oxygen saturation monitoring technique that has been widely used in medical practice for years. A probe is placed over a tooth; the probe contains two light-emitting diodes: red light and infrared light. Some of the light is absorbed as it passes through the pulp tissue. A sensor on the other end of the tooth detects the amount of absorbed light. Since oxygenated and deoxygenated hemoglobin absorb different amounts of red and infrared lights, this ratio is used by the oximeter to calculate pulse rate and the oxygen concentration in the blood [14]. Like LDF, the pulse oximeter is an *objective* test, eliminating some of the bias challenges seen in thermal and electrical testing. However, much like LDF, the available pulse oximetry machines are not suitable for private dental offices because they are very expensive [15].

Box 1.1 lists other experimental diagnostic testing mechanisms that have been in research since the 1990s [17–19].

Interpreting Radiographs

Dental radiography is the most objective tool available to the clinician. The decision to expose radiographs (and if so, how many) is based on the information gathered from the previous portions of the diagnostic process. The chief complaint, extraoral and intraoral examinations, and pulp testing should provide the clinician with a preliminary impression of the type of dental problem the patient is presenting with. Many

Box 1.1 Experimental Diagnostic Testing Modalities

Photoplethysmography

Photoplethysmography is an optical measurement technique that can be used to detect blood volume changes in the microvasculature using a light with a shorter wavelength [16].

Transillumination

Transillumination uses a strong light source that identifies color changes that can indicate pulpal pathology [17].

Ultraviolet light photography

Ultraviolet light photography detects the different fluorescence patterns that can allow additional contrast of visible change that are otherwise more difficult to observe [18].

Cholesteric liquid crystals

The use of cholesteric liquid crystals in detecting pulp vitality is based on the principle that teeth with an intact pulp blood supply have a higher tooth-surface temperature compared with teeth that have no blood supply.

Optical reflection vitalometer

The optical reflection vitalometer is a system based on pulse oximetry. The difference from conventional oximetry is that adsorption is measured from reflected light instead of transmitted light. One can see the pulse of the pulp or the oral mucosa. This device may be used in cases of partially erupted or fractured teeth.

Thermographic imaging (Hughes Probeye Camera)

Thermographic imaging is another noninvasive method of recording the surface temperature of the body [19]. It is a highly sensitive method.

clinicians make the mistake of formulating a diagnosis solely on whether a lesion is present or absent on a radiograph. In many instances, an endodontic lesion is present but is not noticeable in a radiograph [20].

Because endodontic diagnosis is a focused examination, the number of radiographs exposed should be limited. In general, two or three periapical radiographs, exposed from different angles, allow adequate visualization of anatomical structures. In addition, at least one vertical bitewing should be exposed. The proximity of caries or a restoration to the pulp of a tooth is best determined with a bitewing radiograph. A vertical bitewing has an added benefit of providing the clinician with an impression of the alveolar crest and the furcation areas of a tooth.

When interpreting radiographs, clinicians often focus on the most obvious findings and overlook other, subtle findings that may be clinically significant. This can have deleterious consequences for both the clinician and the patient. Therefore, it is best to employ a systematic approach to interpreting radiographs. This ensures that radiographs are interpreted thoroughly and consistently every time. Once again, a pattern of broad to narrow, or general to specific, ensures that radiographs are thoroughly interpreted. Table 1.1 outlines the common structures that should be interpreted when evaluating a radiograph.

Tips for an accurate diagnosis

The components that make up the diagnostic data consist of objective and subjective findings. Objective findings are clinician derived and include radiographic interpretations or clinical observations, such as swelling and fever. Subjective findings are patient derived, such as the chief complaint and patient responses to various pulp tests. An accurate diagnosis is made when the clinician correctly interprets and processes these findings. Because the subjective findings are patient derived,

Table 1.1 Interpreting the dental radiograph.

Structure	Interpretation
Caries and quality of existing restoration	Proximity to the pulp
Osseous levels, including the alveolar crest	Bone loss Inconsistency in trabeculation
Lamina dura	Intact or missing
Radiolucency or radiopacity	Location
Widening of the periodontal ligament	Location
Root appearance	Normal or resorbed
Pulp canal space	Normal, calcified, or enlarged Traceable or not

the information obtained can be confusing at times and can mislead the clinician. Different patients perceive pain differently; therefore, responses can appear atypical or unorthodox at times. The following tips are provided to help minimize errors in interpreting test results.

- During testing for percussion sensitivity, it may be difficult for some patients to communicate the level of sensitivity clearly. If typical responses from a patient include "they all hurt" or "none of them hurt," it may be better to perform tests on pairs of teeth at a time, similar to an eye exam with the optometrist. Some patients can provide a clearer response when asked to compare sensations between two teeth, as opposed to responding about sensitivity on one tooth.
- In general, it is best not to inform the patient about which tooth is being tested. This ensures there is no bias in responses.
- Correctly interpreting a patient's response during cold testing can be challenging, especially when testing a necrotic tooth. One solution may be to approach this test differently. Before testing, the clinician should inform the patient that the purpose of the test is to assess the *maximum threshold* to cold. So, rather than placing a cold pellet on the tooth and asking the patient if it is sensitive, the focus should be on the maximum length of time the patient can tolerate the cold pellet. This approach minimizes the possibility of obtaining a false positive response from a necrotic tooth.
- During thermal testing, patients should be asked to rate their levels of sensitivity using a numerical scale. A scale of 1 to 10 works best, where 1 represents no sensation and 10 represents the worst pain. The clinician should first establish a numerical value for the *baseline* response, thereby calibrating the scale for each patient.
- Even though endodontic diagnosis sometimes involve multiple teeth, it is best to perform treatment one tooth at a time. In employing this modular approach to treatment, where the most obvious tooth is treated first, and the other teeth are reevaluated after a short interval, the clinician minimizes the risk of misdiagnosing or overtreating a patient.

Diagnostic terms

When making an endodontic diagnosis, it is important to provide both a *pulpal* and *periradicular* status for the tooth in consideration. The information gathered from the examinations, clinical testing, and radiographic findings is what is required to make an endodontic diagnosis. Tables 1.2 and 1.3 illustrate the classification states that are routinely associated with symptoms.

Since the 1950s, various diagnostic terms have been used to describe, essentially, the same clinical scenario. At a consensus meeting in 2008, the American Association of Endodontists sought to standardize the terminology used for pulpal and periradicular classifications. This was done in the interest of providing a uniform classification system to be used by clinicians, researchers, authors, and educators. The following are the various classification terms approved by the American Association of Endodontists and the American Board of Endodontics to describe different pulpal and periradicular conditions.

Table 1.2 Pulpal classifications.

Condition	Symptoms* Yes	No	Maybe
Normal pulp		¶	
Reversible pulpitis	¶		
Symptomatic irreversible pulpitis	¶		
Asymptomatic irreversible pulpitis		¶	
Pulpal necrosis		¶*	
Previously treated		¶*	
Previously initiated treatment		¶*	

*Symptoms are exhibited when the periodontal ligament is inflamed. Necrotic pulps or pulpless teeth do not exhibit symptoms in the absence of periodontal ligament inflammation.

Table 1.3 Periradicular classifications.

Condition	Symptoms Yes	No	Maybe
Normal		¶	
Symptomatic apical periodontitis	¶		
Asymptomatic apical periodontitis		¶	
Acute alveolar abscess	¶		
Chronic apical abscess			¶

Classification of pulp

Normal pulp

A diagnosis of normal pulp (NP) is made when a tooth does not exhibit any atypical symptoms during testing. The tooth responds positively to pulp testing; however, the sensation is transient and disappears in seconds. When identifying a tooth as a control tooth during pulp testing, that tooth is intended to have a diagnosis of NP.

Reversible pulpitis

Two findings differentiate reversible pulpitis (RP) from a normal pulp: In RP, the suspect tooth is hypersensitive to thermal testing, as compared to a control tooth. In RP, a clinical finding such as caries, deep restoration, failing restoration, or exposed dentin is commonly seen during examination.

Symptomatic irreversible pulpitis

The pulps of these teeth generally have spontaneous pain. The pain may be sharp or dull, of short duration or long, and localized or diffuse. When pulp testing, the pain from testing lingers well after the stimulus is removed. Radiographs might show a finding such as deep caries or a deep restoration. When reviewing the dental history, it is not uncommon to find recent treatment involving a deep restoration, pulp exposure, or a pulp-capping procedure. However, this diagnosis is mainly a symptom-based diagnosis.

Asymptomatic irreversible pulpitis

In asymptomatic irreversible pulpitis, the tooth is not symptomatic; however, the suspect tooth usually shows caries that has extended into the pulp. The tooth may respond normally to thermal testing. Whereas symptomatic irreversible pulpitis is mainly a diagnosis derived from symptoms, asymptomatic irreversible pulpitis is a diagnosis derived from clinical or radiographic findings. Some examples include a tooth that has radiographic evidence of caries extending into the pulp or an asymptomatic tooth that has had a carious pulp exposure.

Pulpal necrosis

In pulpal necrosis, the pulp of a given tooth does not respond to pulp testing. No other associated findings need to be present in order to make this diagnosis.

Previously treated

The classification of a previously treated tooth is different from the others described above because the diagnosis is made by the dental history and radiographic confirmation that the tooth has had endodontic treatment (Figure 1.9).

Previously initiated treatment

Teeth with previously initiated treatment have had endodontic treatment initiated but not completed. Similar to the *previously treated* classification, pulp testing is not needed in order to make this diagnostic. There needs to be a recent dental history that pulpotomy or pulpectomy was performed or a radiographic verification that the pulp of the tooth has been partially treated. The difference between this classification and *previously treated* is that endodontic treatment has not been completed.

Classification of the periradicular area

Normal

The tooth responds normally to percussion and palpation testing. Radiographically, the lamina dura is intact, and the periodontal ligament space is uniform with no indication of periradicular rarefaction.

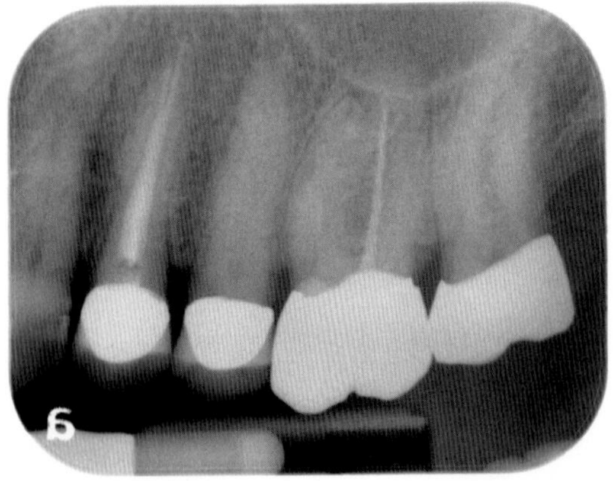

Figure 1.9 Even though endodontic treatment on tooth #14 is incomplete, the pulpal diagnosis would still be previously treated.

Symptomatic periradicular periodontitis

This is perhaps the easiest classification to make for clinicians. The diagnosis is made if the tooth is sensitive to biting pressure, percussion testing, or palpation. However, there is no swelling. Radiographic findings may or may not be present. However, this diagnosis is based solely on the presence of symptoms during testing.

Asymptomatic periradicular periodontitis

In asymptomatic periradicular periodontitis, the tooth responds normally to percussion and palpation testing, but there is radiographic evidence of radiolucency in the periradicular region of a tooth. The radiographic evidence can be subtle, such as widening of the periodontal ligament space, or it can be obvious, such as periradicular lucency. It must be emphasized that the patient does not present with any pain to percussion or palpation testing.

Acute apical abscess

Acute apical abscess is an inflammatory reaction to a pulpal infection, characterized by swelling of the tissues, spontaneous pain, and tenderness of the tooth to pressure and percussion. The patient also often presents with fever, lymphadenopathy, or a general feeling of malaise. The presence of swelling and the other systemic signs of an infection distinguish this stage from *symptomatic periradicular periodontitis*. Radiographic findings may or may not be present; the hallmark finding in this classification is intraoral swelling.

Chronic apical abscess

Chronic apical abscess is an inflammatory reaction to pulpal necrosis or a previously treated tooth, often characterized by slight or no discomfort and an intermittent discharge through a sinus tract. The release of pressure by drainage through a sinus tract is the reason there is little or no discomfort. Radiographically, periradicular radiolucency is seen. The presence of a sinus tract is what separates this classification from asymptomatic apical periodontitis.

Classification of cracks in teeth

The mouth is a dynamic environment that subjects teeth to various destructive forces throughout one's lifetime. Functional and parafunctional forces contribute the most to this destruction and often lead to the development of cracks in teeth. The presence of cracks can lead to changes in the pulp–dentin complex, which can in turn affect pulpal diagnosis. Cracks in teeth are *findings;* to diagnose a tooth as a *cracked tooth* is incomplete within the context of an endodontic diagnosis. There are five distinct types of cracks seen in teeth: craze lines, fractured cusp, cracked tooth, split tooth, and vertical root fracture.

Craze lines

Craze lines are superficial breaks in the crystalline structure of the tooth and are limited to only the enamel layer. Because there is no extension into the dentin, the tooth is completely asymptomatic. Treating a craze line is only necessary where esthetics is the primary concern. To differentiate a craze line from other types of cracks in teeth, transillumination is performed. A craze line allows the light to transmit through completely, whereas a deeper crack blocks the transmission of light in that segment, thus highlighting the location of the crack.

Fractured cusp

As the name implies, fractured cusp involves cracks that are initiated from the cusp of the tooth. It may be a complete or incomplete fracture (Figure 1.10), and it is directed mesiodistally and buccolingually along a buccal or lingual groove. The crack may extend subgingivally.

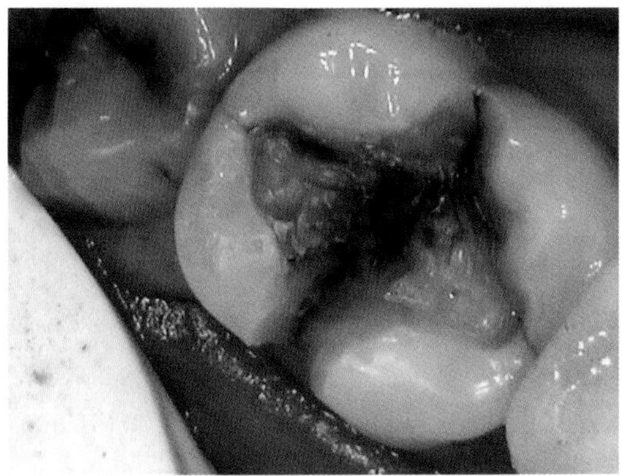

Figure 1.10 After the restoration is removed, inspection of the underlying tooth surfaces reveal an incomplete fracture of the mesiobuccal cusp, extending mesiodistally and buccolingually along a buccal groove.

Treatment involves removing the fractured cusp and placing a suitable restoration. Endodontic treatment is only warranted if the crack is seen extending into the pulp space or if a diagnosis of symptomatic irreversible pulpitis or pulp necrosis is made.

Cracked tooth

A cracked tooth is an incomplete fracture. Clinically, a cracked tooth advances in a mesiodistal direction, extending into one or both marginal ridges (Figure 1.11). A cracked tooth extends more apically than a fractured tooth and therefore has a higher chance of resulting in pulpal or periapical pathology. Treatment can range from restoring the tooth with a full-coverage restoration to extraction, depending on the extent and location of the crack. Root canal treatment is only indicated if the diagnosis confirms a need for it. If the decision is made to keep the tooth and root canal treatment is indicated, the patient should be made aware that the long-term prognosis of a cracked tooth is questionable.

Split tooth

If a cracked tooth is left untreated, it eventually results in a complete fracture, forming two entirely separate segments. This is known as split tooth (Figure 1.12) A split tooth shows mobility. Treatment involves removing the smaller (or more mobile) segment and assessing the structural integrity of the remaining segment for restorability.

Vertical root fracture

Vertical root fracture (VRF) is defined as a complete or incomplete fracture initiated in the root of a given tooth. A VRF occurs exclusively after the tooth has had endodontic treatment (Figure 1.13). The fracture is usually located on one or both proximal surfaces (buccal or lingual) and can extend coronally. Radiographic verification of a VRF can be challenging, because the appearance can mimic that of a failed endodontically treated tooth. However, cone beam computed tomography (CBCT) imaging provides a greater degree of accuracy in identifying VRFs. Clinically, the presence of a sinus tract, along with a narrow, deep periodontal pocket associated with a tooth that has had endodontic treatment usually indicates a VRF. The only predictable treatment of a VRF is extraction of the tooth.

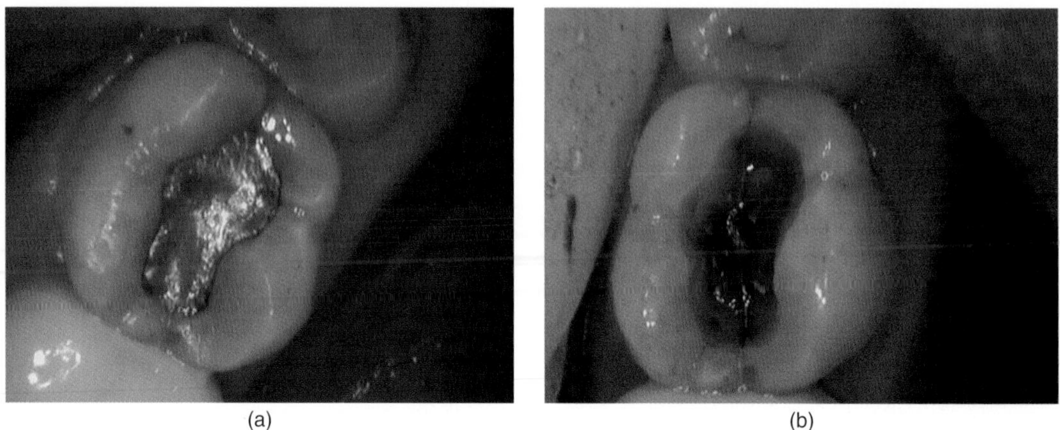

Figure 1.11 A crack is seen advancing in the mesiodistal direction. *A*, With the restoration in place. *B*, With the restoration removed.

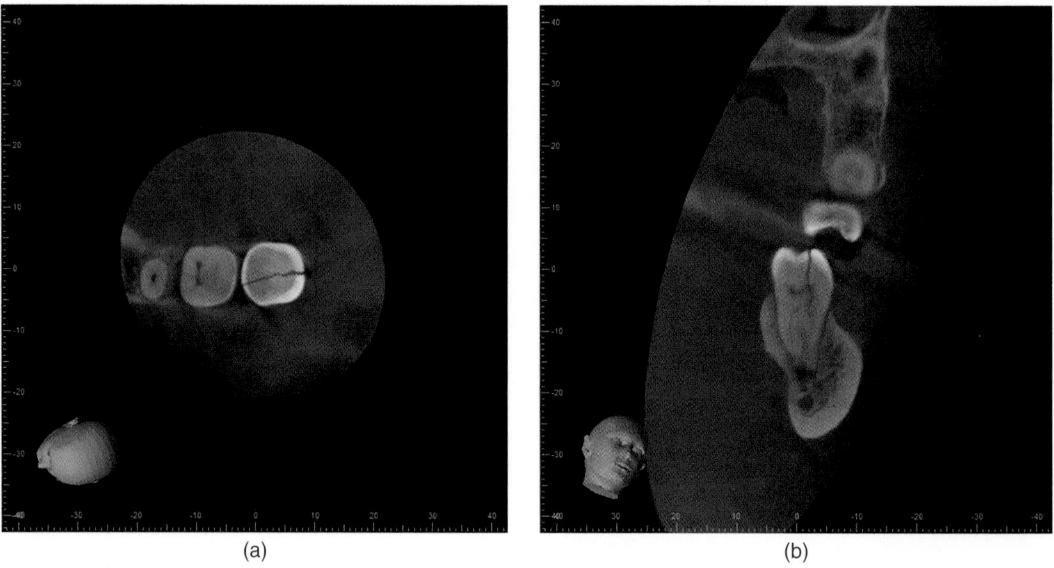

Figure 1.12 A coronal and axial slice from a conebeam volume reveals a crack that has extended apically and formed two separate segments. This is known as a *split tooth*.

Conclusion

The importance of correct diagnosis must not be underestimated. A treatment plan can only be drawn up when a correct and accurate diagnosis has been made. Newer techniques and devices in endodontic diagnosis are ever evolving. Careful attention to these new diagnostic aids and tools combined with an understanding of their usefulness and limitations is necessary if they are to be employed most effectively in clinical dentistry.

**This Taxonomy/statement has been reproduced with permission of the International Association for the Study of Pain® (IASP). The Taxonomy/statement may not be reproduced for any other purpose without permission.*

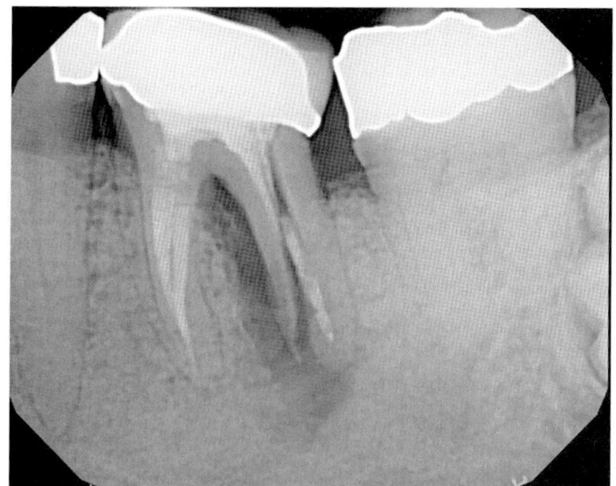

Figure 1.13 This is a more obvious example of a vertical root fracture. In most cases, identifying a vertical root fracture can be challenging without the aid of advanced imaging modalities.

References

1 Merskey H, Bogduk N. *Classification of Chronic Pain*, 2nd edition. Seattle: IASP Press; 1994.

2 Little JW, Falace DA, Miller CS, Rhodus NL. *Dental Management of the Medically Compromised Patient*. 8th edition. St. Louis: Elsevier; 2013.

3 Engstrom S, Berne C, Gahnberg L, Svardsudd K. Efficacy of screening for high blood pressure in dental health care. *BMC Public Health* 2011; 11: 194–201.

4 Krell KV, Rivera EM. A six year evaluation of cracked teeth diagnosed with reversible pulpitis: treatment and prognosis. *J Endod* 2007; 33: 1405–1407.

5 Barthel C, Rosenkranz B. Pulp capping of carious exposures: treatment outcome after 5 and 10 years: a retrospective study. *J Endod* 2000;26: 525–528.

6 *Glossary of Endodontic Terms*, 8th edition. Chicago: American Association of Endodontists; 2012. Sinus tract, p. 46.

7 Ingle JI, Bakland L. *Ingle's Endodontics*. 5th edition. London: BC Decker; 2002.

8 Jones VR, Rivera EM, Walton RE. Comparison of carbon dioxide versus refrigerant spray to determine pulpal responsiveness. *J Endod* 2002; 28: 531–534.

9 Weine FS. *Endodontic therapy*. St. Louis: CV Mosby, 1972, p. 46.

10 Cohen S, Burns RC. *Pathways of the pulp*. St. Louis: CV Mosby; 1976, p. 17.

11 Chen E, Abbott PV. Evaluation of accuracy, reliability, and repeatability of five dental pulp tests. *J Endod* 2011; 37: 1619–1623.

12 Evans D, Reid J, Strang R, Stirrups D. A comparison of laser Doppler flowmetry with other methods of assessing the vitality of traumatised anterior teeth. *Endod Dent Traumatol* 1999; 15: 284–290.

13 Emshoff R, Emshoff I, Moschen I, Strobl H. Laser Doppler flow measurements of pulpal blood flow and severity of dental injury. *Int Endod J* 2004; 37: 463–467.

14 Jafarzadeh H, Rosenberg PA. Oximetry: review of a potential aid in endodontic diagnosis. *J Endod* 2009; 35: 329–333.

15 Dastmalchi N, Jafarzadeh H, Moradi S. Comparison of the efficacy of a custom-made pulse oximeter probe with digital electric pulp tester, cold spray and rubber cup for assessing pulp vitality. *J Endod* 2012; 38: 1182–1186.

16 Schmitt JM, Webber RL, Walker EC. Optical determination of dental pulp vitality. *IEEE Trans Biomed Eng* 1991; 38: 346–352.

17 Hill CM. The efficacy of transillumination in vitality tests. *Int Endod J* 1986; 19(4): 198–201.

18 Foreman PC. Ultraviolet light as an aid to endodontic diagnosis. *Int Endod J 29843*; 16(3): 121–126.

19 Kells BE, Kennedy JG, Biagioni PA, Lamey PJ. Computerized infrared thermographic imaging and pulpal blood flow: Part 1. A protocol for thermal imaging of human teeth. *Int Endod J* 2000; 33: 442–447.

20 Bender IB, Seltzer S. Roentgenographic and direct observation of experimental lesions in bone I. *J Am Dent Assoc* 1961; 62: 152–60.

Questions

1 What is the best way to verify thermal sensitivity on a tooth?

A Use an ice cube.
B Use a cold refrigerant spray, such as Endo-Ice.
C Ask the patient to breathe in air through his or her mouth.
D Take the patient's word for it.

2 A given tooth with irreversible pulpitis always has an associated lingering response to cold.

A True
B False

3 Which of the following statements is or are true?

i. A necrotic pulp does not respond to cold testing.
ii. A necrotic pulp always shows periapical radiolucency.
iii. It is possible for a tooth exhibiting irreversible pulpitis to also show acute alveolar abscess.

A Both i and ii are correct.
B Only i is correct.
C Only ii is correct.
D All of the statements are correct.
E None of the statements are correct.

4 If a clinician is certain of a diagnosis based on clinical findings alone, it is acceptable to forgo exposing a radiograph.

A True
B False

5 Electric pulp testing is more accurate than thermal testing in assessing pulp vitality.
A True
B False

6 Which of the following findings is always associated with a diagnosis of asymptomatic irreversible pulpitis?
A Spontaneous pain
B Swelling
C Recent pulpectomy procedure
D Radiographic evidence of caries extending into the pulp chamber

7 Antibiotics should be prescribed to a patient who presents with swelling, fever, and lymphadenopathy.
A True
B False

8 Which of the following findings negatively affects the prognosis of a tooth?
A A crack
B Swelling
C Presence of a sinus tract
D Lingering pain to hot fluids

9 Percussion testing is done to identify inflammation in the periodontal ligaments of a given tooth.
A True
B False

10 Teeth with the following pulpal diagnosis do not respond to thermal testing.
A Pulpal necrosis
B Previously treated
C Normal pulp
D All of the above
E Only a and b

CHAPTER 2

Imaging technologies

Reza Farshey[1,2]

[1] *Private practice, Chevy Chase, Maryland, USA*

[2] *Clinical Assistant Professor, University of Maryland School of Dentistry*

Dental imaging is the most objective clinical tool available to the clinician during an examination. There have been many improvements, both in quality and in radiation hygiene, since the discovery of x-rays by Wilhelm Roentgen in 1896. Even so, x-ray imaging in the health care arena is not without controversy. Patients presenting for evaluation today have an increased level of knowledge and awareness of the harmful effects of radiation compared to two decades ago. The information (or misinformation) is readily available for the patient to acquire. An op-ed in a *New York Times* article is just one example of how information is accessible to the public. [1] Therefore, the clinician should maintain a factual knowledge of the risks and benefits of various x-ray modalities to present to a concerned patient.

A concern within the medical community is that certain healthcare professionals default to obtaining the best imaging module when an inferior one with a lower radiation level would have achieved the same result. An example in dentistry is obtaining routine cone-beam computed tomography (CBCT) scans on patients simply as a diagnostic tool. Part of this flawed rationale stems from a fear of missing a clinical finding. However, there is also a sense that the radiation levels are too low to be detrimental to the health of the patient.

According to the National Council on Radiation Protection and Measurements (NCRP), radiation from medical imaging is the single biggest source of controllable radiation exposure for the public. The NCRP has adopted a new acronym to help emphasize the importance of optimization in imaging. The concept of as low as reasonably achievable (ALARA) has been modified to as low as diagnostically acceptable (ALADA). The purpose is to emphasize the importance of ordering the image with the least radiation while achieving its diagnostic purpose. [2] Stated differently, the clinician should order the image with the lowest radiation levels that allow him or her to make a correct diagnosis.

Digital radiography

Digital radiography has many advantages over wet film radiography. The most significant advantage is lower radiation exposure for patients [3]. Secondly, images are viewed on a computer monitor. Thirdly, the ability to share pertinent findings on a large computer screen is a more effective patient education tool. And lastly, with digital radiography, the need for processing chemicals is eliminated (Figure 2.1).

There are two types of digital radiography systems on the market: The direct digital systems use an intraoral sensor to produce an instantaneous digital image on a computer monitor. The indirect photo-stimulable phosphor (PSP) systems use a plate, which resembles a dental film, to capture an image. The plate is then placed into a scanner, which produces a digital image within a few minutes.

Direct digital radiography

Direct radiography systems incorporate solid-state technology, such as charge-coupled devices (CCD) or complementary metal oxide semiconductors (CMOS) to acquire a high-resolution image. The sensor is connected to a computer via USB to display and store the image data. Advances in digital radiography have focused on making the sensors less bulky and increasing the spatial resolution of the displayed image. Wet film has a spatial resolution of 16 lp/mm, which increases to about 20 to

Current Therapy in Endodontics, First Edition. Edited by Priyanka Jain.
© 2016 John Wiley & Sons, Inc. Published 2016 by John Wiley & Sons, Inc.

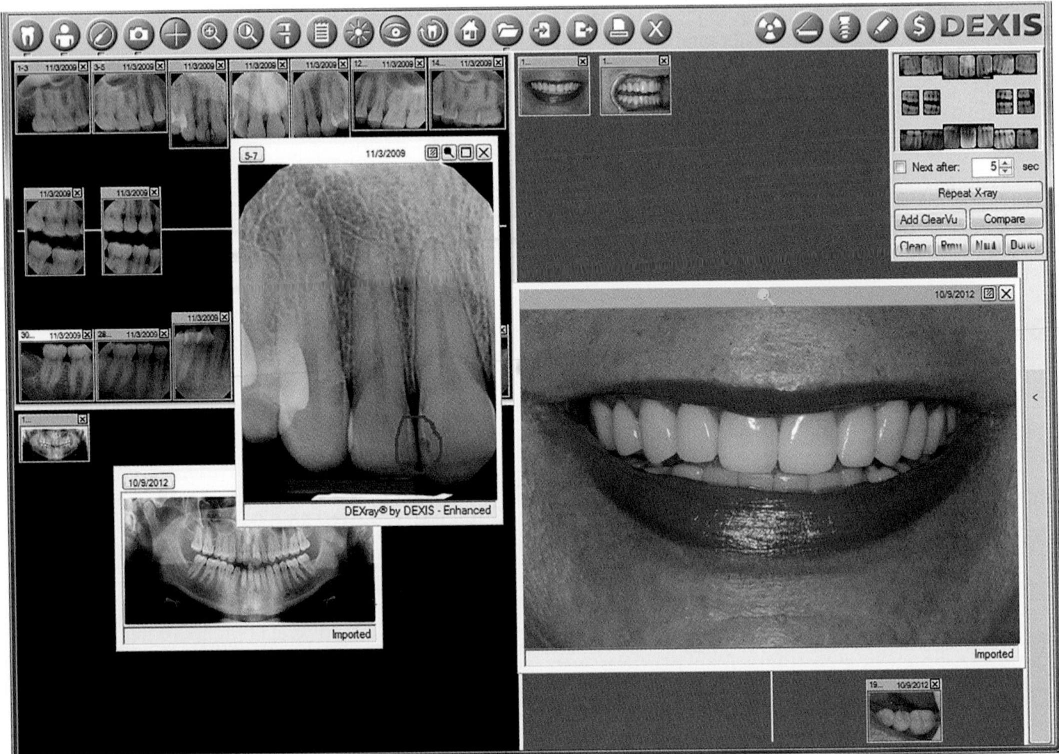

Figure 2.1 A digital image is viewable instantly on a large computer monitor. With available image enhancement tools, patients can more easily visualize important findings, such as caries or a periapical radiolucency.

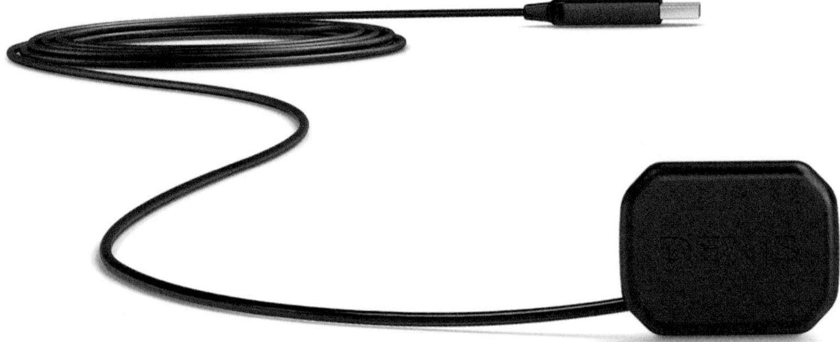

Figure 2.2 The Dexis Platinum Sensor features a beveled corner design to enhance patient comfort. The attached wire connects to a computer via USB to yield high-resolution images instantly. (Image courtesy of Dexis LLC, Hatfield, PA, USA.)

24 lp/mmwith magnification. [4] Newer digital imaging systems have similar or higher spatial resolution. However, the sensor with the highest spatial resolution is not always the best sensor. The human eye is only capable of identifying 10 to 13 lp/mm without any visual aids. [5] Choosing the right system should therefore be based on a number of factors. The cost, warranty, longevity, thickness of the sensor, image quality, and functionality of the software are just a few factors that need to be considered when choosing a sensor (Figure 2.2).

Indirect digital radiography

The PSP system uses a reusable, film-like plate. The image is captured by the thin plate and processed using a laser scanner. PSP resembles wet film radiography in technique. There are no bulky sensors, or wires for the dental staff to be concerned with. Even though the scanning process takes some time to produce the images, obtaining the image is still faster than wet film radiography.

PSP is easy to use, is comfortable for the patient, and requires minimal staff training to incorporate into a practice because most conventional RINN kit holders work well with PSP. The thin screen needs to be replaced from time to time. Most manufacturers claim the screens to last between 500 and 1000 uses. However, independent studies quantifying the maximum number of uses for the PSPs are limited. One study claims the screens become nondiagnostic after 50 uses, [6] and another study found the number to be 200. [7] However, due to the low replacement cost of the thin plates, the discrepancy over the maximum number of uses should not be a major factor in the decision to transition from wet film to digital imaging. PSPs are, in general, more cost effective in the long run than direct digital sensors (Figure 2.3).

Digital imaging is a key component of the modern dental practice. Because the technology has advanced to the point where direct and indirect digital systems are better alternatives to wet film radiography, the decision to transition should be easy.

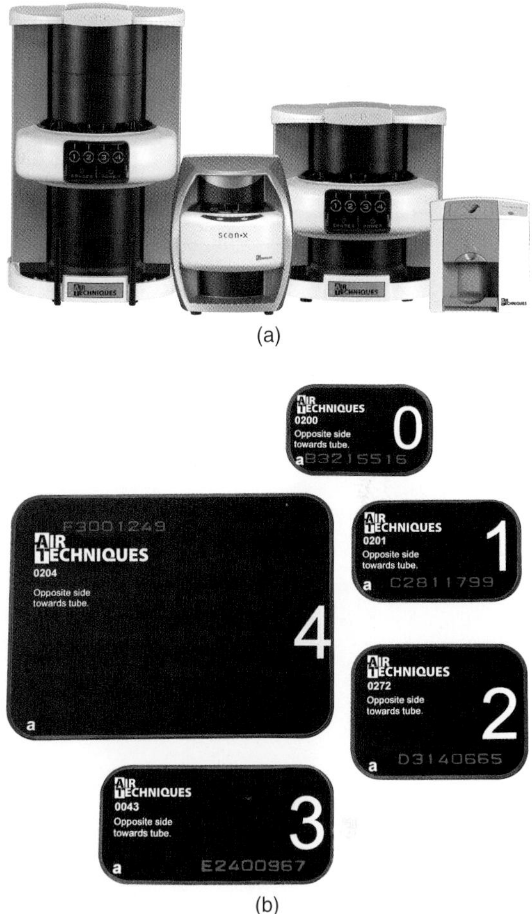

Figure 2.3 ScanX from Air Techniques is an example of a photo-stimulable phosphor system. *A*, The scanning units come in various sizes to handle larger tasks. *B*, The imaging plates come in various sizes similar to a wet film. (Image courtesy of Air Techniques, Melville, NY, USA.)

Cone-beam technology

Cone-beam imaging technology is most commonly referred to as cone-beam computed tomography (CBCT) or cone-beam volumetric tomography (CBVT). The first CBCT unit for dental use was approved by the U.S. Food and Drug Administration in March of 2001. [8] Since that time, there has been an exponential growth in this technology. The number of CBCT device manufacturers in the market today is estimated to be around 50. [9] As the benefits of CBCT imaging gain universal acceptance, through exposure in continuing education courses and scientific articles, the trend will continue as more practitioners choose to acquire one.

Incorporating CBCT imaging into the dental practice will also see an increased liability for clinicians from the perspective of insurance carriers. For example, a clinician is responsible for interpreting the entire imaging area in a CBCT volume, not just the areas pertaining to his or her specialty. Therefore, a clinician can be exposed to unfamiliar findings. It is recommended to consider submitting every CBCT scan to an oral and maxillofacial radiologist (OMR) for an overread. [10, 11] (Figure 2.4).

The technology

A cone-shaped x-ray beam is projected onto a flat panel detector (FPD) while the C-arm rotates around the patient. The volume of data is captured by the FPD and transferred to a computer. A software program, proprietary to each manufacturer, reconstructs the final images for the viewer. The areas of interest are presented in the three anatomic planes: axial, sagittal,

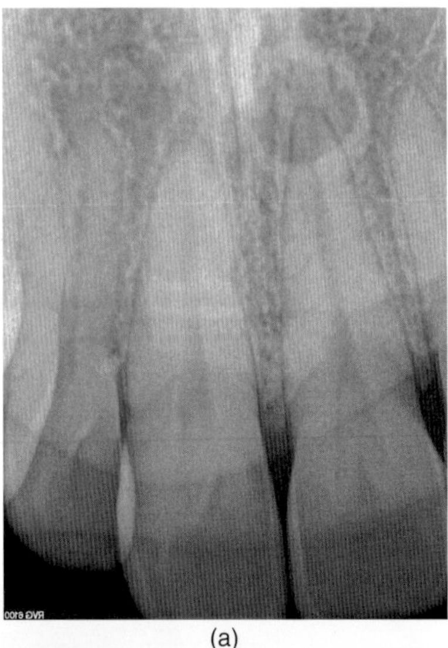

(a)

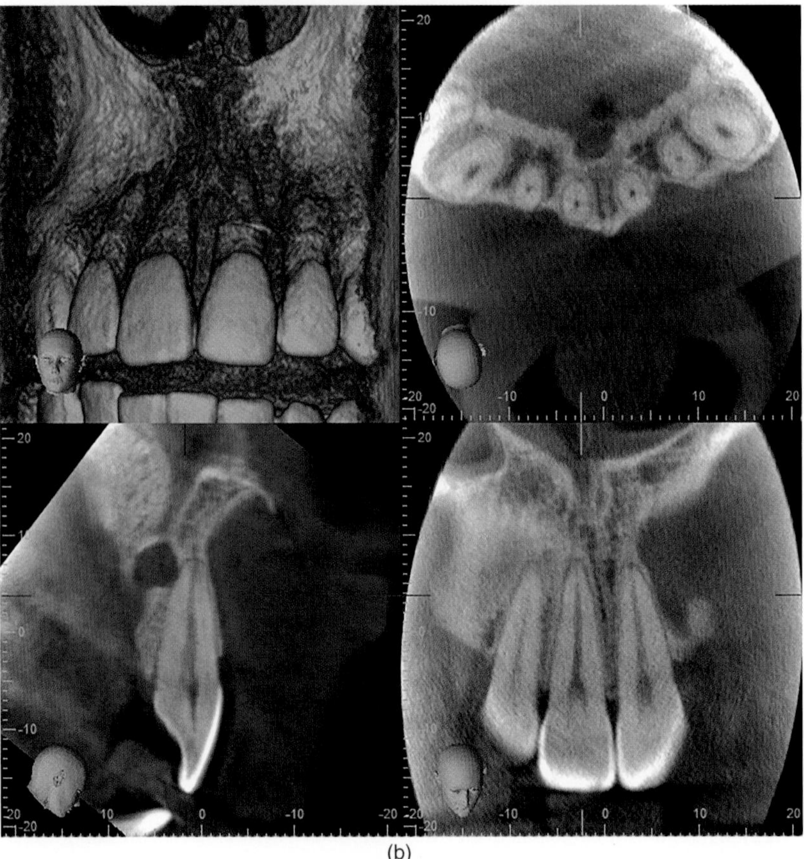

(b)

Figure 2.4 *A,* Periapical lucency is seen associated with the right maxillary central incisor. *B,* A cone-beam computed tomography scan of the area depicts a well-defined circular low-density area palatal to the root of the tooth. An overread from an oral and maxillofacial radiologist confirms a diagnosis of nasopalatine duct cyst.

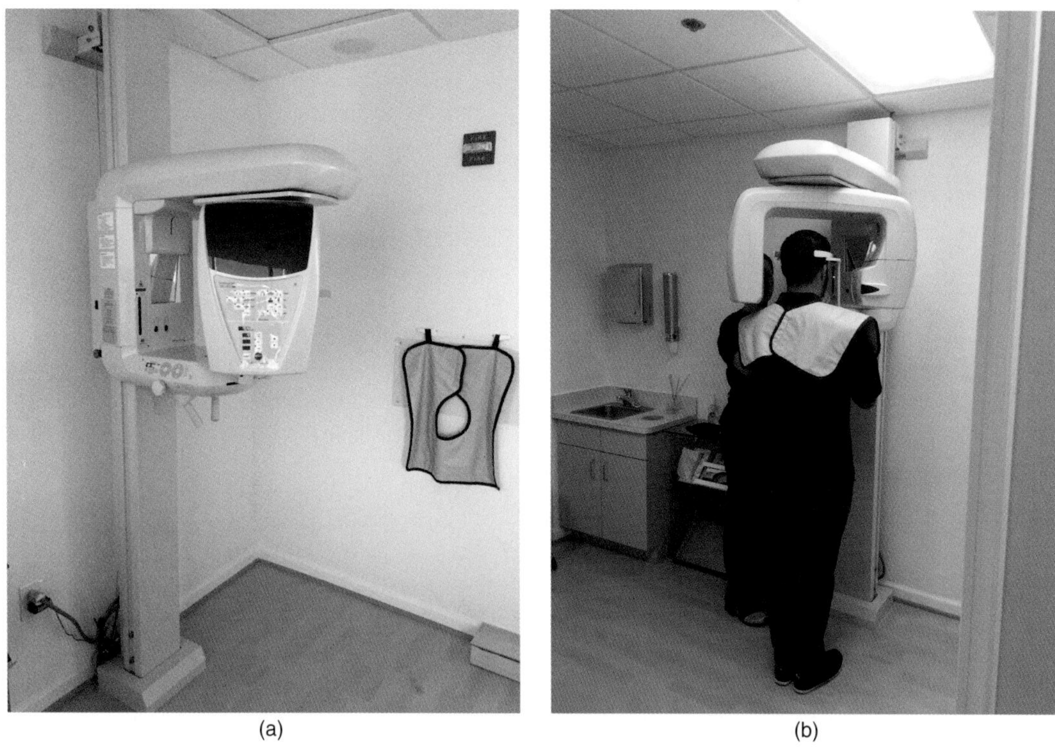

Figure 2.5 *A* and *B*, The Veraviewepocs 3De (J. Morita Manufacturing Corp., Kyoto, Japan) cone-beam computed tomography machine has a footprint similar to that of a panoramic machine.

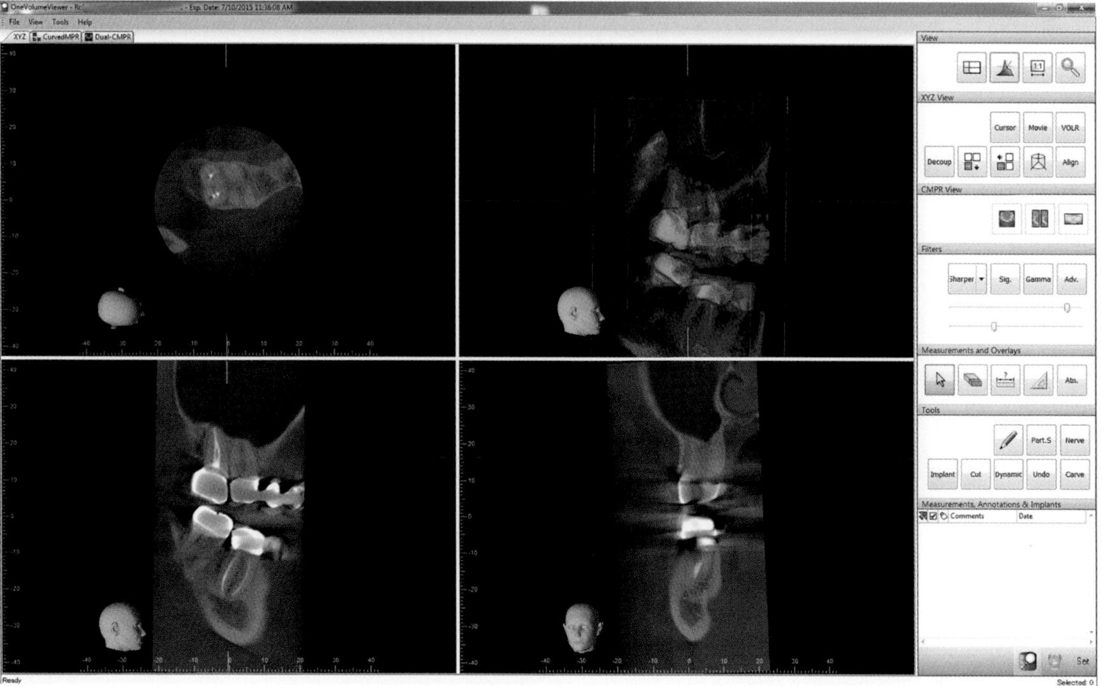

Figure 2.6 One Volume Viewer (J. Morita Manufacturing Corp., Kyoto, Japan) is a versatile viewing program designed to give the clinician maximum functionality in an easy and intuitive interface.

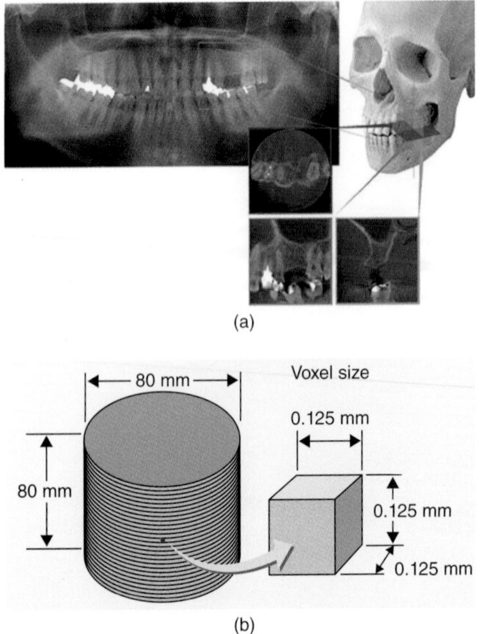

Figure 2.7 *A,* A panoramic scout image is used to define the region of interest for 3D imaging: Axial plane (red box), sagittal plane (blue box), and coronal plane (green box). *B,* An isotropic (symmetrical) voxel provides a highly accurate image that is free of distortion. (images courtesy of J. Morita Manufacturing Corp., Kyoto, Japan)

and coronal. The axial and proximal (sagittal in anterior region, coronal in posterior region) views are of particular value because they cannot be visualized with conventional radiography. (Figures 2.5–2.7).

The volume acquired by a CBCT is composed of tiny isotropic cubes, known as voxels. Just as a pixel is a minimum unit for a digital photo, a voxel (volumetric pixel) is a minimum unit for 3D data. The voxels populate a cylindrical shaped area, known as the field of view (FOV). Generally speaking, a smaller voxel size yields a higher resolution because more voxels can fit within the FOV. The dimension of the FOV depends on a number of factors, such as the size of the FPD and the projection geometry of the x-ray beam. The x-ray beam is collimated to limit the radiation exposure to the area within the FOV. Therefore, a smaller FOV yields a lower effective radiation dose to the patient. [12] Also, a smaller FOV yields a higher resolution because the associated voxels tend to be smaller. For these reasons, it is recommended that a small FOV CBCT be used for endodontic applications (Figure 2.8) [13, 14].

Advantages

The obvious advantage of CBCT over conventional radiography is the ability to visualize an area of interest in three dimensions. Having the axial and proximal views on hand enables clinicians to enhance their

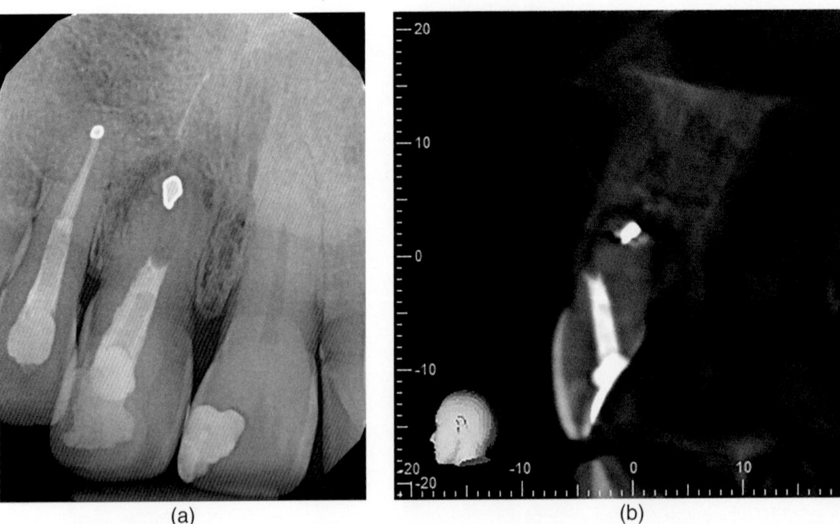

Figure 2.8 A comparison of a periapical (PA) radiograph *(A)* and a proximal slice from a cone-beam computed tomography scan of the same area *(B)* highlights the advantages of 3D imaging in endodontic diagnosis. The proximal slice shows a transported and perforated root canal treatment that is not evident in the PA radiograph.

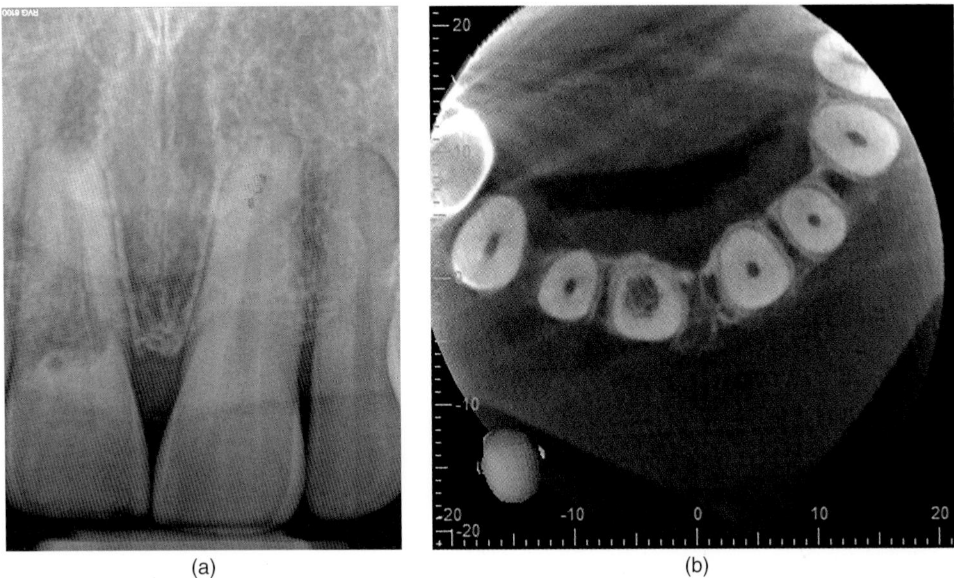

Figure 2.9 *A*, Right maxillary central incisor exhibits an apparent resorptive lesion at midroot level. *B*, An axial slice from a cone-beam computed tomography scan provides the necessary information on the type of resorption (internal or external) and the prognosis of the tooth.

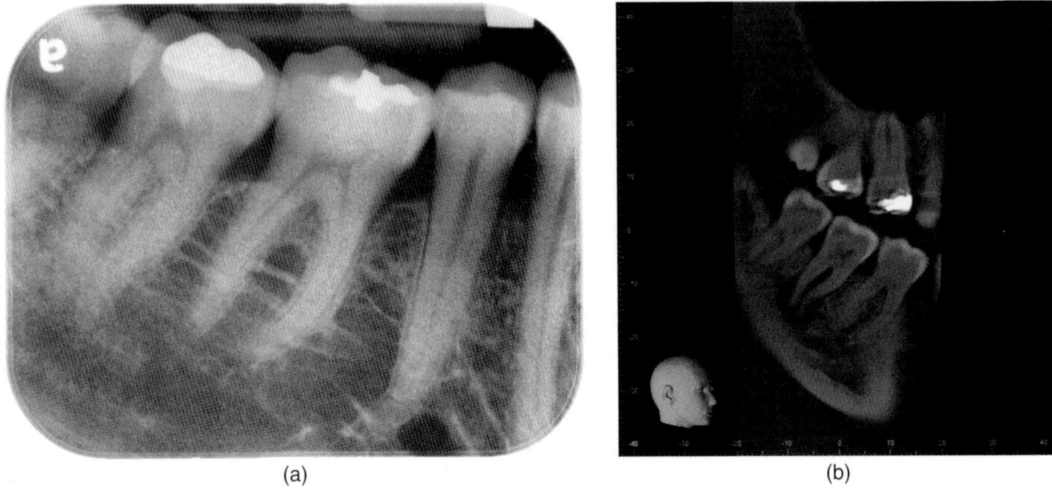

Figure 2.10 *A*, Posteroanterior radiograph of the mandibular right second molar depicts a normal presentation of bone. *B*, A sagittal slice of a cone-beam computed tomography scan of the same area depicts a well-defined low-density finding in the periapical region of the tooth.

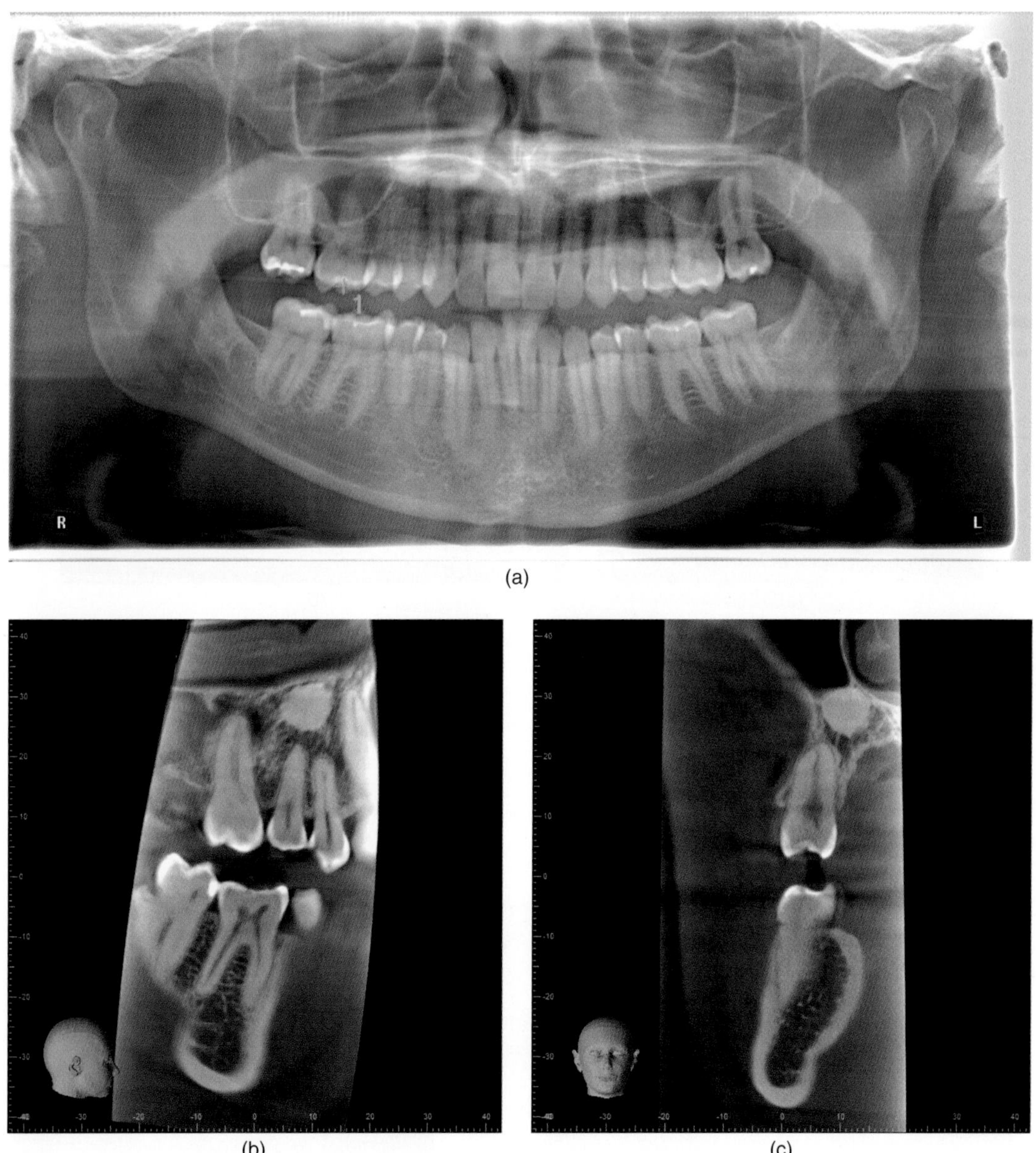

Figure 2.11 *A,* A panoramic radiograph fails to show a radiopaque finding apical to the area of the maxillary right bicuspids. Sagittal *(B)* and coronal *(C)* slices from a cone-beam computed tomography scan of the same area depict the high-density mass clearly. An overread provided by an oral and maxillofacial radiologist identified the high-density mass as idiopathic osteosclerosis.

clinical findings to provide a more accurate diagnosis. Findings such as an unobturated fourth canal in an upper molar, periapical (PA) lesions, and vertical root fractures (VRF) are identified more accurately using CBCT imaging compared to a PA radiograph [15–17].

However, because of the higher radiation levels, CBCT imaging should only be advocated as a secondary imaging modality, where indicated. Regarding the use of CBCT in endodontic practice, the most recent position statement released by the American Association of

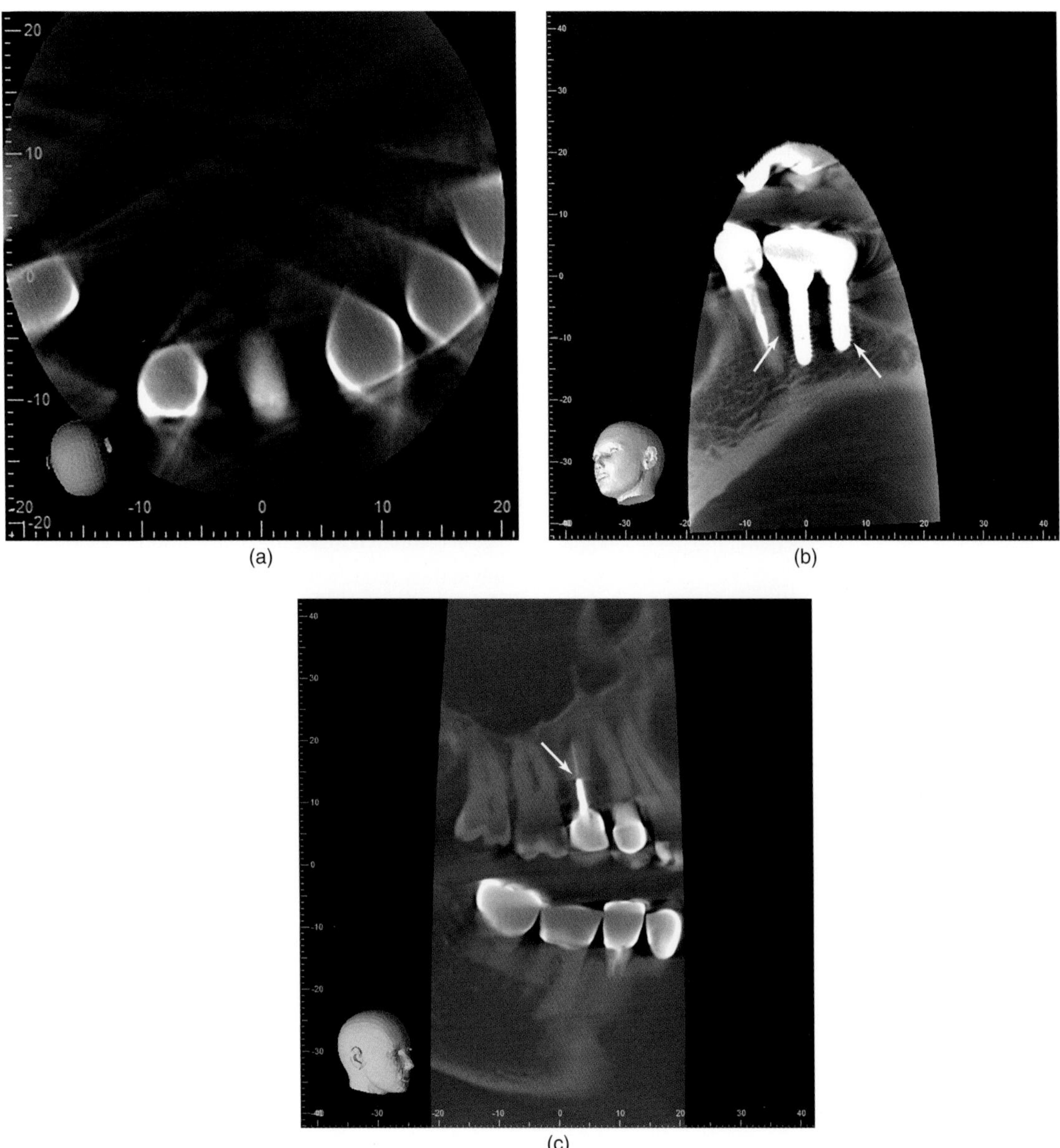

Figure 2.12 *A*, Scatter artifact is seen as light and dark lines extending radially from metallic sources. *B* and *C*, Beam hardening artifacts from cone-beam computed tomography imaging can resemble bone loss or root fracture.

Endodontists (AAE) and the American Association of Oral and Maxillofacial Radiology (AAOMR) states: "CBCT should not be used routinely for endodontic diagnosis or for screening purposes in the absence of clinical signs and symptoms" (Figures 2.9–2.11) [18].

Limitations

The quality of CBCT images can be adversely affected by the presence of high-density structures within the scanned area. Metallic posts, crowns, bridges, implants, and gutta-percha filling materials create artifacts that pose difficulty for the clinician in interpreting findings. [19] The most common artifacts affecting endodontic diagnosis are *beam hardening* and *scatter*. These artifacts can complicate imaging interpretation by masking the area of interest or by mimicking endodontic complications. Beam hardening causes dark bands to appear between two dense objects. Often, this dark band can look like a root fracture (refer to Figure 2.12c) Scatter artifact refers to the linear *streaking* that is seen projecting radially from a high-density source.

Artifacts present a major challenge to a clinician viewing an area of interest. Improvements in reconstruction software have reduced some of these artifacts. However, artifacts continue to be a concern [20], and the clinician should make every attempt to keep the FOV small and away from metallic sources, if possible. Enhanced reconstruction methods aiming to further reduce artifacts are an area of active research by manufacturers of CBCT machines and their respective software developers [21] (Figure 2.12C).

Radiation levels

Many parameters affect the radiation dose produced by a CBCT machine. The kVp, mA, the exposure time, and the size of the FOV affect the radiation dose delivered. However, radiation risk is best measured based on the *effective dose* received by the patient. Effective dose, measured in micro-Sieverts (μSv), is based on the radiation dose to specific tissues and organs within the FOV.

In the head and neck region, the organs used to calculate the effective dose include the thyroid, esophagus, bone marrow, bone surface, salivary glands, skin, and other tissues, as specified by the International Commission on Radiological Protection [22]. However, not all of these tissues are exposed to radiation equally. Therefore, based on the location of the scan (maxillary or mandibular, anterior or posterior), the amount of the tissue in the FOV is adjusted for and weighted according to the tissue's radiation sensitivity. The weighted tissues and organs dosages are added to yield the effective dosage.

To put it more simply, a CBCT machine with identical exposure settings will yield a higher effective dosage of radiation to the patient in the mandibular posterior region compared to the maxillary anterior region. This is due to the presence of more sensitive tissues and organs in the path of the x-ray beam in the mandibular posterior scan. Therefore, it is very difficult to compare the dosages of available units on the market [23]. However, all other factors being equal, the smaller the FOV for a given unit, the lower the radiation dose applied [24]. Table 2.1 lists the radiation dosages for common imaging modalities in dentistry and medicine, compared to background radiation [3, 25].

Table 2.1 Radiation doses for common imaging modalities in dentistry and medicine, compared to background radiation.

Activity	Effective dose in μSv	Dose as days of equivalent background Radiation
1 Day background radiation, sea level	7–8	1
1 Digital periapical radiograph	6	1
4 Dental bitewing radiographs, F-speed film	38	5
Full mouth series, F-speed film	171	21
Kodak CBCT focused field, anterior	4.7	0.71
Kodak CBCT focused field, maxillary posterior	9.8	1.4
Kodak CBCT focused field, mandibular posterior	38.3	5.47
J. Morita 3D Accuitomo	20	3
NewTom 3G, ImageWorks	68	8
Chest xray	170	25
Mammogram	700	106
Medical CT, head	2,000	243
Spiral CT, abdomen	10,000	1,515
Federal occupation safety limit per year	50,000	7,575

CBCT, cone-beam computed tomography; CT, computed tomography

The future

Research into improving CBCT imaging is focused on many aspects of the technology. Improvements in the hardware, such as the flat-panel detector (FPD) and beam quality enhance resolution while reducing radiation exposure. Improvements in stability during patient positioning, and the overall harmonics of the machine, improve image quality by minimizing vibration or motion artifacts. Decreasing the exposure time also minimizes motion artifact and reduces radiation exposure. Lastly, improved software reconstruction filters aim to enhance image quality and reduce or eliminate artifacts.

References

1 Redberg RF, Smith-Bindmanjan R. We are giving ourselves cancer. *New York Times*, January 30, 2014. http://mobile.nytimes.com/2014/01/31/opinion/we-are-giving-ourselves-cancer.html

2 Ludlow JB, Timothy R, Walker C, Hunter R, Benavides E, Samuelson DB, Scheske MJ. Effective dose of dental CBCT: A meta analysis of published data and additional data for nine CBCT units. *Dentomaxillofac Radiol* 2015; 44(1): 20140197.

3 White SC, Pharoah MJ. *Oral Radiology: Principles and Interpretation*. 6th ed. St. Louis: Mosby; 2009.

4 Nair MK, Nair UP. Digital and advanced imaging in endodontics: a review. *J Endod* 2007; 33: 1–6.

5 Udupa H, Mah P, Dove SB, McDavid WD. Evaluation of image quality parameters of representative intraoral digital radiographic systems. *Oral Surg Oral Med Oral Pathol Oral Radiol* 2013; 116: 774–783.

6 Bedard A, Davis TD, Angelopoulos C. Storage phosphor plates: how durable are they as a digital dental radiographic system? *J Contemp Dent Pract* 2004; 2(5): 57–60.

7 Ergün S, Güneri P, Ilgüy D, Ilgüy M, Goyacioglu H. How many times can we use a phosphor plate? A preliminary study. *Dentomaxillofac Radiol* 2009; 38(1): 42–47.

8 Danforth RA. Cone beam volume tomography: a new digital imaging option for dentistry. *J Calif Dent Assoc* 2003; 31: 814 –815.

9 Nemtoi A, Czink C, Haba D, Gahleitner A. Cone beam CT: a current overview of devices. *Dentomaxillofac Radiol* 2013; 42(8): 201–204.

10 Holmes SM. iCAT Scanning in the dental office. *The Fortress Guardian. A Newsletter from Fortress Insurance Company* 2007;9(3):2–3.

11 Turpin DL. Befriend your oral and maxillofacial radiologist. *Am J Orthod Dentofacial Orthop* 2007; 131: 697.

12 Roberts JA, Drage NA, Davies J, Thomas DW. Effective dose from cone beam CT examinations in dentistry. *Brit J Radiol* 2009; 82: 35–40.

13 Venskutonis T, Plotino G, Juodzbalys G, Mickevicienè L. The importance of cone-beam computed tomography in the management of endodontic problems: a review of the literature. *J Endod* 2014; 40(12): 1895–1901.

14 Roberts JA, Drage NA, Davies J, Thomas DW. Effective dose from cone beam CT examinations in dentistry. *Brit J Radiol* 2009; 82: 35–40.

15 Estrela C, Bueno M, Leles CR, Azevedo B, Azevedo JR. Accuracy of cone beam computed tomography and panoramic and periapical radiography for detection of apical periodontitis. *J Endod* 2008; 34: 273–279.

16 Bernardes RA, de Moraes IG, Húngaro Duarte MA, Azevedo BC, de Azevedo JR, Bramante CM. Use of cone beam volumetric tomography in the diagnosis of root fractures. *Oral Surg Oral Med Oral Pathol Oral Radiol Endod* 2009; 108: 270–277.

17 Matherne RP, Angelopoulos C, Kulild JC, Tira D. Use of cone-beam computed tomography to identify root canal systems in vitro. *J Endod* 2008; 1: 87–89.

18 American Association of Endodontists; American Academy of Oral and Maxillofacial Radiology. Use of cone beam-computed tomography in endodontics. Joint Position Statement of the American Association of Endodontists and the American Academy of Oral and Maxillofacial Radiology. *Oral Surg Oral Med Oral Pathol Oral Radiol Endod* 2011;111(2):234-237.

19 Neves FS, Freitas DQ, Campos PS, Ekestubbe A, Lofthag-Hansen S. Evaluation of cone-beam computed tomography in the diagnosis of vertical root fractures: the influence of imaging modes and root canal materials. *J Endod* 2014; 40: 1530–1536.

20 Bechara B, McMahan CA, Moore WS, Noujeim M, Teixeira FB, Geha H. Cone beam CT scans with and without artefact reduction in root fracture detection of endodontically treated teeth. *Dentomaxillofac Radiol* 2013; 42(5): 20120245.

21 Schulze R, Heil U, Gross D, Bruellmann DD, Dranischnikow E, Schwanecke U, Schoemer E. Artefacts in CBCT: a review. *Dentomaxillofac Radiol* 2011; 40: 265–273.

22 Clarke R, Valentin J; International Commission on Radiological Protection Task Group. ICRP publication 109. Application of the Commission's Recommendations for the protection of people in emergency exposure situations. *Ann ICRP* 2009;39(1):1–110.

23 Rottke D, Patzelt S, Poxleitner P, Schulze D. Effective dose span of ten different cone beam CT devices. *Dentomaxillofac Radiol* 2013; 42(7): 20120417.

24 Palomo JM, Rao PS, Hans MG. Influence of CBCT exposure conditions on radiation dose. *Oral Surg Oral Med Oral Pathol Oral Radiol Endod* 2008; 6: 773–782.

25 Ludlow JB, Davies-Ludlow LE, Brooks SL, Howerton WB. Dosimetry of 3 CBCT devices for oral and maxillofacial radiology. *Dentomaxillofac Rad* 2006; 35: 219–226.

Questions

1 With recent advances in x-ray technology, radiation exposure is not as concerning as it once was.
- A True
- B False

2 When examining a patient, a clinician should
- A Obtain a standard number of radiographs every time
- B Obtain a CBCT of the area
- C Avoid obtaining radiographs completely
- D All of the above
- E None of the above

3 Wet film radiography has higher radiation levels than digital radiography.
- A True
- B False

4 Small-field CBCT machines are most suitable for endodontic applications because of
- A Lower levels of radiation exposure
- B Higher resolution of the area of interest
- C Both a and b
- D None of the above

5 CBCT imaging is superior to conventional radiography in
- A Identifying cracks
- B Identifying periapical radiolucencies
- C Highlighting root anatomy
- D All of the above
- E None of the above

6 Beam-hardening artifact occurs during CBCT scanning due to the presence of metal in the area being imaged.
- A True
- B False

CHAPTER 3

Rotary instruments

Priyanka Jain
Dubai, UAE

Endodontic therapy essentially is directed toward one specific set of aims: to cure or prevent periradicular periodontitis [1]. The last two decades have been witness to phenomenal growth in endodontic technology. The introduction of these new technologies has resulted in endodontics becoming easier, faster, and, most importantly, better.

The technical demands and level of precision required for successful performance of endodontic procedures have always been achieved by careful manipulation of hand instruments within the root canal space and by adherence to the biological and surgical principles essential for disinfection and healing. To improve the speed and efficiency of the treatment, there has been a resurgence of mechanized and automated systems for preparing and sealing the root canal system.

The clinical endodontic breakthrough has been progressing from using a series of stainless steel hand files and rotary Gates Glidden drills to integrating NiTi files for shaping canals. Use of automated NiTi instruments was an important and logical development and step to improve the efficiency of the treatment. This chapter includes pertinent information on the most recent rotary NiTi instruments as they have become widely used adjuncts in root canal treatment. The role of root canal irrigants is also briefly reviewed.

Cleaning and shaping

A wide spectrum of possible strategies exists for attaining the goal of removing the canal contents and eliminating infection. At one end of the spectrum is a minimally invasive approach of removing canal contents and accomplishing disinfection that does not involve the use of a file. This is the noninstrumentation technique, which consists of a pump, a hose, and a special valve that is cemented into the access cavity to provide oscillation of irrigation solutions at a reduced pressure [2]. Clinical results in support of this method have not been convincing [3]. At the other end of the spectrum is a treatment procedure that removes all intraradicular infection by extracting the tooth in question. Endodontic therapy takes place along this spectrum of treatment strategies.

Three major elements determine the predictability of successful endodontics. The first is the knowledge, the second is the skill, and the third is the desire. Shaping and cleaning of the root canal system is considered a decisive link in the endodontic chain, because shaping determines the efficacy of subsequent procedures. This includes mechanical debridement, the creation of space for the delivery of medicaments, and optimized canal geometries for adequate obturation [4]. Chemomechanical preparation of the root canal includes both mechanical instrumentation and antibacterial irrigation and is principally directed toward the elimination of microorganisms from the root canal system. This is a critical stage in canal disinfection.

From a biological perspective, the goals of chemomechanical preparation are to eliminate microorganisms from the root canal system, to remove pulp tissue that may support microbial growth, and to avoid forcing debris beyond the apical foramen, which may sustain inflammation. Mechanical instrumentation is one of the important steps in reducing bacteria in the infected root canal. Clinical experience, handling properties, usage safety, and case outcomes should decide the choice of a particular design. NiTi rotary instruments have become a mainstay in clinical

Current Therapy in Endodontics, First Edition. Edited by Priyanka Jain.
© 2016 John Wiley & Sons, Inc. Published 2016 by John Wiley & Sons, Inc.

endodontics because of their exceptional ability to shape root canals with fewer procedural complications and errors.

The technical goals of canal preparation are directed toward shaping the canal so as to achieve the biological objectives and to facilitate placement of a root filling. In 1974, Schilder introduced the concept of "cleaning and shaping" root canals. "Cleaning" refers to removing all contents of the root canal system before and during shaping, "shaping" refers to a specific root canal cavity form with four design objectives:

- The opening should be a continuously tapering funnel from the access cavity to the apical foramen.
- The root canal preparation should maintain the path of the original canal.
- The apical foramen should remain in its original position.
- The apical opening should be kept as small as practical.

The following sections describe the instrument systems most widely used for root canal preparation. The basic strategies apply to all NiTi rotary instrument systems, regardless of the specific design or brand. These instruments can be differentiated into active and passive instruments (Box 3.1). However, three design groups will be analyzed separately: Group I: the LightSpeed; Group II: rotary instruments with 2% (.04) and 6% (.06) tapers, which includes the ProFile and many other models; Group III: rotary instruments with specific design changes, such as the ProTaper (Dentsply Maillefer) and RaCe (FKG, La Chaux-de-Fonds, Switzerland); and Group IV: thermomechanically treated NiTi instruments.

Physical and chemical properties of nickel–titanium alloys

Metallurgy

The NiTi alloy was first used at the beginning of the 1960s by W. H. Buehler in a space program of the Naval Ordnance Laboratory at Silver spring, Maryland, USA. The alloy was called Nitinol, an acronym for the elements from which the material was composed: ni for nickel, ti for titanium, and nol from the Naval Ordnance Laboratory. NiTi alloys are unique in that applied stress (i.e., bending) causes a reversible rearrangement of the nickel and titanium atoms at the molecular level [5]. The NiTi alloy used to manufacture endodontic instruments is composed of approximately 56% nickel and 44% titanium by weight and is generically known as 55 Nitinol [5].

NiTi alloys are softer than stainless steel, are not heat treatable, have a low modulus of elasticity but a greater strength, and are tougher and more resilient. A study found that size #15 NiTi instruments were two to three times more flexible than stainless steel instruments [6]. NiTi instruments showed superior resistance to angular deflection: they fractured after 2 ½ full revolutions (900 degrees) compared with 540 degrees for stainless steel instruments.

Nitinol belongs to a category of alloys called "shape-memory alloys," which have some extraordinary qualities. NiTi behaves like two different metals, because it can exist in one of two crystalline forms. The alloy normally exists in an *austenitic* crystalline

Box 3.1 Root canal instruments

Active Instruments

Active instruments have active cutting blades and are similar to the K-flexo file
They tend to straighten the canal curvature
Examples: Flexmaster, RaCe, ProTaper.Hero, K3

Passive Instruments

Passive instruments perform a scraping or burnishing action rather than a real cutting action.
They have less tendency to straighten the canal.
Examples: ProFile, GT, LightSpeed

phase that transforms to a *martensitic* structure on stressing at a constant temperature. In this martensitic phase, only a light force is required for bending. If the stress is released, the structure recovers to an austenitic phase and its original shape. This phenomenon is called a stress-induced thermoelastic transformation.

These alloys are mainly characterized by two properties that distinguish them from other metal alloys and are of interest in endodontics: superelasticity and high resistance to cyclic fatigue. These two properties allow continuously rotating instruments to be used successfully in curved root canals.

These properties can be explained by specific crystal structures of the austenite and martensite phases of the alloy [5]. Heating the metal above 212 °F (100 °C) can lead to a phase transition, and the shape memory property forces the instrument back to a preexisting form. When this file is placed in a curved canal, the atoms rearrange into a closely packed hexagonal array, and the alloy is transformed into the more flexible martensite crystal structure. This molecular transition enables these files to bend easily and around severe curves without permanent deformation. After release of stresses, the metal returns to the austenitic phase and the file regains its original shape. This stress-induced martensitic transformation is a unique property of NiTi alloys and makes this material one of the few alloys suitable for use in rotary endodontic instruments [5, 7]. The superelasticity of NiTi allows deformation of as much as 8% strain to be fully recoverable, in comparison to a maximum of less than 1% with alloys such as stainless steel [5].

Use and fracture of nickel–titanium instruments

All endodontic instruments have the potential to break within the canal following improper application. Despite the increased flexibility of NiTi instruments, separation is still a concern. Fracture can occur without any visible signs of previous permanent deformation, apparently within the elastic limit of the instrument [8–11].

NiTi engine-driven rotary systems require that the instrument be activated before it is inserted into the canal, where it mostly operates in flexed conditions. Two distinct fracture mechanisms have been described in the literature: torsional load and flexural cyclic fatigue [12–14].

The phenomenon of repeated cyclic metal fatigue may be the most important factor in instrument separation [15–17]. When instruments are placed in curved canals, they deform, and stress occurs within the instrument. The half of the instrument shaft on the outside of the curve is in tension, and the half on the inside is in compression. Consequently, each rotation causes the instrument to undergo one complete tension–compression cycle.

Torsional loading during rotational use is another variable to consider. Torsional load is transferred into the instrument through friction against the canal wall, and cyclic flexural fatigue occurs with rotation in curved canals. These two factors work together to weaken the instrument. Torsional fracture occurs when an instrument tip is locked in a canal while the shank continues to rotate, thereby exerting enough torque to fracture the tip. Torsional fracture can also occur when instrument rotation is sufficiently slowed in relation to the cross-sectional diameter. These are characterized by plastic deformation such as straightening, reverse winding, or twisting.

In contrast, flexural fracture occurs when the cyclic load leads to metal fatigue. Repeated bending of instruments in curved canals causes metal fatigue, leading to instrument fracture. As a general rule, flexible instruments are not very susceptible to torsional load but are resistant to cyclic fatigue. Instruments fracture most commonly at the point of maximum flexion of the shaft, which clinically often corresponds to the midpoint of the canal curvature [18]. In addition to this, the greater the amount and the more peripheral the distribution of metal in cross section, the stiffer the file. Therefore, a file with greater taper and larger diameter is more susceptible to fatigue failure. Cyclic fatigue occurs not only in the lateral aspect, when an instrument rotates in a curved canal, but also axially, when an instrument is bound and released by canal irregularities [18].

To avoid flexural fracture, instruments should be discarded after substantial use. Increased severity of angle and radius of root canal curvature around which the instrument rotates decreases instrument life spans [18].

Other factors that can influence the incidence of fracture in NiTi rotary instruments are lubrication, instrument motion, and speed of rotation. A crown-down approach is recommended to reduce torsional loads (and thus the risk of fracture) by preventing a large portion of the tapered rotating instrument from engaging root dentin (taper lock) [19]. A gentle pecking up and down motion or a light touch is recommended for all current NiTi instruments to avoid forcing the instrument into taper lock. This not only prevents screwing in of the file, it also distributes stresses away from the instrument's point of maximum flexure, where fatigue failure would likely occur (Figure 3.1) [20].

The fracture of rotary NiTi can also be reduced by creating a glide path for the instrument tip by manual preflaring (Figure 3.2). Electropolishing of instruments has also been introduced by some manufacturers (e.g., RaCe) to help reduce the number of surface defects.

Clinicians must fully understand the factors that control the forces exerted on continuously rotating NiTi instruments. To minimize the risk of fracture and prevent taper lock, they should not try to force motor-driven rotary instruments in an apical direction. The incidence of instrument fracture can be reduced to an absolute minimum if clinicians use adequate procedural strategies enhanced by a detailed knowledge of anatomical structures.

Importance of speed and torque

Speed refers not only to revolutions per minute but also to the surface feet per unit that the tool has with the work to be cut [21]. Endodontic motors all use a wide range of speed: 150 rpm to 40,000 rpm. The greater the speed, the greater the cutting efficiency, but with higher speed comes the disadvantages of loss of tactile sensation, breakage of instruments preceded by flute distortion, change in anatomical curvature of canal, and loss of control [22]. Torque is another parameter that might influence the incidence of instrument locking, deformation, and separation.

Torque (also called *moment*) is the term used about forces that act in a rotational manner. Examples of torque are turning a dial, flipping a light switch, or tightening a screw. Torque is the ability of the hand piece to withstand lateral pressure on the revolving tool without decreasing its speed or reducing its cutting efficiency and is dependent upon the type of bearing used and the amount of energy supplied to the handpiece [21]. Theoretically, an instrument used with a high torque is very active, and the incidence of instrument locking and consequently deformation and separation would tend to increase, whereas a low torque would

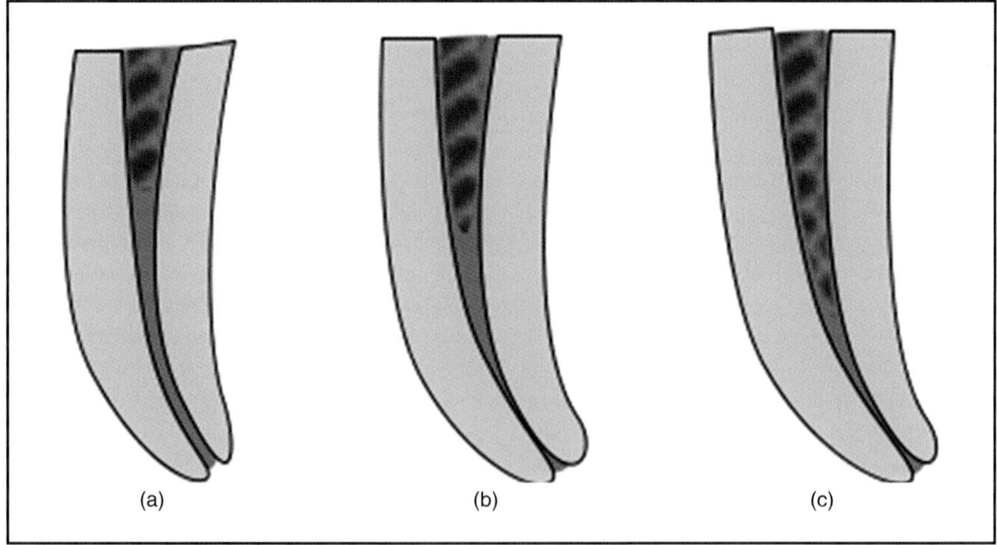

Figure 3.1 Motion for rotary instruments. *A*, Brushing technique. File is moved laterally so as to avoid threading. This motion is most effective with stiffer instruments with a positive rake angle, like ProTaper. *B*, Up-and-down motion. In this a rotary file is moved in an up-and-down motion with a very light touch so as to dissipate the forces until desired working length is reached or resistance is met. *C*, Taking file in the canal till it meets resistance. Gentle apical pressure is used till the file meets resistance and then withdrawn. The instrument is inserted again with a similar motion, e.g., RaCe files.

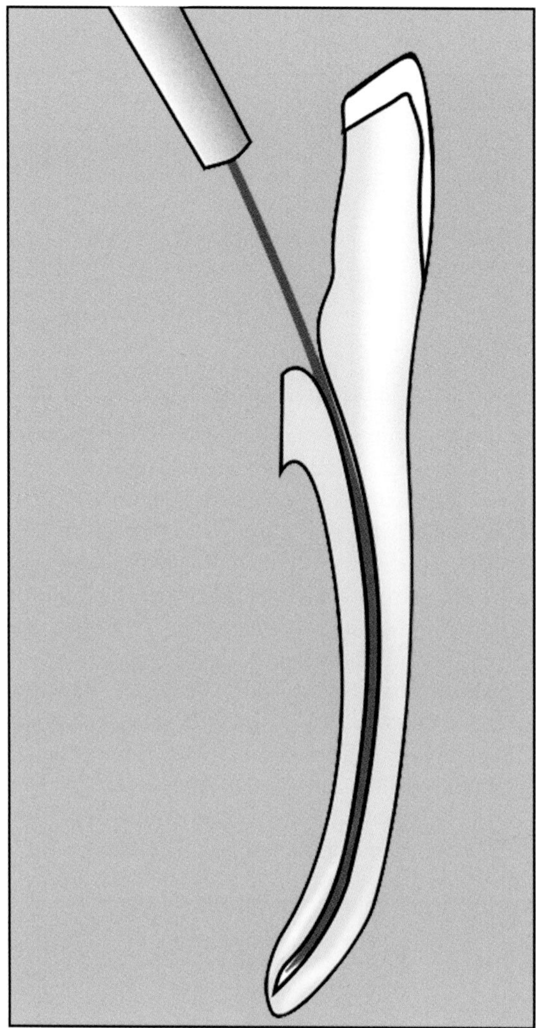

Figure 3.2 Creating a glide path.

reduce the cutting efficiency of the instrument, and instrument progression in the canal would be difficult.

The torque generated during the canal preparation depends on a variety of factors, especially the contact area [23].The size of the surface area contacted by an instrument is influenced by the instrumentation sequence or the taper of the instrument in use [24]. In straight canals where the resistance to dentin removal is low, the high torque provided by the motor can lead to fracture of the blocked instrument, especially because the clinician usually has no time to stop or retract the instrument. Hence, use of slow-speed, high-torque NiTi rotary instruments leads to many iatrogenic errors. The ideal configuration is slow-speed and low-torque or preferably right-torque motors, because each instrument has a specific ideal (right) torque.

Motors and devices

A handpiece is a device for holding rotating instruments, transmitting power to them, and positioning them intraorally. Both speed and torque in a handpiece can be modified by the incorporation of gear systems.

More than 100 years ago, the first endodontic handpiece was developed with the aim of reducing the treatment time and simplifying the preparation procedure. Ideas in the 1980s were transformed into the canal finder and canal leader, with the special combination of 90-degree and an up-and-down filing movement to help reduce fracture. This was the first endodontic handpiece with a partially flexible motion. This was an attempt to make the root canal anatomy one main influencing factor on the behavior of the instrument inside the canal. Further examples of handpieces with modified working motions were the Excalibur handpiece, which was designed to function with laterally oscillating instruments, and the Endoplaner, which used an upward filing motion.

The discovery of NiTi alloys enabled a steadily accelerating development of NiTi files that—first developed and designed for hand instrumentation—enabled a whole range of permanent rotating systems now available in a wide range of types and brands. The combination of the old idea of 360-degree rotation with the new technology met with great success, and progress continues to be made.

Newer motors have been developed for rotary instruments since the simple electric motors of the first generation in the early 1990s. Electric motors with gear reduction are more suitable for rotary NiTi systems because they ensure a constant rpm level; however, they also deliver torques much higher than those required to break tips. A rotary endodontic system incorporates three key elements into its operation: torque-sensing, which monitors how much twisting force the file is encountering; autoreversing, which reverses the rotation of the file if the file exceeds the torque limit; and constant file rotational speed, which many file manufacturers recommend. All these features help to reduce the chance of files breaking in the canal.

Torque-controlled motors, which have been used for several years, increase operational safety and reduce the risk of instrument fracture. These motors have individually adjusted torque limits for each file so that the motor will stop rotating and reverse the direction of rotation when the instrument is subjected to torque levels equal to the torque values set on the motor. Thus instrument failure could be avoided. They can be grouped as first-generation motor without torque control, fully electronically controlled second-generation motor with sensitive torque limiter, third-generation simple torque-controlled motor, and fourth-generation motor with built-in apex locator and torque control (Figure 3.3). Torque limits and speed control allow the dentist to adjust the unit's feel and develop the appropriate degree of finesse during rotary endodontic procedures.

The latest development with regard to torque control is the incorporation of gear systems within the handpiece that regulates torque depending on the size of the rotary instrument (Endoflash [KaVo], NiTi Control [Anthogyr]). This obviates the need for torque-control motors (Table 3.1).

Table 3.1 Available motors for root canal preparation using NiTi instruments.

Motor	Torque	NiTi Systems
Nouvag TCM Endo	Low torque	All systems
Endostepper	Right torque	All systems
E-master	Right torque	Only Flex-Master
K3-etcm	Low torque	K3
Quantec ETM		Quantec, K3
ENDOflash	Low torque	All systems
ENDOadvance	Low torque	All systems
Tascal-handpiece	Undefined	LightSpeed
Endo-mate TC	Low torque	All systems

Preparation techniques

In general, most NiTi devices require preflaring of the upper portion of the root canal before further preparation because, due to their extreme flexibility, NiTi instruments are not designed for initial negotiation of the root canal or for bypassing ledges [25–27]. Coronal widening with Peeso and Gates Glidden reamers provides straight line access and allows more control during the preparation of the middle and apical third.

The delicate and final preparation is usually performed with a coronal–apical (crown-down) or apical–coronal (step-back) approach, depending on the system used. The aim of apical widening in root canal preparation is to fully prepare apical canal areas for optimally effective irrigation and overall antimicrobial activity. This can be achieved in three phases: pre-enlargement, apical enlargement, and apical finishing [28].

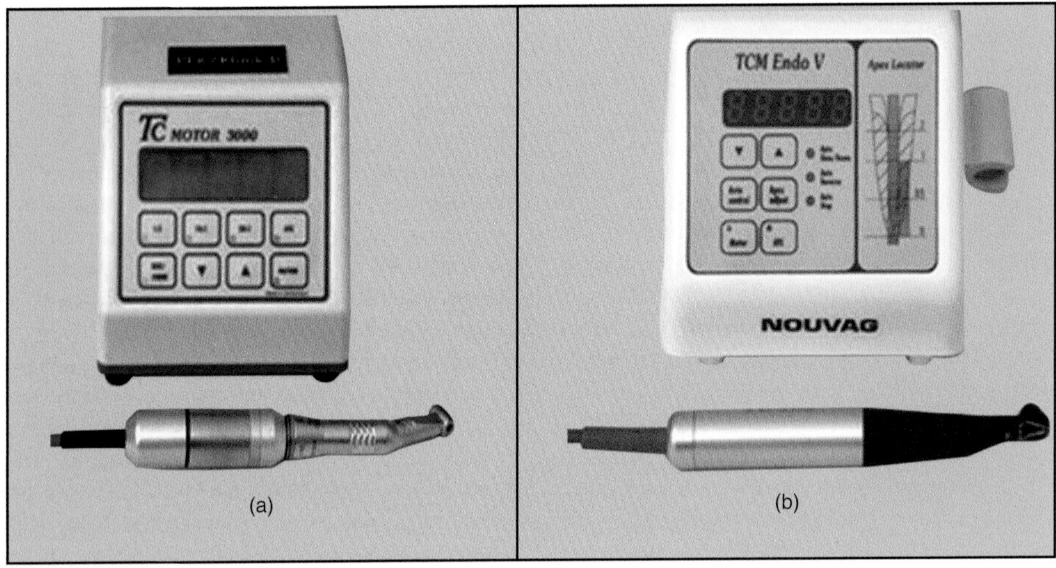

Figure 3.3 Examples of motors. *A*, First-generation motor without torque control. *B*, Newest-generation motor with built-in apex locator and torque control.

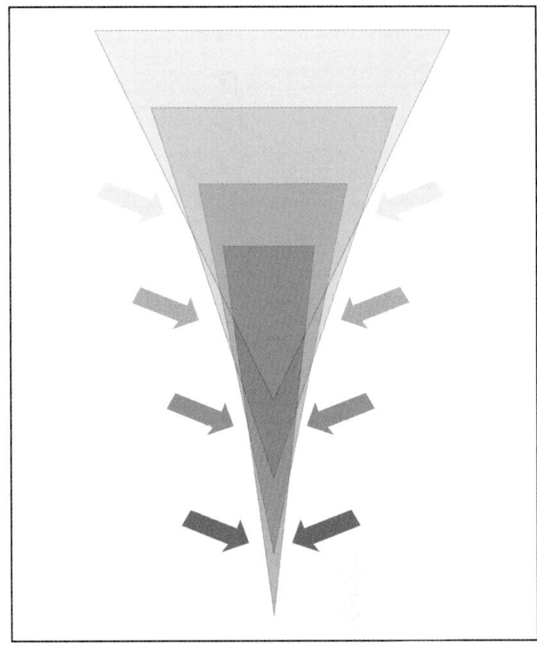

Figure 3.4 Crown-down approach. Arrows indicate corresponding cutting area.

Crown-down versus step-back approach

Most rotary techniques make use of the crown-down approach to minimize torsional loads [23] and to reduce the risk of instrument fracture (Figure 3.4). The step-back technique involves preparing the apical region of the root canal first, followed by coronal flaring to facilitate obturation. But when employed in curved canals, this technique often results in iatrogenic damage to the natural shape of the canal due to the inherent inflexibility of the stainless steel files. Following apical enlargement, instrument length may be reduced with increasing instrument size.

During the step-down approach there is less constraint to the files and better control of the file tip, and therefore it is expected that apical zipping is less likely to occur. Pre-enlarging the coronal region of the canal before completing apical preparation provides several advantages, including straighter access to the apical region, enhanced tactile control, and improved irrigant penetration and suspension of debris.

A crown-down approach is considered safer than step-back because it results in less tip contact, less force, and less torque compared with step-back [29]. Over the years, several modifications of these techniques have been proposed, such as the hybrid techniques combining an initial crown-down with a subsequent step-back (modified double flare).

Continuous reaming motion

The use of automated handpiece systems for canal preparation is accelerating with the introduction of NiTi engine-driven files. Although some variations exist, NiTi files are generally used in a very-low-speed torque-control handpiece system and a full 360-degree file rotation. This continuous rotating movement results in less straightening of the canal.

Hybrid technique

The idea of the hybrid concept is to combine instruments of different file systems and use different instrumentation techniques to manage individual clinical situations to achieve the best biomechanical cleaning and shaping results and the fewest procedural errors. The hybrid concept combines the best features of different systems for safe and quick results and reduces the shortcomings of individual instruments. Although many combinations are possible, the most popular and useful ones involve coronal pre-enlargement followed by different additional apical preparation sequences. However, clinicians must keep in mind that anatomic variations in each canal must be addressed individually with specific instrument sequences. The recommended sequence of steps in the order of preparation are presented in Figure 3.5.

The benefits of working in this order include less risk of iatrogenic contamination, more visibility and control over the area of dentinal wall removal, better access for irrigants, and fewer procedural errors. The instruments can be used in a manner that promotes their individual strengths and avoids their weaknesses; for example, the hand instruments create a patent glide path, tapered rotary instruments efficiently enlarge coronal canal areas, and less-tapered instruments allow additional apical enlargement.

Extreme canal curvatures and ribbon-shaped canals cannot be managed effectively and efficiently with tapered NiTi rotaries. NiTi hand files used in a step-back approach are probably the best option for such cases. In addition, C-shaped canals should only be hand instrumented because their anatomy is unpredictable.

Some hybrid procedures work better than others, but the main deciding factor remains the root canal's

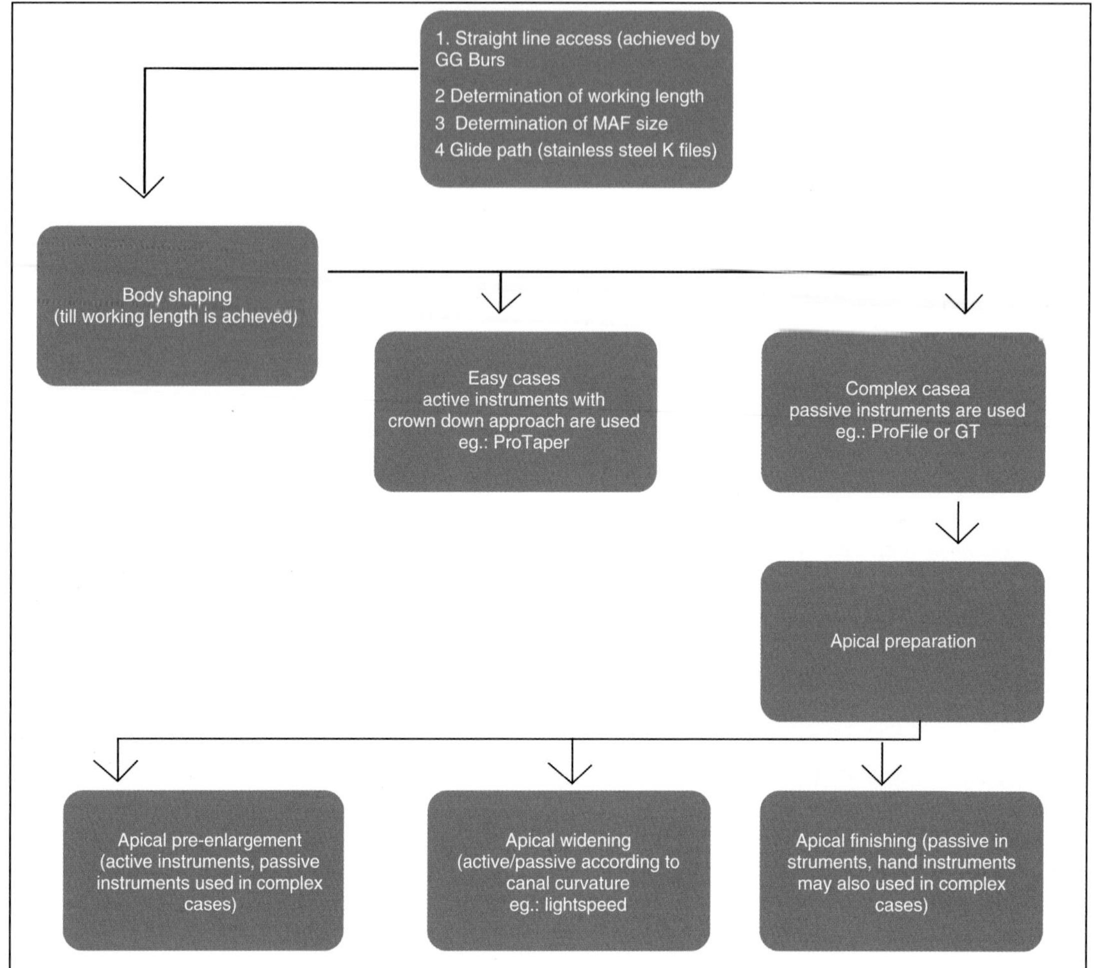

Figure 3.5 Recommended steps for hybrid technique.

anatomy and an adequate preparation goal. Instrument systems can be combined in a hybrid concept based on an understanding of where each instrument performs its cutting action in the canal and when and how to use each instrument to its best ability. The aim of hybridizing NiTi rotary techniques, therefore, is to increase apical size using a fast and safe clinical procedure.

Design features of rotary instruments

Tip design and transition angle

It is important to remember that the cutting efficiency of the tip depends on the transition angle (TA) (Roane et al) [28]. The TA is formed by an instrument axis and is tangent to the last spiral of the same instrument. It is difficult to define a precise value of the TA for each instrument because multiple factors, such as shape of the cutting surfaces and the pitch, can influence the end result.

A rotary cutting instrument may have a cutting or noncutting tip according to the type of machining used for this part of the instrument. Instruments with machined (rounded and noncutting) tips are less aggressive than ones with nonmachined (sharp) tips. Unlike the pilot tip, the instrument shaft retains its active cutting blades. Tip design plays an important role in the instrument's capacity to overcome impediments within the canal and for the incidence of clinical damage and complications [31, 32]. A cutting tip gives the ability to enter narrow, calcified canals, but it is much riskier to use in a curved canal as compared to noncutting tip. Recent NiTi rotary files have rounded and noncutting tips that ride on the canal wall rather than gouging into it. Unlike a pilot tip, the instrument shaft retains its active cutting blades.

Taper

Taper is another feature of file design, and it is particularly important concerning system concepts. NiTi alloy has made it possible to engineer instruments with multiple and progressive tapers (4%–12%), thereby allowing better control of root canal shape [33]. The idea behind variable or graduating tapers is that each successive file engages only a minimal aspect of the canal wall. Therefore, frictional resistance is reduced, and less torque is required to properly run the file.

Rake angle

Rake angle is the angle formed by the cutting edge and a cross section taken perpendicular to the long axis of the instrument. The cutting angle, on the other hand, is the angle formed by the cutting edge and a radius when the file is sectioned perpendicular to the cutting edge. It is the angle formed by two intersecting lines. A positive rake angle occurs when the peripheral line segment is located in front of the cutting face; when it is located behind the cutting face, it is a negative rake angle (Figure 3.6) [34].

The more positive the rake angle (closed), the greater the cutting efficiency. Alternately, a neutral or negative rake angle (open) reduces the file's cutting efficiency [35, 36]. Most conventional endodontic files use a negative or substantially neutral rake angle. Positive rake angles cut more efficiently than neutral rake angles, which scrape the inside of the canal. An overly positive rake angle digs and gouges the dentin. This can lead to separation.

Radial land (number and type of working surfaces)

Another critical design feature in rotary instruments is the concept of radial land. A radial land is a surface that projects axially from the central axis, between flutes, as far as the cutting edge. The best way to explain this is the blade support. Blade support can be defined as the amount of material supporting the cutting blades of the instrument. This part of the file is called the radial land. A radial land surface produces a planing or scraping effect on the dentin walls, and a blade surface engraves them. The less blade support (the amount of metal behind the cutting edge), the less resistant the instrument is to torsional or rotary stresses [37].

With radial land surfaces, friction is enhanced, reducing the mechanical resistance of the files. An attempt has been made to lower the friction, thus creating a kind of recessed radial land (Quantec and K3 instruments) [38, 39]. This helps to prevent the propagation of cracks and reduces the chances of separation and deformation from torsional stresses. Rotary files with radial land areas are further subdivided depending on the shape of the grooves, U-shaped or L-shaped, resulting in a U-type or H-type file. The U-type file is constructed by grinding three equally spaced U-shaped grooves around the shaft of a tapered wire, whereas the H-type file consists of a single L-shaped groove (Hedström type) produced in the same way.

It is this combination of a noncutting tip and radial land that keeps a rotary file centered in the canal and reduces the chances of transporting the root canal. An important concept of rotary instrumentation should be remembered. The concept is not of drilling a hole in a root. Rather, it is one of taking a small hole, planing the inside, and making it larger.

Helical or flute angle

The helical angle is the angle that the cutting edge makes with the long axis of the file. Files with a constant helical flute angle allow debris to accumulate, particularly in the coronal part of the file. Additionally, files that maintain the same helical angle along the entire working length will be more susceptible to the effect of screwing-in forces. By varying the flute angles, debris will be removed in a more efficient manner and the file will be less likely to screw into the canal (Figure 3.7) [40].

Pitch is the number of spirals or threads per unit length. The result of a constant pitch and constant helical angles is a pulling down or sucking down into the canal. This is of significance in rotary instrumentation when using files with a constant taper. For example, the K3 file has been designed with constant tapers but with variable pitch and helical angles. This reduces the sense of being sucked down into the canal (Figure 3.8) [40].

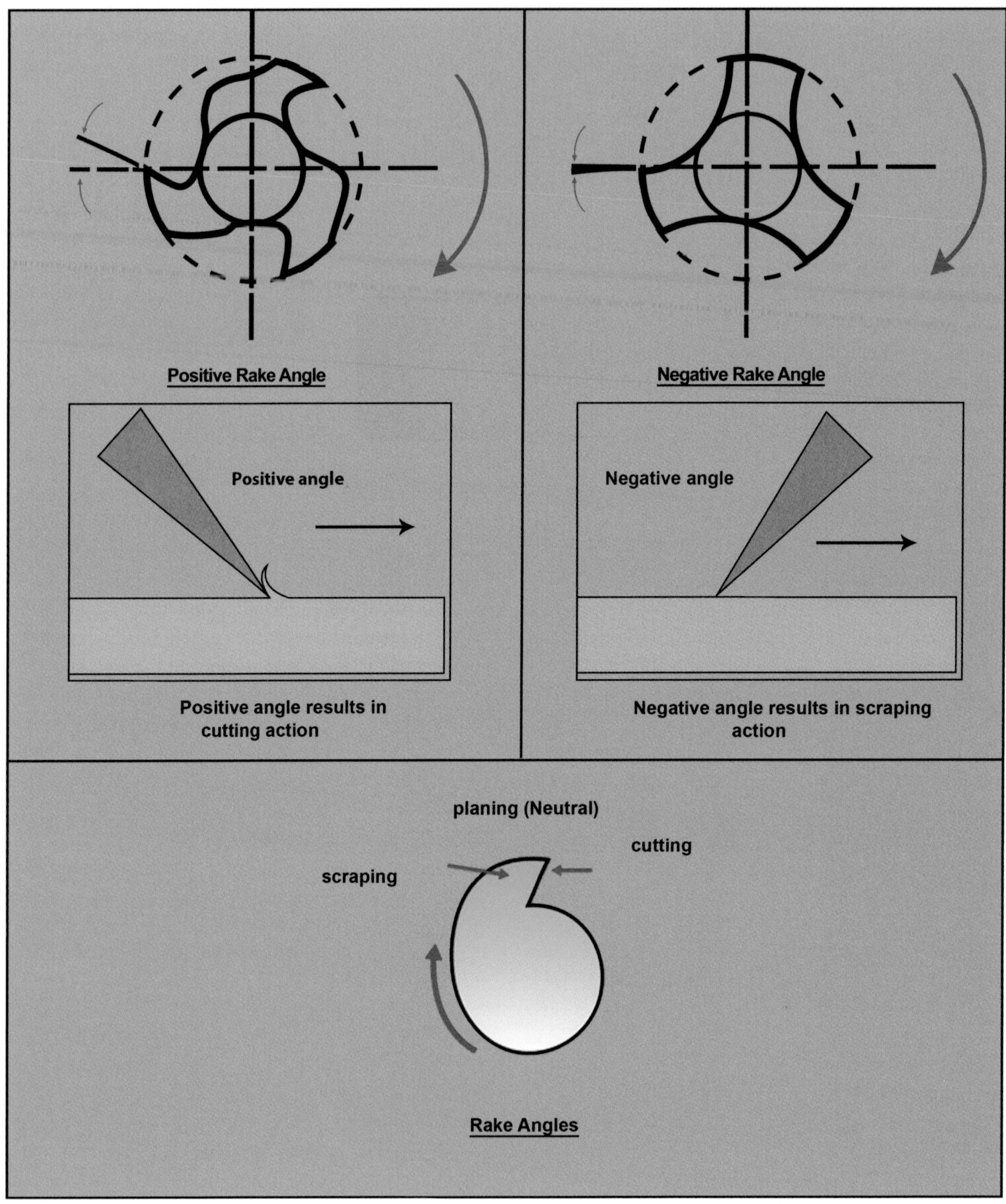

Figure 3.6 Rake angles.

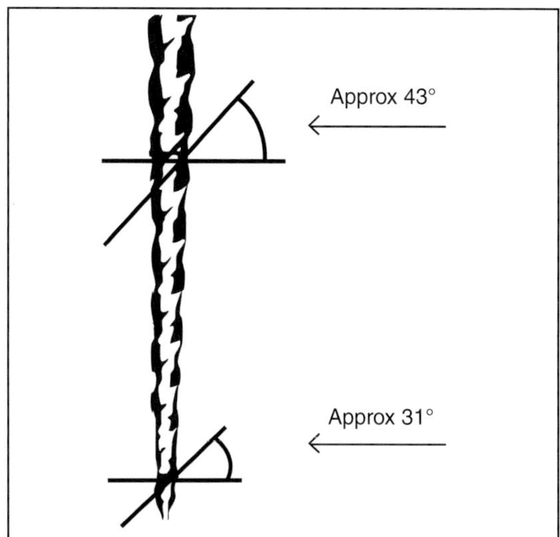

Figure 3.7 Variable helical angle.

The Nickel–Titanium era

The actual number of systems on the market increases the probability of success, but it can also confuse the clinician, who needs constant clinical updates in order to be successful. This part of the chapter talks about the five generations of NiTi filing systems in an attempt to improve clinicians' understanding of the real innovations and advantages behind the NiTi file.

Since the early 1990s, several instrument systems manufactured from nickel–titanium have been introduced into endodontic practice (Table 3.2) [41]. Some of the early systems have been removed from the market or play only minor roles; others, such as LightSpeed (LightSpeed Technologies, San Antonio, TX) and ProFile (Dentsply Tulsa, Dentsply Maillefer), are still widely used. New designs are continually produced, but the extent to which, if any, clinical outcomes depend on design characteristics is difficult to forecast.

Although NiTi systems have similar features, they differ in their cross-sectional and shank design (Figure 3.9). The design of the instruments, including the cutting angle, number of blades, tip design, conicity, and cross section, directly influences the flexibility, cutting efficacy, and torsional resistance of the instrument, as well as its performance in narrow or wider canals. It is beyond the scope of this textbook to describe every system available, but every effort has been made to explain the more commonly used rotary systems.

LightSpeed (LightSpeed Technology, San Antonio, TX, USA)

LightSpeed LS1

The LightSpeed was developed by Dr. Steve Senia and Dr. William Wildey in the early 1990s and is also known as LS1. It refers to simple handling with concomitant rapid rotation speed. The instrument features a design similar to the Gates Glidden (GG) bur. It has a small cutting head with minimal cutting surface; a long, thin, noncutting shaft; and a 0.25- to 2-mm anterior cutting part. This was originally designed to improve on the flexibility of stainless steel files [42].

The files have a noncutting pilot tip (tip length increases with instrument size to compensate for decreasing flexibility) with U-designed blades, radial lands and a neutral rake angle. The diameter of the shaft is increased according to the ISO size. The complete system consists of 25 instruments ranging from ISO 20 to 100. Half sizes are available from 20 to 70 and full sizes from 80 to 100. These instruments are available in lengths of 21, 25 and 31 mm.

Because the cutting head is short, this system tends to produce a round parallel shape. Hence, numerous instrument sizes are used to achieve sufficient conicity. The main advantage of this system clearly is its undefeated ability to manage curves with large instrument sizes because of its shaft flexibility. The main drawback is the high number of instruments per set and the need for a step-back preparation in combination with constant recapitulation to avoid retaining apical debris.

These instruments are mainly used for apical preparation and are used with a slow, continuous apical movement until the blade binds, a momentary pause, and then advancing to the working length with pecking motions. The recommended working speed is 1500 to 2000 rpm, and they should be used with minimal torque (Box 3.2).

There are two recommended motions with this system. If upon introduction of the file in the canal, no resistance is felt, the LightSpeed is advanced to the desired length and gently withdrawn. Alternatively, if resistance is felt upon entering the canal, a very light apical pecking motion should be used until the desired working length is achieved. This prevents blade locking, removes debris coronally, and aids in keeping the blades clean.

The MAR is the smallest LightSpeed size to reach the working length, but it is large enough to clean the apical

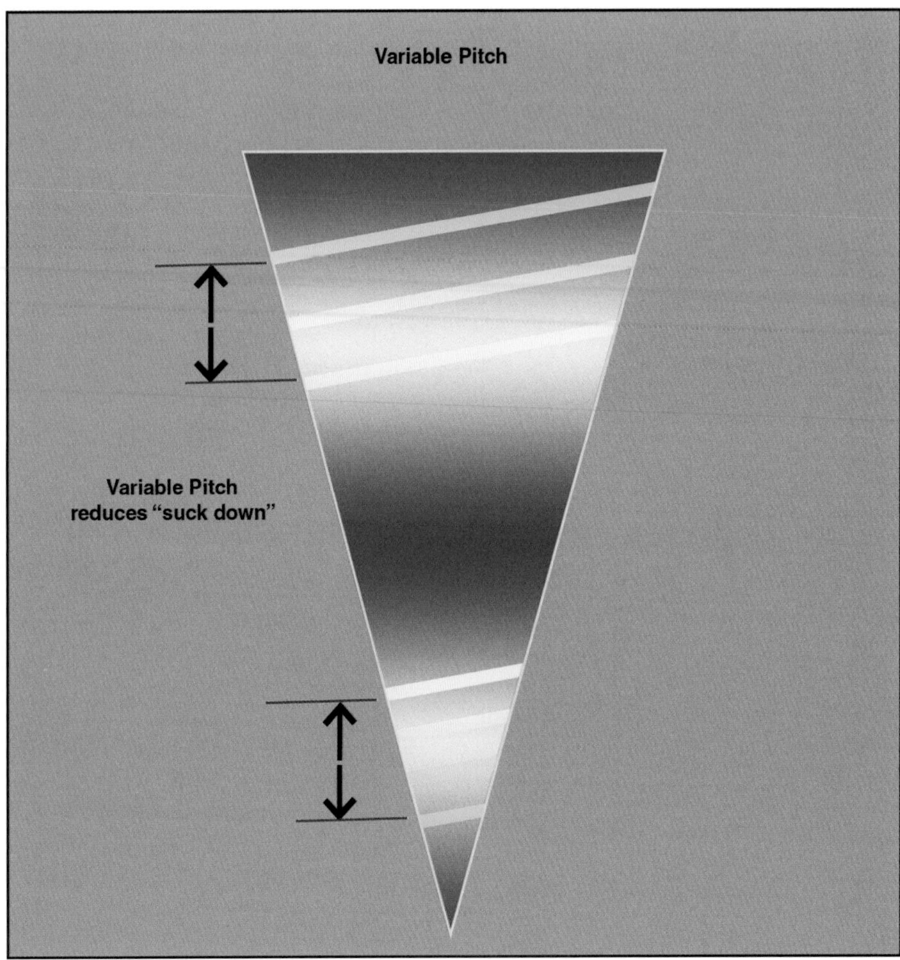

Figure 3.8 Pitch refers to the number of flutes per unit length.

Table 3.2 Categories of Ni Ti instruments.

Generation	Features	Examples
First (mid to late 1990s)	Passive cutting radial lands (helps the file to stay centered in canal curvatures) Requires numerous instruments Fixed tapers along the length of the file	ProFile, GT Files, LightSpeed
Second (2001)	Active cutting edges Requires fewer instruments Some files were electropolished	Flexmaster, Endosequence (electropolished surface), BioRaCe, ProTaper, Hero
Third (2007 (active files)	Thermomechanically treated Decreased incidence of file fracture because cyclic fatigue is reduced	K3, Twisted file, GT Vortex, Hyflex
Fourth	Uses reciprocation Single-file technique	Reciprocating systems: M4, Endo-Express, Endo-Eze Single file systems: Self-adjusting, Wave One, Reciproc
Fifth	Center of rotation is offset Increased flexibility of the file	Protaper Next (PTN), One shape, Revo-S

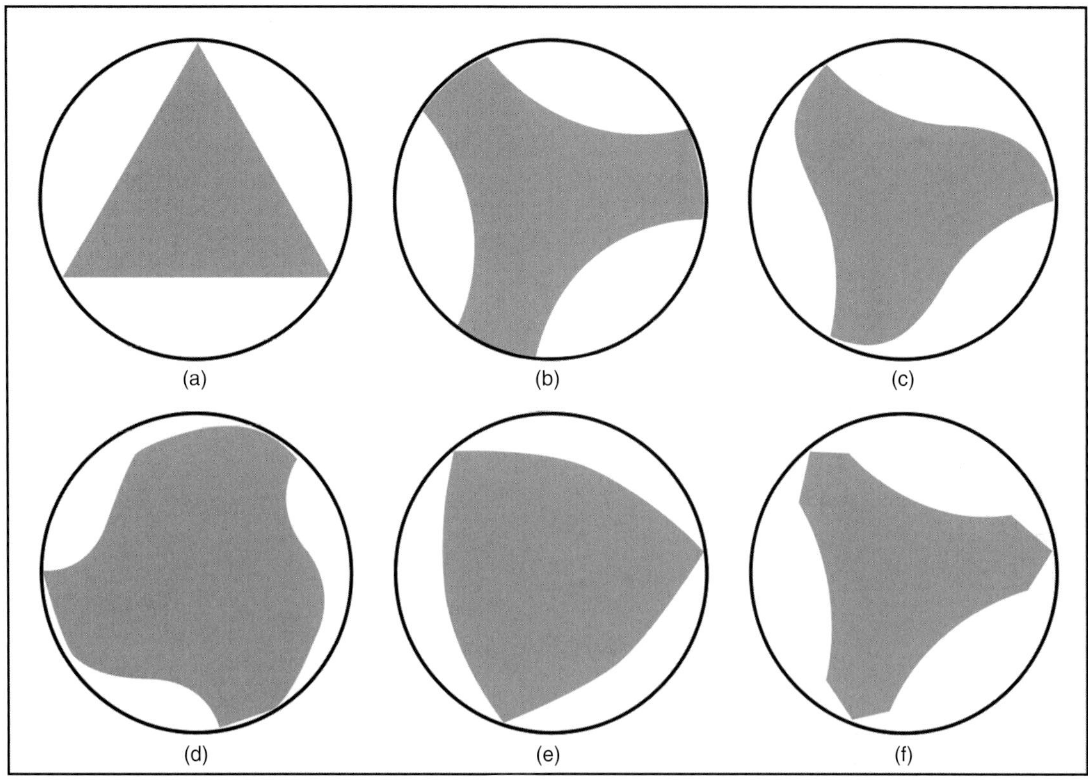

Figure 3.9 Cross-section of different rotary instruments. *A*, K-File RaCe. *B*, ProFile, GT, LightSpeed. *C*, Hero 642. *D*, K3. *E*, ProTaper, Flexmaster. *F*, ProTaper F3.

Box 3.2 LightSpeed preparation sequence*

Step 1. Gauge the minimal diameter of the canal using LightSpeed hand instruments.
Step 2. Use the first LightSpeed instrument size to bind (before reaching the working length) to start the mechanical apical preparation. End with the MAR (the smallest LightSpeed instrument).
Step 3. The next largest instrument in sequence is used 4 mm short of the working length.
Step 4. Instrument and prepare the middle third with 3 or 4 larger sizes.
Step 5. Recapitulate to full working length with the MAR.

*For coronal flaring, use Gates Glidden drill or other small instruments.

area of the canal. It is the first instrument that binds 3 to 4 mm short of the working length. The apical 4 mm of the canal is shaped using larger instruments in the sequence in a step-back manner.

The LightSpeed's predecessor, the Canal Master-U, had the same general design but was used as a hand instrument. LightSpeed's manufacturer still recommends some hand use of its instruments, specifically for determining canal diameter. The LightSpeed system requires a specific instrument sequence to produce a tapered shape that facilitates obturation with a gutta-percha cone or with LightSpeed's proprietary obturation system. Most studies have found that the system has a low incidence of canal transportation and preparation errors [43–49].

LightSpeed LSX (Spade Blade)

Since 2005, further modifications and developments of LightSpeed instruments, called LSX, have been introduced wherein the number of instruments have been reduced to 12 and half sizes are no longer available. It was so named because evaluators felt very safe using it, suggesting that the "X" be added for "extra safe." The blade design provides better tactile feedback than the original. The combination of a short blade, a thin shaft, and NiTi makes the LSX an extremely flexible instrument.

The spade blade has several advantages: There are no flutes to fill with debris. The spade blade has no helical angle (spiral thread) that produces a self-threading tendency. The blade design provides space for cut debris and for bypassing in the unlikely event of instrument separation. However, the blade design indicates an oval rather than a round canal shape.

To significantly reduce stresses, the LSX was designed with a short blade to be used at a high rpm (optimum is 2500 rpm) and was designed with a "safe failure" mode, which means that if it is overstressed, there is an excellent chance that no part of the instrument will be left in the canal (Figure 3.10).

The previous pecking motion of canal preparation is no longer necessary because the LSX does not have flutes to fill with debris. The LS1 required the pecking motion to clear the blade of debris (and reduce the torsional load). With LSX, the clinician slowly advances the instrument apically until a binding sensation is felt. After a pause, the clinician slowly and gently pushes the instrument to the desired length.

Hero 642 (Micro-Mega, Besançon, France)

Hero is an acronym for high elasticity in rotation, and the number 642 represents the varying tapers of 6% (.06), 4% (.04), and 2% (.02). These instruments have a triangular section (refer to Fig. 3.9) with three blade surfaces and are classified as instruments with an open flute angle. A complete set consists of 12 files with varying ISO sizes, tapers, and lengths of cutting segments. In comparison to other NiTi rotary systems, these files have no radial lands but have a triple helix cross section with three equally spaced cutting edges and a positive rake angle.

The new-generation Hero instruments are called Hero Shapers (Figure 3.11). They come in tapers of .06 and .02. The .06 taper instrument shapes the coronal two thirds of the canal and is available in 21-mm and 25-mm lengths. The .04 taper instrument is used to shape the apical third of the canal and is available in lengths of 21 mm, 25 mm, and 29 mm [49]. The Hero shaper instrument handle is metallic and is 11 mm in length to allow use in areas that are more difficult to access. The system also includes a pre-enlargement single instrument called the Endoflare. This has a triangular cross section with three cutting blades like other Hero instruments, a noncutting tip with a 0.25 mm diameter, and a .12 taper. The instrument length is 15 mm, and the shank has a diameter of 0.8 mm to provide flexibility to the instrument. Endoflare is recommended to be used with a brushing-milling movement. This helps in removing coronal constraints and thus helps in improving access to canal entrances.

In clinical practice, the system works in a crown-down manner and is divided into three preparation sequences according to the canal curvature (three-wave concept). For simple cases, the "blue wave" is recommended, intermediate cases are prepared using the "red wave" and difficult cases are treated using the "yellow wave" (Table 3.3) [50].

The Hero series also includes the Hero Apical instruments for apical enlargement and final apical shaping. They come in tapers of .06 (black ring) and .08 (red ring) and are highly flexible. Both have a tip diameter of 0.3 mm. These instruments allow the clinician to create high tapers in the apical third, thereby saving dentin in the middle and coronal third. The file with the .06 taper is followed by the .08 taper. In large roots, both apical files are brought to working length. In narrow roots, .06 taper is brought to working length and .08 taper 1 mm short to the working length. In very narrow, curved roots, .06 taper is brought 1 mm short to working length and .08 is brought 2 mm short to working length.

Quantec (Sybron Endo)

The Quantec system is the product of two previous NiTi rotary systems, the NT system and the McXim system, developed by McSpadden. They were introduced in 1996 and are available in tapers of 0.12, 0.10, 0.08,

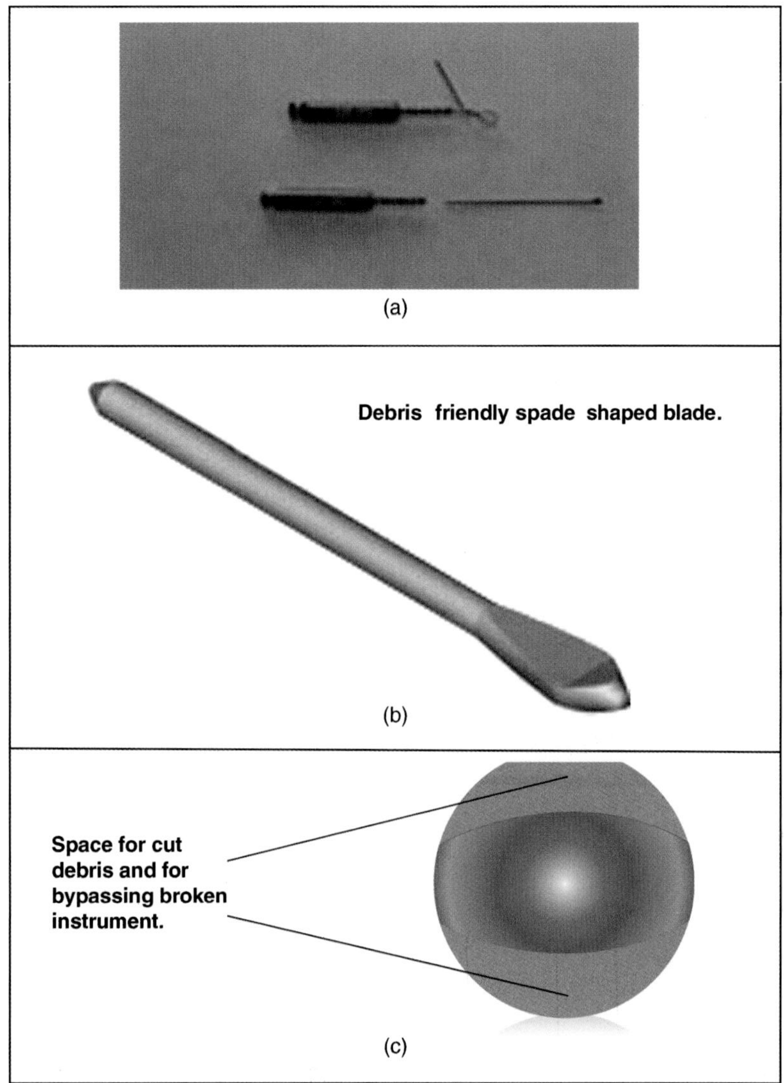

Figure 3.10 LightSpeed LSX. *A*, Safe-failure design. *B*, Absence of flute. *C*, Front view.

0.06, 0.05, 0.04, 0.03, and 0.02 (mm/mm). All have a diameter of 0.25 mm.

Quantec files have a cross-sectional design of S-shape double helical flute, positive rake angle, and two wide radial lands (Figure 3.12). The recessed radial land minimizes surface tension, contact area, and stress on the instrument. Two flutes allow a greater depth of flute. Increasing the flute depth provides more space for debris accumulation, and it potentially reduces file breakage. A variable helical angle reduces the tendency of the file to screw into the canal. The Quantec instrument systems are unique in their positive rake angle, which is designed to shave dentin, unlike conventional files with a negative rake angle, which is designed to scrape dentin.

Quantec files vary in taper along their blanks and are available in noncutting tip (LX, gold handles) or safe-cutting tip (SC silver handles) (Figure 3.13). The Quantec SC files have a negotiating tip that cuts as it moves apically, following canal pathways and minimizing stress. The SC instruments should be used in small, narrow, and tight canals, narrow curvatures, and calcified canals. A 1998 study by Thompson and

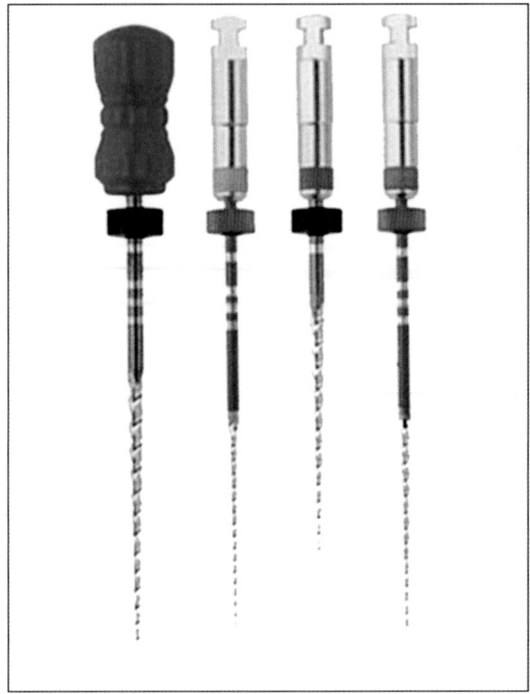

Figure 3.11 Hero Shapers rotary files.

Dummer showed that the major problem with these instruments were the "safe cutting tips" that created canal aberrations such as zips, elbows, perforations, and ledges [51]. The results of this study led to the development of the LX noncutting tip [52].

The LX noncutting tip is a nonfaceted bullet-nosed tip for use in severe canal deflections with a high risk of iatrogenic mishaps. The LX instruments are also recommended for enlarging the body and coronal segments and delicate apical areas. Quantec files are also available with the Axxess handle, which is shorter by 4 mm, providing easier access when vertical space limitation is a concern. When placed into a minihead contra-angle, 7 mm of interocclusal clearance can be gained.

Quantec files use a graduated taper technique to prepare a canal sequence, starting with a larger tapered file and progressing with files of lesser taper until working length is achieved. The technique consists of canal negotiation, canal shaping, and, apical preparation (Box 3.3). The Quantec series were designed for a step-by-step sequence using all the instruments from numbers 1 through 10 in different phases. The files are to be used at 300 rpm to 350 rpm, using each instrument for no longer than 3 to 5 seconds and with a pecking motion. An alternative sequence using crown-down preparation technique has also been proposed by the manufacturer. Accessory files are also available in tapers of .05, .04, .03, .02, and .02 with a .15 tip.

K3 (Sybron Endo)

In a sequence of constant development by their inventor, Dr. McSpadden, the Quantec files were followed by the current K3 system. The overall design of the K3 is similar to that of the ProFile and the Hero in that it includes size .02, .04, and .06 instruments. It has a unique three-cutting-edge design that provides an active file as opposed to the old passive files; active files are the third-generation endodontic files that have greater cutting power and better debris removal.

The most significant and obvious difference between the Quantec and K3 models is the K3's unique cross-sectional design: a slightly positive rake angle for greater cutting efficiency as opposed to the screwing

Table 3.3 Hero shapers preparation sequence.

Technique	Blue sequence (easy cases)	Red sequence (average/ inter mediate cases)	Yellow sequence (difficult cases)	Instrument depth
Coronal Flaring	Endoflare	Endoflare	Endoflare	3 mm
Crown-down technique	30/.06	25/.06	20/.06	2/3 working length
	30/.04	30/.04	20/.04	Working length
		30/.04	25/.04	
			30/.04	
Apical preparation (Hero Apicals)	30/.06	30/.06	30/.06	According to the function and curvature of the root anatomy
	30/.08	30/.08	30/.08	

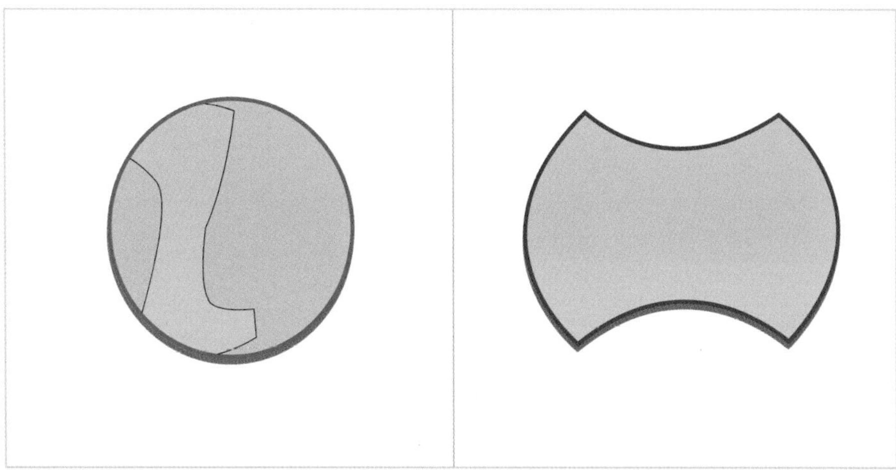

Figure 3.12 Cross section of a Quantec file.

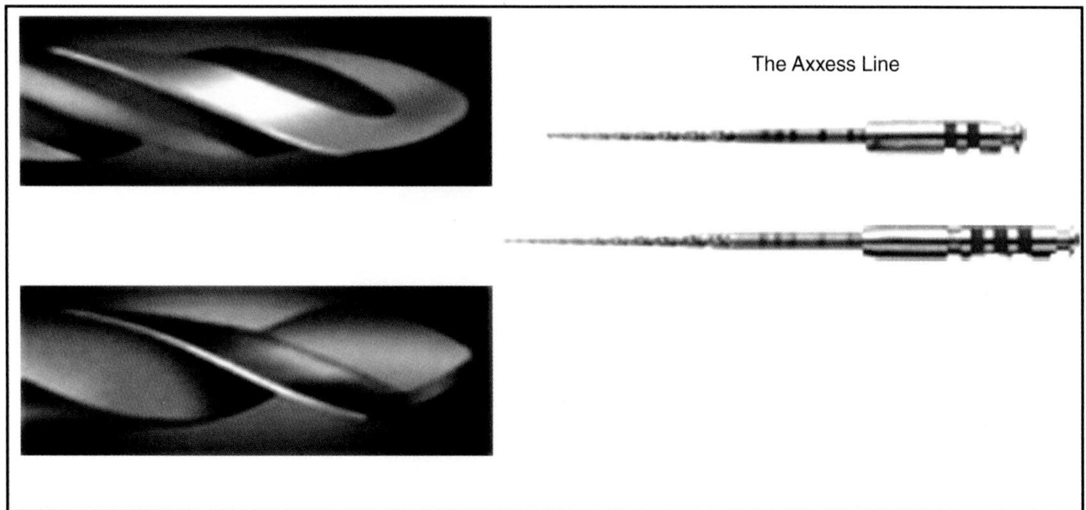

Figure 3.13 Quantec Files. *Top*, LX noncutting (gold handles). *Bottom*, SC safe cutting (silver handles).

action of a U-shaped instrument with a negative rake angle, wide radial lands, and a peripheral blade relief for reduced friction (Figure 3.14). Unlike the Quantec, a two-flute file, the K3 features a third radial land to help prevent screwing in. In the lateral aspect, the K3 has a variable pitch and variable core diameter, which provide apical strength. This complicated design is relatively difficult to manufacture, resulting in some metal flash.

The K3 standard set is composed of 20 instruments, divided into 10 progressively larger sizes (from 15 to 60) with three different tapers: .02, .04 and .06. In addition, the orifice openers (.08 and .10) are used for pre-enlargement of the canal and have a tip size of 25 mm. Each instrument can have a length of 21 mm, 25 mm, or 30 mm. The K3 instruments are recommended to be used at 300 rpm to 350 rpm, using each instrument for no longer than 5 to 7 seconds with a passive, light-pressure movement [53]. Additional flaring can be achieved using a brushing motion with the rotary instruments [54]. Three different procedure techniques are suggested by the manufacturer: the "Procedure pack" sequence, the "G-pack" sequence, and the "VTVT" sequence (Box 3.4).

Box 3.3 Quantec Preparation Sequence

Canal negotiation

Coronal flaring

Use 25/.06 orifice shaper file to a depth just short of the apical third. Instrument should be allowed to progress passively into the canal.

Pre-flaring

Use ISO standard #10 file with .02 taper and then #15 hand file to working length to create a glide path.

Canal Shaping

Crown-down sequence

25/.12 → 25/.10 → 25/.08 → 25/.06 →25/.05 → 25/.04 → 25/.03 → 25/.02

Apical preparation

Gauge working-length diameter by establishing the first standard .02 taper hand file that binds at the length required. If a larger apical resistance form is required, complete preparation using Quantec 40/.02, 45/.02 instruments.

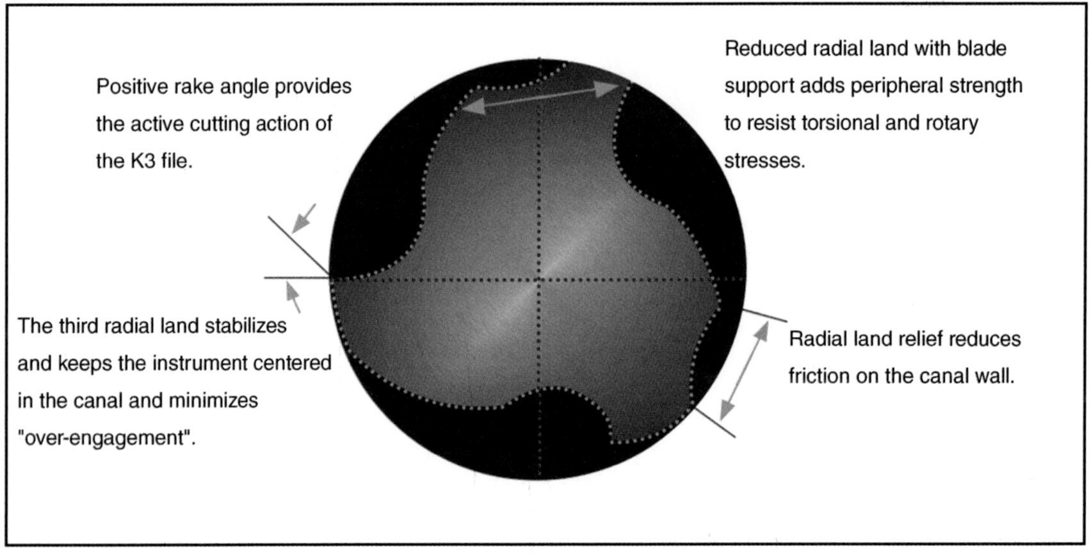

Figure 3.14 K3 file design.

FlexMaster (VDW, Munich, Germany)

FlexMaster instruments are characterized by a convex triangular cross section with sharp cutting edges (similar to a K-type blade), negative rake angle, and no radial lands (refer to Figure 3.9). This makes for a relatively solid instrument core and excellent cutting ability. The overall manufacturing quality is high, with minimal metal flash and rollover. FlexMaster files have flattened passive tips. For curved or narrow canals, files with greater taper are designed to initially enlarge the coronal and the middle portion of the canal. This is the Intro file, which has a .11 taper and a 9-mm cutting part. The 2% tapered files are used to finish the apical area. ISO sizes 20, 25 and 30 instruments have three different tapers: .02, .04, and .06. ISO sizes 35 to 70 are only available as .02 taper.

The instruments are marked with milled rings on the instrument shaft; the manufacturer provides a system

Box 3.4 K3 Preparation sequence

Procedure Pack Sequence

Coronal Flaring
25/.10→25/.08 (orifice opener to resistance)

Crown Down
Size 40 with .06 or .04 taper (EWL) → size 35 with .06 or .04 taper → size 30 with .06 or .04 taper → size 25 with .06 or .04 taper
Selection between .04 and .06 tapers is determined by the canal's anatomy and the filling technique.

G-Pack (Graduating Taper Sequence

Coronal Flaring
25/.12 → 25/.10 (orifice opener to resistance) → EWL

Crown Down
25/.08 → 25/.06 → 25/.04 → 25/.02
For canals that differ in size and shape, additional sizes of K3 instruments may be required.

VTVT (Variable Tip and Variable Taper) Sequence

Coronal Flaring
.10/25→.08/25 (orifice opener to resistance)→EWL

Crown Down
35/.06 → 30/.04 → 25/.06 → 20/.04
For canals that differ in size and shape, additional sizes of K3 instruments may be required.

EWL, Estimated working length

box that indicates sequences for narrow, medium, and wide canals. Studies indicate that the FlexMaster allows centered preparations in both constricted and wider canals [55].

The FlexMaster is not currently available in the United States.

RaCe (FKG, Dentaire, La-Chaux-de-Fonds, Switzerland)

The RaCe system was introduced in 1999 and stands for *r*eamer with *a*lternating *c*utting *e*dges. The cutting edges show twisted areas (a feature of conventional files) alternating with straight areas, thus reducing the torque and the tendency to screw into the root canal. The surface of the RaCe is treated by electropolishing to improve resistance to corrosion and fatigue (Figure 3.15). RaCe files are available in sizes from ISO 15 to 60 in tapers of .02, .04, .06, .08, and .10.

RaCe files are characterized by a triangular cross section except for .02 taper, which have a square cross section. The two largest files are size 35 with a .08 taper (35/.08) and 40/.10; these are also available in stainless steel. The tips are round and noncutting, ensuring excellent centering in the canal, decreasing the risk of deviations and ledging. The instruments are marked by color-coded handles and milled rings. RaCe instruments are recommended to be used between 300 rpm and 600 rpm, with light apical pressure in a pumping–pecking motion [56]. They can be used in three different operative sequences: two step-back techniques and one crown-down technique (Table 3.4). BioRaCe differs from other RaCe instruments in regard to tapers, sizes, and sequence. The major goal of BioRaCe is to achieve apical preparation sizes (with few instruments) that can effectively disinfect the canal.

The fatigue and number of uses of each instrument can be controlled according to the complexity of the canal with SMD (Safety MemoDisc) (Figure 3.16) [57]. Each SMD has eight petals. After each use, the

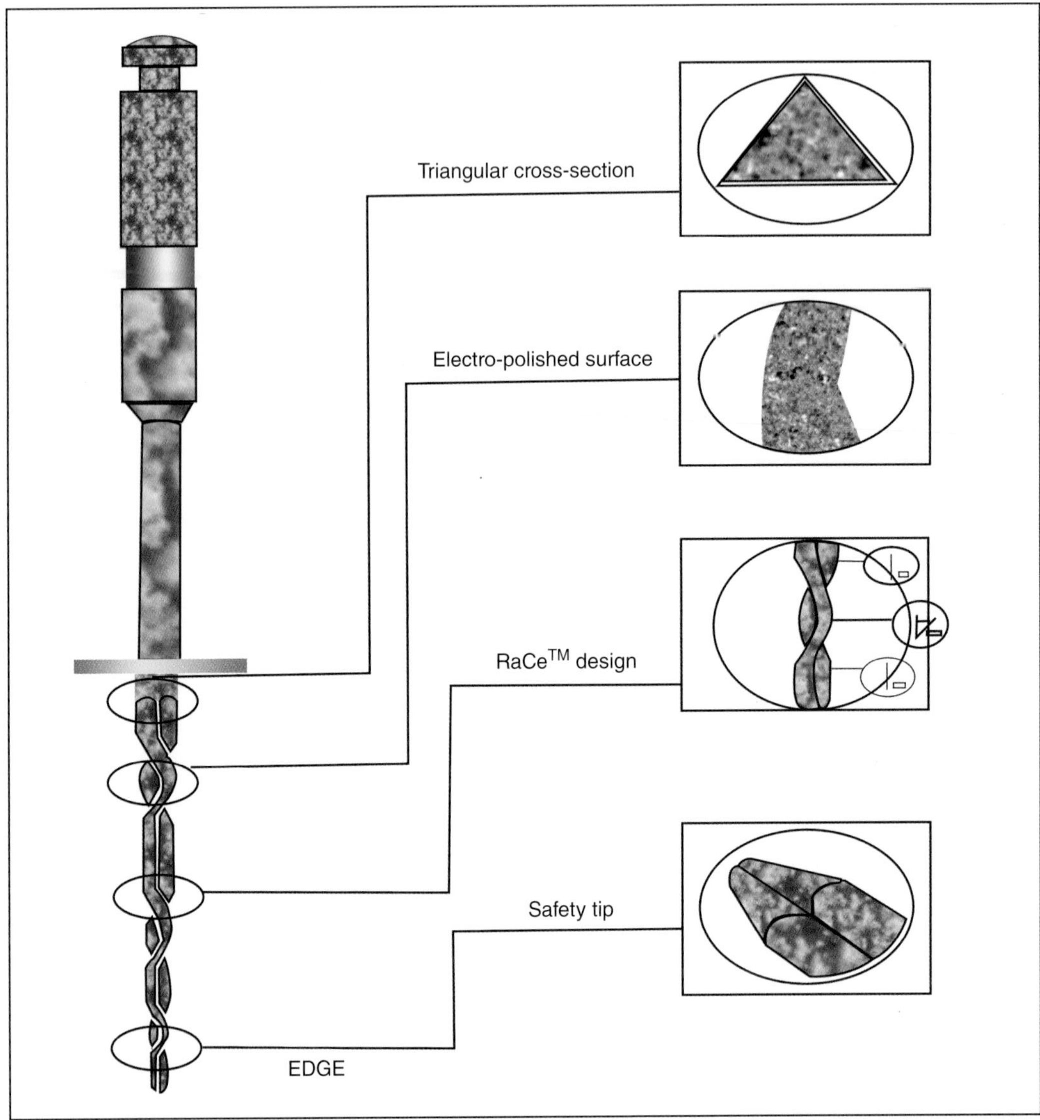

Figure 3.15 RaCe design characteristics.

practitioner pulls off several petals. The petals indicate the possibility of further use. The SMDs are sterilizable and therefore stay on the instruments. One petal corresponds to simple cases, that is, straight, slightly curved, and/or wide canals. Two petals correspond to moderately complex cases, that is, more curved or narrow canals. Four petals correspond to complex cases, that is, canals with extreme curvature or S-shaped, very narrow, or calcified canals. When all petals have been removed, the instrument is discarded.

The RaCe system is distributed in the United States by Brasseler.

Mtwo (VDW, Munich, Germany)

The Mtwo system has been available since 2005. The set includes eight files with tapers ranging from .04 to .07 and sizes from ISO 10 to 40. The number of grooved rings on the handle identifies the instrument taper. The instruments are available in 21 mm, 25 mm, and 31 mm lengths and are also produced with an extended

Table 3.4 Available RaCe instruments.

Type	Use
Basic Set consists of five NiTi files and includes two 19-mm long highly tapered PreRaCe for coronal shaping, and three 25-mm long less-tapered RaCe for apical finishing. Easy RaCe RaCe Xtreme (used only with step-back technique	Treatment of simple and medium canals Enlargement of difficult and curved canals
Scout RaCe	To prepare the glide path of straight canals, canals with severe curvature, or S-type canals Set of three instruments
RaCe ISO 10	For use in calcified or very narrow canals when manual K files of ISO 06 or 08 cannot progress farther, Set of three instruments
BioRaCe	Designed to achieve the biological aim of the root canal treatment without compromising efficiency Set of six files
iRaCe	Allows the clinician to achieve working length with fewer than three rotary files, It is a simplified version of the BioRaCe
BT-RaCe (Booster Tip)	Sterile-packed and single-use set of three files
D-RaCe	To remove different filling materials such as gutta-percha, carriers, paste, and resin-based materials Set of two instruments

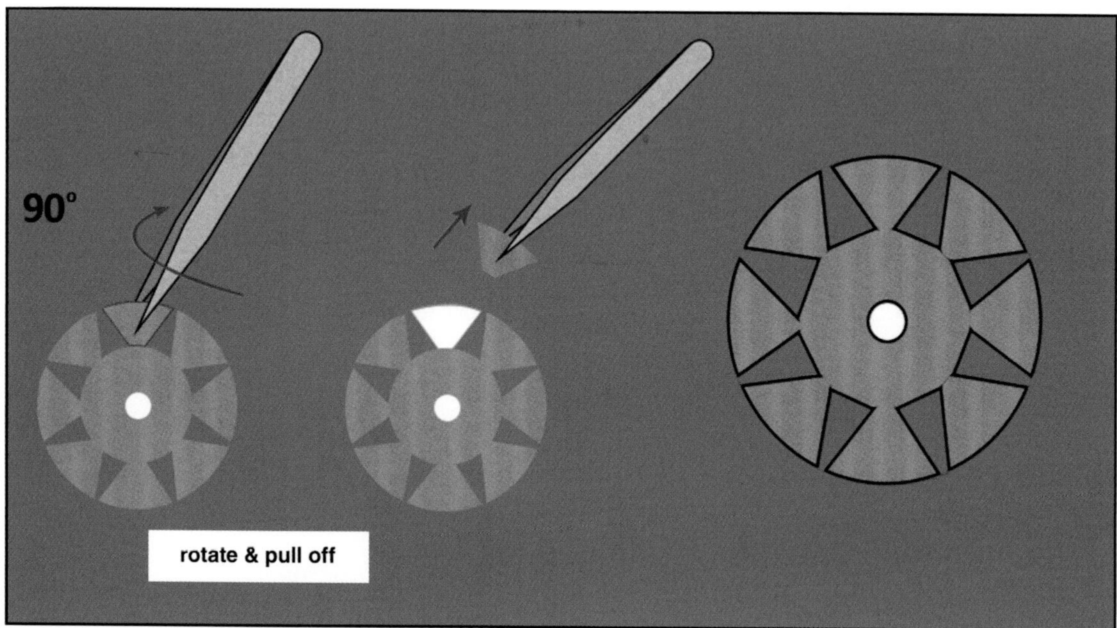

Figure 3.16 Safety memo disc (SMD) showing how petals are used.

cutting portion of 21 mm as well as the conventional 16-mm cutting part, allowing the instrument to cut in the coronal portion of the canals efficiently, on the cavity access walls, where dentin interferences are often located.

They have an S-shaped cross-sectional design and a noncutting safety tip (Figure 3.17). Two symmetrical blades characterize Mtwo cross section. This geometrical design reduces the contact lengths of the blades on the dentinal walls, thus reducing the production of debris and smear layer and increasing the available volume for irrigating solutions and upward elimination of debris.

Mtwo files are further characterized by a positive rake angle with two cutting edges. These instruments also have an increasing pitch from tip to shaft to eliminate screwing and binding in continuous rotation. All instruments are used at working length.

The Mtwo NiTi rotary instruments are used at 300 rpm and in a simultaneous technique without any early coronal enlargement: the crown-down technique is used, but smaller instruments are used before bigger ones, as is done in the step-back technique, and thus the entire length of the canal is approached at the same time [58]. The system permits three different approaches to root canal preparation after the basic sequence has been completed with a 25/.06 Mtwo instrument. The first sequence allows clinicians to achieve enlarged apical diameters; the second leads to a .07 taper that can facilitate vertical condensation of gutta-percha;

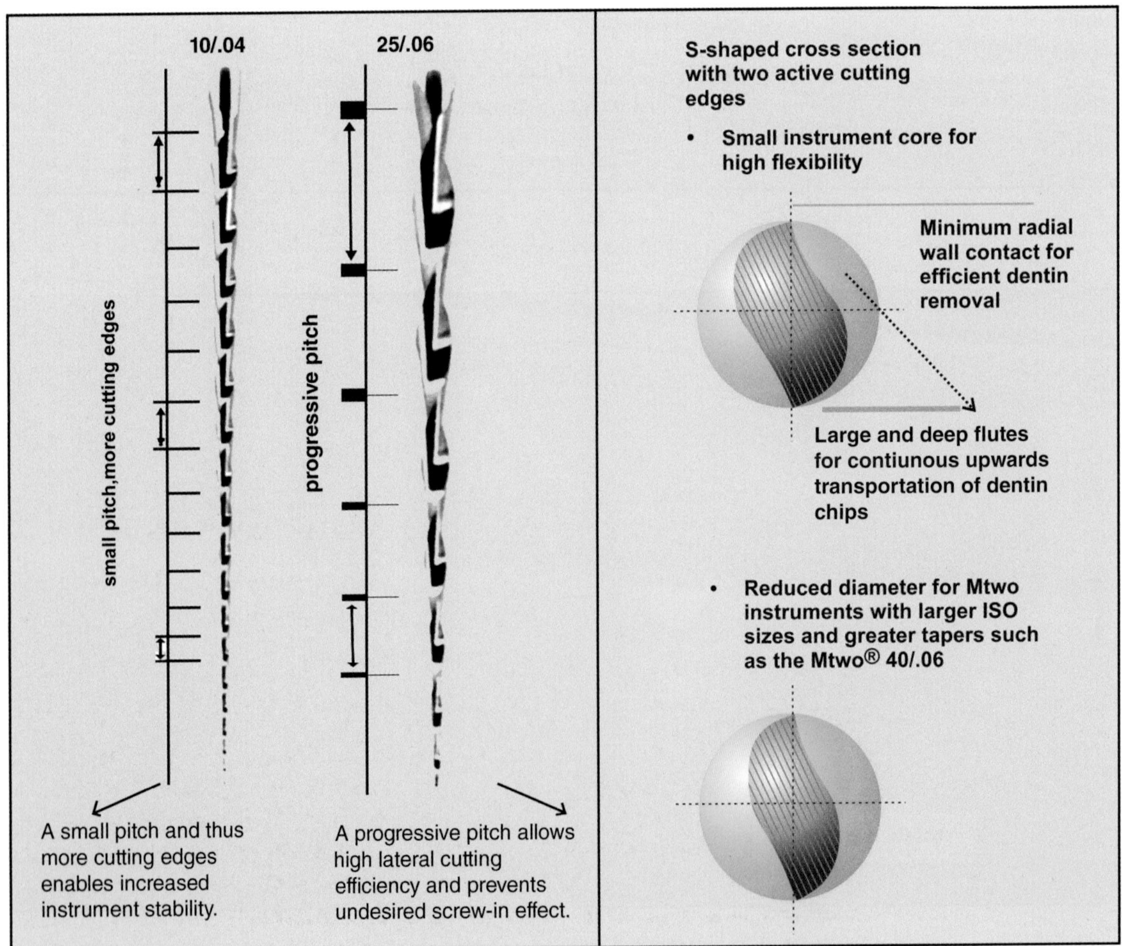

Figure 3.17 Mtwo file characteristics.

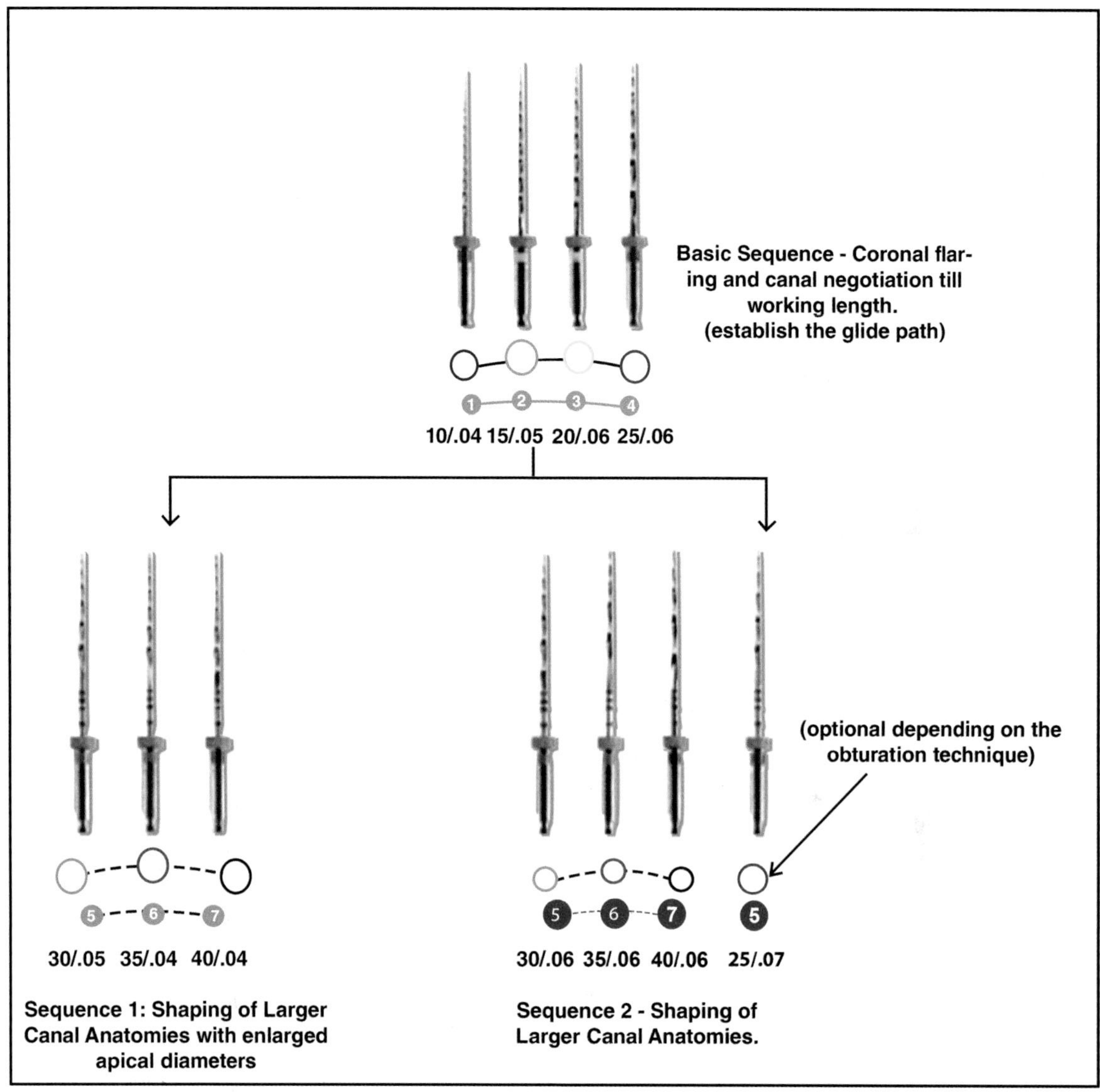

Figure 3.18 Mtwo preparation sequence. All the files in sequence 1 and sequence 2 are to working length.

the third implies the use of the Mtwo apical files (Figure 3.18).

Mtwo A and Mtwo R

The system is further updated with three rotary files specifically designed for apical preparation, the Mtwo A, and two files for retreatment, the Mtwo R. The three apical files are Mtwo A1, A2, and A3, and they vary in tip size and taper. The innovative feature of these instruments is the high taper of the last apical millimeter to maintain the apical anatomy while obtaining larger apical diameters, while the rest of the coronal portion is a 2% ISO taper. This enhanced taper in the apical zone also provides resistance against the condensation pressures of obturation and acts to prevent extrusion of the filling material [59].

The Mtwo R instruments are specifically designed for the retreatment of obturating materials. The retreatment files are Mtwo R 15/.05 and Mtwo R 25/.05, presenting an active tip that allows clinicians to easily penetrate in the obturation material.

ProFile System (Denstply Maillefer, Ballaigues, Switzerland)

Introduced by Dr. Ben Johnson in 1994, the ProFile has an increased taper compared with conventional hand instruments. The ProFile first was sold as a series of 29 hand instruments in .02 taper, but it soon became available in .04 and .06 and a ProFile Orifice Shaper. It is recommended that coronal flaring with Orifice Shapers and initial scouting of the canal be performed (Table 3.5) [60, 61]. All share the same cross-sectional geometry (refer to Figure 3.9) of having three radial lands. Instruments are used between 150 and 300 rpm while allowing the instrument to progress passively into the canal in a crown-down manner. A light pecking motion is recommended, withdrawing and advancing the instrument until it will not proceed further. Cross sections of a ProFile instrument shows a U-shape design with radial lands, a negative rake angle, a noncutting pilot tip, and a parallel central core to enhance flexibility.

ProFile series 29 NiTi rotary instruments feature a constant 29% increase in the tip diameter between the file sizes. This constant percentage increase offers a smooth progressive enlargement of the canal. The .02 taper series is designed for use in extremely curved canals. The .04 series was designed for subsequent carrier-based obturation techniques, and .06 instruments provide a fuller shape over the length of the canal.

ProTaper (Progressively Tapered) (Denstply Maillefer, Ballaigues, Switzerland)

The ProTaper system is based on a unique concept and comprises six instruments: three shaping files and three finishing files. This system was designed by Dr. Cliff Ruddle, Dr. John West, and Dr. Pierre Machtou. The unique design factor is the varying tapers along the instruments' long axes. The three shaping files have tapers that increase coronally, and the reverse pattern is seen in the three finishing files. SX (ISO size 19) has a progressive taper (.03–.19), whereas S1 and S2 (ISO size 17 and 20) have tapers ranging from .02 to .11 and from .04 to .115, respectively. The finishing files (ISO size 20, 25, and 30) F1 (.07–.05), F2 (.08–.055), and F3 (.09–.05) have decreasing tapers (Figure 3.19) [62].

The Shaping X (auxiliary shaping) file is used to optimally shape canals in shorter roots, to relocate canals away from external root concavities, and to produce more shape in the coronal aspects of canals in longer roots using a brushing motion. S1 is designed to prepare the coronal one third of a canal, whereas, S2 enlarges and prepares the middle one third. Although both instruments optimally prepare the coronal two thirds of a canal, they do progressively enlarge its apical one third. The finishing files, or F1, F2, and F3 instruments, finish the apical one third. Generally, only one finishing instrument is required to prepare the apical one third of a canal (Figure 3.20).

The cross section of the ProTaper resembles a modified K-type (convex triangular) file with sharp cutting edges and no radial lands (refer to Figure 3.9). This reduces the contact areas between the file and the dentin. The cutting efficiency is improved by balancing the pitch and helix angle. The cross section of finishing file F3 is slightly relieved for increased flexibility. The finishing files have noncutting tips, and the shaping files have partially active tips. The instruments are used at a constant speed of 300 to 350 rpm in a gear-reduction handpiece. Compared with other rotary instruments, the shaft is 15% shorter to facilitate access to posterior teeth. The instruments are coded by colored rings on the handles. The auxiliary shaping file has no identification ring on its handle.

In 2006, The ProTaper Universal was introduced by adding two new finishing files, F4 (ISO size 40) and F5

Table 3.5 ProFile preparation sequence.

Use	Small Canals	Medium Canals	Large Canals
Coronal flaring (orifice shapers)	40/.06 30/.06	50/.07 40/.06	60/.08 50/.07
Crown-down sequence	25/.06 → 20/.06 → 25/.04	30/.06 → 25/.06 → 30/.04	30/.06 → 30/.06 → 35/.04
Apical preparation	20/.04 → 25/.04	25/.04 → 30/.04	30/.04 → 35/.04

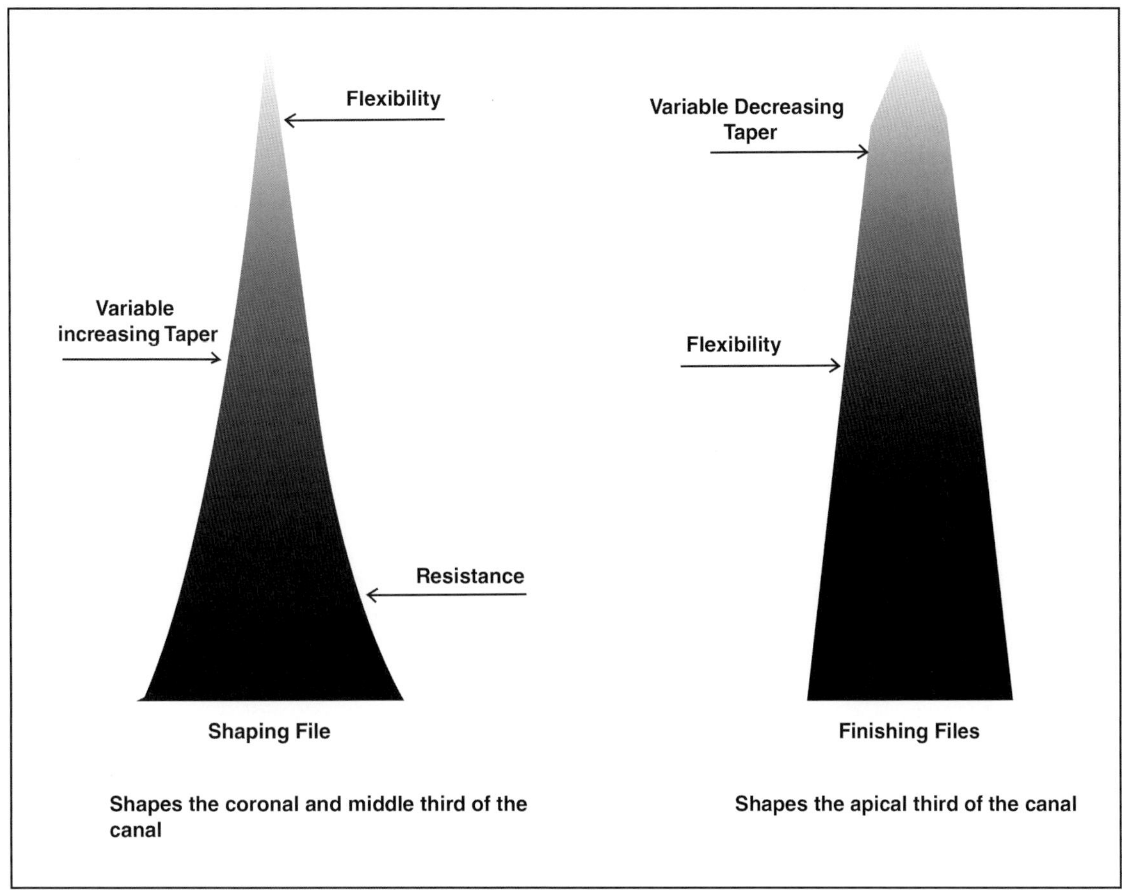

Figure 3.19 Differences between ProTaper shaping files and finishing files.

(ISO size 50), for apical preparation. The other modification was the safe rounded tip instead of the partially active tip in the previous system.

GT Rotary System (Greater Taper) (Denstply Maillefer)

The GT file was introduced by Dr. Buchanan in 1994. This instrument also incorporates the U-shaped file design. The GT system was first produced as a set of four hand-operated files and later as engine-driven files. The instruments had a variable pitch and an increasing number of flutes in progression to the tip. Instrument tips were noncutting and rounded.

ProSystem GT

In 2001, the GT set was modified to accommodate a wider range of apical sizes. The current set includes instruments of three apical diameters: GT20, GT30, and GT40 according to ISO size and with varying tapers of .10, .08, .06, and .04. In addition, accessory files with a .12 taper are available in sizes 35, 50, 70, and 90. The recommended rotational speed for GT files is 350 rpm, and the instrument should be used with minimal apical force to avoid fracturing the tip. The instruments are selected according to the canal anatomy: small canals, GT20; medium canals, GT30; and large canals, GT40. They are used in a crown-down manner in a sequence of larger taper to smaller taper.

Summary

The preceding descriptions covered only a limited selection, the most popular and widely used rotary instruments. New files are continually added to the armamentarium, and older systems are updated. Thus

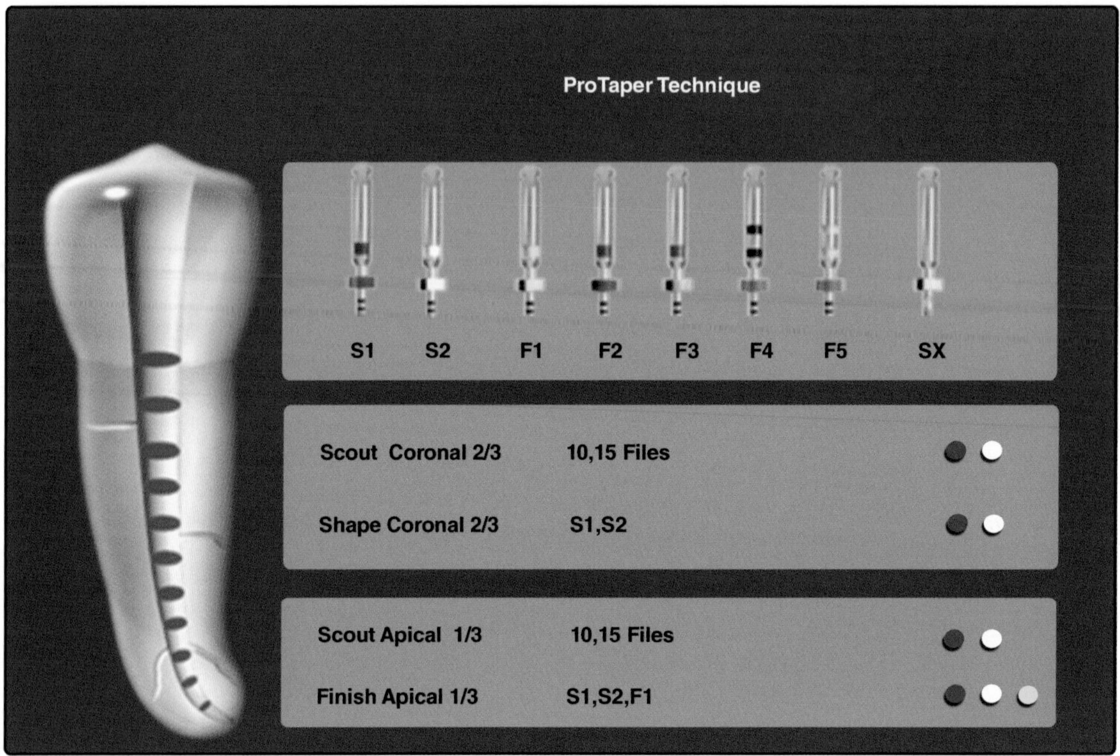

Figure 3.20 ProTaper instrument sequence.

it is next to impossible to keep track of file designs. To summarize, most systems include files with tapers greater than the .02 stipulated by the ISO norm. The LightSpeed is different from all other systems, the ProTaper and RaCe have some unique features, and most other systems have increased tapers. Minor differences exist in tip designs, cross sections, and manufacturing processes.

Advances in Nickel–Titanium Metallurgy (Thermomechanical Treatment of Nickel–Titanium Instruments)

At the beginning of 2000, a series of studies [63–66] found that changes in the transformation behavior via heat treatment was effective in increasing the flexibility of NiTi endodontic instruments. Since then, heat-induced or heat-altering manipulations have been used to influence or alter the properties of NiTi endodontic instruments, which are the main reasons for pursuing the use of NiTi instruments in endodontics. New forms of NiTi have been created by heating the alloy during the manufacturing process, resulting in a combination of heat-treatment and hardening [7]. Because the martensitic form of NiTi has remarkable fatigue resistance, instruments in the martensite phase can easily be deformed and yet recover their shape on heating above the transformation temperatures. The explanation for this may be that heating transforms the metal temporarily into the austenitic phase and makes it superelastic, which makes it possible for the file to regain its original shape before cooling down again.

Proprietary thermomechanical treatment is a complicated process that integrates hardening and heat treatment into a single process. Enhancement in these areas of material management have led to the development of the next generation of endodontic instruments. The new manufacturing processes aims at respecting the molecular structure of the alloy for maximum strength, as opposed to grinding that creates microfracture points during the production of the instruments [67]. M-wire and R-phase treated wire represent the next generation of NiTi alloys with improved flexibility and fatigue resistance [68–71].

Studies have also demonstrated that the centering ability is improved and transportation is reduced while using these new-generation files [72]. Because heat treatment affects the physical properties of NiTi alloys, autoclaving could modify their physical properties; however, up to seven sterilization cycles have not significantly affected the flexibility or fracture resistance of M-wire (ProFile Vortex), R-phase (TF) or CM-wire NiTi instruments [73].

M-wire NiTi (Dentsply Tulsa Dental Specialties)

M-wire was introduced in 2007 using a proprietary thermal cycling process (applying a series of heat treatments to NiTi wire blanks). The manufacturer claims that this material has greater flexibility and an increased resistance to cyclic fatigue when compared to traditional NiTi alloys. M-wire technology significantly improves the resistance to cyclic fatigue by almost 400% compared to commercially available NiTi files [74]. Three file systems fabricated from M-wire NiTi, currently in use, are the ProFile Vortex, Vortex Blue, GT Series X, and ProTaper Next files.

R-phase NiTi (Sybron Endo)

R-phase is an intermediate phase with a rhombohedral structure that can be formed either during the martensite-to-austenite or the austenite-to-martensite transition. In 2008, instruments were developed by transforming a raw NiTi wire in the austenite phase into the R-phase through a thermal process (Figure 3.21).

R-phase technology offers the following advantages: It overcomes many of the limitations of ground file technology and opens up new opportunities for improved file design, such as twisting. It optimizes the molecular phase structure, thus resulting in improved properties of nickel–titanium. It employs a crystalline structural modification that maximizes flexibility and resistance to breakage.

The Twisted File (TF) and K3XF file are based on R-phase NiTi technology, and the manufacturer claims the files have reduced stiffness and more fracture

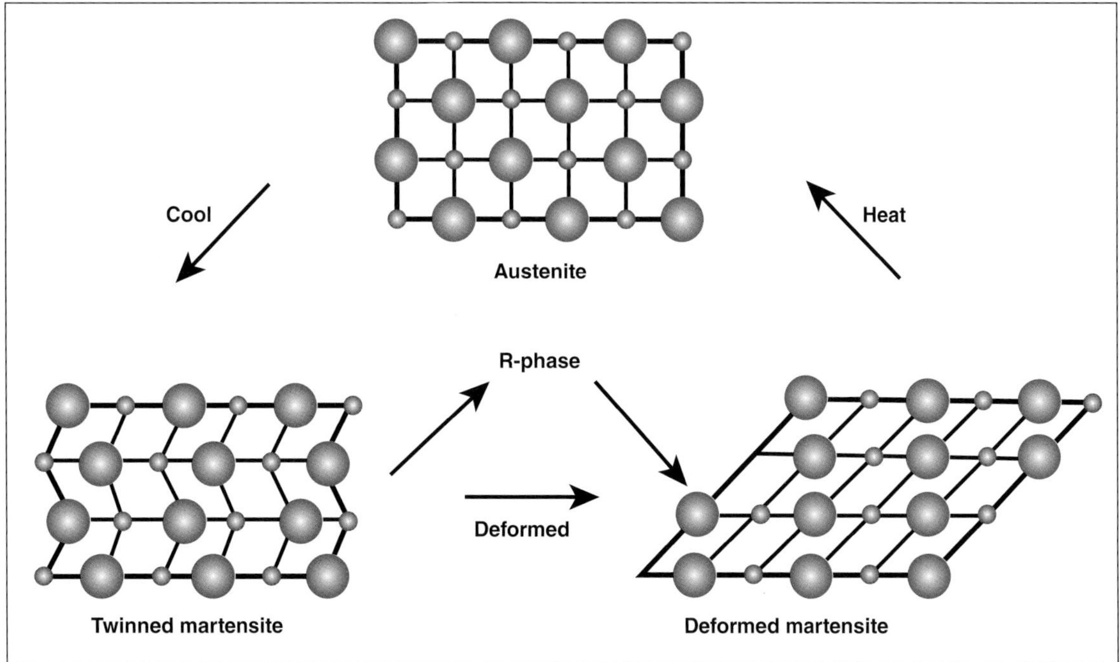

Figure 3.21 R-Phase diagram. Force and temperature-dependent transitions for austenite to martensite, including the intermediary R-phase. The proportion of alloy that is in R-phase depends on heat treatment of the raw wire.

resistance compared to standard NiTi files. The R-phase shows good superelasticity and shape-memory effects. In 2013, TF Adaptive was introduced based on the same concept.

Controlled-Memory (CM) (D&S Dental, Johnson City, TN, USA)

Introduced in 2010, CM NiTi files are manufactured using a special thermomechanical process that controls the memory of the material, making the files extremely flexible but without the shape memory of other, conventional NiTi files. This allows the instrument to be precurved before it is placed into the root canal. Sterilization of these files returns them to their original shape. Both HyFlex (Coltène Whaledent) and Typhoon (TYP) (Clinician's Choice Dental products, USA) are made from CM wire.

ProFile GT Series X (GTX) (Tulsa Dental)

Designed by Dr. L. Stephen Buchanan, the first commercially available endodontic rotary system using the new M-wire technology was GTX in 2008. The design principles of the ProFile GT instrument were mostly followed in the ProFile GTX, with the main differences being subtle changes in the longitudinal design and a different approach to instrument use, emphasizing the use of the #20/.06 rotary. (Table 3.6)

The design features of GTX include fewer cutting flutes and wider, more open blade angles that significantly reduce core mass. Flutes hold more debris, reducing the number of strokes needed to shape the canal. This decreases the number of file rotations and reduces cyclic fatigue that can lead to file separation. Wider flutes make fewer continuous rotations around the instrument from the tip to the end of the cutting zone. Open blade angles reduce the chance of threading. The result is a faster-cutting instrument with increased flexibility to follow curved canals. The instruments also have variable-width lands, which virtually eliminate the taper lock in the canal, and a 1-mm maximum shank diameter (Figure 3.22). This permits rapid cutting without transportation, thus enhancing the overall cutting efficiency of GTX [75].

The design change offers three advantages: a reduction in the number of instruments to an eight-file set, a reduction in the number of files needed to cut a given preparation, and a reduction in the possibility of file separation caused by choosing a too-large shaping objective when canals contain hidden curves.

The GTX set currently includes tip sizes 20, 30, and 40 in tapers ranging from .04 to .10 (Figure 3.23) [76]. The recommended rotational speed for GT and GTX files is 300 rpm, and the instruments should be used with minimal apical force and a slight pecking action. In canals with very large apical diameters, one of the .12 GT Accessory files should be used.

ProFile Vortex (Dentsply Tulsa)

In 2009, ProFile Vortex rotary files were introduced (Figure 3.24). These instruments yield increased flexibility and resistance to fatigue compared to traditional NiTi wire [77]. The major change lies in the nonlanded cross section, whereas tip sizes and tapers are similar to existing ProFiles. Manufactured using M-wire, Profile Vortex files also have varying helical angles. This geometry promotes more-efficient cutting and decreased threading-in effects. Files are also able to navigate the canal curvatures predictably and safely. They have a rectangular cross section and a recommended rotary

Table 3.6 GT series X sequence.

	No. of Instruments	Available Lengths
	8	21, 25, and 31
	Preparation Sequence	
Use	Small Canals	Medium and Large canals
Canal negotiation	ISO #15 K-file, WL established	ISO #15 K-file, WL established
Shaping	20/.06	20/.06 → 20/.04 → 20/.06
Apical finishing	30/.06	30/.08 or 40/.08

WL, working length

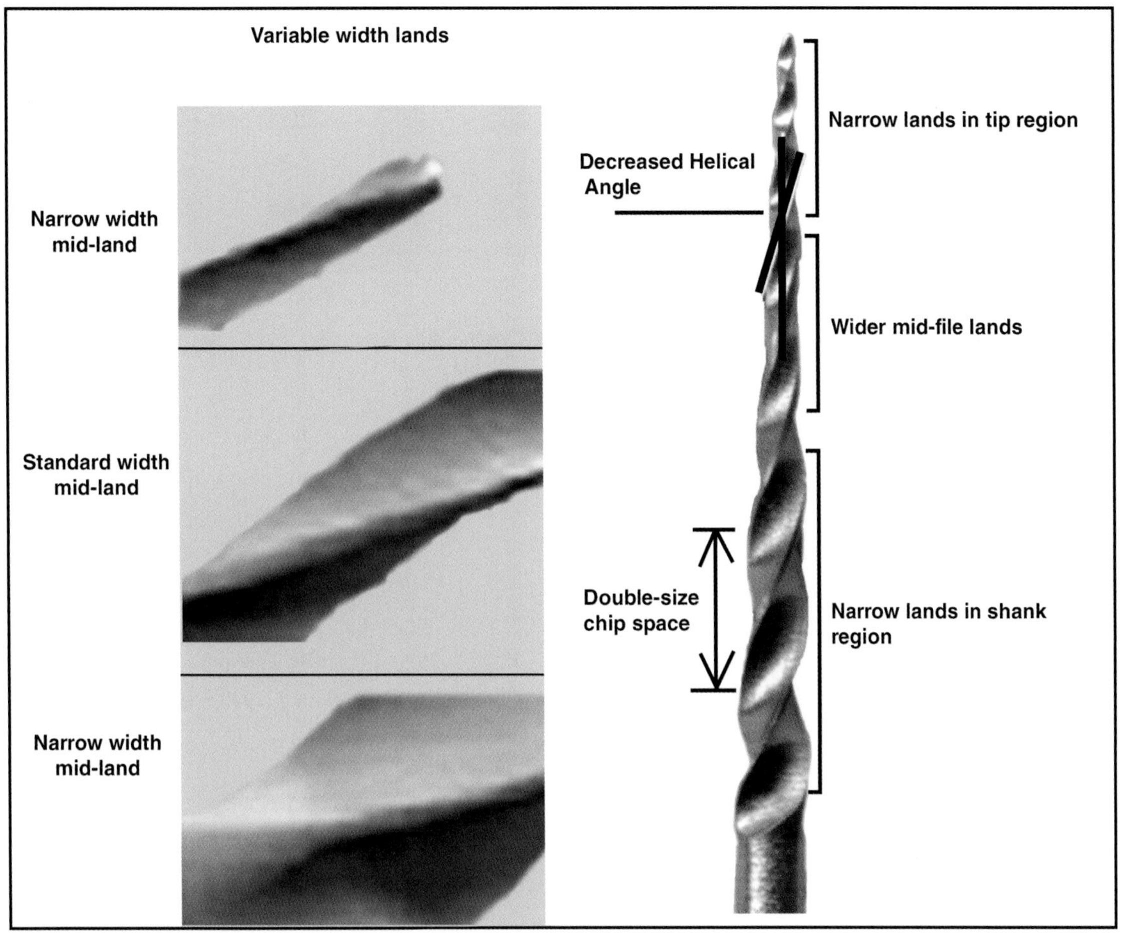

Figure 3.22 GT Series X File design. At the tip and shank ends, the land widths are half the size of the lands in the middle region of the flutes, allowing rapid and efficient cutting.

speed of 500 rpm [78]. They are available in ISO tip sizes from 15 to 50 and in .04 or .06 taper.

Vortex Blue (Dentsply Tulsa)

In 2012, Vortex Blue was manufactured using an advanced thermomechanical process that shows greater resistance to cyclic fatigue, greater torque strength [7], improved flexibility, and reduced shape memory while conforming to natural curvatures. The distinctive color of Vortex Blue is an optical effect, created by light rays interacting with a titanium oxide layer on the surface of the file, that is a result of the proprietary manufacturing process (Figure 3.25).

The files stay centered in the canal due to the reduced shape-memory effect. The relatively hard titanium oxide surface layer on the Vortex Blue instrument compensates for the loss of hardness compared with ProFile Vortex M-wire [77] while improving the cutting efficiency and wear resistance [77]. These files are available in tapers of .04 and .06 from sizes 15 to 50 and in lengths of 21 mm, 25 mm, and 30 mm. Vortex Blue is rectangular in cross section and has a recommended rotary speed of 500 rpm [78].

ProTaper Next (PTN) (Dentsply Tulsa)

Introduced in 2013, PTN files are the convergence of three significant design features, including progressive tapers on a single file as in the ProTaper Universal M-wire technology, which allows more-flexible instruments, increased fatigue resistance, and the fifth

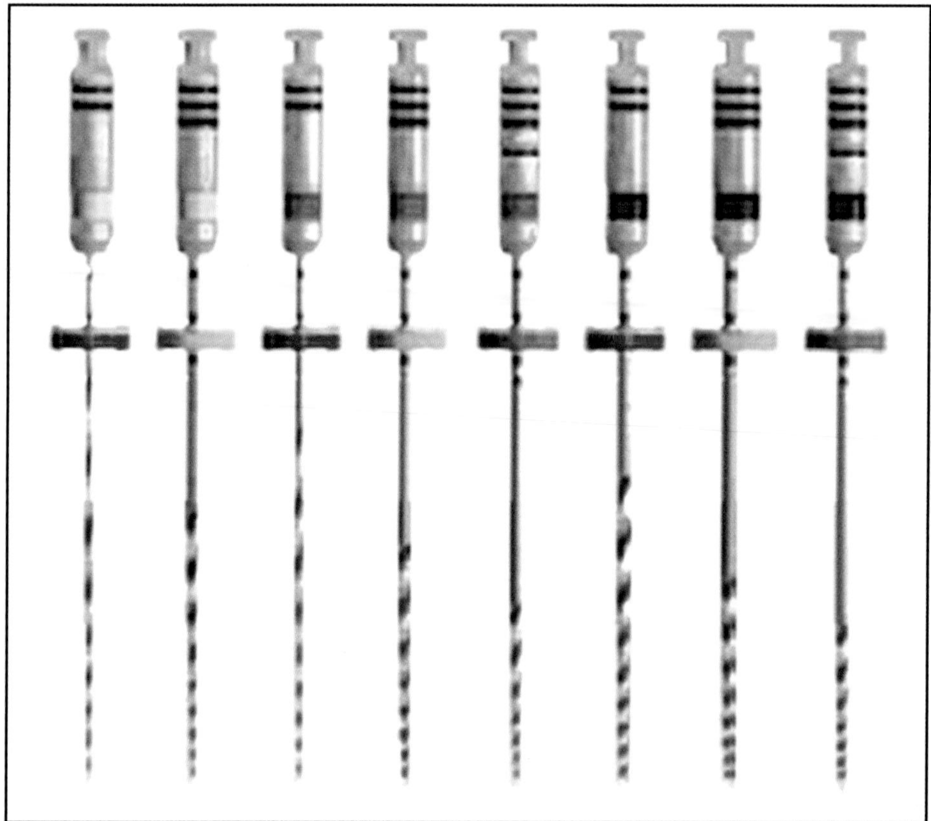

Figure 3.23 GT Series X instrument system.

generation bilateral symmetrical offset rectangular cross-sectional design. This offset feature gives the file a unique asymmetric rotary movement, termed *swaggering*, due to which only two points of the rectangular cross section touch the canal wall at a time (Figure 3.26) [79]. The exception is the ProTaper X1, which has a square cross section in the last 3-mm segment to give the instrument a bit more core strength in the narrow apical part.

The offset design provides three distinct advantages: The swaggering effect limits the undesirable taper lock and hence serves to minimize the engagement between the file and the dentin. The offset affords more cross-sectional space for auguring debris removal in a coronal direction, which leads to improved cutting efficiency as the blades remain in contact with the surrounding dentin walls. The offset allows the file to cut a bigger envelope of motion compared to a similarly sized file with a symmetrical mass and axis of rotation. Therefore, a smaller and more flexible PTN file can cut the same size preparation as a larger and stiffer file with a centered mass and axis of rotation. This allows the clinician to use fewer instruments in preparing a root canal, at the same time maintaining adequate shape and taper.

Five PTN files are available in different lengths for shaping canals, namely X1, X2, X3, X4, and X5. In sequence, these files have yellow, red, blue, double black, and double yellow identification rings on their handles, corresponding to sizes and tapers of 17/.04, 25/.06, 30/.07, 40/.06, and 50/.06.

Both the X1 and X2 have an increasing and decreasing percentage tapered design over the active portion of the instruments. The last three finishing instruments are the X3, X4, and X5, which have a decreasing percentage taper from the tip to the shank. They can be used to either create more taper in a root canal or prepare larger root canal systems. The ProTaper

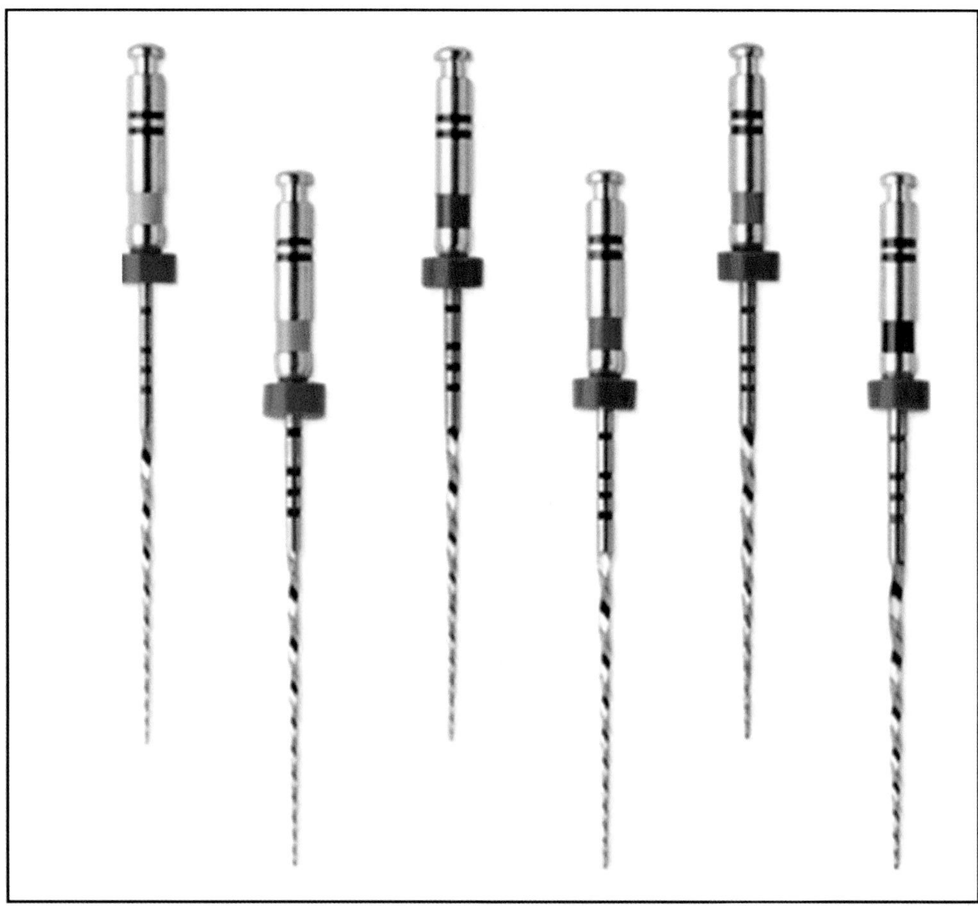

Figure 3.24 ProFile (Image courtesy of Dentsply, Tulsa, OK, USA.)

Universal SX shaper file is recommended for preflaring the orifice (Figure 3.27). For very long and severely curved root canals, as well as large-diameter root canals and root canals for retreatment, canal preparation can be initiated with the ProTaper Next X2, X3, X4, or X5 directly.

The PTN files are used at 300 rpm and are used with a deliberate outward brushing motion (never in a pecking motion) when progressively shaping canals [80]. All files are used in exactly the same way, and the sequence always follows the ISO color progression and is always the same regardless of the length, diameter, or curvature of a canal. This motion creates lateral space and enables the file to progress and improve contact between the file and dentin.

Sequence ESX System (Brasseler USA, Savannah, GA, USA)

Sequence ESX is an advanced rotary file system that aims to improve two specific challenges: system simplicity and cutting efficiency using fewer files. The ESX system was inspired by the original EndoSequence system (Brasseler USA, Savannah, GA, USA) [81–83]. The core design features of EndoSequence files, namely the triangular cross section, their patented asymmetrical Alternating Contact Points (ACP), and the electropolished NiTi metal wire, have been retained for the ESX. Both file systems use a recommended speed of 500 to 600 rpm.

There are three significant differences between the two file systems: The ESX file has incorporated a new patented BT-Tip (booster tip), which helps

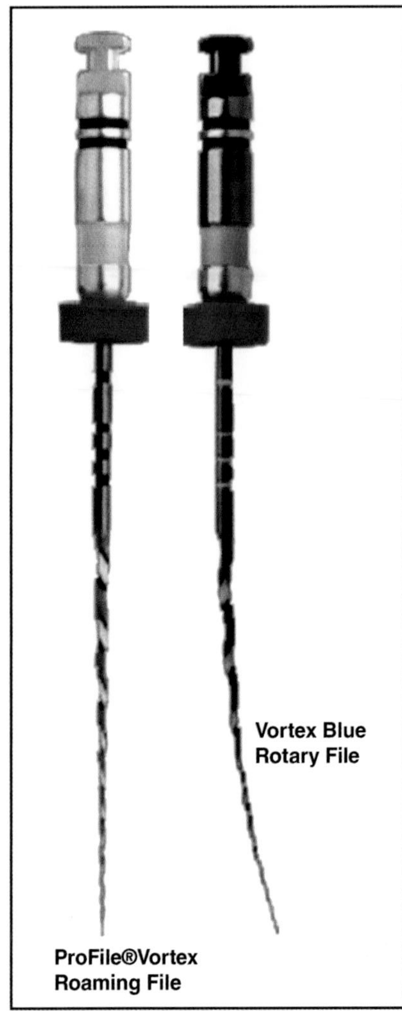

Figure 3.25 Vortex Blue.

guide the file while simultaneously reducing canal ledging, the use of a unique operator motion called Single Stroke and Clean (SSC) technique, which drastically reduces torque exerted on each file, and a more-efficient protocol requiring fewer files to achieve the same results.

There are four ESX finishing files: 25, 35, 45, and 55, all in .04 taper and with booster tip. This tip uses flat transition angles from the rounded noncutting tip to advance to the triangular shank. This change in tip design helps in creating a guiding motion with the benefit of reduced potential for ledging.

The SSC operator motion recommended for ESX files reduces the torque exerted on the file. The technique involves using the ESX rotary file for one engagement and filling of the flutes, followed by immediately removing and cleaning the file. This guiding tip and SSC technique (file motion based on chip space) allows the clinician to reduce the number of files required to instrument any root canal.

The Basic ESX File System consists of an Expeditor (15/.05) file, and finishing files. The protocol is to hand instrument the canal to the full working length and then to use the Expeditor to file down to the same length using the SSC motion. If significant engagement is met, then a size 25/.04 finishing file is used to the same length using the SSC motion. A size 35/.04 is used as the master finishing file when the Expeditor experiences moderate engagement to length, and a size 45/.04 is used when the Expeditor experiences minimal engagement to length. A size 55 is also provided for cases where the operator observes inadequate cleaning after the size 45 finishing file has reached the apex.

In more-challenging cases with significant curvatures or calcifications, an Advanced ESX protocol is recommended. This method uses three additional files before using the Expeditor: The ESX Orifice Opener (20/.08) and two ESX Scouting Files (15/.04 and 15/.02) are used alone or with hand instrumentation to achieve the required working length before employing the Expeditor.

EdgeFile X-3 Heat-Treated FireWire (Edge Endo, Johnson City, TN, USA)

The EdgeFile is made of an annealed heat-treated (AHT) nickel–titanium alloy brand named FireWire, which increases cyclic fatigue resistance and torque strength. Due to this proprietary processing, EdgeFile X3 files may be slightly curved. This is not considered a manufacturing defect and can easily be straightened with the fingers. This is not necessary to do, however, because once it is inside the canal, the EdgeFile X3 follows and conforms to the natural canal anatomy and curvatures. These rotary files are for single-patient use and are constant tapered. XR Retreatment Files are also available as R1 (25.12), R2 (25./08), R3 (25./06), and R4 (25./04).

Twisted Files (Sybron Endo, Orange, CA, USA)

The Twisted File system is manufactured from a proprietary process of heating, cooling in the rhombohedral

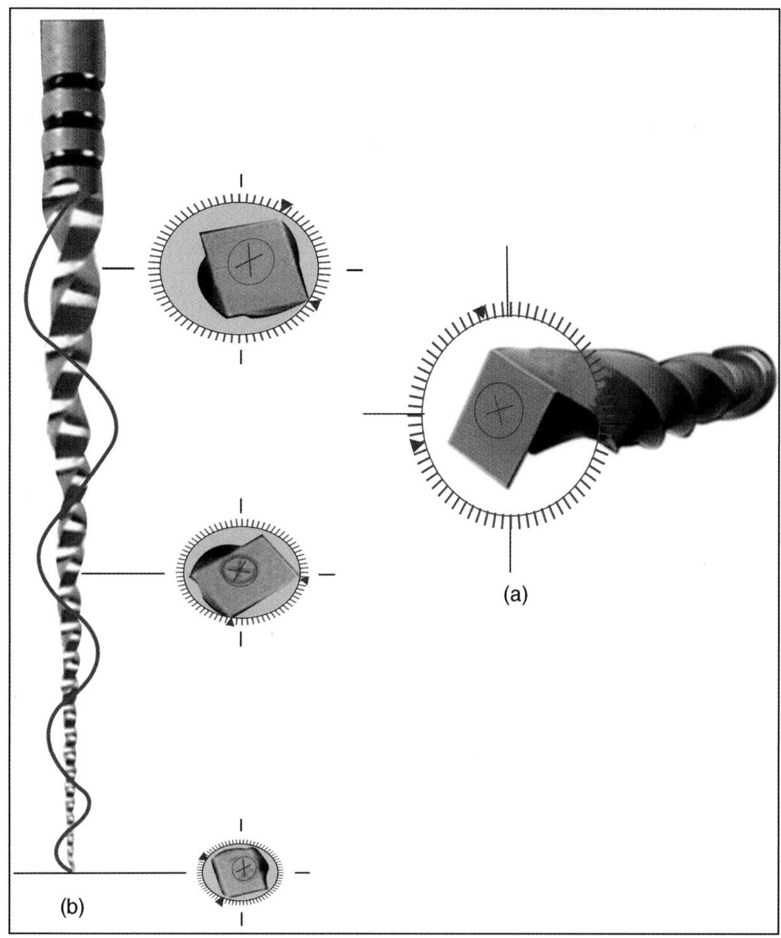

Figure 3.26 ProTaper Next. *A*, Cross section. *B*, Swaggering effect. Three unique elements are used in the design of this ProTaper NEXT file: a rectangular cross section, an asymmetric rotary motion, and M-wire NiTi alloy.

crystalline phase configuration (an intermediate phase between austenite, the phase at rest, and martensite, the phase present during function R phase), which allows the twisting of the file. This makes Twisted File distinct from all the other systems. The shape of the other rotary files is machined by milling, a mechanical process. This unique procedure lends particular resistance to TF, as well as an extraordinary flexibility.

In addition, in twisted files, having been made by twisting and not by polishing/milling, all the microcracks are eliminated, resulting in a more resistant, higher-strength file. The manufacturing process is completed by applying an advanced surface-conditioning treatment that helps to maintain the surface hardness of the material and sharpness of the edges. TF optimizes the strength and flexibility of NiTi, creating a highly durable and flexible file while maintaining the canal curvature even in extreme cases [84]. TF offers three to four times greater resistance to torsion and cyclic fatigue relative to ground files. Owing to its unique machining, TF untwists before separating in the canal, thereby giving the clinician timely warning to replace the file and significantly decreasing the risk of accidents while working with the rotary files.

With regard to file design, Twisted File has a triangular cross section that enhances flexibility and generates less friction inside the canal walls due to a lack of

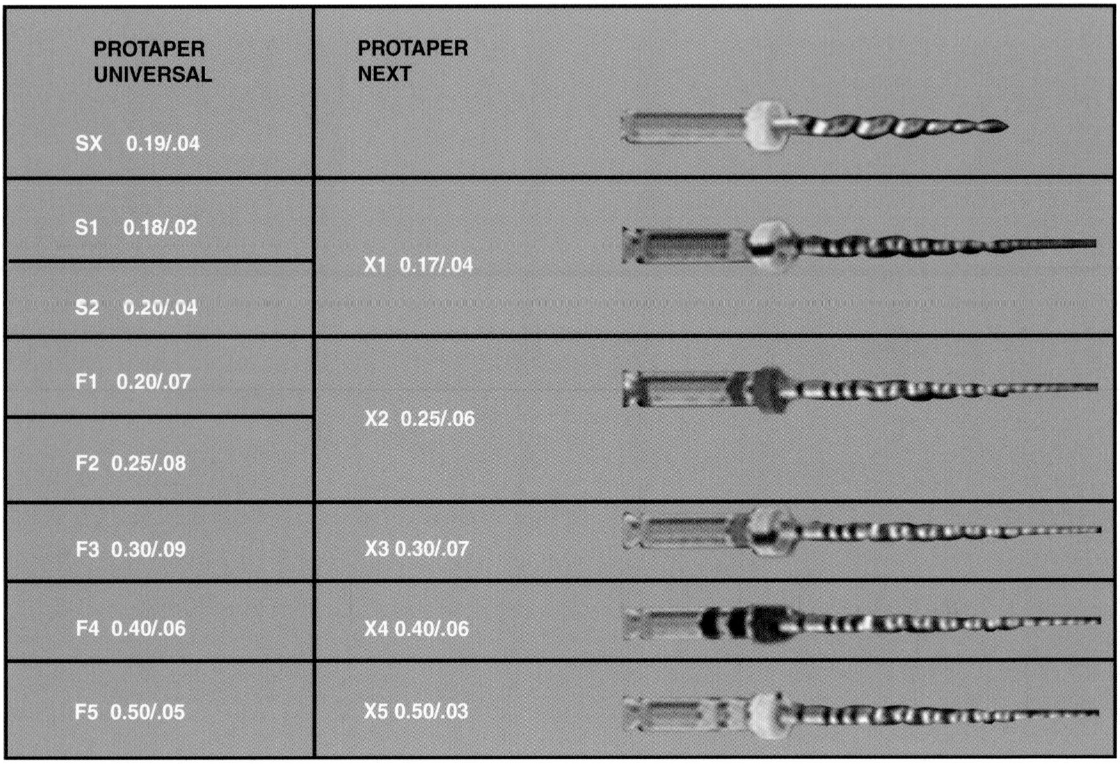

PROTAPER UNIVERSAL	PROTAPER NEXT
SX 0.19/.04	
S1 0.18/.02	X1 0.17/.04
S2 0.20/.04	
F1 0.20/.07	X2 0.25/.06
F2 0.25/.08	
F3 0.30/.09	X3 0.30/.07
F4 0.40/.06	X4 0.40/.06
F5 0.50/.05	X5 0.50/.03

Figure 3.27 ProTaper Universal (PTU) versus PTN. (Image courtesy of Dentsply, Tulsa, OK, USA.)

peripheral lands. It has a variable pitch that minimizes the "screw-in" effect and allows debris to be effectively channeled out of the canal. The file is made from one piece of nickel–titanium, giving it more structural integrity and minimizing the wobble during rotation. The tip of a Twisted File is inactive, which allows it to follow the route of the canal easily and to minimize canal transportation [85].

Twisted File is available in five tapers – .12, .10, .08, .06, and .04 – with a fixed 25 tip size and in 23-mm and 27-mm lengths (Figure 3.28). There are two colored rings on the file: The lower one (closer to the active part) shows the apical diameter (ISO standard) and the upper one shows the taper size. The file also has laser markings that can be used in lieu of rubber stoppers. Recommended speed is 500 rpm, and it can be used with or without torque control and autoreverse.

Twisted File can be used in a crown-down sequence or as a single file system. It eliminates the need for orifice openers. The file is inserted passively and gently and must always be in motion, either being inserted or withdrawn, but never held stationary in the canal. (Table 3.7).

TF Apical was introduced in 2014. Available lengths remain the same and they come in sizes 40/.04, 35/.06, and 30/.06.

Twisted File Adaptive (Sybron Endo)

Since 2007, with the development of heat-treated Twisted File technology (Axis, Sybron Endo, Coppel, TX, USA) and M-wire (Dentsply Maillefer, Ballaigues, Switzerland), instruments produced with the newly treated alloys have been commercialized by aiming at improving their mechanical properties. A third factor has become important in this search for stronger and better instruments, namely movement kinematics [86]. The Twisted File (TF) Adaptive technique has been introduced to maximize the advantages of reciprocation while minimizing its disadvantages (Figure 3.29).

Introduced in 2013, the idea behind TF Adaptive was to combine a twisted design, thermal treatment of alloy, continuous rotation, and reciprocation in an

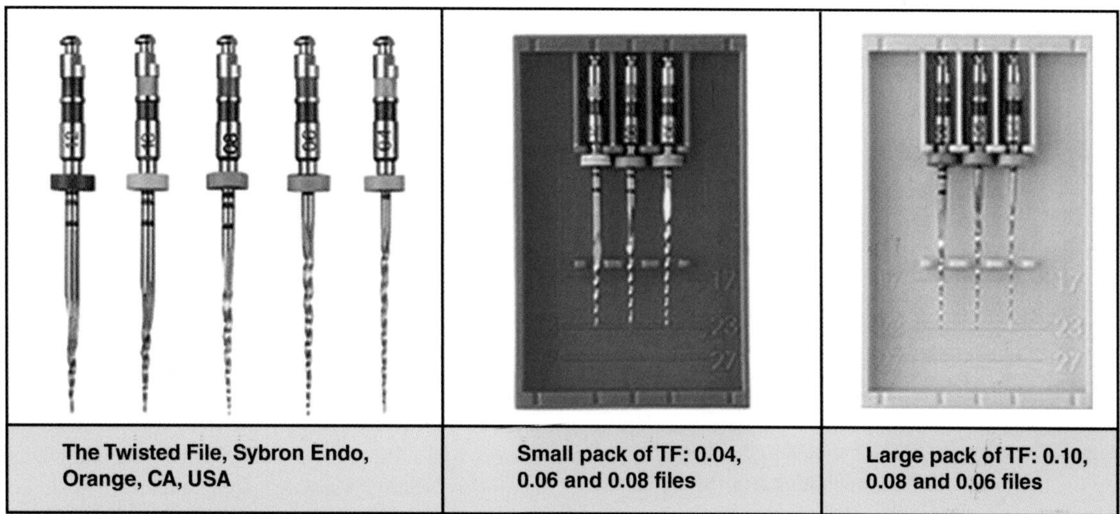

Figure 3.28 Twisted File (TF) rotary system.

Table 3.7 Twisted file preparation sequence.

Use	Small and curved canals with constricted roots	Medium canals	Large canals
Coronal flaring	Establish glide path and working length		
Shaping and Finishing	25/.08 (to resistance) → 25/.06 (to WL)	25/.10 → 25/.08 (to WL)	25/.12 → 25/.10 (to WL)

WL, working length

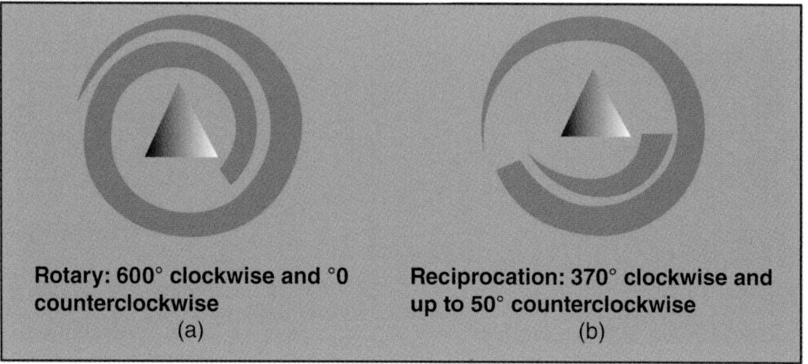

Figure 3.29 Adaptive motion. *A*, File motion when minimal or no load is applied. *B*, File motion when it engages dentin and load is applied.

innovative new system to allow simple, predictable, and safe instrumentation to be achieved. The concept is the provision of a motor that automatically detects the stress generated during instrumentation (the more complex the case, the higher the stress). Adaptive motion technology is based on a patented, smart algorithm designed to work with the TF Adaptive file system. This technology allows the TF Adaptive file to adjust to intracanal torsional forces depending on the amount of pressure placed on the file. This means the file is in either a rotary or reciprocation motion depending on the situation. The result is exceptional debris removal and less chance of file pull-in and debris extrusion.

When the TF Adaptive instrument is not (or very lightly) stressed in the canal, the movement can be described as a continuous rotation [87], allowing better cutting efficiency and removal of debris and reducing the tendency of screwing in. On the contrary, while negotiating the canal, due to increased instrumentation stress and metal fatigue, the motion of the TF Adaptive instrument changes into a reciprocation mode, with specifically designed clockwise and counterclockwise angles. These angles are not constant, but vary depending on the anatomical complexities and the intracanal stress placed on the instrument. This adaptive motion therefore helps to reduce the risk of intracanal failure without affecting performance, because the best movement for each clinical situation is automatically selected by the adaptive motor.

The TF Adaptive system relies on only three files and is color coded similar to a traffic light signal sequence: start with green, continue or stop with yellow, and stop with red (Figure 3.30) [88]. The red file is mainly for apical widening. Due to this system's recent introduction, limited research is available.

K3XF (Sybron Endo)

Introduced in 2011, K3XF uses R-phase technology to improve on their original K3 system. The file design includes a positive rake angle and variable helical flute angles, which aid in removing debris from the canal. It also has a third radial land, which provides better centering ability, variable pitch, superior flexibility, and resistance to fatigue. The recommended rotational speed is 350 to 500 rpm. They are available in lengths of 17 mm, 21 mm, and 25 mm with tapers of .04, .06,

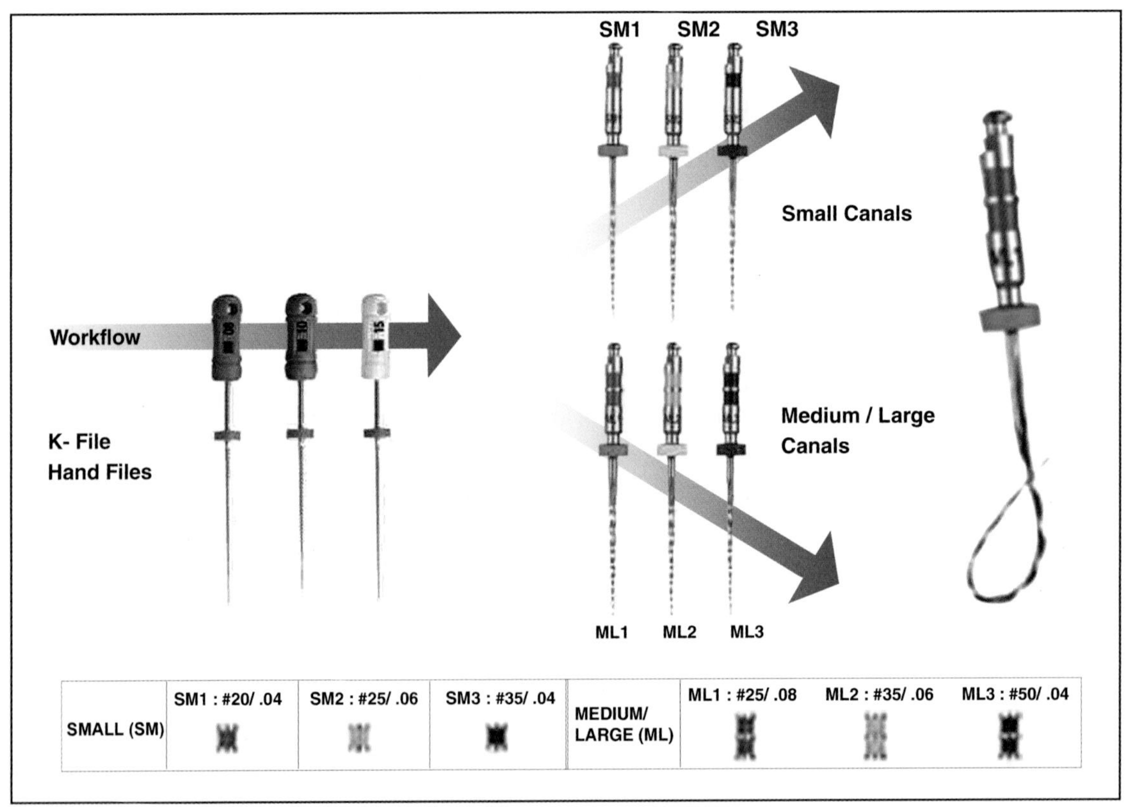

Figure 3.30 TF Adaptive File system uses a color-coded identification system for efficiency and ease of use. Just like a traffic light, start with green and stop with red.

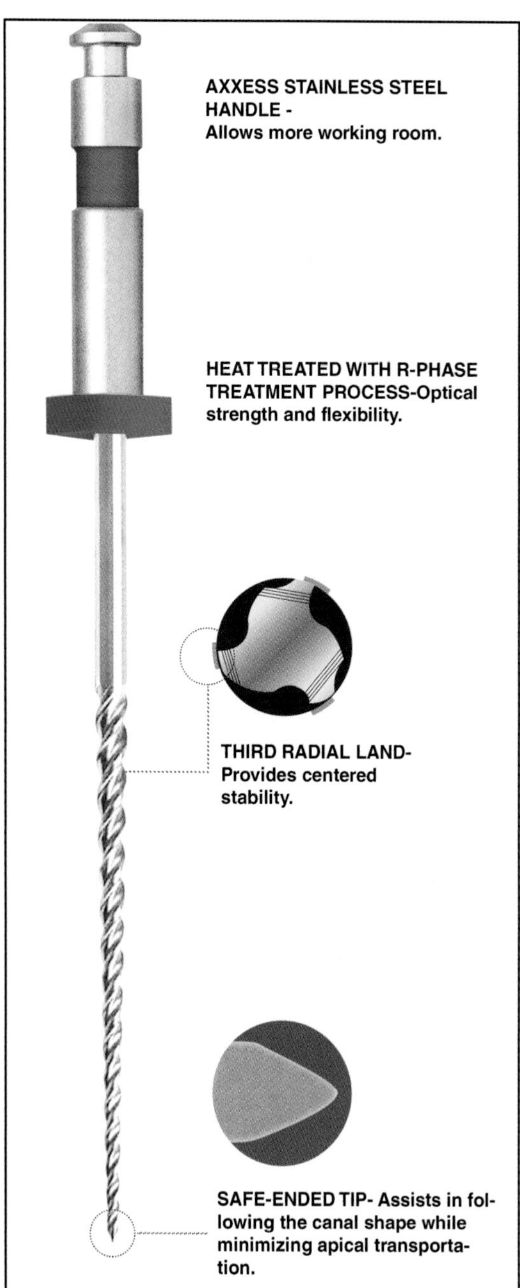

Figure 3.31 K3XF File.

.08, and .10 in sizes of 21, 30, and 40. The files have a noncutting tip for added safety [89]. They also have a stainless steel Axxess handle to ensure better posterior access (Figure 3.31).

Hyflex CM (Coltène/Whaledent, Altstätten, Switzerland)

The Hyflex CM (controlled memory) is a modification of an H-file with S-shaped cross section instead of the single-helix teardrop cross section of an H-file. HyFlex NiTi files are manufactured using a unique thermomechanical process that controls the material's memory, making the files extremely flexible but without the shape memory of conventional NiTi files. These files demonstrate martensitic properties at room temperature [7], which is not observed with conventional NiTi metal.

This gives the file the ability to follow the anatomy of the canal very closely, without creating undesirable lateral forces on the outer canal wall, reducing the risk of ledging, transportation, or perforation. HyFlex CM NiTi files are up to 300% more resistant to cyclical fatigue compared to other NiTi files, which substantially helps reduce the incidence of file separation [90, 91]. They have normal torsional strength [92]. During heat treatment (e.g., during autoclaving) the instruments return back to their original shape (Figure 3.32).

HyFlex instruments made from CM wire were commercialized in 2011. They exhibit a lower percentage by weight of nickel (52% nickel by weight) than the common 54.5% to 57% nickel by weight of most commercially available NiTi rotary instruments [93]. The recommended rotational speed is 500 rpm. These instruments can be used in a crown-down manner, step-back technique, or the manufacturer's recommended single-file technique. They are also available as HyFlex NT NiTi rotary files and as HyFlex GPF glide path rotary files.

HyFlex NT endodontic rotary NiTi file is designed to work in specific clinical situations, such as calcified canals, straight canals, retreatments, and removing gutta-percha. HyFlex NT files are available in .06 and .04 tapers in 21-mm, 25-mm, and 31-mm lengths [94]. Some instruments (20/.02, 20/.06, 30/.04, and 40/.04) have triangular cross section with three blades and three flutes; others (.04/20 and .04/25) have quadrangular cross section with four blades and four flutes (Figure 3.33).

Typhoon Infinite Flex NiTi (TYF CM) (Clinical Research Dental, London, ON, Canada)

Introduced in 2011, Typhoon Infinite Flex files are also made from controlled-memory wire with an efficient

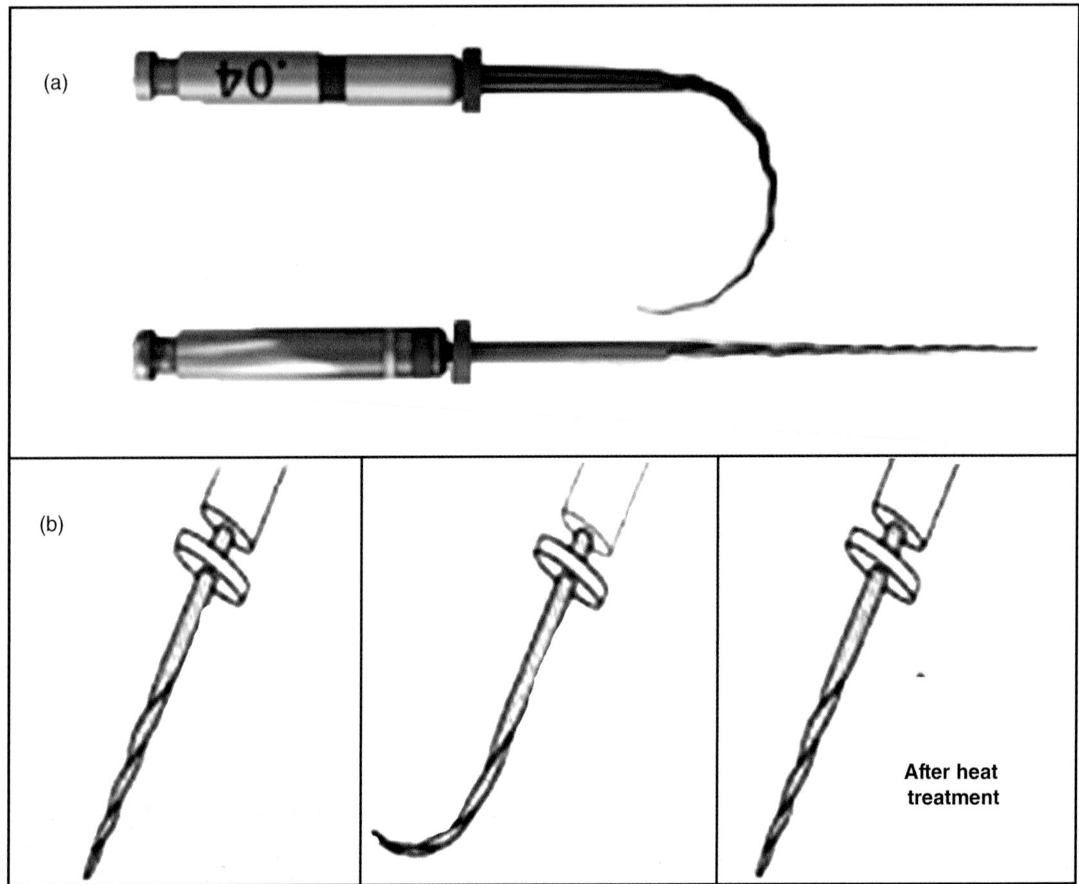

Figure 3.32 Hyflex CM. *A*, Hyflex CM NiTi File. *B*, After heat treatment (autoclaving).

cutting design (Figure 3.34). The instrument has increased torsional strength with increased resistance to cyclic fatigue and is more likely to unwind than separate. The files have a triangular cross section and a variable pitch, further increasing their flexibility and minimizing the stress on the file. The recommended rotational speed is 400 rpm. To further reduce the stress on the instrument and in order to preserve dentin in the cervical portion of the root, Typhoon Infinite Flex files have a 12-mm cutting zone instead of the traditional 16 mm. These files can also be used in a hybrid fashion with some traditional NiTi files for the curvier apical portion of the root [95, 96].

The canal preparation is achieved in a crown-down sequence, and for most canal shapes the files should be used in the order 35/.06 > 30/.04 > 25/.06 > 20/.04. This technique uses alternating tapers to prevent taper lock. For larger canals, files are also available as .04 taper files up to size 50.

Rotation versus reciprocation

Endodontic instruments have been used in rotational or axial reciprocation or a combination of both movements. Most available NiTi files are mechanically driven in continuous rotation. Reciprocation is defined as any repetitive back-and-forth motion and has been used clinically to drive stainless steel files since 1958. Initially, all reciprocating motors and related handpieces rotated files in large equal angles of 90 degrees clockwise and counterclockwise rotation. Over time, smaller, yet equal, angles of clockwise/counterclockwise rotation (true reciprocation) were used in systems such as M4

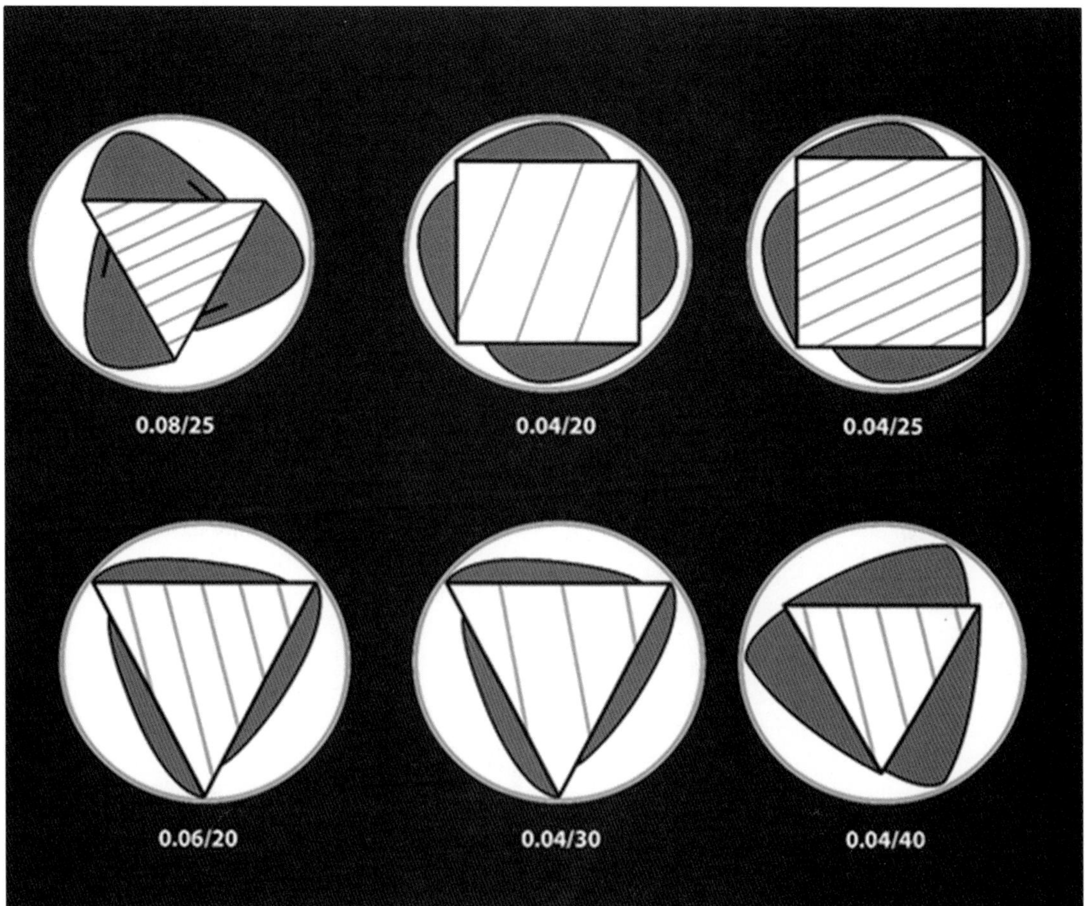

Figure 3.33 Cross sections of Hyflex NiTi files.

(SybronEndo), Endo-Eze AET (Ultradent Products), and Endo-Express (Essential Dental Systems). These systems have certain recognized limitations, including decreased cutting efficiency, more required inward pressure, and a limited capacity to auger debris out of a canal.

The greater tactile touch and efficiency gained with continuously rotating NiTi files must be balanced with the inherent risks associated with torque and cyclic fatigue failures. To decrease this risk, files were designed for use in a mechanical reciprocating movement, turning a specific distance clockwise, then rotating counterclockwise. The clockwise and counterclockwise rotations are usually not equivalent (modified reciprocation), so the file advances through a partial clockwise rotation with each reciprocation cycle. This mimics manual movement and reduces the risks associated with continuously rotating a file through canal curvatures.

The angles of rotation are unequal and lower than the angle at which the elastic limit of the metal composing the instrument develops. Consequently, torsional stress would be reduced and safety would be enhanced. The major breakthrough was changing the mode of action of rotary NiTi from 360 degree rotation to reciprocation. Yared in 2007 described the use of a ProTaper F2 file in a reciprocating handpiece [97].

Reciprocating motion can also extend cyclic fatigue life when compared to continuous rotation [98–100]. However, the term *reciprocating motion* includes several possible movements and angles, each of which can influence performance and strength of NiTi instruments.

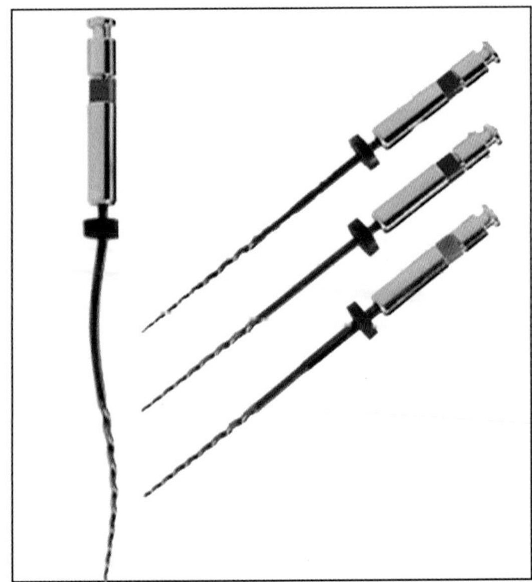

Figure 3.34 Typhoon Infinite Flex NiTi files.

The reduction of instrumentation stress (both torsional and bending) is the main advantage of reciprocating movements.

Two systems have been introduced based on this concept: WaveOne developed by Dentsply and Reciproc developed by VDW. One key difference from their rotary counterparts is that the principal movement is in a counterclockwise direction and cut is in a counterclockwise direction. Both are based on multiple reciprocation motion to complete 360 degrees rotation (Table 3.8). Although reciprocating files have the potential to advance endodontic instrumentation, research to date has not indicated they are superior to files used in continuous rotation.

Wave One (Dentsply)

Introduced in 2011, the Wave One is a single-file, single-use system using a reciprocating motion rather than a rotary motion, in a specially designed handpiece and motor. The instruments are designed to work with a reverse cutting action. The cross-section of the instruments is a modified convex triangle in the apical segment and a convex triangle in the coronal segment (Figure 3.35) [101]. The files are manufactured with M-Wire (Dentsply Tulsa Dental, Tulsa, OK, USA) NiTi alloy, improving strength and resistance to cyclic fatigue [102].

There are three files in the WaveOne single-file reciprocating system, which are available in lengths of 21, 25, and 31 mm. The Small (yellow) has a tip size ISO 21 and a continuous taper of 6%; the Primary (red) has a tip size ISO 25 and an apical taper of .08 that reduces toward the coronal end. The Large (black) has a tip size ISO 40 and an apical taper of .08 that reduces toward the coronal end [78, 103]. The files have noncutting modified guiding tips (Figure 3.36). The plastic color coding in the handle becomes deformed once it is sterilized, preventing the file from being placed back into the handpiece. Therefore, this system is marketed as single-use only. The single use has the added advantage of reducing instrument fatigue, which is an even more important consideration with WaveOne files, because one file does the work performed by three or more rotary NiTi files (Box 3.5).

The WaveOne motor (e3) is operated by a rechargeable battery with a 6:1 reducing handpiece. The counterclockwise movement of the file is greater than the clockwise movement. Counterclockwise movement advances the instrument, engaging and cutting the dentin. Clockwise movement disengages the instrument from the dentin before it can lock into the canal. Three reciprocating cycles complete one complete reverse rotation, and the instrument gradually advances into the canal with little apical pressure required. Because these files have their own unique reverse design, they can only be used with the WaveOne motor with its reverse reciprocating function.

Table 3.8 Files and systems for rotation and reciprocation.

Motion	System	Material
Reciprocation (clockwise and counterclockwise)	ProTaper F2 file (Yared 2007)	NiTi
Multiple reciprocation (360 degrees rotation)	Wave One (Dentsply) Reciproc (VDW)	M-wire
Rotary	ProTaper (Dentsply) Hyflex (Coltène/Whaledent)	NiTi

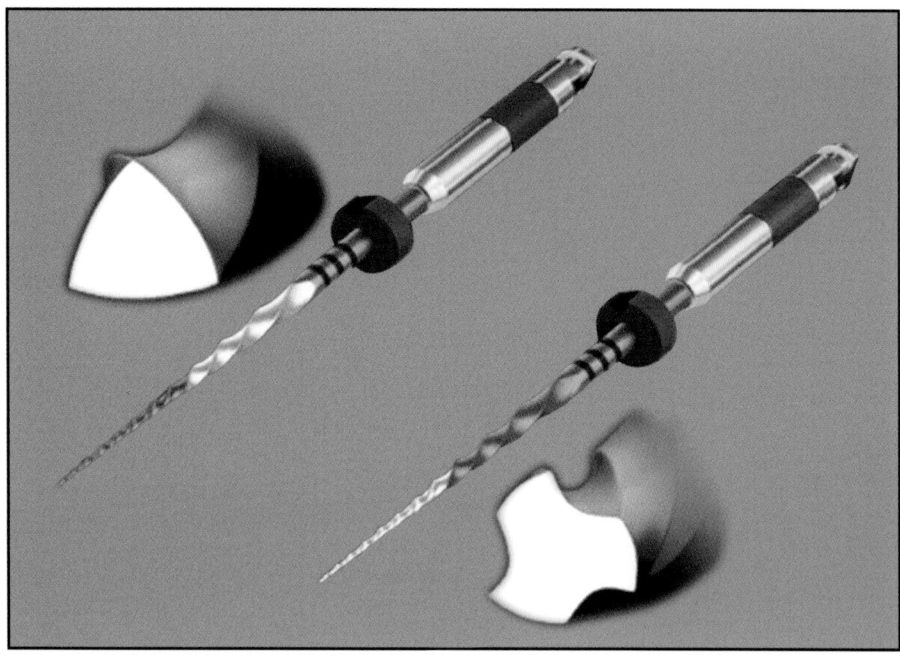

Figure 3.35 WaveOne file cross section. This image depicts two different cross sections on a single WaveOne file. The more distal cross section improves safety and inward movement.

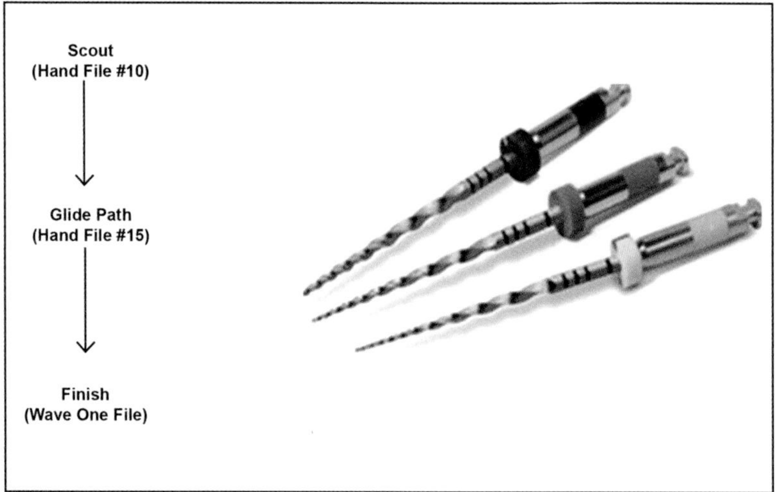

Figure 3.36 WaveOne Rotary Files and their sequence of use.

The files are used with a progressive up and down movement no more than three to four times, and only a little force is required. The main drawback of this system is that the files only shape the canal, extremely quickly in many instances, but they do not clean the root canal.

Reciproc (VDW, Munich, Germany)

Introduced in 2011, Reciproc (made from M-Wire), also used in a reciprocal motion, is also single-file, single-use system. The counterclockwise angle is greater than the clockwise one, which allows the instrument

Box 3.5 WaveOne Preparation Sequence

Small WaveOne (21/.06)

Used mainly for small canals and when the primary file does not progress apically through a smooth, reproducible glidepath
This file is designed to work in smaller-diameter, longer-length, or more apically curved canals.

Primary WaveOne (25/.08)

Invariably used first in any canal

Large WaveOne (40/.08)

Used to complete the shape in larger-diameter canals
Designed to work in canals that are typically straighter

Shaping Technique

Take hand file (#10) into canal to resistance (approximately two thirds of canal length).

Introduce appropriate WaveOne file to approximately two thirds of canal length.

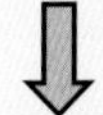

Take hand file to length.

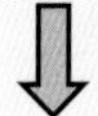

Introduce WaveOne file to length.

to continuously progress toward the apex of the root canal. In general, reciprocating root canal preparation is an evolution of the balanced force technique that allows shaping of even severely curved canals with hand instruments to larger apical diameters [103].

Reciproc files are available in different sizes: R25 with a taper of .08, R40 with a taper of .06, and R50 with a taper of .05. They are marked with ISO color of the instrument for easy identification. The files possess sharp cutting edges and have a continuous taper over the first 3 mm of their working part followed by a decreasing taper to the shaft. An S-shaped cross section is used for the entire working part of the instrument. The creation of a glide path is not required in the majority of the canals before using a Reciproc instrument in reciprocation. Hence it is claimed that the incidence of procedural errors resulting from the use of small hand files in narrow canals is reduced [104].

This new alloy shows improved elastic properties and a better cyclic fatigue behavior compared with the conventional NiTi alloy, and the Vickers hardness of the M-wire alloy is much higher compared to the NiTi alloy (Liu et al 2009) [102]. Reciproc files are available in lengths of 21, 25, and 31 mm.

In the counterclockwise movement phase, the Reciproc instrument is active and cutting dentin; in the subsequent clockwise movement the instrument is released and by a slight apically oriented pressure pushed farther into the channel until the desired preparation length is reached.

Reciproc and Wave One systems are the direct full-sequence counterparts of the single-file reciprocating systems, within the range of current rotary full-sequence NiTi systems. An additional advantage specific to the Reciproc system is its efficiency in removing obturating materials, including plastic carrier-based obturations.

Self-Adjusting File (ReDent Nova, Ra'anana, Israel)

The Self-Adjusting File (SAF) system is a new approach to shaping root canal systems. It does not use solid metal files [106–108]. Instead it relies on the gentle abrasive action of a flexible mesh lattice to prepare the root canal walls (Figure 3.37). The SAF offers the

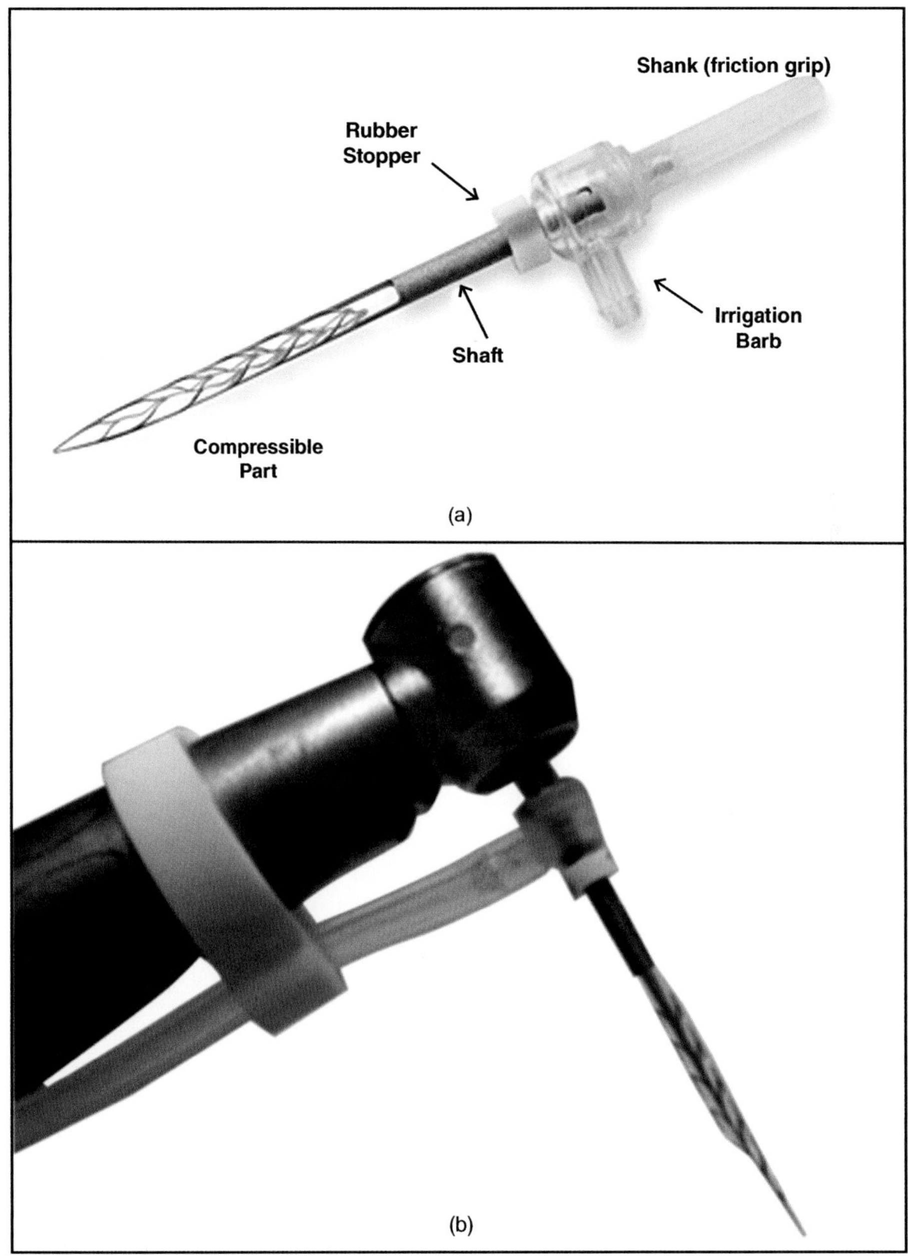

Figure 3.37 *A*, Self-adjusting file design. *B*, VATEA irrigation device attached with silicon tube on the shaft of the file. The SAF instrument is activated with a transline vibrating handpiece adapted with a RDT3 head.

ability to instrument and prepare complex-shaped root canal anatomies, the opportunity to provide continuous and efficient irrigation and debridement, the potential for eliminating file breakage within the canals because there is no file rotation when cleaning and shaping, and the opportunity to simplify and reduce the number of required dental instruments [106–111].

The SAF is a hollow file designed as a compressible, thin-walled pointed cylinder (1.5 or 2.0 mm) composed of 120-μm thick NiTi lattice. Its surface is treated to render it abrasive, which allows it to remove dentin with a back-and-forth grinding motion [112].The file can be compressed when inserted into any root canal previously negotiated and prepared up to an ISO size 20. The compressed file then adapts itself three-dimensionally to the shape of the root canal [113]. The file is operated with transline (in and out) vibrating handpieces with 3000 to 5000 vibrations per minute. The vibrating movement combined with intimate contact along the entire circumference and length of the canal removes a layer of dentin with a grinding motion. The hollow design allows continuous irrigation throughout the procedure. A special irrigation apparatus called VATEA (ReDent Nova) is used. This is attached by a silicon tube to the irrigation hub on the shaft of the file (Figure 3.37b), and continuous irrigation flow at low pressure and low flow rates is delivered. The instruments are extremely flexible and available in 21-, 25-, and 31-mm lengths.

The SAF technique does not employ forced apical extrusion of the irrigant fluid. Therefore, homeostatic balance is maintained and the irrigant is not passed out of the foramen. SAF is extremely durable, flexible, and pliable and can mechanically endure use under its recommended mode of operation with a minimal loss of efficacy. It does not impose its shape on the canal but rather complies with the canal's original shape both circumferentially and longitudinally.

TRUShape 3D Conforming files (Dentsply Tulsa Dental Specialties)

Tru 3-D Conforming files allow the clinician to preserve more dentinal structure while removing pulp and debris along the entire root (removes 36% less dentin). The file's S-shape design conforms to areas of the canal larger than the nominal file size by creating a predictable shape with up to 32% less apical transportation. This creates an envelope of motion that better disrupts biofilms for improved bacterial reduction (Figure 3.38). As a result, TRUShape 3D Conforming files preserve more dentinal structure while removing pulp and debris along the entire root canal. These files look and feel different from conventional files. They clean irregular geometries better than traditional ISO rotary files by contacting up to 75% of canal walls. They are available in lengths of 21 mm, 25 mm, and 31 mm in tapers of .06 and in tip sizes of 20, 25, 30, and 40.

TRU Shape Orifice modifiers are also available as 20/.08 in 16-mm length. They are designed to modify the orifice and create an ideal receptacle for the introduction of the files. Their main features are an active cutting cross section, a fluted length of about 7 mm, a maximum fluted diameter of 0.75 mm to facilitate conservative radicular access, and blue wire NiTi for strength and flexibility.

Table 3.9 summarizes the various rotary systems discussed.

Glide-path rotary instruments

Preflaring is the pre-enlargement of canals needed to decrease the fracture risk of NiTi instruments inside the canal. With preflaring, the taper lock on the instrument tip is decreased and a glide path is created that facilitates the penetration of the subsequent rotary instruments regardless of the technique used. According to John West, a glide path is defined as a smooth radicular tunnel from the orifice of the canal to the physiologic terminus of the root canal. A glide path is achieved when the file forming it can enter from the orifice and follow the smooth canal walls uninterrupted to the terminus. Without the endodontic glide path, the rationale of endodontics cannot be achieved.

Traditionally, preflaring and glide paths were achieved with manual steel instruments, K-files #10, #15, and #20, used sequentially. Despite the introduction over the years of rotary instruments specifically designed for preflaring, the manual technique continues to offer undeniable advantages: greater tactile control, lower risk of endodontic fracture, and the option of precurving the instrument in order to pass ledges and false channels. These files, unfortunately, also present several drawbacks due to their relative stiffness and a cutting tip that in curved and/or calcified canals can cause ledges or transportation.

This led to the introduction of the first generation for mechanical preflaring in NiTi: the PathFiles. The benefits of using a rotary instrument to create a glide path are numerous. The flexibility of NiTi is well tested and proved to prevent ledge formation and transportation when compared to stainless steel. Also, the rotary action of the file severs and moves vital pulp tissue out of the canal in the coronal direction and prevents compaction

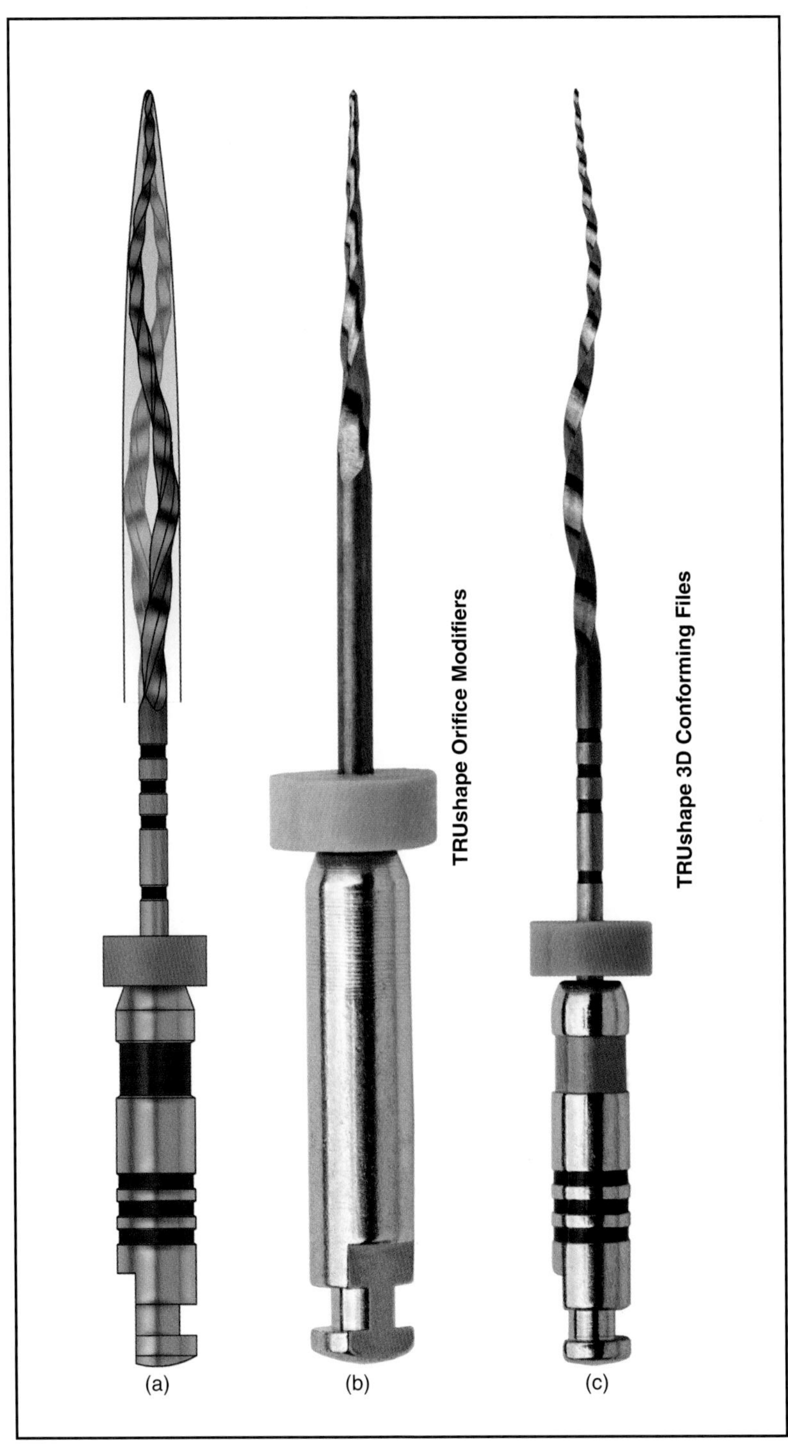

Figure 3.38 TRUshape 3D Conforming File. (Image courtesy of Dentsply, Tulsa, OK, USA.)

Table 3.9 Characteristics of rotary systems.

System	Tapers	Tip design and sizes	Cross Section	Recommended rpm	Available lengths	Instruments per set	Other features
LightSpeed Instruments (LightSpeed, San Antonio, TX)	Specific instrument sequence produces a tapered shape	Non-cutting tip sizes 20–140, including half sizes	Triple-U shape	750–2000, with step-back technique	21 mm, 25 mm, 31 mm	25	Radial land, thin flexible noncutting shaft, and short cutting head (1–2 mm)
Hero 642 (Micro-Mega)	Fixed taper 2%, 4%, 6%	Non cutting tips 2% (sizes 20–45) 4% and 6% (sizes 20–30)	Triple helix	300–600 with minimal axial force, crown-down technique	21 mm and 25 mm	12	Variable pitch Files have short cutting portion (12–16 mm), with positive rake angle for cutting efficiency. No radial land
K3 (Sybron Endo)	Fixed taper 2%, 4%, 6%	Non cutting tips sizes 15–60	Asymmetrical, variable core diameter	300–350 with minimal axial force, crown-down/ modified double flare technique	21 mm, 25 mm, 30 mm	27	Positive rake angle, three radial lands, peripheral blade relief, variable pitch
ProTaper (Dentsply Maillefer)	Variable taper along the length of the instrument	Non cutting tips in sizes 19–30	Convex triangular	150–350, with crown-down technique	19 mm, 21 mm, 25 mm	6: 3 finishing and 3 shaping	No radial land. F3, F4, F5 have U flutes for increased flexibility Pitch and helical angle are balanced to prevent instruments from screwing into canals.
GT Files (Dentsply Maillefer)	Fixed taper 4%, 6%, 8%, 10%, 12% (Accessory)	Non cutting tips Sizes 20, 30, 40 12% in tip sizes 35, 50, 70, 90	Triple-U shape	150–350, with crown-down technique and no pecking motion	18 mm, 21 mm, 25 mm	4: GT 20, GT 30, GT 40, GT Accessory	Files have a short cutting portion, variable pitch, and radial lands.
Profile (Dentsply Maillefer)	Orifice Openers	Non cutting 20–80	Triple U shape	150–350, with crown-down/ modified double flare technique	19 mm	6	20-degree helix angle and constant pitch Radial lands and neutral rake angle
	4%	15–90			21 mm, 25 mm, some 31 mm	2% and 6%: 6 4%: 9	
	6%	15–40					
	2%	15–45					
	Series 29	13–100			21 and 25mm		
	Shapers (5%–8%)	20–80			19mm	6	

Flex Master (VDW, Munich, Germany)	2%, 4%, 6% Intro file has 11% taper	Non cutting 15–70 15–40	Convex triangular	150–300	21 and 25mm 2% and 4% are also available in lengths of 28 mm	22	Sharp cutting edge and no radial land Individual helical angle for each instrument size
RaCe (FKG, La Chaux-de-Fonds, Switzerland)	2%	Modified 15–60	Triangular shape (except RaCe 15/.02 and 20/.02, which have a square shape)	300–600, with step-down/ crown-down technique	2%: 19 mm 4%–10%: 25 mm	15	Alternating cutting edge No radial lands
	4% 6% 8% 10%	25–35 30, 40 35 40					
Quantec SC (cutting), LX (noncutting) (Sybron Endo)	2%	15–60 (SC/LX)	Triple helix	300–350			Double helical flute Positive rake angle Two wide radial lands
	3%–6% 8%–12%	25 (SC/LX) 25 (LX)					
Mtwo (VDW, Munich, Germany)	4%–7%	Non cutting tips sizes 10–40	S-shape	Not specified, simultaneous technique		8	Positive rake angle No radial land

Antimicrobial activity.

of pulp tissue in the apical direction. The primary function of these instruments is not to shape the canal but to remove tissue from the canal and create a glide path.

PathFiles (Dentsply)

The PathFile rotary system was introduced in 2009 and consists of three NiTi .02 tapered rotary instruments. PathFile No.1 (purple ring) has an ISO 13 tip size, PathFile No. 2 (white ring) has an ISO 16 tip size, and PathFile No.3 (yellow ring) has an ISO 19 tip size. These can be used to enlarge the glide path after initially negotiating and establishing a glide path with a number 10 K-file. The gradual increase of the tip diameter facilitates the progression of the files without needing to use strong axial pressure. The tip is rounded and noncutting to prevent ledging and zip. The files have a square cross section, which increases the resistance to cyclic fatigue, ensures flexibility, and improves cutting efficiency [114]. The distance between two following blades has been optimized to increase the strength of the instruments. They are available in lengths of 21 mm, 25 mm, and 31 mm. These are used with a rotation speed of 300 rpm.

X-Plorer Canal Navigation NiTi Files (Clinician's Choice Dental Products, New Milford, CT, USA)

Introduced in 2010, X-Plorer system consists of three instruments. They are each available in lengths of 21 mm and 25 mm. The unique design features of these instruments are their cutting surfaces, tapers, and cross sections. The cutting surface is limited to the apical 10 mm of the file, which decreases surface contact and torsion and increases tactile feedback.

G-Files (Micro-Mega, Besançon, France)

The G-File glide-path instruments were introduced in 2011 and consist of two files, which are available in 21-mm, 25-mm, and 29-mm lengths. The tip sizes are ISO 12 and ISO 17, and the noncutting tip is asymmetrical to aid in the progression of the file. The files have a .03 taper along the length. The cross section of the file has blades on three different radii to aid in the removal of debris and to reduce torsion. The files also have an electropolished surface to improve efficiency.

ProGlider (Dentsply Tulsa Dental Specialties)

The ProGlider is a single-file rotary glide-path instrument based on the M-wire alloy. The system was introduced to increase the glide-path diameter, as an alternative to using a series of three PathFiles. The principal features of the instrument are a semiactive tip and size ISO 16 with a .02 taper. The active component is 18 mm, compared to 16 mm in the PathFiles, centered, and square cross section with variable helical angles. These are available in 21-, 25-, and 31-mm length and are used in continuous rotation of 300 rpm.

Disinfectants and lubricants

Studies have demonstrated that mechanical enlargement of canals must be accompanied by copious irrigation in order to facilitate maximum removal of microorganisms so that the prepared canal becomes as bacteria-free as possible [115, 116]. The desired attributes of a root-canal irrigant include the ability to dissolve necrotic and pulpal tissue, bacterial decontamination and a broad antimicrobial spectrum, the ability to enter deep into the dentinal tubules, biocompatibility and lack of toxicity, the ability to dissolve inorganic material and remove the smear layer, ease of use, and moderate cost [117].

A large number of substances currently in use as root canal irrigants include acids (citric and phosphoric), chelating agent (ethylenediaminetetraacetic acid [EDTA]), proteolytic enzymes, alkaline solutions (sodium hypochlorite, sodium hydroxide, urea, and potassium hydroxide), oxidative agents (hydrogen peroxide and Gly-Oxide), local anesthetic solutions, chlorhexidine, and normal saline [118]. They can be grouped as tissue-dissolving agents such as NaOCl; antibacterial agents, including bactericidal (CHX) and bacteriostatic (MTAD); chelating agents such as EDTA; and natural agents, such as green tea, triphala, and others. Table 3.10 summarizes the characteristics of currently available irrigants.

The most widely used irrigant that satisfies most of the requirements is 0.5% to 6.0% sodium hypochlorite (NaOCl) because of its bactericidal activity and ability to dissolve vital and necrotic organic tissue [119, 120]. However, even though it is a highly effective antimicrobial agent, it does not remove the smear layer from the

Table 3.10 Characteristics of few currently used intracanal irrigants.

Irrigant	Antimicrobial activity	Ability to remove smear layer	Biocompatibility	Ability to dissolve pulp tissue
NaOCl	+	–	–	+
CHX	+	–	+	–
EDTA	–	+	+	+/–
MTAD	+	+	+	+/–
Tetraclean	+	+	+	+/–
ECA	+	+	+	+
Ozonated water		+		+
PAD	+	+	+	+

+, Good, –, Poor

dentin walls [121–123]. Chelating agents (EDTA or citric acid) assist in softening and dissolving inorganic dentin particles, thereby preventing the accumulation of debris on the root canal walls [124]. but these solutions have relatively limited antiseptic capacities [125].

Chlorhexidine was developed in the late 1940s in the research laboratories of Imperial Chemical Industries Ltd. (Macclesfield, England). Despite its usefulness as a final irrigant, chlorhexidine cannot be advocated as the main irrigant in standard endodontic cases because chlorhexidine is unable to dissolve necrotic tissue remnants and because chlorhexidine is less effective on gram-negative than on gram-positive bacteria.

Hydrogen peroxide as a canal irrigant helps to remove debris by the physical act of irrigation, as well as through effervescing of the solution. However, although it is an effective antibacterial irrigant, hydrogen peroxide does not dissolve necrotic intracanal tissue, and it exhibits toxicity to the surrounding tissue. Alcohol-based canal irrigants have antimicrobial activity too, but they do not dissolve necrotic tissue.

The combination of NaOCl and EDTA has been used worldwide for antisepsis of root-canal systems. The concentration of NaOCl used for root-canal irrigation ranges from 2.5% to 6%. It has been shown, however, that tissue hydrolyzation is greater at the higher end of this range.

All the irrigation solutions at our disposable have their share of limitations, and the search for an ideal root canal irrigant continues with the development of newer materials and methods. To date, none of these irrigants are ideal, and hence, in current endodontic practice, dual irrigants such as sodium hypochlorite with EDTA or chlorhexidine are often used as initial and final rinses to make up for the shortcomings that are associated with the use of a single irrigant. Quite a bit of literature is already available in textbooks on the more traditionally used irrigants. The following text reviews the advantages and shortcomings of some of the newer irrigating agents and their use in the future.

BioPure MTAD (Dentsply Tulsa)

BioPure MTAD was introduced by Torabinejad and colleagues as an alternative to EDTA to remove the smear layer. It is a *m*ixture of a *t*etracycline isomer (3% doxycycline), an acetic *a*cid (4.25% citric acid), and Tween 80 *d*etergent (MTAD) and was designed to be used as a final root canal rinse before obturation [32].

In comparison to other solutions, MTAD is effective in removing the smear layer along the whole length of the root canal and in removing organic and inorganic debris. MTAD does not erode dentin as EDTA does, it has sustained antibacterial properties (against *Enterococcus faecalis*), and the detergent is postulated to coagulate microscopic debris into suspension for removal. Its recommended use is as a final irrigant before obturation: The root canal is flooded with 1 mL of the irrigant and allowed to soak for 5 minutes, and the remaining 4 mL is then delivered with continuous irrigation and suction [126].

Because this irrigant is based on a tetracycline isomer, there may be problems with staining, resistance, and sensitivity. MTAD can be a useful irrigant due to its antimicrobial properties and less cytotoxicity, but its effectiveness against fungi and its value in the apical one third need to be assessed further.

Tetraclean (Ogna Laboratori Farmaceutici, Muggiò, Italy)

Tetraclean, like MTAD, is a mixture of an antibiotic doxycycline (50 mg/mL), an acid (citric acid), and a detergent (polypropylene glycol) [127]. Citric acid acts as a chelating agent, assisted by a weak action of the antibiotic, and the surfactant makes its penetration in the root canal system easier. It has low surface tension, which enables a better adaptation of the mixtures to the dentinal walls [127]. Tetraclean shows a high action against both strictly anaerobic and facultative anaerobic bacteria and caused a high degree of biofilm disaggregation at each time interval when compared with MTAD [128].

QMix (Dentsply Tulsa)

QMix is a combination of chlorhexidine with EDTA and a surfactant solution to improve penetration in dentinal tubules. It has been on the market for a short time, so there is limited research available yet. It removes smear layer at least as effectively as 17% EDTA, and it has proven to be a highly effective antimicrobial agent. QMix is an irrigation solution used as a final rinse. Research shows it is capable of penetrating biofilms due to its unique blend of antibacterial substances and their combined synergistic effect. This is available as a premixed, ready-to-use, colorless and odorless solution that is free of antibiotics. No evidence of tooth staining has been observed in laboratory conditions following use of this solution.

The proprietary formula is based on an advanced chemical design to minimize any undesirable reactions with other root canal irrigants. The manufacturer recommends 60 to 90 seconds of continuous irrigation as the final rinse of the root canal before root filling.

Electrochemically activated solution

Electrochemically activated (ECA) solutions are produced from water and low-concentrated salt solutions [129]. The ECA technology represents a new scientific paradigm developed by Russian scientists at the All-Russian Institute for Medical Engineering in Moscow.

The principle of ECA is transferring liquids into a metastable state via an electrochemical unipolar (anode or cathode) action through the use of a flow electrolytic module (FEM). The FEM consists of an anode, a solid titanium cylinder with a special coating that fits coaxially inside the cathode, and a hollow cylinder with another special coating. The electrodes are separated by a ceramic membrane. The FEM is capable of producing solutions that have bactericidal and sporicidal activity, are essentially noncorrosive for most metal surfaces, and are safe to human tissue [129].

Anolyte solution (produced in the anode chamber) has been termed a superoxidized water or oxidative potential water [130, 131]. Depending on the type of device that incorporated the FEM elements, the pH of anolyte solution varies; it may be acidic (anolyte), neutral (anolyte neutral), or alkaline (anolyte neutral cathodic). Acidic anolyte was used initially, but in recent years the neutral and alkaline solutions have been recommended for clinical application.

Studies demonstrated that freshly generated superoxidized solution is highly active against all microorganisms, giving a 99.999% or greater reduction in 2 minutes or less [130, 132]. That allowed investigators to treat it as a potent microbicidal agent. It is nontoxic when in contact with vital biological tissues [129]. The quality of debridement was better in the coronal and middle parts of canal walls, and only scattered debris was noted in the apical part. Solovyeva and Dummer studied the cleaning effectiveness of root canal irrigation with ECA solution and found that it was more effective than NaOCl in removing the smear layer [129].

ECA solutions have shown better clinical effect and were associated with lower incidence of allergic reaction compared to other antibacterial irrigants tested [133]. ECA is showing promising results due to ease of removal of debris and smear layer and because it is nontoxic and efficient in the apical one third of the canal. It has the potential to be an efficient root canal irrigant.

Ozonated water

Ozone is a chemical compound consisting of three oxygen atoms (O_3, triatomic oxygen), a higher energetic form than normal atmospheric oxygen (O_2), with the molecules being different in structure. Ozone is produced naturally from electrical discharges following thunderstorms and from ultraviolet rays emitted from the sun. Ozone is a powerful bactericide that can kill microorganisms effectively [134]. As a result of cavitation, a forced collapse of bubbles causes implosions that impact on surfaces, further causing surface deformation and removal of surface material. In the root canal environment, such shockwaves could potentially disrupt bacterial biofilms, rupture bacterial cell walls, and remove smear layer and debris [135]. However, ozonated water was not able to neutralize *Escherichia coli* and lipopolysaccharides inside the root canal. There is a need for further studies before it can be used as a root canal irrigant.

Photo-activated disinfection (PAD)

This makes use of photodynamic therapy (PDT) for the inactivation of microorganisms and was first shown by Oscar Raab. PDT is based on the concept that nontoxic photosensitizers can be preferentially localized in certain tissues and subsequently activated by light of the appropriate wavelength to generate singlet oxygen and free radicals that are cytotoxic to cells of the target tissue [136]. PAD is not only effective against bacteria, but also against other microorganisms including viruses, fungi, and protozoa [137–140].

Methylene blue has been used in PDT for targeting various gram-positive and gram-negative oral bacteria. Methylene blue alone (PS) fully eliminated all bacterial species with the exception of *E. faecalis* (53% killing); methylene blue in combination with red light (PAD) was able to eliminate 97% of *E. faecalis* biofilm bacteria in root canals [141].

Along with methylene blue, tolonium chloride has been also used as a photosensitizing agent. It is applied to the infected area and left in situ for a short period. The agent binds to the cellular membrane of bacteria, which will then rupture when activated by a laser source emitting radiation at an appropriate wavelength. Tolonium chloride dye is biocompatible and does not stain dental tissue.

FotoSan is one of the most recent PAD devices introduced in endodontics. The manufacturer's protocol indicates that, after canal preparation, the canal have to be inoculated with the methylene blue solution, which is left in situ for a fixed period of time (60 seconds) to permit the solution to come into contact with the root canal and irradiation have to be carried out for 30 seconds in each canal.

Further clinical are needed to verify the efficacy of PAD in aiding cleansing and disinfecting of endodontic space and to confirm if there is need for new irrigating solutions or devices for endodontic use.

Irrigant delivery systems

Manual

For the solution to be mechanically effective in removing all the particles, it has to reach the apex, create a current (force), and carry the particles away. The effectiveness and safety of irrigation depends on the means of delivery. Various methods and systems have been developed to provide effective delivery (Box 3.6).

One of the advantages of syringe irrigation is that it allows comparatively easy control of the depth of needle penetration within the canal and the volume of irrigant that is flushed through the canal (Figure 3.39) [142, 143].

Brushes are adjuncts that have been designed for debridement of the canal walls or agitation of root canal

Box 3.6 Irrigation Systems

Manual

Manual dynamic: hand-activated, well-fitting gutta-percha cone
Syringe irrigation with needles
Brushes: NaviTip FX

Machine Assisted

Pressure alteration devices: EndoVac, RinsEndo
Ultrasonics
Sonic: EndoActivator
Rotary brushes
Continuous irrigation during instrumentation

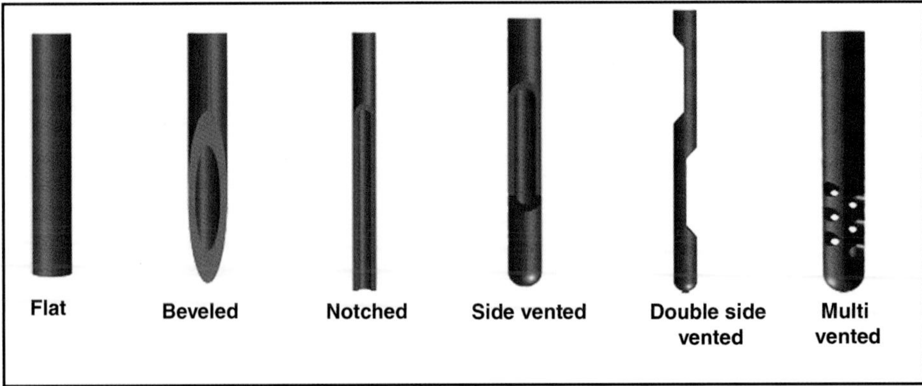

Figure 3.39 Different types of needles used for irrigation in endodontics.

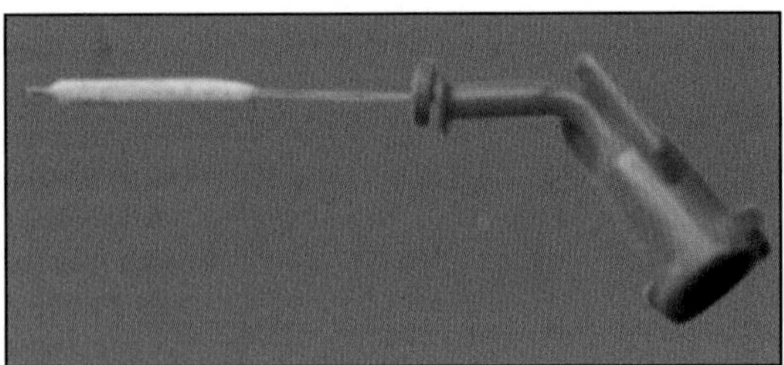

Figure 3.40 sNaviTip FX.

irrigant. They might also be indirectly involved with the transfer of irrigants within the canal spaces. NaviTip FX (Figure 3.40) (Ultradent Products, South Jordan,UT) is a 30-gauge irrigation needle covered with a brush. A hand-activated, well-fitting, root-filling material (e.g., a 40/.06 taper gutta-percha point) is a simple method used to disrupt the vapor lock in the apical region of the root canal. Research has shown that gently moving a well-fitting gutta-percha master cone up and down in short 2- to 3-mm strokes within an instrumented canal can produce an effective hydrodynamic effect and significantly improve the displacement and exchange of any given reagent.

Sonics

Vibringe (Vibringe BV, Amsterdam, Netherlands)

Vibringe is a new sonic irrigation system that combines battery-driven vibrations (9000 cpm) with manually operated irrigation of the root canal. It employs a traditional two-piece syringe with a rechargeable battery with sonic activation (Figure 3.41).

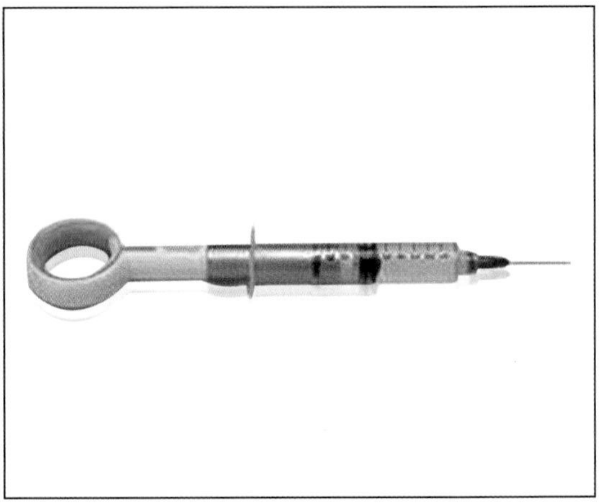

Figure 3.41 Vibringe Irrigator.

EndoActivator (Advanced Endodontics, Santa Barbara, CA, USA)

EndoActivator is a new type of irrigation facilitator. It is based on sonic vibration (up to 10,000 cpm) of a plastic tip in the root canal (Figure 3.42). The system has three different sizes of polymer tips that are easily attached (snap on) to a portable handpiece that creates the sonic vibrations. EndoActivator does not deliver new irrigant to the canal, but it facilitates the penetration and renewal of the irrigant in the canal [144]. Studies have indicated that the use of EndoActivator facilitates irrigant penetration and mechanical cleansing compared with needle irrigation, with no increase in the risk of irrigant extrusion through the apex [145, 146].

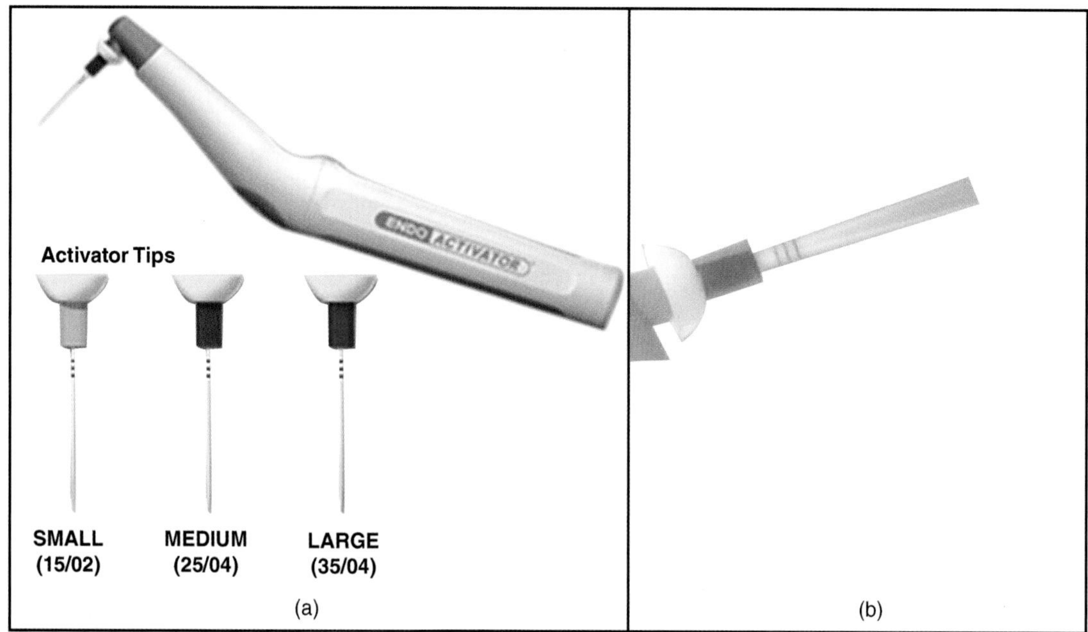

Figure 3.42 *A*, EndoActivator. *B*, Sonic Motion.

Ultrasonics

Ultrasonic irrigation can be used as an intermittent irrigation or a continuous ultrasonic irrigation. In intermittent flushed ultrasonic irrigation, the irrigant is delivered to the root canal by a syringe needle. The irrigant is then activated with the use of an ultrasonically oscillating instrument.

Ultrasonic handpieces pass sound waves to an endodontic file and cause it to vibrate at about 25,000 vibrations per second. Two types of ultrasonic irrigation are available: active ultrasonic irrigation (AUI) and passive ultrasonic irrigation operating without simultaneous irrigation (PUI). Active ultrasonic irrigation is the simultaneous combination of ultrasonic irrigation and instrumentation. It has been almost discarded in the clinical practice.

The literature indicates that it is more advantageous to apply ultrasonics after completion of canal preparation rather than as an alternative to conventional instrumentation [147,148]. PUI irrigation allows energy to be transmitted from an oscillating file or smooth wire to the irrigant in the root canal by means of ultrasonic waves [147]. The latter induces acoustic streaming and cavitation of the irrigant. PUI is more effective than syringe-needle irrigation at removing pulpal tissue remnants and dentin debris due to the much higher velocity and volume of irrigant flow that are created in the canal during ultrasonic irrigation.

Cavitation and acoustic streaming of the irrigant contribute to the biological and chemical activity for maximum effectiveness. Ultrasound creates both cavitation and acoustic streaming. The cavitation is minimal and is restricted to the tip [149]. Ultrasonic files must have free movement in the canal without making contact with the canal wall to work effectively [148]. Acoustic streaming significantly produces cleaner canals when activated with ultrasonic energy in a passive manner. However, ultrasonics cannot effectively get through the apical vapor lock [150–152].

F File (Plastic Endo, LLC, Lincolnshire, IL, USA)

An endodontic polymer-based rotary finishing file was developed to overcome the drawbacks of sonics and ultrasonics, namely, they are time consuming and expensive, and there is lack of awareness of the benefits. The F File is a single-use plastic rotary file with a unique file design with a diamond abrasive embedded into a nontoxic polymer. The F File safely removes dentinal wall debris and agitates the NaOCl without enlarging the canal further.

Pressure-alteration devices

Positive pressure versus apical negative pressure

There are two dilemmas associated with conventional syringe-needle delivery of irrigants. It is difficult for the irrigants to reach the apical portions of the canals because of air entrapment, when the needle tips are placed too far away from the apical end of the canals. Conversely, if the needle tips are positioned too close to the apical foramen, there is an increased possibility of irrigant extrusion from the foramen that might result in severe iatrogenic damage to the periapical tissues [153]. Pressure-alternation devices were developed to provide a plausible solution to this problem. The first technique was noninstrumentation technology by Lussi and colleagues [154]. This technique did not enlarge root canals because there was no mechanical instrumentation of the canal walls. Although noninstrumentation technology was successful *in vitro*, the technique was not considered safe in *in vivo* animal studies and did not proceed to human clinical trials.

RinsEndo System (Dürr Dental, Bietigheim, Germany)

In the RinsEndo system, 65 mL of a rinsing solution oscillating at a frequency of 1.6 Hz is drawn from an attached syringe and transported to the root canal via an adapted cannula. There is a higher risk of apical extrusion of the irrigant with this method.

EndoVac (Discus Dental, Culver City, CA, USA)

EndoVac represents a novel approach to irrigation because, instead of delivering the irrigant through

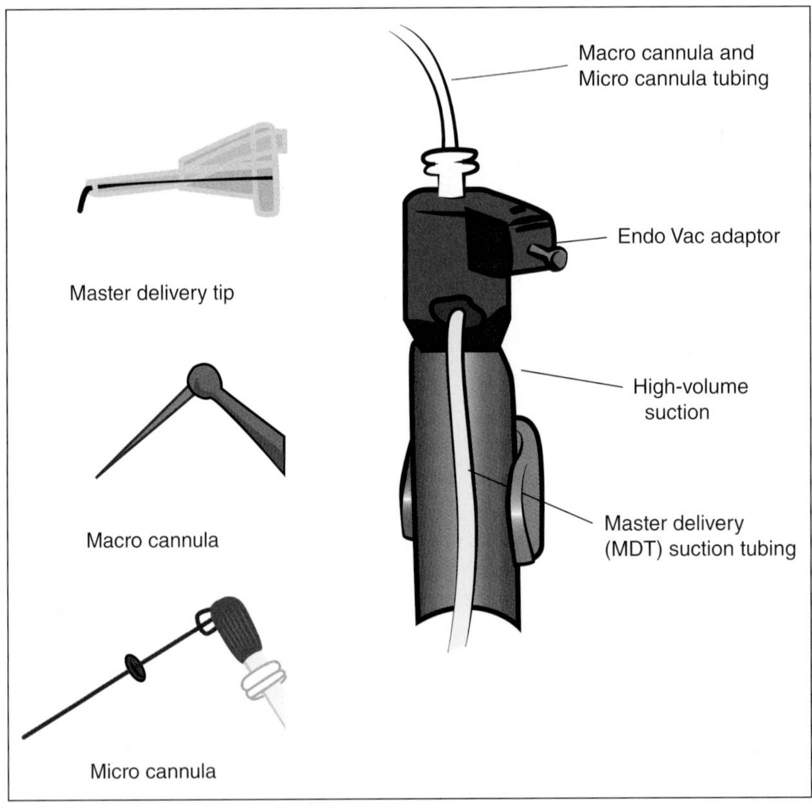

Figure 3.43 EndoVac.

the needle, the EndoVac system is based on a negative-pressure approach whereby the irrigant placed in the pulp chamber is sucked down the root canal and back up again through a thin needle, thereby avoiding undue extrusion into the periapex.

The EndoVac system is composed of three basic components: a master delivery tip, the macro cannula, and the micro cannula. The master delivery tip delivers irrigant to the pulp chamber and evacuates the irrigant simultaneously. The macro cannula is used to suction irrigant from the chamber to the coronal and middle segments of the canal (Figure 3.43).

During irrigation, the master delivery tip delivers irrigant to the pulp chamber and siphons off the excess irrigant to prevent overflow, as compared with needle irrigation. Both the macro cannula and micro cannula exert negative pressure that pulls fresh irrigant from the chamber, down the canal to the tip of the cannula, into the cannula, and out through the suction hose. Thus, a constant flow of fresh irrigant is delivered by negative pressure to working length. This also results in less postoperative pain than a conventional needle irrigation protocol.

Conclusion

A rotary armamentarium can be expensive, and the cost is also high in maintaining a supply of files. All of the systems have advantages and limitations. It is up to the practitioner to determine which system best fits their individual needs and their level of experience to provide the best possible endodontic care for their patients. These instruments and devices should be used with careful attention to detail and to the technical and clinical aspects of endodontic therapy depending on the case. The clinician should integrate his or her knowledge about anatomy with the clinical information. These should be considered as specialist tools to improve the quality of treatment.

References

1 Trope M. The vital tooth: its importance in the study and practice of endodontics. *Endod Top* 2003; 5:1.

2 Lussi A, Messerli L, Hotz P, Grosrey J. A new non-instrumental technique for cleaning and filling root canals. *Int Endod J* 1995; 28:1–6.

3 Attin T, Buchalla W, Zirkel C, Lussi A. Clinical evaluation of the cleansing properties of the noninstrumental technique for cleaning root canals. *Int Endod J* 2002; 35: 929–933.

4 Peters OA. Current challenges and concepts in the preparation of root canal systems: a review. *J Endod* 2004; 30: 559–567.

5 Thompson SA. An overview of nickel titanium alloys used in dentistry. *Int Endod J* 2000; 33(4): 297–310.

6 Walia HM, Brantley WA, Gerstein H. An initial investigation of the bending and torsional properties of nitinol root canal files. *J Endod* 1988; 14: 346–351.

7 Shen Y, Zhou HM, Zheng YF, Peng B, Haapasalo M. Current challenges and concepts of the thermo mechanical treatment of nickel–titanium instruments. *J Endod* 2013; 39(2): 163–172.

8 Zuolo ML, Walton RE. Instrument deterioration with usage: nickel–titanium versus stainless steel. *Quintessence Int* 1997; 28: 397–402.

9 Dieter GE. *Mechanical metallurgy*. 3rd ed. New York: McGraw-Hill, 1986. pp. 119, 138, 185–188, 382–387, 394.

10 Cohen S, Burns RC. *Pathways of the pulp*, 6th ed. St. Louis: CV Mosby, 1994. p. 206.

11 Peters OA, Barbakow F. Dynamic torque and apical forces of ProFile .04 rotary instruments during preparation of curved canals. *Int Endod J* 2002; 35: 379–389.

12 Sattapan B, Nervo GJ, Palamara JEA, Messer HH. Defects in rotary nickel-titanium files after clinical use. *J Endod* 2000; 26: 161–165.

13 Ullmann C, Peters OA. Effect of cyclic fatigue on static fracture loads in ProTaper nickel–titanium rotary instruments. *J Endod* 2005; 31: 183–186.

14 Serene TP, Adams JD, Saxena A. *Nickel–titanium instruments: Applications in endodontics*. St. Louis: Ishiyaku Euro-America, 1994.

15 Sotokawa T. An analysis of clinical breakage of root canal instruments. *J Endod* 1988; 14: 75–82.

16 Pruett JP, Clement DJ, Carnes DL. Cyclic fatigue testing of nickel–titanium endodontic instruments. *J Endod* 1997; 23: 77–85.

17 Yared GM, Bou Dagher FE, Machtou P. Failure of ProFile instruments used with high and low torque motors, *Int Endod J* 2001; 34: 471–475.

18 Li UM, Lee BS, Shih CT, Lan WH, Lin CP. Cyclic fatigue of endodontic nickel–titanium rotary instruments: static and dynamic tests. *J Endod* 2002; 28: 448–451.

19 Marzouk MA, Simonton AL, Gross RD. *Operative Dentistry: Modern Theory and Practice*. St. Louis: Ishiyaku EuroAmerica; 1997. p. 71.

20 Gabel WP, Hoen M, Steiman HR, Pink FE, Dietz R. Effect of rotational speed on nickel–titanium file distortion. *J Endod* 1999; 25: 752–754.

21 Blum JY, Cohen A, Machtou P, Micallef JP. Analysis of forces developed during mechanical preparation of

extracted teeth using ProFile NiTi rotary instruments. *Int Endod J* 1999; 32: 24–31.

22 Schrader C, Peters OA. Analysis of torque and force during step-back with differently tapered rotary endodontic instruments *in vitro*. *J Endod* 2005; 31: 120–123.

23 Al-Omari MAO, Dummer PMH, Newcombe RG. Comparison of six files to prepare simulated root canals. Part 1. *Int Endod J* 1992; 25: 57–66.

24 Cymerman JJ, Jerome LA, Moodnik RM. A scanning electron microscope study comparing the efficacy of hand instrumentation with ultrasonic instrumentation of the root canal. *J Endod* 1983; 9: 327–331.

25 Czonstkowsky M, Wilson EG, Holstein FA. The smear layer in endodontics. *Dent Clin North Am* 1990; 34: 13–25.

26 Walmsley AD, Williams AR. Effects of constraint on the oscillatory patterns of endosonic files. *J Endod* 1989; 15: 189–194.

27 Ahmad M. Effect of ultrasonic instrumentation on *Bacteroides intermedius*. *Endod Dent Traumatol* 1989; 5: 83–86.

28 Roane JB, Sabala CL, Duncanson MG. The "balanced force" concept for instrumentation of curved canals. *J Endod* 1985; 11(5): 203–211.

29 Powell SE. A comparison of the effect of modified and nonmodified instrument tips on apical canal deformation (Part I). *J Endod* 1986; 12: 293–300.

30 Powell SE. A comparison of the effect of modified and nonmodified instrument tips on apical canal deformation (Part II). *J Endod* 1988; 14: 224–228.

31 Hülsmann M, Peters OA, Dummer PMH. Mechanical preparation of root canals: shaping goals, techniques and means. *Endod Topics* 2005; 10: 30–76.

32 Park JB, Lakes RS. *Biomaterials: An introduction*. 2nd ed. New York: Kluwer Academic Publishers; 1992. pp. 297–300.

33 Senia SE, Johnson B, McSpadden J. The crown-down technique: a paradigm shift. Interview by Donald E. Arens. *Dent Today* 1996; 15(8): 38–47.

34 Camps J, Pertot WJ. Torsional and stiffness properties of Canal Master U stainless steel and nitinol instruments. *J Endod* 1994; 20(8): 395–398.

35 Schafer E, Tepel J. Relationship between design features of endodontic instruments and their properties. Part III. Resistance to bending and fracture. *J Endod* 2001; 27: 299–303.

36 McSpadden J. La preparazione canalare con tecnica Quantec. 18th National Congress SIE. Verona, 1997.

37 McSpadden J. New technology in endodontics. Third world conference of endodontics IFEA. Rome, 1995.

38 Sanghavi Z, Mistry K. Design features of rotary instruments in endodontics. *J Ahmedabad Dent Coll Hosp* 2011; 2(1): 6–11.

39 Walsch H. The hybrid Concept of nickel–titanium rotary instrumentation. *Dent Clin North Am* 2004; 48: 183–202.

40 Wildey WL, Senia ES. A new root canal instrument and instrumentation technique: a preliminary report. *Oral Surg Oral Med Oral Pathol* 1989; 67: 198–207.

41 Glosson CR, Haller RH, Dove SB, del Rio C. A comparison of root canal preparations using NiTi hand, NiTi engine driven, and K-Flex endodontic instruments,. *J Endod* 1995; 21: 146–151.

42 Peters OA, Kappeler S, Bucher W, Barbakow F. Maschinelle Aufbereitung gekrümmter Wurzelkanäle: Messaufbau zur Darstellung physikalischer Parameter. *Schweiz Monatsschr Zahnmed* 2001; 111: 834–842.

43 Shabahang S, Torabinejad M. Effect of MTAD on *Enterococcus faecalis*–contaminated root canals of extracted human teeth,. *J Endod* 2003; 29: 576–579.

44 Shadid DB, Nicholls JI, Steiner JC. A comparison of curved canal transportation with balanced forces versus LightSpeed. *J Endod* 1998; 24: 651–654.

45 Thompson SA, Dummer PM. Shaping ability of Hero 642 rotary nickel–titanium instruments in simulated root canals. Part 2. *Int Endod J* 2000; 33: 255–261.

46 Thompson SA, Dummer PM. Shaping ability of Light-Speed rotary nickel–titanium instruments in simulated root canals. Part 1. *J Endod* 1997; 23: 698–702.

47 Plotino G, Grande NM, Butti A, Buono L, Somma F. Modern endodontic NiTi systems: morphological and technical characteristics (part 2). *Endod Ther* 2004; 5(2): 22–25.

48 Calas P. Hero shapers: the adapted pitch concept. *Endod Top* 2005; 10(1): 155–162.

49 Preparation of the Root Canal System 2 Rotary Instrumentation http://www.tupeloendo.com/pdfs/Selected-Literature/Instrumentation-2-Rotary-Instrumentation .pdf

50 Kosa DA, Marshall G, Baumgartner JC. An analysis of canal centering using mechanical instrumentation techniques. *J Endod* 1999; 25: 441–445.

51 Mounce RE. The K3 rotary nickel–titanium file system. *Dent Clin North Am* 2004; 48(1): 137–157.

52 Gambarini G. The K3 rotary nickel titanium instrument system. *Endod Top* 2005; 10(1): 179–182.

53 Hübscher W, Barbakow F, Peters OA. Root canal preparation with FlexMaster: canal shapes analysed by micro-computed tomography. *Int Endod J* 2003; 36: 740–747.

54 Baumann MA. Reamer with alternating cutting edges – concept and clinical applications. *Endod Top* 2005; 10(1): 176–178.

55 FKG Dentaire. FKG RaCe and SMD rotary endodontic system. (Brochure). La Chaux-de-Fonds, Switzerland: FKG Dentaire (n.d.).

56 Foschi F, Nucci C, Montebugnoli L, Marchionni S, Breschi L, Malagnino VA, Prati C. SEM evaluation of canal wall dentine following use of M*two* and ProTaper NiTi rotary instruments. *Int Endod J* 2004; 37(12): 832–839.

57 Serota KS, Nahmias Y, Barnett F, Brock M, Senia ES. Predictable endodontic success: the apical control zone. *Dent Today* 2003; 22(5): 90–97.

58 Lloyd A. Root canal instrumentation with ProFile instruments. *Endod Top* 2005; 10(1): 151–154.
59 Hsu YY, Kim S. The ProFile system. *Dent Clin North Am* 2004; 48(1): 69–85.
60 Ruddle CJ. The ProTaper advantage: shaping the future of endodontics. *Dentistry Today* 2001 Oct: 1–9.
61 Kuhn G, Tavernier B, Jordan L. Influence of structure on nickel–titanium endodontic instrument failure. *J Endod* 2001; 27: 516–520.
62 Kuhn G, Jordan L. Fatigue and mechanical properties of nickel–titanium endodontic instruments. *J Endod* 2002; 28: 716–720.
63 Hayashi Y, Yoneyama T, Yahata Y, Miyai K, Doi H, Hanawa T, et al. Phase transformation behaviour and bending properties of hybrid nickel–titanium rotary endodontic instruments. *Int Endod J* 2007; 40: 247–253.
64 Yahata Y, Yoneyama T, Hayashi Y, Ebihara A, Doi H, Hanawa T, Suda H. Effect of heat treatment on transformation temperatures and bending properties of nickel–titanium endodontic instruments. *Int Endod J* 2009; 42: 621–626.
65 American Association of Endodontists. Rotary instrumentation: an endodontic perspective. *Colleagues for Excellence Newsletter* Winter 2008: 1–8.
66 Bhagabati N, Yadav S, Talwar S. An *in vitro* cyclic fatigue analysis of different endodontic nickel–titanium rotary instruments. *J Endod* 2012 Apr;38(4): 515–518.
67 Sonntag D, Peters OA. Effect of prion decontamination protocols on nickel–titanium rotary surfaces. *J Endod* 2007 Apr; 33(4): 442–446.
68 Aasim SA, Mellor AC, Qualtrough AJ. The effect of pre-soaking and time in the ultrasonic cleaner on the cleanliness of sterilized endodontic files. *Int Endod J* 2006 Feb; 39(2): 143–149.
69 Ha JH, Kim SK, Cohenca N, Kim HC. Effect of R-phase heat treatment on torsional resistance and cyclic fatigue fracture. *J Endod* 2013 Mar; 39(3): 389–393.
70 Yamamura B, Cox TC, Heddaya B, Flake NM, Johnson JD, Paranjpe A. Comparing canal transportation and centering ability of EndoSequence and Vortex rotary files by using micro-computed tomography. *J Endod* 2012 Aug; 38(8): 1121–1125.
71 Casper RB, Roberts HW, Roberts MD, Himel VT, Bergeron BE. Comparison of autoclaving effects on torsional deformation and fracture resistance of three innovative endodontic file systems. *J Endod* 2011 Nov; 37(3): 1572–1575.
72 Johnson E, Lloyd A, Kuttler S, Namerow K. Comparison between a novel nickel–titanium alloy and 508 nitinol on the cyclic fatigue life of ProFile 25/.04 rotary instruments. *J Endod* 2008; 34: 1406–1409.
73 Buchanan S. The technique for GT Series X rotary shaping files. *Endo Tribune U.S* 2007; 12: 8–9.
74 http://www.scribd.com/doc/35935026/GT-Series-XBrochure
75 Gao Y, Gutmann JL, Wilkinson K, Maxwell R, Ammon D. Evaluation of the impact of raw materials on the fatigue and mechanical properties of ProFile Vortex rotary instruments. *J Endod* 2012 Mar; 38(3): 398–401.
76 http://www.tulsadentalspecialties.com
77 Ruddle CJ, Machtou P,West JD. The shaping movement: fifth-generation technology. *Dentistry Today* http://dentistrytoday.com/endodontics/8865-the-shaping-movement-fifth-generation-technology
78 Blum JY, Machtou P, Ruddle C, Micallef JP. Analysis of mechanical preparations in extracted teeth using ProTaper rotary instruments: value of the safety quotient. *J Endod* 2003; 29: 567–575.
79 Koch KA, Brave DG. Real World Endo Sequence File. *Dent Clin North Am* 2004; 48(1): 159–182.
80 Koch K, Brave D. The EndoSequence file: a guide to clinical use. *Compend Contin Educ Dent* 2004; 25(10A): 811–813.
81 Koch K, Brave D. Endodontic synchronicity. *Compend Contin Educ Dent* 2005; 26(3): 218, 220–224.
82 Gergi R, Rjeily JA, Sader J, Naaman A. Comparison of canal transportation and centering ability of Twisted files, Pathfile-ProTaper system, and Stainless steel hand K-files by using computed tomography *J Endod* 2010; 36(5): 904–907.
83 El Batouty KM, Elmallah WE. Comparison of canal transportation and changes in canal curvature of two nickel–titanium rotary instruments. *J Endod* 2011; 37(9): 1290–1292.
84 Gambarini G, Gergi R, Naaman A, Osta N, Al Sudani D. Cyclic fatigue analysis of twisted file rotary NiTi instruments used in reciprocating motion. *Int Endod J* 2012; 45(9): 802–806.
85 Gambarini G. Influence of a novel reciprocation movement on the cyclic fatigue of twisted files (TF) instruments. Healthcare learning website. www.healthcare-learning.com April 2014.
86 Kerr Dental. TF Adaptive NiTi Endo File System. http://tfadaptive.com/
87 Kerr Dental.K3 XF NiTi Endo Files. https://www.kerrdental.com/kerr-endodontics/k3-xf-niti-endo-files-shape
88 Shen Y, Qian W, Abtin H, Gao Y, Haapasalo M. Fatigue testing of controlled memory wire nickel–titanium rotary instruments. *J Endod* 2011; 37: 997–1001.
89 Shen Y, Qian W, Abtin H, Gao Y, Haapasalo M. Effect of environment on fatigue failure of controlled memory wire nickel–titanium rotary instruments. *J Endod* 2012; 38: 376–380.
90 Peters OA, Gluskin AK,Weiss RA, Han JT. An *in vitro* assessment of the physical properties of novel Hyflex nickel–titanium rotary instruments. *Int Endod J* 2012; 45: 1027–1034.
91 Zinelis S, Eliades T, Eliades G. A metallurgical characterization of ten endodontic Ni-Ti instruments: assessing the

clinical relevance of shape memory and superelastic properties of Ni-Ti endodontic instruments. *Int Endod J* 2010; 43: 125–134.

92 Coltene Endo. Changing the DNA of NiTi. www.hyflexcm.com/DevDownloads/30464A_HYFLEX-CM_bro.pdf

93 http://www.clinicalresearchdental.com/products.php?product=Typhoon-Infinite-Flex-NiTi-Files*

94 Reddy SA, Hicks ML. Apical extrusion of debris using two hand and two rotary instrumentation techniques. *J Endod* 1998; 24: 180–183.

95 Yared G. Canal preparation using only one Ni-Ti rotary instrument: preliminary observations. *Int Endod J* 2008; 41: 339–344.

96 Kim HC, Kwak SW, Cheung GS, Ko DH, Chung SM, Lee W. Cyclic fatigue and torsional resistance of two new nickel–titanium instruments used in reciprocation motion: Reciproc versus WaveOne. *J Endod* 2012 Apr; 38(4): 541–544.

97 Castelló-Escrivá R, Alegre-Domingo T, Faus-Matoses V, Román-Richon S, Faus-Llácer VJ. *In vitro* comparison of cyclic fatigue resistance of ProTaper, WaveOne, and Twisted Files. *J Endod* 2012 Nov; 38(11): 1521–1524.

98 Webber J, Machtou P, Pertot W, Kuttler S, Ruddle C, West J. The WaveOne single-file reciprocating system. *Roots* 2011. http://www.endoexperience.com/documents/WaveOne.pdf

99 Yared G. Canal preparation with only one reciprocating instrument without prior hand filing: a new concept. http://www.endodonticcourses.com.

100 Liu J. Characterization of new rotary endodontic instruments fabricated from special thermomechanically processed NiTi Wire. PhD dissertation, Ohio State University, 2009; http://etd.ohiolink.edu/view.cgi/Liu%20Jie.pdf?osu1244643081

101 Metzger Z, Teperovich E, Zary R, Cohen R, Hof R. The self -adjusting file (SAF). Part 1: Respecting the root canal anatomy: A new concept of endodontic files and its implementation. *J Endod* 2010; 36: 679–690.

102 Hof R, Perevalov V, Eltanani M, Zary R, Metzger Z. The self-adjusting file (SAF). Part 2: mechanical analysis. *J Endod* 2010; 36: 691–696.

103 Metzger Z, Teperovich E, Cohen R, Zary R, Paque F, Hulsmann M. The self-adjusting file (SAF). Part 3: removal of debris and smear layer: a scanning electron microscope study. *J Endod* 2010; 36: 697–702.

104 Peters OA, Boessler C, Paque F. Root canal preparation with a novel nickel–titanium instrument evaluated with micro-computed tomography: canal surface preparation over time. *J Endod* 2010; 36: 1068–1072.

105 Metzger Z, Zari R, Cohen R, Teperovich, E, Paque F. The quality of root canal preparation and root canal obturation in canals treated with rotary versus self-adjusting files: a three-dimensional micro-computed tomographic study. *J Endod* 2010; 36: 1569–1573.

106 Ruckman JE, Whitten B, Sedgley CM, Svec T. Comparison of the self-adjusting file with rotary and hand instrumentation in long-oval-shaped root canals. *J Endod* 2013; 39: 92–95.

107 Cantatore G, Berutti E, Castellucci A. The PathFile: a new series of rotary Nickel Titanium instruments for mechanical pre-flaring and creating the glide path. www.endoexperience.com/documents/pathfile-italy.doc

108 Lin LM, Skribner JE, Gaengler P. Factors associated with endodontic treatment failures. *J Endod* 1992; 18(12): 625–627.

109 Molander A, Reit C, Dahlen G, Kvist T. Microbiological status of root-filled teeth with apical periodontitis. *Int Endod J* 1998; 31(1): 1–7.

110 Torabinejad M, Walton RE. *Endodontics: Principles and practice*. St. Louis: Saunders Elsevier; 2009.

111 Becker TD, Woollard GW. Endodontic irrigation. *Gen Dent* 2001; 49(3): 272–276.

112 Carson KR, Goodell GG, McClanahan SB. Comparison of the antimicrobial activity of six irrigants on primary endodontic pathogens. *J Endod* 2005; 31(6): 471–473.

113 Clegg MS, Vertucci FJ, Walker C, Belanger M, Britto LR. The effect of exposure to irrigant solutions on apical dentin biofilms *in vitro*. *J Endod* 2006; 32(5): 434–437.

114 Mentz TCF. The use of sodium hypochlorite as a general endodontic medicament. *Int Endod J* 1982; 15(3): 132–136.

115 Ohara PK, Torabinejad M, Kettering JD. Antibacterial effects of various endodontic irrigants on selected anaerobic bacteria. *Dent Traumatol* 1993; 9(3): 95–100.

116 Shih M, Marshall FJ, Rosen S. The bactericidal efficiency of sodium hypochlorite as an endodontic irrigant. *Oral Surg Oral Med Oral Pathol* 1970; 29(4): 613–619.

117 Hülsmann M, Heckendorff M, Lennon A. Chelating agents in root canal treatment: mode of action and indications for their use. *Int Endod J* 2003; 36(12): 810–830.

118 Zehnder M, Schmidlin P, Sener B, Waltimo T. Chelation in root canal therapy reconsidered. *J Endod* 2005; 31(11): 817–820.

119 Torabinejad M, Khademi AA, Babagoli J, Cho Y, Johnson WB, *et al.* A new solution for the removal of the smear layer. *J Endod* 2003; 29(3): 170–175.

120 Giardino L, Ambu E, Becce C, Rimondini L, Morra M. Surface tension comparison of four common root canal irrigants and two new irrigants containing antibiotic. *J End* 2006; 32(11): 1091–1093.

121 Giardino L, Ambu E, Savoldi E, Rimondini R, Cassanelli C, Debbia EA. Comparative evaluation of antimicrobial efficacy of sodium hypochlorite, MTAD, and Tetraclean against *Enterococcus faecalis* biofilm. *J Endod* 2007; 33(7): 852–855.

122 Solovyeva AM, Dummer PMH. Cleaning effectiveness of root canal irrigation with electrochemically activated anolyte and catholyte solutions: a pilot study. *Int Endod J* 2000; 33(6): 494–504.

123 Selkon JB, Babb JR, Morris R. Evaluation of the antimicrobial activity of a new super-oxidized water, Sterilox, for the disinfection of endoscopes. *J Hosp Infect* 1999; 41(1): 59–70.
124 Hata G, Uemura M, Weine FS, Toda T. Removal of smear layer in the root canal using oxidative potential water. *J Endod* 1996; 22(12): 643–645.
125 Shetty N, Srinivasan S, Holton J, Ridgway GL. Evaluation of microbicidal activity of a new disinfectant: Sterilox 2500 against *Clostridium difficile* spores, *Helicobacter pylori*, vancomycin-resistant *Enterococcus* species, *Candida albicans* and several *Mycobacterium* species. *J Hosp Infect* 1999; 41(2): 101–105.
126 Legchilo AN, Legchilo AA, Mostovshchikov IO. Preparation of suppurative wounds for autodermatoplasty with electrochemically activated solutions. *Surgery* 1: 57–58.
127 Broadwater WT, Hoehn RC, King PH. Sensitivity of three selected bacterial species to ozone. *J Appl Microbiol* 1973; 26(3): 391–393.
128 Baysan A, Lynch E. The use of ozone in dentistry and medicine. *Prim Dent Care* 2005; 12(2): 47–52.
129 Dougherty TJ, Gomer CJ, Henderson BW, Jori G, Kessel D, *et al.* Photodynamic therapy. *J Natl Cancer Inst* 1998; 90(12): 889–905.
130 Bonsor SJ, Nichol R, Reid TMS, Pearson GJ. Microbiological evaluation of photo-activated disinfection in endodontics (an *in vivo* study). *Br Dent J* 2006; 200(6): 337–341.
131 Schlafer S, Vaeth M, Horsted-Bindslev P, Frandsen EVG. Endodontic photoactivated disinfection using a conventional light source: an *in vitro* and *ex vivo* study. *Oral Surg Oral Med Oral Pathol* 2010; 109(4): 634–641.
132 Gambarini G, Plotino G, Grande NM, Nocca G, Lupi A, et al. *In vitro* evaluation of the cytotoxicity of Fotosan light-activated disinfection on human fibroblasts. *Med Sci Monit* 2011;17(3):21–25.
133 Kömerik N, Curnow A, MacRobert AJ, Hopper C, Speight PM, Wilson M. Fluorescence biodistribution and photosensitising activity of toluidine blue o on rat buccal mucosa. *Lasers Med Sci* 2002; 17(2): 86–92.
134 Soukos NS, Chen PSY, Morris JT, Ruggiero K, Abernethy AD, et al. Photodynamic therapy for endodontic disinfection. *J Endod* 2006; 32(10): 979–984.
135 Boutsioukis C, Verhaagen B, Versluis M, Kastrinakis E, Wesselink PR, van der Sluis LW. Evaluation of irrigant flow in the root canal using different needle types by an unsteady computational fluid dynamics model. *J Endod* 2010; 36(5): 875–879.
136 Al-Hadlaq SM, Al-Turaiki SA, Al-Sulami U, Saad AY. Efficacy of new brush-covered irrigation needle in removing root canal debris: a scanning electron microscopic study. *J Endod* 2006; 32(12): 1181–1184.
137 Ruddle C. Endodontic disinfection: tsunami irrigation. *Endod Prac* 2008; 5: 8–17.
138 Townsend C, Maki J. An *in vitro* comparison of new irrigation and agitation techniques to ultrasonic agitation in removing bacteria from a simulated root canal. *J Endod* 2009; 35: 1040–1043.
139 Desai P, Himel V. Comparative safety of various intracanal irrigation systems. *J Endod* 2009; 35: 545–549.
140 Richman RJ. The use of ultrasonics in root canal therapy and root resection. *Med Dent J* 1957; 12:12–18.
141 Tilk MA, Lommel TJ, Gerstein H. A study of mandibular and maxillary root widths to determine dowel size. *J Endod* 1979; 5: 79–82.
142 Ahmad M, Pitt Ford TR, Crum LA, Walton AJ. Ultrasonic debridement of root canals: acoustic cavitation and its relevance. *J Endod* 1988; 14: 486–493.
143 Walker TL, del Rio CE. Histological evaluation of ultrasonic and sonic instrumentation of curved root canals. *J Endod* 1989; 15: 49–59.
144 Burleson A, Nusstein J, Reader A, Beck M. The *in vivo* evaluation of hand/rotary/ultrasound instrumentation in necrotic, human mandibular molars. *J Endod* 2007; 33(7): 782–787.
145 Carver K, Nusstein J, Reader A, Beck M. *In vivo* antibacterial efficacy of ultrasound after hand and rotary instrumentation in human mandibular molars. *J Endod* 2007; 33(9): 1038–1043.
146 Lussi A, Nussbächer U, Grosrey J. A novel noninstrumented technique for cleansing the root canal system. *J Endod* 1993; 19: 549–553.

Questions

1 What strength of sodium hypochlorite (bleach) is used for canal irrigation?
A 1%
B 2%
C 5%
D 10%
E 20%
F 50%

2 What is a hermetic seal, as applied to endodontics?
A Airtight
B Waterproof
C Saliva can't pass
D Microorganisms can't pass
E All of these

3 Rotary instruments should not be used
A To negotiate a canal
B To enlarge a canal
C with a light touch

4 Which of the following files are manufactured by a twisting process?
A ProFiles
B Reciproc

C Twisted Files
D Hyflex

5 The distinctive blue color of Vortex Blue is a result of light rays interacting with a titanium oxide layer on the surface of the file.
A True
B False

6 Which of the following are examples of single file rotary systems?
A Wave One
B Reciproc
C Typhoon
D Both a and b
E All of the above

7 The functions of the irrigation solution are the following, except:
A Lubrication
B Debridement
C Sterilization
D Disinfection

8 MTAD is
A Bacteriostatic
B Bactericidal
C Both a and b

9 ProTaper F2 file is an example of
A Rotation
B Reciprocation
C Both a and b

10 All NiTi instruments are best used in a step-back manner only
A True
B False

CHAPTER 4

Determination of working length

Priyanka Jain
Dubai, UAE

The triad in endodontic therapy comprises total debridement of the pulpal space, proper cleaning and shaping of the canal space, and three-dimensional obturation of the root canal.

As stated in the previous chapter, the most important segment of endodontic treatment in the canal preparation is the calculation of the working length [1–3]. Therefore, the procedure should be performed with skill, using techniques that have been proven to give accurate results. The significance of accurate working length is threefold: it determines where the instruments are placed in canal, it limits the depth to which the root filling is placed if calculated properly, and it plays an important role in the success of the treatment and conversely can lead to failure if calculated improperly.

Grove in 1930 stated that "the proper point to which root canals should be filled is the junction of the dentin and the cementum and that the pulp should be severed at this point of its union with the periodontal membrane." Working length in endodontics is defined as "the length from a coronal reference point to the point at which the canal preparation and obturation should terminate" [4].

In order to define an apical end point during a course of root canal treatment, it is important to know the anatomy of the apical portion of the root. The extent of the apical limit of the root canal preparation is still debatable based upon different clinical opinions regarding the distance between the end point of the canal preparation and the periodontal tissues. In current endodontic practice, various methods are used to determine working length. This chapter talks about the more recent ones.

Anatomic considerations in determining the working length

Each time we need to determine working length, we are faced with various challenges and factors influencing our decision of where to locate the apical terminus. There is an ongoing debate regarding the extent of the apical limit of root canal preparation. This controversy is based upon different clinical opinions regarding the distance between the end point of the root canal preparation and the periodontal tissues (Box 4.1).

In the 1900s the popular opinion was that dental pulp extended through the tooth and ended at the apical foramen, and the narrowest diameter of the apical portion of the root was at the site where the canal exits the tooth at the extreme apex (Figure 4.1). These views fostered the then-existing technique to calculate working length to the tip of the root on the radiographs – that is, the radiographic apex – as the correct site to terminate the canal. In the 1920s considerable study of the apex of the tooth led Grove, Hatton, Blayney, and Coolidge to offer reports that contradicted this position. Kuttler did the most comprehensive study in 1955 on the microscopic anatomy of the root tip [5]. His study is one of the most important sets of proper standards for sophisticated successful endodontic treatment even today.

Cementodentinal junction

The cementodentinal junction (CDJ) is considered by a majority of schools across the world as the ideal end point for the preparation, because it represents the point at which the root canal system terminates and the periodontium (presence of cementum) begins.

Current Therapy in Endodontics, First Edition. Edited by Priyanka Jain.
© 2016 John Wiley & Sons, Inc. Published 2016 by John Wiley & Sons, Inc.

Box 4.1 Apical anatomy definitions*

Anatomical apex: The end of the root as determined morphologically. It is the junction between the cementum and dentin.
Apical constriction or *Minor apical foramen* or *Physiological apex:* The apical portion of the root canal system with the narrowest diameter. It is usually 0.5- to 1.0 mm short of the center of the anatomical apical foramen.
Cementodentinal junction: The region where the dentin and cementum meet. Its position can range from 0.5 to 3.0 mm from the anatomical apex.
Major apical foramen: Main apical opening of the root canal.
Radiographic apex: The end of the root as determined radiographically. Its location can vary due to root morphology and distortion of the radiographic image.

*Adapted from American Association of Endodontists. *Glossary of Endodontic Terms*, 7th edition. Chicago: American Association of Endodontists, 2003.

However, this junction is strictly histological and is impossible to locate clinically. It is also a highly irregular reference point, because in some cases the CDJ can be up to 3 mm higher on one wall of the root canal as compared to the other [6].

Radiographic apex

The radiographic apex was believed to commonly coincide with apical foramen and was easy to detect radiographically; therefore, it was considered the end of the root canal. Although it was commonly used many years ago, a number of excellent clinicians still use the radiographic apex as the site of canal termination. Those who believe this concept state that it is impossible to locate the CDJ clinically and that the radiographic apex is the only reproducible site available in this area. However, the position of the radiographic apex depends on several factors, such as the angulation of the tooth, position of the film, holding device for the film (finger, x-ray holder), length of the x-ray cone, horizontal and vertical positioning of the cone, and anatomic structures adjacent to the tooth, as well as several other factors. Thus the reliability is questionable.

Apical foramen

It is a proven fact that in a root canal anatomy, root canals always deviate from the long axis of their roots, and the major apical foramen (foramen of the main root canal) almost never coincides with the principal axis of the root.

However, several investigators have shown that less than 50% of the time, the apical foramen coincides with the anatomical apex [5]. Such variations are not easily detectable in two-dimensional radiography, even with minimum distortion. Deposition of the cementum at the root apex also leads to discrepancy between the apical foramen and the root tip, and this discrepancy increases with age [5, 7]. Deviation of the major apical foramen can also occur as a result of pathological changes (external root resorption) [8]. Therefore, it is a fact that the anatomical foramen is neither at the anatomical nor at the radiographic apex.

Apical constriction

Another anatomic consideration to be discussed is the apical constriction. This is the naturally narrowest area of the canal located in its last few millimeters. This is a highly variable part of the root canal system and is not present in all teeth. It has been classified into simple, diverging, multiple, and parallel constrictions. The apical constriction and dentinocemental junction were viewed as a single area for a long time and located at an average of 1 mm from the root apex. These estimations have led clinicians to teach and believe that the working length is 1 mm from the radiographic apex junction. This technique is no longer reliable for three main reasons: The dentinocemental junction is very rarely located at the apical constriction, the thickness of the cementum varies greatly from one tooth to another and between patients, and the thickness of the cementum changes with physiology (increases with aging) and pathology (apical resorption related to canal infection).

Although the apical foramen can demonstrate considerable morphological variation, it is still a more

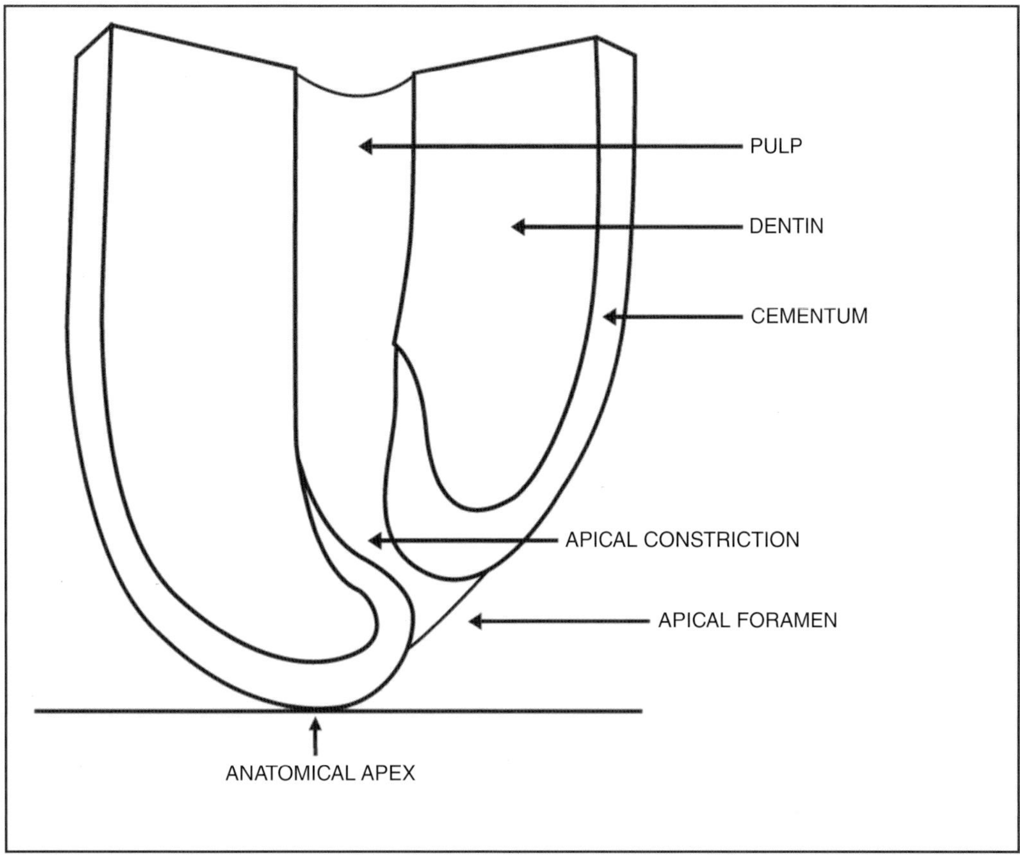

Figure 4.1 Anatomy of the apical root.

consistent anatomical reference point than the apical constriction or radiographic apex [8]. The use of the major foramen is more reproducible for accuracy studies [9]. Owing to numerous inconsistencies, variations with regard to the apical constriction, and CDJ and their interrelationship, the apical foramen may be a more useful and reliable apical reference point in determining working length. Facts in favor of this approach are that it is on an average 0.5 to 1.0 mm short of the radiographic apex and is a more-practical landmark to use when terminating a root canal preparation.

The pathological and microbiological status of the dental pulp and periapical tissues is also an extremely important decision-making factor for where, when, why, and how to locate the apical terminus. In cases with necrotic and/or infected pulp with no periapical lesion, researchers recommend that the apical terminus be located at the physiological foramen. This location preserves integrity of the apical morphology, and it neither violates the apical foramen nor challenges the periodontal ligament, thus enabling optimal healing. It has also been suggested that the apical terminus be located at the anatomical foramen, sometimes identified as the apex, or even at the radiographic apex.

In cases with apical periodontitis there is controversy about the location of the apical terminus. A conservative approach states that all preparation of the root canal system should end at the physiological foramen, because any manipulations beyond this endpoint will lead to either clinical or histological failure. Another approach suggests that preparation and obturation in such cases should always be terminated at the anatomical or radiological foramen, the radiographic apex of the tooth.

With periapical pathosis associated with pathological inflammatory apical root resorption, it is particularly difficult to decide where to locate and how to determine the endodontic terminus. Literature suggests that it should be either 0.5 mm short or 1.0 mm long of the apex. To date, there is no accurate technique for such cases.

In an ideal situation, the root canal should be prepared and obturated to a point as close to the apical foramen as possible yet still within sound tooth structure. The objective of determining the working length is to enable the root canal to be prepared as close to the apical constriction as possible. It is not possible to determine if one concept is superior to the other. Each operator will strive to justify his or her approach. A compromise may be accepted by most practitioners, one in which the foramen is located at canal length (L), so the working length is L – 0.5 mm and the patency of the canal is checked frequently with small files (sizes 6, 8, 10).

Limitations of traditional working length assessment

Traditional methods for establishing working length (Box 4.2) have been the use of anatomical averages and the knowledge of the anatomy, tactile sensation, and moisture on a paper point and radiography.

Patient's response to pain is probably the oldest method used. However, due to numerous interfering factors, it is very unreliable in clinical practice. This technique is also extremely subjective owing to the individual pain threshold of each patient. Moreover, it is impossible to apply this method when local anesthesia is performed.

Tactile feedback from instruments is also a very subjective technique. This method clearly has its limitations in cases where the canal is sclerosed or the anatomical landmark has been obliterated by resorption. Furthermore, topography of the apical constriction can vary due to morphological irregularities, tooth type, and age (generally leading to shorter length values) or wide foramen in immature teeth, which leads to longer working length. All these coupled with the fact that there will be considerable variation in the clinician's ability to accurately feel the apical constriction makes this technique questionable and unreliable.

Another method used for determining length is the paper point measurement technique (PPT) described by Rosenberg. PPT is dependent on having achieved apical patency [9, 10]. This technique is particularly useful toward the end of preparation or on roots with a very wide canal in which the apex locator can sometimes be unreliable (discussed later in the chapter). This method consists of placing a feathered-tip paper point in the prepared canal, knowing that the canal has been cleared of all its contents. A minute amount of blood or tissue fluid at the end of the point indicates that it has been inserted beyond the foramen. Although this technique is useful when managing teeth with open apices or abnormal apical anatomy, it cannot be used in cases where it is impossible to dry the canal or achieve apical patency. PPT lacks the ability to determine morphological details and pathological states within the root canal and in the apical tissues. Furthermore, neither scientific nor clinical evidence is available in the literature to verify the effectiveness of this technique.

Radiographic methods

Conventional radiography

Film radiography

Radiographs are probably the most common and oldest method used for determining working length. Although radiographs are important in endodontic treatment, primarily for assessing canal curvature and root form, they have limitations regarding determining working length. The most commonly employed radiographic method for determining working length is that of Ingle [11]. Ingle's method depends on estimating the distance between the file tip and the radiographic apex and adjusting it until the file tip is 0.5 to 1 mm short of the radiographic apex. Other radiographic methods described in the literature are discussed in brief.

Best (1960) described a method that depends on securing a 10-mm steel pin to the labial surface of the tooth parallel to its long axis before obtaining the radiograph. The radiograph is related to a gauge allowing the clinician to determine the length of the tooth [12, 13].

Bergman's method is based on calculating the real tooth length based on the radiographic appearance of a 25-mm probe that has an acrylic stop that allows it to penetrate 10 mm in the canal [12, 13]. Bramante introduced a technique that used stainless steel probes of different gauges and lengths bent at one end to form a right angle. A radiograph is obtained with the probe in place, then the tooth length could be calculated (similar to Bergman's method) or the distance between the probe end and the radiographic apex could be used to determine the adjustment needed (similar to Ingle's method).

Box 4.2 Methods of Determining Working Length

Conventional

Grossman's formula
Radiographic method
- Ingle's method
- Best's method
- Bregman's method
- Bramante's method

Weine's method
Kuttler's method
Digital tactile sense
Apical periodontal sensitivity
Paper point method
Radiographic grid
Endometric probe
Patient's pain response

Recent

Electronic method
Direct digital radiography
Xeroradiography
Subtraction radiography
Digital image processing
Laser optical storage
Tomography
Fourth-generation direct digital radiography

The rationale for using this technique is based on the suggestion that the apical constriction may be located at 1 mm short of the radiographic apex. However, in some cases, the apical foramen can even be located as far as 3 mm short of the radiographic apex, thus increasing chances of overinstrumentation. Furthermore, the apical foramen and the radiographic apex do not always coincide [5, 14]. When the apical foramen exits to the sides of the root or in a buccolingual direction, it becomes difficult to view on the radiograph [6].

Xeroradiography

Invented by Chester F. Carlson in 1937, xeroradiography records images produced by x-rays but differs from conventional radiography in that it does not require wet chemicals or a darkroom for processing. In endodontics, this imaging permits better visualization of pulp chamber morphology, root canal configuration, and root outline, which is especially useful in imaging maxillary molars and premolars, in which zygomatic arch and maxillary sinus superimpositions will hinder accurate visualization of dental structures. Xeroradiographic images differ from conventional radiographs in three ways: they exhibit high edge contrast due to edge enhancement (the boundaries between structures are clear), which facilitates perception of anatomic details; the image is on paper and can be viewed under reflective light; and the choice of a negative or a positive image is possible.

Limitations of conventional radiography

The radiographic technique, coupled with the clinician's knowledge of dental anatomy and root canal systems, can be a very useful method. Although the image obtained provides valuable information regarding the shape and curvature of the root apex, it also has limitations and often provides an illusory image. It is only a two-dimensional representation of a three-dimensional structure, which is subject to error, and some anatomical landmarks could be superimposed on each other. For example, the superimposition of the zygomatic arch over the roots of maxillary molars or mandibular torus over the roots of mandibular premolars will impede the proper location of the radiographic apex on those teeth. Dense bone can also make the visualization of root canal files difficult by obscuring the apex. Newer digital radiography systems might overcome this problem by image manipulation [15].

The presence of apical resorption can also create a problem while using this technique. Because root resorption can alter the apical constriction, Weine (2004) suggested subtracting an extra 0.5 mm from the working length in teeth exhibiting radiographic evidence of apical resorption. This can ensure that both the instrumentation and the filling materials will be kept confined within the root canal space [16].

Variables such as radiographic technique, angulations, and inadequate radiographic exposure play an important role in assessing length because they can result in distorted radiographic images. It is sometimes necessary to take several radiographs, which exposes the patient to unnecessary radiation levels; for example, identification of buccal and lingual canals may be challenging because of superimposition of those over each other in a radiographic straight-angle image. Radiographs are also technique sensitive and require exposing the patient to ionizing radiation. The interpretation of the radiographic image can be very subjective and an important factor in the accuracy of the technique [10]. Other disadvantages include the need for chemical solutions, the time required to process the radiographs, the need for radiographs that cannot be modified, and the control and maintenance of radiographs during and after treatment [15, 17].

However, it is not always possible to accurately determine the tooth's length radiographically because of anatomical variations in the apical foramen, which is not visualized in the radiograph. In addition, roots often present different degrees of curvature or superposition of anatomical structures. Presence of periapical pathology, degree of pathological or physiological resorption, and presence of permanent successor tooth are also factors complicating the working length determination of primary teeth [18]. Clinically, the radiographic apex is used as reference point. However, because the apex does not always coincide with the actual position of the apical foramen, there is a difference between apparent tooth length and actual tooth length in the majority of the cases [19].

Digital radiography

How it works

The main purpose of a radiographic capturing device, whether it is digital sensor or conventional film, is to capture the dispersion pattern of the x-ray photon density pattern as it emerges from the tissues, which is a function of the tissues and the radiation source. These x-ray photons cannot be focused into a sharp image (the way light can be focused through a camera lens), so the image captured by a conventional film or a digital sensor will never have a sharp, in-focus appearance like a photograph focused through a lens. Hence, radiographic images are always subject to a certain degree of geometric unsharpness, thereby limiting the resolution of the image captured.

The ability to capture the emerging photon pattern accurately can be improved upon. This is dependent on the size of the sensor's capture units. Smaller capture units add more resolution, and hence more detail and clarity to the image processed. The capture units of conventional radiographic films are the grain size of the film. Faster films have larger grain size, thus resulting in the loss of image sharpness. This is one of the main reasons digital radiography is a step ahead of the conventional radiographic system.

Current progress in this field is targeted toward reducing the exposure time and obtaining direct digital images. Digital imaging incorporates computer technology in the capture, display, enhancement, and storage of direct radiographic images. It offers some distinct advantages over conventional film. One advantage of digital intraoral radiograph is the reduction of radiation dosage by up to 22% of F-speed film. Digital radiography requires only approximately 23% of the x-ray dosage of D-speed film [20]. However, like any emerging technology, it presents new and different challenges for the practitioner to overcome.

Advantages and disadvantages

The main advantages of digital radiography include immediate observation of radiographic images; elimination of chemical processing and associated errors; reduction in radiation dose; data storage; transfer of images electronically, thus encouraging communication between practitioners; and image enhancement and manipulation. Digital radiography is a fast technique, allowing paralleling and reduction in radiation dose per image, besides being comfortable for the patient and yielding data that can be quickly analyzed by software [21, 22].

On the other hand, limitations include cost of the device, reduced resolution of the image, quality of the printed image, thickness of the available sensor and its rigidity, and lack of training to use the technique. Digital images can be distorted or amplified due to geometrical variations such as angulation, distance between sensor and tooth, and distance between x-ray source and tooth.

It is important to note that all the studies and research on the image quality compared the performance of different systems and attributed variations to differences in image clarity. However, evaluation of image clarity also depends on the observer's perception and experience. Image manipulation is one of the main advantages of digital radiography [15, 23]; however, enhancement does not always result in better interpretation when compared to conventional films [24–28]. Although digital images are instantly available, their manipulation takes time and requires experience [29, 30].

Types of systems

A new radiographic system called *direct digital radiology* (DDR) digitizes ionizing radiation and produces high-resolution computer monitor images with reduced radiographic exposure. The system consists of a conventional x-ray–generating device that replaces the radiographic film, hence the term *filmless radiography.* Two of the earlier models of the DDR system are radiovisiography (RVG), developed by Dr. Francis Mouyan, a French dentist, and video imaging x-ray application (VIXA).

Continuous development and improvements have been achieved and new digital systems have been introduced [31]. Digital images can be acquired directly using capturing devices that may be either solid-state receptors such as charge-coupled devices (CCD) or complementary metal oxide semiconductors (CMOS). Semidirect capture is achieved via photo-stimulable phosphor (PSP). The indirect capture is acquired by flatbed scanner or digital camera.

RVG, a CCD-based digital system, has been compared with conventional films for determining working length. This device has three components: The *radio* part consists of a hypersensitive intraoral sensor (instead of the conventional x-ray film) and a conventional x-ray unit. The second component, the *vision*, consists of a video monitor and display-processing unit. The third component is the *graphic*, a high-resolution video printer that instantly provides a hard copy of the screen image, using the video signal. RVG allowed a substantial reduction in the duration of endodontic procedures, because it effectively eliminated the film-processing time. In the same way, the zoom function had the potential to improve the diagnostic performance by magnifying areas such as the apical zone.

The image quality of a PSP-based system (Vistascan; Dürr Dental GmbH, Bissingen, Germany) was found to be superior to a CCD-based system (Sidexis; Sirona Dental Systems GmbH, Bensheim, Germany). The latter required lower radiation but was associated with more retakes [32].

Tomography (micro computed tomography [μCT])

Tomography is a radiographic technique that produces images of "slices" of teeth in thin sections. These sections are then reassembled to generate a three-dimensional image. Dental anatomy including buccolingual curvatures, shapes of the root canal spaces, and location of the apical foramen (which is important in determining or calculating the working length) can be visualized in three dimensions. This method provides the additional advantage of eliminating angled radiographs, because all angled views are captured in just one exposure [33, 34]. This innovation was achieved because new hardware and software was available to evaluate the metric data created by μCT, thus allowing geometrical changes in prepared canals to be determined in more detail [33].

Videography and intraoral cameras

Intraoral videography is a nonionizing diagnostic imaging technique that uses miniature color CCD (charge coupled device) chips. They have small fiberoptic probes with video cameras attached to them. These devices are useful in endodontics because they can display canal morphology and perforations by inserting the fiberoptic probe down the canal. The device is connected to a computer that provides enhanced images for teaching and patient education.

Direct digital radiography (DDR)

The DDR system consists of a programmed computerized receiver that processes signals from an intraoral sensor stimulated by x-rays from a standard dental machine. The signals are then transferred to a monitor as a large regular radiograph.

One of the more-recent additions to the fourth generation of RVG systems is the capability of on-screen point-to-point measurements using multiple additive points. This capability allows fast and accurate estimation of working length in roots demonstrating severe apical curvatures The RVG on-screen measurement utility allows rapid additive multiple-point measurement of digital images, automatically tallying the measurement points on the screen to a tenth of a millimeter, because it was expected that multiple measurements along the curve of a canal would be more accurate than a straight-line measurement from the reference point to the apex. It was felt that if measurement points were able to closely follow the curve, a true estimate of the working length would be obtained.

Nonradiographic methods

M.M. Negm in 1982 introduced a novel method of determining the length of root canal without the use of radiographs, called the *apex finder*. This instrument is used to locate the apex and measure the root length. In this method, a fine plastic tapered bared shaft is inserted through a beveled tube into the root canal. Resistance to withdrawal indicates that some barbs have engaged the apical margin; when this resistance is felt, the shaft is marked at the level of the cusp tip. The distance between the mark and the barbs, which caused the resistance, is measured.

Another nonradiographic method is the *audio metric method*. It is based on the principle of electrical resistance of comparative tissue using a low-frequency oscillation sound to indicate when similarity to electrical resistance has occurred by a similar sound response. An instrument is placed in the gingival sulcus and an electric current is given until a sound is produced. This is then repeated by placing an instrument through the root canal until the same sound is heard. Thus, one can determine the length of the tooth.

Electronic apex locators

An electronic apex locator (EAL) is an electronic device used in endodontics to determine the position of the apical foramen and thus determine the length of the root canal space. An electronic method for determining root length was first investigated by Cluster (1918) [35]. The idea was revisited in 1942 by Suzuki, who studied the flow of direct current through the teeth of dogs. He took these principles and constructed a simple device that used direct current to measure the canal length. It worked on the principle that the electrical resistance of the mucous membrane and the periodontium registered 6.5 kilo-ohms in any part of the periodontium regardless of the person's age or the shape and type of teeth [36]. He further stated that it is possible to use this value of resistance in estimating the root length. The device by Sunada in his research became the basis for most EALs.

Although the term "apex locator" is commonly used and has become accepted terminology, it is a misnomer [37]. It may be more appropriate to use other terms such as "electronic root canal length-measuring instruments" or "electronic canal length measuring devices" [38–42].

These devices measure the change in electrical impedance at the canal terminus. This is the reason they are most accurate at showing when a file is in the canal (not patent), and when a file is out of the canal (patent). The location at which these two point meet is the point of patency, or the canal terminus.

Operating principle of apex locators

An understanding of physics and current electricity is essential to appreciate the operating principles of EAL. Direct current (DC) is a fixed amount of current per unit of time, whereas the amount of an alternating current (AC) alternates with time. A structure of two conductive materials with an insulator between them forms an electrical device called a *capacitor*. This is able to store charge. When a capacitor is connected to a DC voltage source, electrons (negative charge) move from one plate to another, making one plate acquire a negative charge and the other a positive charge. When the voltage source is disconnected, the capacitor retains the stored charge, and a voltage remains across it. The amount of charge that a capacitor can store is called *capacitance* and is dependent on the nature of the insulating material between the plates, the distance between the conductors, and their surface areas.

All apex locators function by using the human body to complete an electrical circuit. These features can be compared to an endodontic file in the root canal, surrounded by periodontium. The tooth can be compared to a capacitor. Root canals are surrounded by dentin and cementum that are insulators to electric current and the periodontal ligament (PDL); the AC and the file in the root canal are all conductors of electricity. Therefore, an endodontic file and the PDL surrounding the radicular dentin act as conductors in a capacitor. The dentin and the cementum within the root canal acts as the insulator of the system (Figure 4.2).

Therefore, an electric circuit is formed that runs through a clip on a file, through the root canal, out the PDL, and finally through the mucosa and onto a clip on the patient's lip. The circuit is now complete, and the electrical resistance of the EAL and the resistance between the file and oral mucosa are now equal, which results in the device indicating that the apex has been reached.

An understanding of this can help the clinician to maximize their use and avoid errors. The classification presented here is based on the type of current flow and its opposition, as well as the number of frequencies involved (Table 4.1, Table 4.2, and Box 4.3).

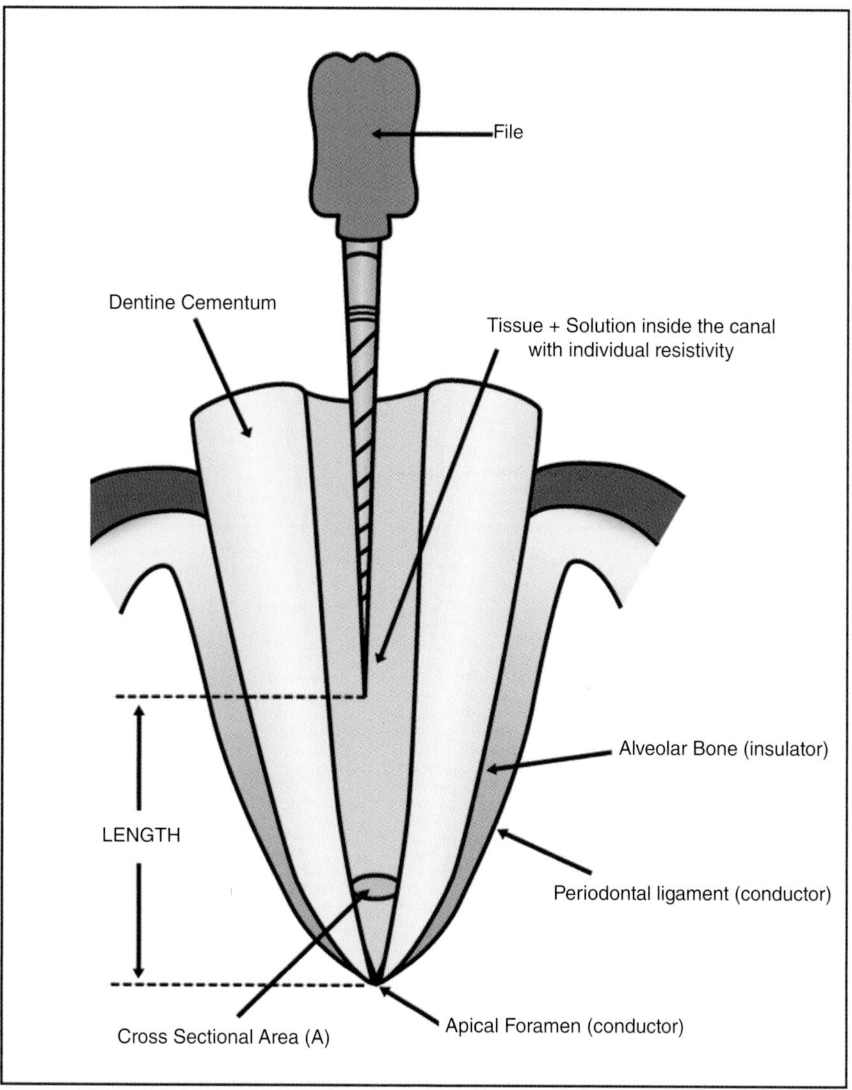

Figure 4.2 Diagrammatic representation of an endodontic instrument, the root canal system, and the electrical features [43]. The resistance is 6.5 kΩ when a file touches the periodontal ligament space at the apical foramen.

Box 4.3 Advantages and Disadvantages of Apex Locators

Advantages

Electronic apex locators reduce the number of radiographs required to determine working length [39, 77]. Thus, by decreasing the total number of required radiographs, the patient's exposure to radiation is also reduced.

They provide a greater precision in locating the apical foramen compared to the radiographic method [78, 79].

These devices can be used at any stage, and, if required, they can be used repeatedly during instrumentation to verify whether the working length remains stable or not and can be adjusted accordingly.

Electronic apex locators are very helpful in multirooted teeth, where the radiographic method the radiographic method can be complicated for measuring working length.

Endodontic procedures can take less time with the use of an electronic apex locator [80].

Locators are extremely useful in patients with acute gag reflex, in whom taking radiographs can be challenging.

Electronic apex locators can be used in pregnant women because they do not produce radiation.

The devices can be used when a dense zygomatic arch overlaps the apices of upper molars.

They can be used to detect perforations.

The technique is fast and easy and accurate.

Disadvantages

Electronic apex locators are devices the endodontist must have on hand.

The accuracy is influenced by the electrical conditions in the root canal.

They give inconsistent readings in teeth with open apices.

Some patients have sensed electrical impulses when apex locators are used, although this is not common [39].

Patients with cardiac pacemakers must consult with their physician before these devices are used on them [75].

They are relatively expensive.

The technique requires the clinician to be familiar with the device and learn how to interpret the readings. A period of learning is a must for their efficient use.

Table 4.1 Generations of apex locators.

Generation	Mechanism	Examples
First (direct current)	Measures resistance	Root canal meter/Endodontic meter (Onuki Medical Co., Tokyo, Japan)
Second	Measures impedance	Sono Explorer Mark II (Hayashi Dental Supply, Tokyo, Japan) Formatron 1V (Parkell Dental, Farmingdale, NY, USA) Digipex 1, II, III (Mada Medical Products, Carlstadt, NJ, USA)
Third	Uses two different frequencies at the same time to measure the difference in impedance	Root ZX (J. Morita, Tokyo, Japan) Neosono Ultima EZ (Satelec Inc, Mount Laurel, NJ, USA) Apex Finder (Micro-Mega, Besançon, France) Just II (Yoshida & Co., Tokyo, Japan) Endex/Apit (Osada Electric Co., Tokyo, Japan) Apex Finder AFA, Model #7005 (Sybron Endo/Analytic Technologies, Orange, CA, USA) Mark V Plus (Moyco/Union Broach, Bethpage, NY, USA)
Fourth	Uses two or more frequencies to measure the impedance ratio between two currents	Raypex 4 (VDW, Munich, Germany) Elements Diagnostic Unit (Sybron Endo, Orange, CA, USA) Propex (Dentsply) iPex (NSK, Japan) Neosono MC (Amadent, USA)

Table 4.1 *(Continued)*

Generation	Mechanism	Examples
Fifth	Measures the capacitance and the resistance of the circuit separately	Propex II (Dentsply, York, PA, USA) Raypex 5 (VDW, Munich, Germany) i-Root (S-Denti Co., Seoul, South Korea)
Sixth	Adapts to the root canal's moisture characteristics	Adaptive (Optica Laser, Sofia, Bulgaria)

Table 4.2 Characteristics of different generations of apex locators.

Generation	Advantages	Disadvantages
First: resistance type	Easy to operate and has a digital readout Able to detect perforation The device comes with a built-in pulp tester	Requires a dry environment Results are not accurate or reliable in the presence of metallic restorations Requires calibration Patient sensitivity is a concern because direct current is applied Requires a lip clip and a file that fits snugly Contraindicated in patients with pacemakers Unreliable in teeth with perforations
Second: impedance type	Able to operate in the presence of electrolytes No patient sensitivity because alternating current is used Able to detect perforations	Requires calibration Cannot use files and requires an insulated/coated probe Does not have a digital readout Difficult to operate
Third: frequency dependent	Easy to operate Operates in the presence of fluids and electrolytes Analog readout Low-voltage electrical output	Requires calibration for each canal Device is sensitive to the amount of fluid present Needs to be fully charged before it can be used
Fourth: ratio type	Reduced electrical noise	Requires a relatively dry or partially dried canals
Fifth	Best accuracy in the presence of fluids and exudates Can be connected to the computer	Difficult to use in dry canals; may need additional insertion of liquids
Sixth	Eliminates the necessity of drying or moistening the canal	

Generations of electronic apex locators

Resistance-based (first-generation) apex locators

First-generation apex location devices, also known as resistance apex locators, measure opposition to the flow of direct current or resistance on the tooth under investigation. The Root Canal Meter/Endodontic Meter (Onuki Medical Co., Tokyo, Japan) was developed in 1969. It used the resistance method and alternating current and worked at a frequency of 150 Hz. Endodontic Meter and the Endodontic Meter S II (Onuki Medical Co.) used a current of less than 5 μA [43].

These devices were found to be unreliable when compared with radiographs, with many of the readings being significantly longer or shorter than the accepted working length [44]. They were found to be accurate under dry conditions, but electrolytic substances like sodium hypochlorite caused a decrease in their efficiency and measurements. Also, the capacitance component of the circuit was not taken into consideration when designing these apex locators. Furthermore, the patient often felt pain due to high currents in the machines [45]. It also gave inaccurate readings in obstructed canals, in teeth with caries or defective restorations, and in cases of perforations.

Other examples in this generation are Neosono D, MC, and Ultima EZ (Amadent), Apex Finder (EIE: old version). Today, most resistance-based electronic apex locators are off the market.

Impedance-based (second-generation) apex locators

Impedance-based apex locators, also known as single-frequency impedance apex locators, measure opposition to the flow of alternating current or impedance instead of resistance. Impedance is composed of resistance and capacitance. These devices operate on the principle that there is electrical impedance across the walls of the root canals (due to the presence of the transparent dentin), which is greater apically than coronally. At the level of the cementodentinal junction (CDJ), the level of impedance drops dramatically. Impedance-based locators were introduced to overcome the problems of the first generation. Theoretically, they would be more accurate; however, the impedance and therefore the capacitance of the root canal was dependent on many variables and varied between different root canals, thus requiring individual calibration between each tooth.

This property was used to measure distance in different canal conditions by using different frequencies. The change in frequency method of measuring was developed by Inoue in 1971 and introduced in the Sono-Explorer (Hayashi Dental Supply, Tokyo, Japan), which calibrated at the periodontal pocket of each tooth. This measures two impedances and identifies the canal terminus when the readings approach each other. The frequency of this impedance is directed to a speaker that produces an auditory tone generated by means of low-frequency oscillation. The most important disadvantage of this device was the need for individual calibration. This consisted of an insulated file that was introduced in the gingival crevice, and the sound produced was named the "gingival crevice sound." Then the conventional endodontic file was inserted into the root canal, and when the sound produced by this file became "identical" with the gingival crevice sound, the rubber stop was aligned with the reference point, and the measurement was taken. The Sono-Explorer Mark III, introduced later, used a meter to indicate distance to the apex [46].

To decrease the variable capacitance feature of the circuit, a high-frequency (400 kHz) wave-measuring device, the Endocater (Yamaura Seisokushu, Tokyo, Japan), was introduced by Hasegawa and colleagues (1986). This device consisted of an insulated file. The sheath, however, caused problems because it would not enter narrow canals, could be rubbed off, and was affected by autoclaving. Furthermore, the device gave inaccurate readings when used in canals containing electrolytes [38, 47].

A number of second-generation apex locators were designed and marketed, but all suffered similar problems of incorrect readings with electrolytes in the canals and also in dry canals. Some of them are the Apex Finder and the Endo Analyzer (the combined pulp tester and apex locator) (Analytic/Endo, Orange, CA, USA), which are self-calibrating with a visual indicator but have had variable reports of accuracy. These devices adjust their sensitivity to compensate for the intracanal environment and indicate on the display when the device should be switched from a "wet" to a "dry" mode or vice versa.

The Digipex I, II and III (Mada Equipment Co., Carlstadt, NJ, USA) also combined a pulp vitality tester with an apex locator. Czerw and colleagues (1995) found the Digipex II to be as reliable as the Root ZX in an *in vitro* study [41]. The Exact-A-Pex (Ellmann International, Hewlett, NY, USA) is another example that uses an audio signal and a light-emitting-diode (LED) display [31]. This device always duplicated the canal length as determined by visualizing the tip of a file at the foramen of extracted teeth (Czerw *et al.*, 1994). The *Formatron IV* (Parkell Dental, Farmingdale, NY, USA) is a small, simple device with an LED display [48]. It uses an alternating current and measures impedance to measure the distance of the file tip to the apex; it has also had variable results in terms of accuracy. Himel (1993) found it to be accurate to ± 0.5 mm from the radiographic apex 65% of the time and within 1 mm 83% of the time. Some of the other apex locators in this generation include Dentometer (Dahlin Electromedicine, Copenhagen, Denmark) and Endo Radar (Elettronica Liarre, Imola, Italy).

The major disadvantage of second-generation electronic apex locators is that the root canal has to be reasonably free of electroconductive materials to obtain accurate readings. The presence of tissue and electroconductive irrigants in the canal changes the electrical characteristics and leads to inaccurate, usually shorter measurements [49].

Third-generation electronic apex locators

The major disadvantage encountered with second-generation EALs was the need for a relatively large insulated probe to be used in the canal instead of a small, uninsulated endodontic file. In an effort to improve the accuracy and reliability of root canal length determination under normal clinical conditions, third-generation EALs employed multiple AC frequencies to determine the distance between an endodontic instrument and the end of the canal, unlike second-generation EALs, which only use a single AC of known frequency. Third-generation devices work by monitoring changes in impedance of the tooth at different frequencies: a high one at 8 kHz and a low one at 400 Hz. In the coronal portion of the canal, the impedance difference between the frequencies is constant. As the file is advanced through apical constriction, the difference in the impedance value increases and reaches a maximum value at the apical area [38, 50]. All apex locators are equipped with a display screen or some indicators and a type of alarm that visually and audibly indicate both the proximity and the location of the apical foramen.

Because the magnitude of impedance depends on the measurement of the frequency, the use of two frequencies gives the opportunity of observing the difference between the two results as the needle advances in the root canal. Therefore, this is a *comparative-impedance method* because it measures the impedance difference, which can be converted into length information. Because the impedance of a given circuit may be substantially influenced by the frequency of the current flow, these devices are also known as *frequency-dependent apex locators.* These devices have more powerful microprocessors and are able to process the mathematical quotient and algorithm calculations required to give accurate readings. The accuracy of third-generation EALs tends to be unaffected by the presence of electrolytes in the root canal space. They have also demonstrated functional reliability with no statistically significant difference in measurements between teeth with necrotic or vital pulpal diagnoses [51]. Third-generation EALs enjoy widespread use and acceptance today (Figure 4.3).

Endex (Osada Electric Co., Los Angeles, CA, and Tokyo, Japan) made the original third-generation apex locator. It was first described by Yamaoka and colleagues [52]. In Europe and Asia, it is available as APIT. It uses a low AC but requires calibration for each canal.

The Root ZX (J. Morita, Tokyo, Japan) is an example of a self-calibrating third-generation apex locator based on the ratio method. The ratio method works on the principle that two electric currents with different wave frequencies will have measurable impedances that can be measured and compared as a ratio regardless of the type of electrolyte in the canal. Kobayashi and Suda (1994) showed that the ratio of different frequencies have definitive values and that the ratio rate of change did not change with different electrolytes in the canal [51]. The change in electrical capacitance at the apical constriction is the basis for the mechanism of the Root ZX and its reported accuracy.

Root ZX is based on two electric currents, which have a frequency of either 8 kHz or 400 Hz. Since its introduction in 1992, it has become the benchmark to which other apex locators are compared. It produces more stable readings in the presence of electrolytes and in the presence or absence of blood or other discharges, in contrast to the second-generation EALs, which are more accurate when the root canals are dry. Root ZX

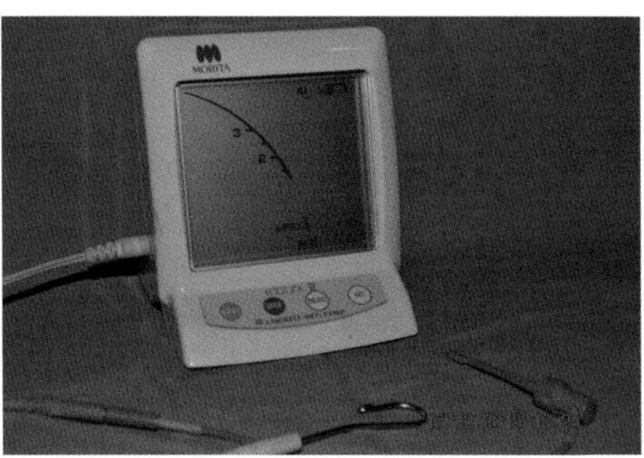

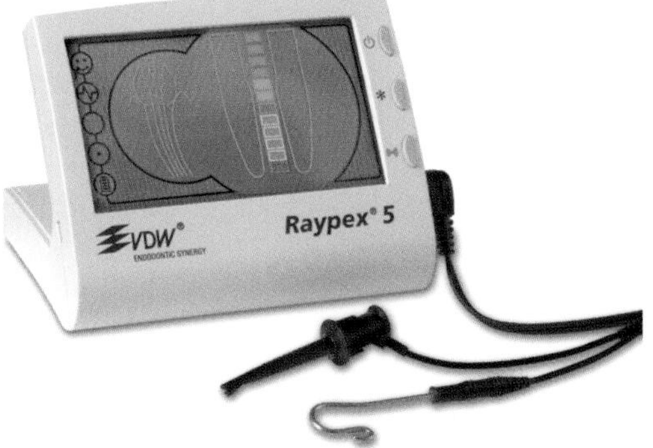

Figure 4.3 *A,* Third-generation apex locator. *B,* Fourth-generation apex locator.

has been researched and studied extensively in the literature. The results give a combined accuracy of 90% to within 0.5 mm of the apical foramen or the CDJ, depending on the reference point used, with many studies reporting 100% accuracy if 1.0 mm is accepted [53].

The Root ZX mainly detects the change in electrical capacitance that occurs near the AC [50]. A microprocessor in the device calculates the ratio of the two impedances. The quotient of the impedances is displayed on a liquid crystal display meter panel and represents the position of the instrument tip in the canal. This device has the advantage of not having to be calibrated for each patient and makes it one of the most efficient and versatile to use.

The Root ZX has been combined with a handpiece to measure canal length when a rotary file is used [54]. This is marked as the Tri Auto ZX (J. Morita Co., Kyoto, Japan) with an integrated hand-piece which uses nickel–titanium (NiTi) rotary instruments that rotate at 240 to 280 rpm [55]. The Tri Auto ZX has a reported accuracy of 95%, similar to that of the Root ZX, and has some additional safety features such as auto-reverse when working length is reached [56–62].

The Dentaport ZX (J. Morita Co., Kyoto, Japan, and J. Morita Mfg. Co., Irvine, CA, USA) is composed of two modules: the Root ZX and the Tri Auto ZX. The handpiece uses NiTi rotary instruments that rotate at 50 to 800 rpm.

Other apex-locating handpieces are the ultrasonic system called SOFY ZX (J. Morita Co., Kyoto, Japan) and the Endy 7000 (Ionyx SA, Blanquefort Cedex, France). The SOFY ZX uses the Root ZX to electronically monitor the location of the file tip during all instrumentation procedures [63]. The device minimizes the danger of over-instrumentation.

The Apex Finder AFA (all fluids allowed) (EIE/Analytic Endodontics, Orange, CA, USA) has five signal frequencies and reads four amplitude ratios (EIE Analytic Endodontics 2002). The unit is self-calibrating and can measure with electrolytes present in the canal. This was only able to detect the apical constriction in 76.6% of necrotic canals, but it was effective for 93.9% of vital canals [64–66]. The principle behind this device, however, is similar to the impedance ratio-based devices. It detects the canal terminus by determining a sudden change in the dominant characteristic (capacitive or resistive) of the impedance.

Neosono Ultima EZ (Satelec Inc., Mount Laurel, NJ, USA)

The Neosono Ultima EZ is known in the Southern Hemisphere as the DatApex (Dentsply Maillefer, Ballaigues, Switzerland). It is the successor to the Sono Explorer line of apex locators and uses a number of frequencies to sample the canal, using the best two for its reading. This unit was found to be 100% accurate in the ±0.5 mm range in an *in vitro* model with dry and wet canals with sodium hypochlorite, and it was the least susceptible to operator influence [67]. The unit is mounted with a root canal graphic showing the file position and has an audible signal. The ability to set the digital readout at 0.5 or 1.0 mm permits measurements of wide open canals as well. This is also available with an attached pulp tester, called the Co-Pilot.

There are several other third generation apex locators in use world-wide. These include the Justwo or Justy II (Yoshida Co., Tokyo, Japan), the Mark V Plus (Moyco/Union Broach, Bethpage, NY, USA), and the Endy 5000 (Loser, Leverkusen, Germany).

Fourth-generation apex locators

Fourth-generation devices measure and compare the complex electrical characteristic features of the root canal at two or more frequencies of electrical impulses [7, 36]. They measure resistance and capacity separately, rather than the resultant impedance (Figure 4.3). There can be different combinations of values of capacitance and resistance that determine the same impedance (and thus the same apical constriction reading). Separate measurements of primary components permit better accuracy. In addition, the device named *Elements* uses a lookup matrix rather than making any internal calculations.

It is important to note that although the fourth-generation devices use different frequencies, only one frequency is used at a time (unlike third-generation EALs, which use both simultaneously). The manufacturers claim that by doing this and by then calculating the standard deviation of the differences between the two frequencies, they increase the accuracy of the device [7]. This also eliminates the need for a filter (source for the noise).

The fourth-generation apex locators are marketed by Sybron Endo and include the Apex Locator and the Elements Diagnostic Unit. Both are ratio-type apex locators that determine the impedance at five frequencies, and both have built-in electronic pulp testers. The Ray-Pex 4 and 5 (Forum Engineering Technologies, Rishon Lezion, Israel) are also examples of this generation.

Elements Diagnostic Unit and Apex Locator do not process the impedance information as a mathematical algorithm, but instead they take the resistance and capacitance measurements and compare them with a database to determine the distance to the apex [7]. Introduced in 2003, these use a composite waveform of two signals, 0.5 and 4 kHz, compared with the Root ZX at 8 and 0.4 kHz. The signals go through a digital-to-analog converter to be converted into an analog signal, which is then amplified and passed to the patient circuit model, which is assumed to be a resistor and capacitor in parallel. The feedback signal waveforms are then fed into a noise-reduction circuit. This reduces error and produces consistently more accurate-readings [7]. A significant disadvantage of this generation is that they need to perform in relatively dry or in partially dried canals [49].

When using the Elements Diagnostic Unit, the clinician should withdraw the file to the 0.5-mm mark instead of the 0.0-mm mark to achieve the accurate identification of the apical constriction that they assumed should be 0.5 mm short of the external (major) foramen. Therefore, taking the file to the 0.0 mark on the display and then withdrawing it 0.5 mm appears to be the most accurate way to use this device. (Figure 4.4)

Fifth-generation electronic apex locators

Fifth-generation EALs were developed in 2003 and measure the capacitance and resistance of the circuit separately. Hence they are also known as dual-frequency ratio type apex locators (Figure 4.5). The device is supplied by a diagnostic table that includes the statistics of the values at different positions to identify the position of the file. Devices employing this method experience considerable difficulties while operating in dry canals; therefore, additional insertion of irrigants or lubricants are required [68]. During clinical work it was noticed that the accuracy of electronic root canal length measurement varies with the pulp and periapical condition [69]. Thus, pulp condition and periapical diseases should be considered to evaluate the accuracy of apex locators. Some examples in this generation are E-Magic Finder Apex Locator, I-Root EMF 100 Deluxe (Meta Biomed, Chongju, South Korea), and Joypex 5 (Denjoy, Changsha City, China).

Sixth-generation electronic apex locators

So far, five generations of instruments have been created that constantly evolve and are being improved. Currently, fourth- and fifth-generation devices are

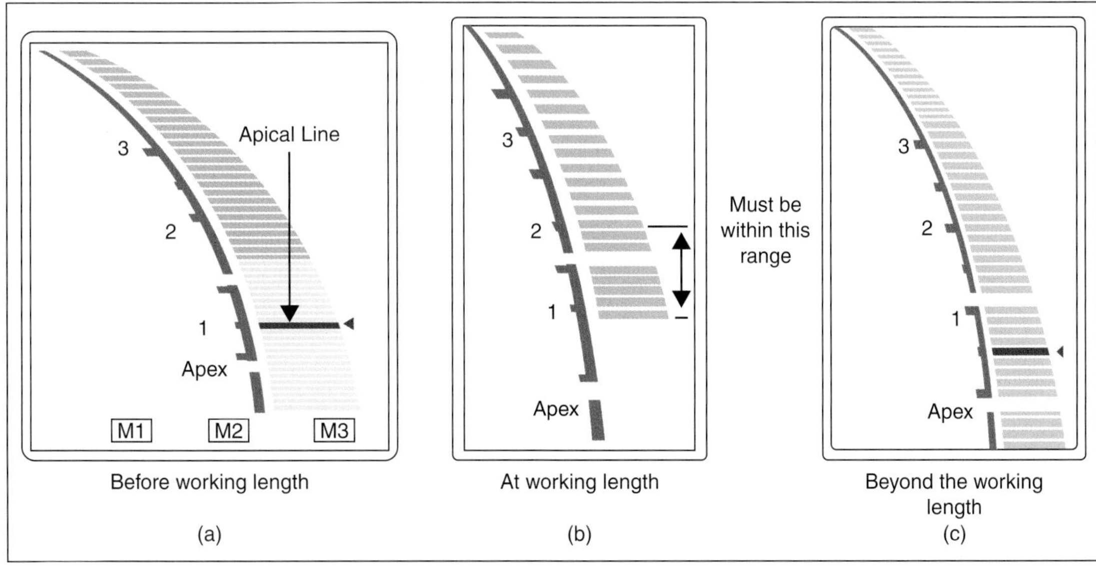

Figure 4.4 Clinical use of an apex locator.

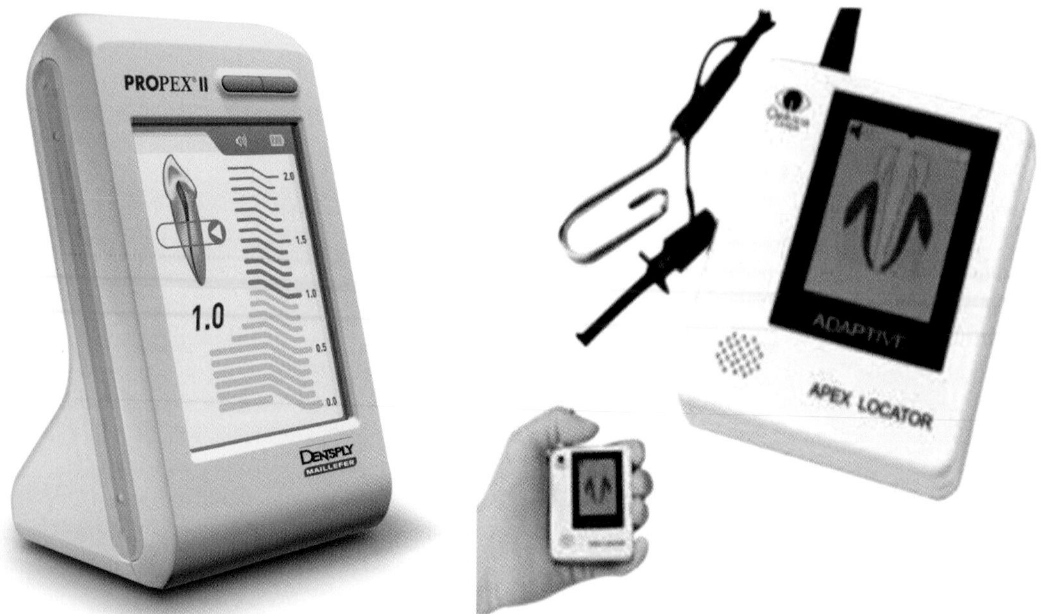

Figure 4.5 *A*, Fifth-generation apex locator. *B*, Sixth-generator apex locator.

mostly employed. This combines Prof. Sunada's method for "dry" canal measurement and a method of Prof. Kobayashi's for "wet" root canal measurement. The adaptive apex locator overcomes the disadvantages of the fourth-generation popular apex locator's low accuracy in working in wet canals, as well the disadvantages of fifth generation's difficulty in working in dry canals and necessity of compulsory additional wetting. The purpose is to adapt to the manner of measuring in accordance with the actual characteristic features of the environment to measure [69].

The adaptive apex locator continuously defines humidity of the canal and immediately adapts to dry or wet canal. This way it can be used in dry and in wetted canals, in canals with blood or exudates, and in canals in which the pulp has not yet been extirpated. Measurement with the adaptive apex locator has made it possible to eliminate the necessity of drying or moistening the canal, as well as to achieve a high degree of measurement precision in the presence of blood, liquid, or sodium hypochlorite or while manipulating dry canals

Due to modern technology, the sixth-generation adaptive apex locator is a pleasant, small device no larger than a dentist's palm. The device is the first "talking" apex locator. Depending on the constantly measured moistness, and entirely on its own, the device adapts the measuring method for either a dry or a wet canal.

Other uses of apex locators

All modern apex locators are able to detect root perforations to clinically acceptable limits and are equally able to distinguish between large and small perforations [70]. Suspected periodontal or pulpal perforation during pinhole preparation can be confirmed by all apex locators, because a patent perforation will cause the instrument to complete a circuit and indicate the instrument is beyond the apex [11]. Furcation perforations may be detected if "Apex" is registered immediately upon file insertion into a would-be canal. Strip perforations can be detected and their position measured when "Apex" is reached well short of the estimated working length. Apical perforations may be detected when a sudden change in working length is noted when reverifying working length. Once an apical perforation occurs, the "Apex" may register at a location that was previously short of the initial greater foramen "Apex" reading. Another use for an EAL is post perforation detection [71].

Any connection between the root canal and the periodontal membrane such as root fracture, cracks, and internal or external resorption will be recognized by the apex locator [72]. They can be used to detect horizontal fractures, and some are also helpful in root canals of teeth with incomplete root formation, requiring apexification [73].

EALs can be used safely in pacemaker patients because most modern pacemakers are shielded to block outside electromagnetic interference, and direct wiring of the apex locator to the pacemaker does not occur clinically [74, 75]. However, manufacturers still warn against using an EAL in cardiac pacemaker patients because electrical stimulation to such patients could interfere with the pacemaker's function [71]. An appropriate consult with the patient's cardiologist is *mandatory*.

Multiple-function apex locators are becoming more common, and several have vitality testing functions. Combination electronic apex locators and electric handpieces are also becoming common (described earlier in the chapter) and are able to achieve excellent results with the same accuracy as the stand-alone units [75–80].

Variables affecting the accuracy of apex locators

New generations of EALs could be confidently used for working length measurement in the presence of tissue fluids or different electrolytes. Intact vital tissue, inflammatory exudate, or blood can conduct electric current and can cause inaccurate readings; hence, their presence should be minimized during the use of these devices [63]. Other conductors that can cause inaccurate readings are metallic restorations, caries, saliva, and instruments in a second canal. Care must be taken if any of these variables exist. Type of alloy used for endodontic files does not seem to affect accuracy, with the same measurements being obtained in the same root canal using stainless steel and nickel–titanium instruments [81].

Lack of patency, the accumulation of dentin debris, and calcifications can affect accuracy of working length determination with electronic apex locators [39, 71]. Preflaring does not seem to affect the accuracy of these devices. Even in mechanically enlarged canals, small or large files gave the same electronic reading [61]. Canal patency is more important, because dentin debris may disrupt the electrical resistance between the inside of the canal and the periodontal ligament. Constant recapitulation and irrigation ensures accurate electronic length readings during instrumentation [82].

The size of the apical foramen also has an influence on electronic length determination. As the width of the major foramen increases, the distance between file tip and foramen also increases, and thus the size of the root canal diameter should be estimated first and then a snug-fitting file should be chosen for determining the root canal length because small files can affect the reliability of the measurements [83].

In a study with Root ZX, in teeth with large canals, it was not necessary to match the canal diameter with a corresponding file. A small file is just as likely to find the apical constriction as a large file in wide-diameter canals. In that same study, the apex locator identified the apically constricted area of the canal even in the absence of an anatomic apical constriction [71]. In canals with simulated apical root resorption, it was concluded that the Root ZX can be used to accurately determine the working length as "Apex," even in the absence of an apical constriction [84].

Immature or "blunderbuss" apices tend to give short measurements electronically due to the instruments not touching the apical dentine walls [73]. Other methods for determining length should be considered. The apical extent of the root canal system of primary teeth is difficult to determine. Adjunctive methods should supplement the use of EALs.

Recommended working length technique: combination of EAL and radiographic method

Accurate determination of the working length is a crucial part of successful root canal treatment. In addition to radiographic measurements, electronic working length determination has become increasingly important. The electronic method reduces many of the problems associated with radiographic measurements. Its most important advantage over radiography is that it can measure the length of the root canal to the apical foramen, not to the radiographic apex [43].

Guidelines recommend a combination of electronic and radiographic methods for determining working length [85]. This is in line with several studies that have recommended that an EAL reading should be radiographically confirmed to reduce the chances of erroneous working length determination.[72, 73, 82, 83, 86] This recommendation is further supported by the complexity and variability of the apical part of the root canal, which makes it obligatory to use multiple techniques in the same canal to determine working length. The higher accuracy of the combined method is nearly 96%.

"Digital radiography uses sensors to produce electronic radiographic images that can be viewed on a monitor and that allow for a reduction in radiation exposure; sensors can be integrated with intraoral digital cameras and patient management database software" (American Association of Endodontists, 2003). As a result, to reduce the radiation dose, the use of digital radiographs instead of conventional radiographs in combination with EALs is advised for determining the working length [77]. EALs are not meant to replace radiographs but to add to the information provided by them.

Conflicts in the length measurements given by the two techniques have also been reported. If the radiographic image of the indicated EAL length appeared to be well short of the radiographic apex, the EAL reading should be chosen because this should be closer to the vicinity of the AC. This is recommended but is not mandatory. If the radiographic length is short by more than 3 mm of the desired position, the length should be adjusted and confirmed by another radiograph. It might also be helpful to use tactile sensation in such situations.

Another advantage of the combined method is the reduction in the number of radiographs needed for determining the working length, meaning clinical time and radiation hazards are reduced, specially while treating maxillary molars. EALs cannot help the clinician determine canal width, canal curvature, or the number of canals. However, EALs offer the advantage of measuring the canal to the level of its terminus instead of its radiographic apex. Meanwhile, the radiographic method has the advantages of being able to inspect root anatomy and document it in patient records. The canal lengths measured on cone-beam computed tomography (CBCT) images were highly correlated with electronic lengths. More studies are required before implementing CBCT as a method for determining working length.

Clinical troubleshooting of apex locators

The first thing to check if your EAL is not functioning are the batteries and/or power source, because some units do not operate effectively when the charge falls below 50%. As with any electronic device, short circuits will render the unit inoperative. Presence of any dentinal shelves or considerable debris in the canals will give an erratic or a premature reading. Often in roots with severe curvatures, the length is shortened slightly during routine shaping, and thus confirming the length at this stage will enhance the accuracy of the readings.

The current generation of EALs requires the measuring electrode (usually a K-file) to not touch any metallic restorations or be in contact with electrolyte solutions in the coronal pulp chamber. Often, solutions in the pulp chamber can cause a short circuit. This is especially important in multirooted teeth, because the canals must be isolated from one another. If isolation from a metallic restoration is a problem, you can paint the upper part of the K-file with nail varnish, thus providing an insulating barrier. Another alternative is to fill the access cavity with a nonconducting gel.

To check for perforations, place the tip of the K-file into the catch. If you get a reading that the apex has been reached, there is a possibility of a perforation. This can be confirmed with radiographs. At the mid-root level, a similar reading might indicate a horizontal root fracture or even a large lateral canal.

To confirm whether the apical constriction has been reached, audible signals generated by the EAL are very helpful, because it is often difficult to ensure that the file is not touching metallic restorations and at the same time observe the graphical display on the unit. The file is slowly advanced until the audible signal changes to a higher frequency, which then changes to a continuous signal on advancing the file further. This can be taken as the file position beyond the apex. The file can be slowly withdrawn until the sound returns to a low pitch.

It is important to calibrate your EAL because each unit is unique, and even EALs from the same manufacturer can give slightly different readings. When working on an upper tooth whose roots are very close to the maxillary sinus, caution needs to be exercised because the file can penetrate into the sinus and thus give an inaccurate reading. Therefore, it is advisable to confirm the length electronically at least twice. A radiograph should be taken if you are repeatedly getting variable length. Figure 4.6 summarizes the troubleshooting of apex locators.

Determining working length in teeth with open apices

The term *open apex* is often used to describe an exceptionally wide apical foramen, in which preparation of an apical "stop" is difficult, if not impossible, to achieve.

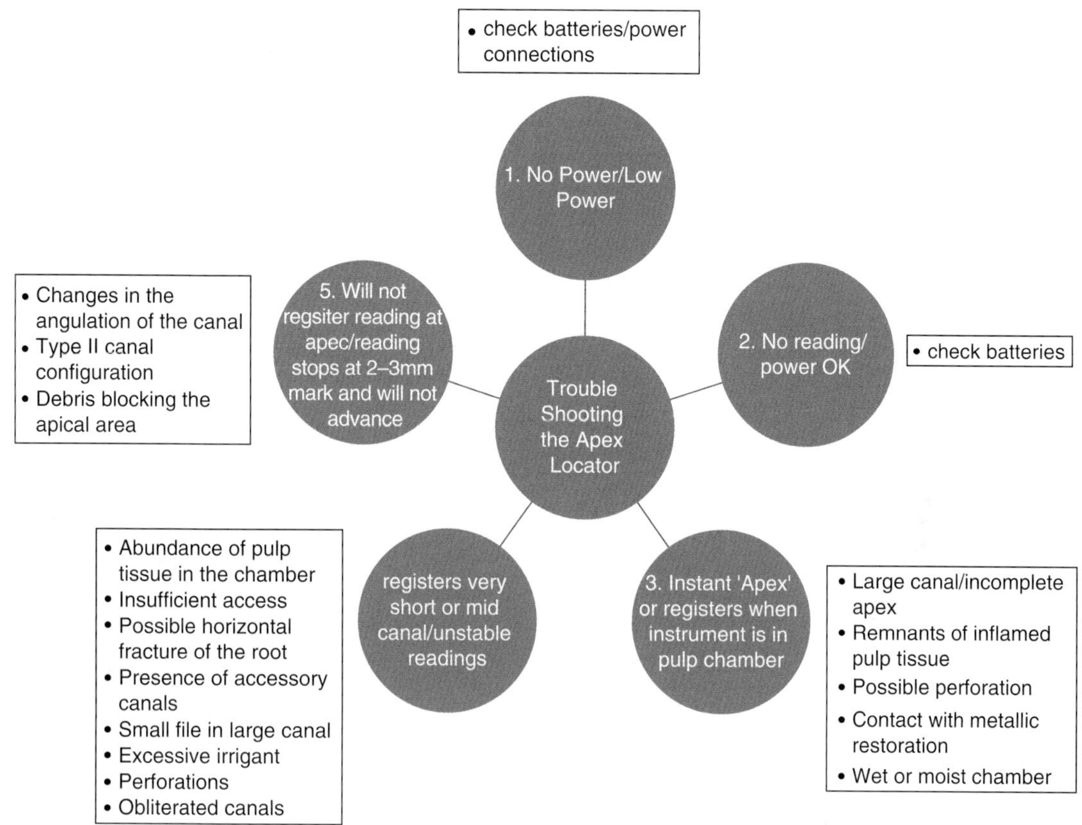

Figure 4.6 Troubleshooting the apex locator.

This may be due to trauma, extensive apical resorption, root end resection, or over-instrumentation. In such teeth, the radiographic interpretation of canal length is even more difficult due to the altered apical anatomy and the missing periodontal ligament space at the apex [87, 88]. Apex locators are of little use in such situations, because the wide root canals associated with open apices adversely influence the function of apex locators [58, 84, 89, 90].

The apical constriction is considered to be the narrowest region of the apical portion of the root canal system. However, it is not always present in cases of root resorption associated with pulp and periapical pathosis or in teeth with open apices. The European Society of Endodontology recommends using an EAL followed by confirming the canal length with an undistorted radiograph during root canal treatment.

As mentioned earlier, if the instrument in the canal appears to be more than 3 mm from the radiographic apex, the working length needs to be adjusted. The paper point technique using the tactile method may be used in such cases (Figure 4.7). It was found to be comparable to radiography and unaffected by the size of the apex or the presence of periapical pathology. The technique involved using a size 30 paper point placed in the canal and advanced until resistance was felt. A shortcoming of the technique is that if periapical soft tissues extend into the canal, the method can underestimate the working length. This technique requires the canal to be completely dry and the periapical tissues to be relatively moist. In open apices, the control of moisture is difficult because the contact area to the inflamed periapical tissues is large, and excess moisture is common, which can result in measurement errors.

Additionally, there is the potential for overfill when the level of the apical terminus, affected by pathological resorption, is uneven. To overcome this problem, Williams and colleagues proposed a tactile method

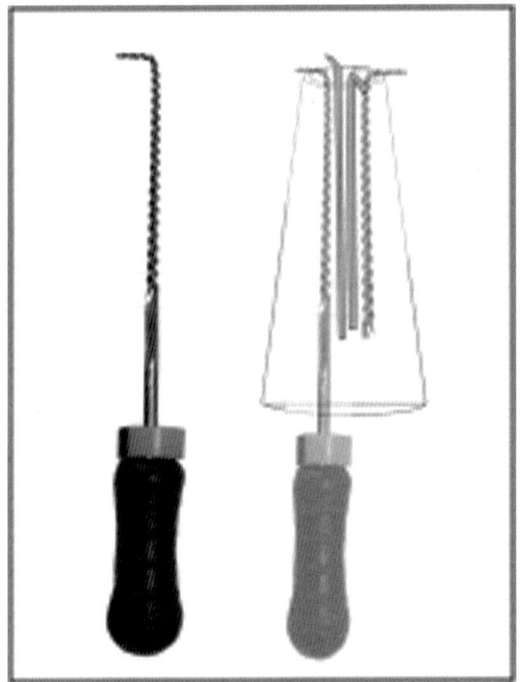

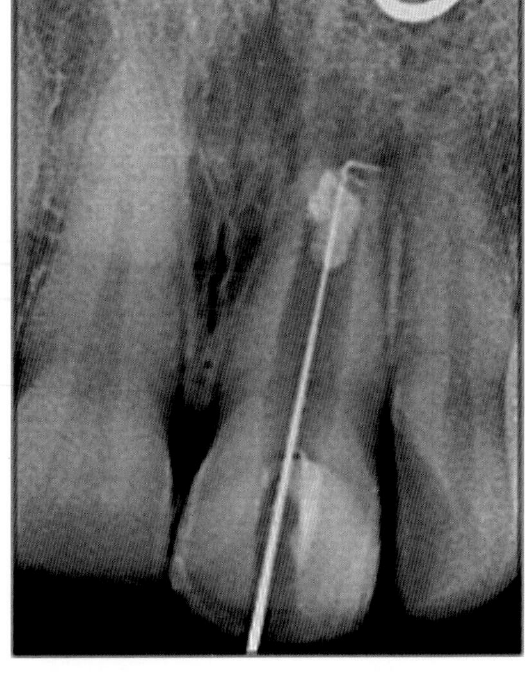

Figure 4.7 Determining working length in an open apex [91].

involving the use of a size 25 K-file bent at the tip, with its orientation marked with a silicone ring [87]. The file was bent to facilitate ease of use. This method may be restricted to relatively straight canal curvatures. Clinical trials are needed to further assess this method, especially in curved canals.

More research is necessary on how best to image the very fine detail of root apices. Clinically, owing to their limitations, the use of EALs and radiographs should be supplemented with other methods, especially when treating very wide apical terminations.

Short note on reference points

A reference point that will not change between the treatments should be selected. Whereas one point of measurement of a working length refers to the end of the preparation, another point may vary considerably. In anterior teeth, this point is usually the incisal edge, but in broken-down teeth, length may be measured either from the adjacent teeth or from the projecting portion of the remaining structure. In posterior teeth, buccal canals are measured to the buccal cusp tip, and the palatal canal may use either cusp tip as a reference. In addition to recording the working length of the canal, the reference point from which it is measured should be similarly recorded.

Stop attachments should be placed on the instruments perpendicular to the long axis of the instrument. Care should be taken that they are not pushed up the shaft during use because this can give an inaccurate or elongated working length, thus leading to apical perforation and problems thereafter.

Conclusion

Technological evolution is the hallmark of all scientific and clinical effort. No individual technique is truly satisfactory in determining the working length. Electronic devices find their usefulness when root canals are covered by anatomical structures or there are pathological processes on the tooth. The use of electronic devices can reduce radiographic exposure for the patient, because the operator may need fewer radiographs to correctly determine the working length. Modern apex locators can determine the position of the

CDJ with 90% accuracy but still have limitations. It is important to note that an electronic device is not an absolute substitute for radiographs and should be used as an adjunct. Knowledge of the apical anatomy, use of radiographs, and the proper use of apex locators will help the clinician in achieving good results.

References

1 Coolidge ED. Past and present concepts in endodontics. *J Am Dent Assoc* 1960; 16: 676–688.

2 Ingle Jl, Taintor JF. Endodontics. 3rd ed. Philadelphia: Lea & Febiger; 1985. pp. 184–195.

3 Blayney JR. Some factors in root canal treatment. *J Am Dent Assoc* 1924; 11: 840–850.

4 American Association of Endodontists. *Glossary of endodontic terms*, 7th edition. Chicago: American Association of Endodontists, 2003.

5 Kuttler Y. Microscopic investigation of root apexes. *J Am Dent Assoc* 1955; 50: 544–552.

6 Gutierrez J H, Aguayo P. Apical foraminal openings in human teeth. Number and location. *Oral Surg Oral Med Oral Pathol Oral Radiol Endod* 1995; 79: 769–777.

7 Gordon MPJ, Chandler NP. Electronic apex locators. *Int Endod J* 2004; 37: 425–437.

8 Malueg L, Wilcox L, Johnson W. Examination of external apical root resorption with scanning electron microscopy. *Oral Surg Oral Med Oral Pathol Oral Radiol Endod* 1996; 82: 89–93.

9 Cox VS Brown CE Jr., Bricker SL, Newton CW. Radiographic interpretation of endodontic file length. *Oral Surg Oral Med Oral Pathol* 1991; 72: 340–344.

10 Rosenberg DB. The paper point technique, Part 1. *Dent Today* 2003; 22: 80–86.

11 Ingle J, Himel T, Hawrish C Glickman GN, Serene T, Rosenberg PA, *et al.* Endodontic cavity preparation. In: Ingle J, Bakland L, eds. *Endodontics*. Hamilton, Ontario: BC Decker; 2002. pp. 517–525.

12 Grossman LI. *Endodontic practice*, 11th edn. Philadelphia: Lea & Febiger, 1988.

13 Cohen S, Burns RC. *Pathways of the pulp*. 4th ed. St Louis: CV Mosby; 1987. pp. 164–169.

14 Pineda F, Kuttler Y. Mesiodistal and buccolingual roentgenographic investigation of 7,275 root canals. *Oral Surg Oral Med Oral Pathol* 1972; 33, 101–110.

15 Radel RT, Goodell GG, McClanahan SB, Cohen ME. *In vitro* radiographic determination of distances from working length files to root ends comparing Kodak RVG 6000, Schick CDR, and Kodak Insight Film. *J Endod* 2006; 32: 566–8.

16 Weine FS. *Endodontic therapy*. 2nd ed. St Louis: CV Mosby; 1976. pp. 206–214.

17 Stavropoulos A, Wenzel A. Accuracy of cone beam dental CT, intraoral digital and conventional film radiography for the detection of periapical lesions. An *ex vivo* study in pig jaws. *Clin Oral Investig* 2007; 11: 101–106.

18 Mello-Moura ACV, Moura-Netto C, Araki AT, Guedes-Pinto AC, Mendes FM. *Ex vivo* performance of five methods for root canal length determination in primary anterior teeth. *Int Endod J* 2010; 43(2): 142–147.

19 Griffiths BM, Brown JE, Hyatt AT, Linney AD. Comparison of three imaging techniques for assessing endodontic working length. *Int Endod J* 1992; 25(60: 279–287.

20 Parks ET, Williamson GF. Digital radiography: an overview. *J Contemp Dent Pract* 2002; 3: 36–40.

21 Loushine RJ, Weller RN, Kimbrough WF, Potter BJ. Measurement of endodontic file lengths: calibrated versus uncalibrated digital images. *J Endod* 2001; 27(12): 779–781.

22 Lim KF, Loh EE-M, Hong YH, Intra-oral computed radiography—an *in vitro* evaluation. *J Dent* 1996; 24(5): 359–364.

23 Gluskin AH. Anatomy of an overfill: a reflection on the process. *Endod Top* 2009; 16: 64–81.

24 Ellingsen MA, Harrington GW, Hollender LG. Radiovisiography versus conventional radiography for detection of small instruments in endodontic length determination. Part 1: *In vitro* evaluation. *J Endod* 1995; 21: 326–331.

25 Ellingsen MA, Hollender LG, Harrington GW. Radiovisiography versus conventional radiography for detection of small instruments in endodontic length determination II. *In vivo* evaluation. *J Endod* 1995; 21: 516–520.

26 Leddy BJ, Miles DA, Newton CW, Brown CE Jr., Interpretation of endodontic file lengths using RadioVisioGraphy. *J Endod* 1994; 20: 542–545.

27 Friedlander LT, Love RM, Chandler NP. A comparison of phosphor-plate digital images with conventional radiographs for the perceived clarity of fine endodontic files and periapical lesions. *Oral Surg Oral Med Oral Pathol Oral Radiol Endod* 2002; 93: 321–327.

28 Fuge KN, Stuck AM, Love RM. A comparison of digitally scanned radiographs with conventional film for the detection of small endodontic instruments. *Int Endod J* 1998; 31: 123–126.

29 Mouyen F, Benz C, Sonnabend E, Lodter JP. Presentation and physical evaluation of RadioVisioGraphy. *Oral Surg Oral Med Oral Pathol* 1989; 68: 238–242.

30 Hedrick RT, Brent Dove S, Peters DD, McDavid WD. Radiographic determination of canal length: direct digital radiography versus conventional radiography. *J Endod* 1994; 20: 320–326.

31 Nair MK, Nair UP. Digital and advanced imaging in endodontics: a review. *J Endod* 2007; 33: 1–6.

32 Farrier SL, Drage NA, Newcombe RG, Hayes SJ, Dummer PM. A comparative study of image quality and radiation exposure for dental radiographs produced using a charge-coupled device and a phosphor plate system. *Int Endod J* 2009; 42: 900–907.

33 Peters OA, Laib A, Rüegsegger P, Barbakow F. Three-dimensional analysis of root canal geometry by high-resolution computed tomography. *J Dent Res* 2000; 79: 1405–1409.

34 Gluskin AH, Brown DC, Buchanan LS. A reconstructed computerized tomography comparison of Ni-Ti rotary GT files versus traditional instruments in canals shaped by novice operators. *Int Endod J* 2001; 34: 476–484.

35 Cluster C. Exact methods for locating the apical foramen. *J Nat Dent Assoc* 1918; 5: 815–819.

36 Sunada I. New method for measuring the length of the root canal. *J Dent Res* 1962; 41: 375–387.

37 American Association of Endodontists. *Glossary: Contemporary Terminology for Endodontics.* 6th ed. Chicago: American Association of Endodontists; 1998.

38 Fouad AF, Krell KV, McKendry DJ, Koorbusch GF, Olson RA. A clinical evaluation of five electronic root canal length measuring instruments. *J Endod* 1990; 16: 446–449.

39 Nahmias Y, Aurelio JA, Gerstein H. Expanded use of the electronic canal length measuring devices. *J Endod* 1983; 9: 347–349.

40 Donnelly JC. A simplified model to demonstrate the operation of electronic root canal measuring devices. *J Endod* 1993; 19: 579–580.

41 Czerw RJ, Fulkerson MS, Donnelly JC. An *in vitro* test of simplified model to demonstrate the operation of electronic root canal measuring devices. *J Endod* 1994; 20: 605–606.

42 Czerw RJ, Fulkerson MS, Donnelly JC, Walmann JO. *In vitro* evaluation of the accuracy of several electronic apex locators. *J Endod* 1995; 21: 572–575.

43 Neekofar MH, Ghandi MM, Hayes SJ, Dummer PMH. The fundamental operating principles electronic root canal measuring devices. *Int Endod J* 2006; 39: 595–609.

44 Kobayashi C. Electronic canal length measurement. *Oral Surg Oral Med Oral Pathol Oral Radiol Endod* 1995; 79: 226–231.

45 Tidmarsh BG, Sherson W, Stalker NL. Establishing endodontic working length: a comparison of radiographic and electronic methods. *NZ Dent J* 1985; 81: 93–96.

46 Kim E, Lee SJ. Electronic apex locator. *Dent Clin North Am* 2004; 48: 35–54.

47 Lauper R, Lutz F, Barbakow F. An *in vivo* comparison of gradient and absolute impedance electronic apex locators. *J Endod* 1996; 22: 260–263.

48 Pallares A, Faus V. An *in vivo* comparative study of two apex locators. *J Endod* 1994; 20: 576–579.

49 Himel VT, Cain C. An evaluation of two electronic apex locators in a dental student clinic. *Quint Int* 1983; 24: 803–809.

50 Fouad AF, Krell KV. An *in vitro* comparison of five root canal length measuring instruments. *J Endod* 1989; 15: 573–577.

51 Stare Z, Šutalo J, Galić N. The "Effect of Apical Foramen and Electrode Diameter on the Accuracy of Electronic Root Canal Measuring Devices." *Proceedings of the 8th International IMEKO Conference on Measurement in Clinical Medicine,* September 16–19, 1998, Dubrovnik, Croatia, 5-33, 5-36.

52 Yamaoka M, Yamashita Y, Saito T. Electric root canal measuring instrument based on a new principle. Thesis. Tokyo: Nihon Univ. School of Dentistry; 1989.

53 Kobayashi C, Suda H. New electronic canal measuring device based on the ratio method. *J Endod* 1994; 20: 111–114.

54 Pagavino G, Pace R, Baccetti T. A SEM study of *in vivo* accuracy of the Root ZX electronic apex locator. *J Endod* 1998; 24: 438–441.

55 Kobayashi C, Yoshioka T, Suda H. A new engine-driven canal preparation system with electronic canal measuring capability. *J Endod* 1997; 23: 751–754.

56 Kobayashi C, Yoshioka T, Suda H. A new ultrasonic canal preparation system with electronic monitoring of file tip position. *J Endod* 1996; 22: 489–492.

57 Meares WA, Steiman HR. The influence of sodium hypochlorite irrigation on the accuracy of the Root ZX electronic apex locator. *J Endod* 2002; 28: 595–598.

58 Ebrahim AK, Yoshioka T, Kobayashi C, Suda H. The effects of file size, sodium hypochlorite and blood on the accuracy of Root ZX apex locator in enlarged root canals: an *in vitro* study. *Aust Dent J* 2006; 51: 153–157.

59 Ebrahim AK, Wadachi R, Suda H. *Ex vivo* evaluation of the ability of four different electronic apex locators to determine the working length in teeth with various foramen diameters. *Aust Dent J* 2006; 51: 258–262.

60 Ebrahim AK, Wadachi R, Suda H. Accuracy of three different electronic apex locators in detecting simulated horizontal and vertical root fractures. *Aust Endod J* 2006; 32: 64–69.

61 Katz A, Mass E, Kaufman AY. Electronic apex locator: a useful tool for root canal treatment in the primary dentition. *ASDC J Dent Child* 1996; 63: 414–417.

62 Nguyen HQ, Kaufman AY, Komorowski RC, Friedman S. Electronic length measurement using small and large files in enlarged canals. *Int Endod J* 1996; 29: 359–364.

63 Trope M, Rabie G, Tronstad L. Accuracy of an electronic apex locator under controlled clinical conditions. *Endod Dent Traumatol* 1985; 1: 142–145.

64 Vajrabhaya L, Tepmongkol P. Accuracy of apex locator. *Endod Dent Traumatol* 1997; 13: 180–182.

65 Haffner C, Folwaczny M, Galler K, Hickel R. Accuracy of electronic apex locators in comparison to actual length —an *in vivo* study. *J Dent* 2005; 33: 619–625.

66 Pommer O, Stamm O, Attin T. Influence of the canal contents on the electrical associated determination of the length of the root canals. *J Endod* 2002; 79: 769–777.

67 Lucena-Martín C, Robles-Gijón V, Ferrer-Luque CM, de Mondelo JM. *In vitro* evaluation of the accuracy of three electronic apex locators. *J Endod* 2004; 30: 231–233.

68 Kovacevic M, Tamarut T. Influence of the concentration of ions and foramen diameter on the accuracy of electronic

root canal length measurement: an experimental study. *J Endod* 1998; 24: 346–351.

69 Dimitrov S, Roshkev D. Sixth generation adaptive apex locator. Journal of IMAB (annual proceedings scientific papers 2009, book 2)

70 Fuss Z, Assooline LS, Kaufman AY. Determination of location of root perforations by electronic apex locators. *Oral Surg Oral Med Oral Pathol Oral Rad Endod* 1996; 82: 324–329.

71 J. Morita Manufacturing Corporation. Root ZX Operation Instructions. 1998, Kyoto, Japan: J. Morita Manufacturing Corporation. 1–13.

72 Chong BS, Pitt Ford TR. Apex locators in endodontics: which, when and how? *Dent Update* 1994; 21: 328–330.

73 Hulsmann M, Pieper K. Use of electronic apex locators in the treatment of teeth with incomplete root formation. *Endod Dent Traumatol* 1989; 5: 238.

74 Garofalo RR, Ede EN, Dorn SO, Kuttler S. Effect of electronic apex locators on cardiac pacemaker function. *J Endod* 2002 Dec; 28(12): 831–833.

75 Woolley LH, Woodworth J, Dobbs JL. A preliminary evaluation of the effects of electrical pulp testers on dogs with artificial pacemakers. *J Am Dent Assoc (1939)*, 1974; 89: 1099–1101.

76 Steffen H, Splieth CH, Behr K. Comparison of measurements obtained with hand files or the Canal Leader attached to electronic apex locators: an *in vitro* study. *Int Endod J* 1999; 32: 103–107.

77 Saad AY, al-Nazhan S. Radiation dose reduction during endodontic therapy: a new technique combining an apex locator (Root ZX) and a digital imaging system (RadioVisioGraphy). *J Endod* 2000; 26: 144–147.

78 Green D. A stereomicroscopic study of the root apices of 400 maxillary and mandibular anterior teeth. *Oral Surg Oral Med Oral Pathol* 1956; 9: 1224–1232.

79 Green D. Stereomicroscopic study of 700 root apices of maxillary and mandibular posterior teeth. *Oral Surg Oral Med Oral Pathol* 1960; 13: 728–733.

80 Cash PW. Letter: Endo research challenged. *J Am Dent Assoc (1939)*, 1975; 91: 1135–1136.

81 Thomas AS, Hartwell GR, Moon PC. The accuracy of the Root ZX electronic apex locator using stainless-steel and nickel–titanium files. *J Endod* 2003; 29: 662–663.

82 Rivera EM, Seraji MK. Placement accuracy of electrically conductive gutta-percha. *J Endod* 1994; 20: 342–344.

83 Stein TJ, Corcoran JF. Anatomy of the root apex and its histologic changes with age. *Oral Surg Oral Med Oral Pathol* 1990; 69, 238–242.

84 Goldberg F, De Silvio AC, Manfre S, Nastri N. *In vitro* measurement accuracy of an electronic apex locator in teeth with simulated apical root resorption. *J Endod* 2002 Jun; 28(6): 461–463.

85 Kaufman AY. The Sono-Explorer as an auxillary device in endodontics. *Isr J Dent Med* 1976; 25: 27–31.

86 Kielbassa AM, Muller U, Munz I, Monting JS. Clinical evaluation of the measuring accuracy of Root ZX in primary teeth. *Oral Surg Oral Med Oral Pathol Oral Radiol Endod* 2003; 95: 94–100.

87 ElAyouti A, Weiger R, Lost C. Frequency of overinstrumentation with an acceptable radiographic working length. *J Endod* 2001; 27(1): 49–52.

88 Williams CB, Joyce AP, Roberts S. A comparison between *in vivo* radiographic working length determination and measurement after extraction. *J Endod* 2006; 32(7): 624–627.

89 Herrera M, Abalos C, Planas AJ, Llamas R. Influence of apical constriction diameter on root ZX apex locator precision. *J Endod* 2007; 33(8): 995–998.

90 Tosun G, Erdemir A, Eldeniz AU, Sermet U, Sener Y. Accuracy of two electronic apex locators in primary teeth with and without apical resorption: a laboratory study. *Int Endod J* 2008; 41(5): 436–441.

91 Kaurani M, Kaurani P, Kaur Samra R, Kaur G. Tactile method for estimation of working length in open apex: a case report. *Indian J Dent Sci* 2013; 4(5): 116–119.

Questions

1 How far short of the anatomical apex would one normally prepare the root canal?
A 0 mm
B 0.5 mm
C 1 mm
D 1.5 mm
E 2 mm
F 2 mm

2 A working-length radiograph has a file inserted 17 mm. It is 2.5 mm short of the anatomical apex. What is the true working length?
A 17 mm
B 18.5 mm
C 19 mm
D 19.5 mm

3 An electronic apex locator may be useful when
A The patient is physically impaired
B Anatomic structures overlay the root apex
C A pregnant patient wishes to avoid x-ray exposure
D All of the above

4 The working length of a tooth refers to
A The total length of a tooth from crown tip to root tip
B The measured length of a radiograph of the tooth
C The distance between a reference point on the crown and the apical limit of the tooth
D None of the above

5 The most unreliable technique for determining working length is
A The patient's response
B An apex locator

C Radiography
D Tactile feedback

6 Which of these is the usual reference point for a molar?
A Level of access cavity
B A cusp tip
C A rubber stop
D A graduated seeker file

7 Which of these would *not* sometimes give a false reading on an electronic apex locator?
A Lateral canal
B Root fracture
C Contact with metal restoration
D Fluid in canal
E Pulp stone

CHAPTER 5
Root canal filling

Priyanka Jain[1], Mahantesh Yeli[2], and Kakul Dhingra[3]
[1] *Dubai, UAE*
[2] *SDM College of Dental Sciences and Hospital, Dharwad, India*
[3] *Colaba, Mumbai, India*

Obturation of the radicular space is one of the areas in endodontics that receives the most attention. Obturation of the root canal space has been described in various ways for well over 100 years. It has been over four decades since the late Dr. Herbert Schilder published his article on filling the root canal space in three dimensions, making it one of the pillars of successful endodontic treatment.

In 1967, Grossman described his classic principle of hermetic seal of the canal. Since then, the ultimate goal of endodontic obturation has remained the same: a true hermetic seal. The word *hermetic* means sealed against the escape or entry of air or made airtight by fusion or sealing. Therefore, it is a seal with no coronal, apical, or lateral leakage of any kind whatsoever. It is a seal that will maintain the root canal therapy that has been performed by preventing the ingress of microorganisms, thereby preventing secondary infections. Along with this, an additional objective has been to create a clinical technique so user friendly that it results in a majority of the dentists performing the best possible obturation [1].

Endodontics has witnessed a true evolution in recent years. The main ingredient that creates the seal in all of the obturation techniques (silver points, lateral condensation, and thermoplastic methods) is the sealer. Sealer, along with solid obturating material, acts synergistically to create a hermetic seal. This chapter talks about the evolution of sealers from the conventional zinc oxide eugenol to the current ones like resin-based sealers, MTA-based sealers, and bioceramics. The monoblock concept is also explained in detail. The text also discusses at length the more recent and current obturating core materials and systems in use.

Conventional sealers

The use of a sealer during root canal obturation is essential for success. It enhances the possible attainment of an impervious seal and also serves as a filler for canal irregularities and minor discrepancies between the root canal wall and core filling material. Sealers are often expressed through lateral or accessory canals to assist in microbial control should there be microorganisms left on the root canal walls or in the tubules [2, 3]. They also serve as lubricants, enabling thorough compaction of the core-filling material. A good sealer must be biocompatible, well tolerated by the periradicular tissues, nontoxic, and absorbable when exposed to tissues and tissue fluids. Excessive sealer should not routinely be placed in the periradicular tissues as part of an obturation technique.

Sealers and cements can be classified according to their prime constituent, such as zinc oxide eugenol (ZOE), polyketone, epoxy, calcium hydroxide, silicone, resin, glass ionomer, or resin-modified glass ionomer (Table 5.1). However, many of the sealers are combinations of components, such as zinc oxide eugenol and calcium hydroxide [4]. Epoxy-based and methacrylate-based resin sealers that can be bonded to the root canal dentin (but not to gutta-percha) are also available [5].

Early sealers were modified ZOE cements based on Grossman's or Rickerts's formula that were widely used throughout the world. Their setting reaction is a chelation reaction occurring between eugenol and the zinc ion of the zinc oxide. The decreased setting shrinkage associated with the ZOE-based sealers [6] may be

Current Therapy in Endodontics, First Edition. Edited by Priyanka Jain.
© 2016 John Wiley & Sons, Inc. Published 2016 by John Wiley & Sons, Inc.

Table 5.1 Classification of root canal sealers.

Type	Brand	Manufacturer
Zinc oxide eugenol	Roth Kerr PCS Endomethasone	Roth Inc., Chicago, IL, USA Kerr, Romulus, MI, USA Septodont, Saint-Maur des Fossés, France
Glass ionomer	Ketac-Endo	3M ESPE, St. Paul, MN, USA
Epoxy resin	AH Plus AH 26	Dentsply Maillefer, Ballaigues, Switzerland
Methacrylate resin	First generation: Hydron Second generation: EndoREZ Third generation: Epiphany Fibrefill Fourth generation: Realseal SE Metaseal SE Smartseal	Hydron Technologies, Pompano Beach, FL, USA Ultradent, South Jordan, UT, USA Pentron Clinical Technologies, Wallingford, CT, USA Sybron Endo, Orange, CA, USA Parkell Inc, Stamford, UK
Silicone	RoekoSeal GuttaFlow	Roeko/Coltene/Whaledent, Langenau, Germany
Mineral trioxide aggregate	Endo-CPM-Sealer MTA Obtura MTA Fillapex	EGEO srl, Buenos Aires, Argentina Angelus, Londrina PR, Brazil
Calcium phosphate	Capseal I Capseal II	Sankin Apatite Sealer, Sankin Kogyo, Tokyo, Japan
Calcium-silicate-phosphate–based bioceramic	Endosequence iRoot BP Bioaggregate	Brasseler, USA Innovative Bioceramix, Vancouver, Canada

explained by the fact that the setting reaction at times also occurs with the zinc oxide phase of gutta-percha along with the calcium ions of dentin.

Despite their advantages (easy to handle, antimicrobial, decreased dimensional change, and low shrinkage), sealing properties of ZOE sealers were inferior in comparison to other sealers due to their relatively high solubility, thus leading to a weak adhesion between gutta-percha and the sealer [7].

The challenge, therefore, has been to find a sealer that would simultaneously bond to the canal wall and to the gutta-percha cone or a similar core material. Endodontic science has realized that if it could satisfy such a challenge, we would then have the possibility of creating a true monoblock (explained later in the chapter).

To overcome the problem of microleakage and shortcomings of bonding of material to the tooth structure, Buonocore [8] in 1950 had introduced the acid-etch technique. The ideal product should provide a good adhesion to both dentin and the obturating material, be hydrophilic, and have a dimensional stability of low solubility and shrinkage or expansion of the material. Ease of application along with good radiopacity is also necessary.

Resin cement sealants have been developed, thereby improving the root canal seal and imparting it more strength as compared to the conventional materials [9, 10]. These also include silicon-based sealers, epoxy resin–based sealers, and mineral trioxide aggregate (MTA)-based sealers.

Modern sealers

Epoxy resin–based sealers: AH Plus (Dentsply Maillefer, Tulsa, OK, USA)

AH Plus was introduced to overcome the shortcomings of its precursor, AH 26. Retaining the advantageous properties of AH 26 (high radiopacity, low solubility, little shrinkage, and good tissue compatibility), and eliminating certain disadvantageous properties such as a tendency to discolor and the release of formaldehyde, AH Plus was introduced. AH Plus consists of a paste–paste system (amine and epoxy), delivered in two tubes in a double-barrel syringe called the AH Plus Jet for better mixing.

AH Plus retains the epoxide–amine chemistry of AH 26, which contains radiopaque fillers and aerosol [10]. However, three different types of amines were added to the amine paste, namely 1-adamantane amine N,N′-dibenzyl-5-oxa-nonandiamine-1,9 TCD-diamine. In addition to the diepoxide, the epoxide paste contains radiopaque fillers like calcium tungstate, zirconium oxide, and aerosil.

According to the ISO standard for root canal sealing materials, the film thickness of the sealer should be less than 50 mm. AH Plus sealer, because of its thixotropic nature, is as thin as 26 mm, which is below the required value. [11]. Hence, it has greater adhesion to root dentin. It can also penetrate better into the irregularities of the anatomy of canals due to its creep capacity and long setting time. It has no genotoxic effects or mutagenic effects *in vivo* [11]. Due to its excellent properties, such as low solubility, small expansion, adhesion to dentin, and very good sealing ability, AH Plus is considered a gold standard [1].

GuttaFlow Sealer (Coltène/Whaledent, Altstätten, Switzerland)

Silicone was introduced as a root canal sealer in 1984. These sealers exhibit comparatively little leakage, are virtually nontoxic, and display no antibacterial activity. Silver particles are added as preservative [12–15]. GuttaFlow demonstrates good spreadability with both ethylenediamenetetraacetic acid (EDTA) and sodium hypochlorite (NaOCl). The reason for this is the increase in the surface energy of the root dentinal wall free of the smear layer [15]. A gutta-percha–containing silicone sealer expands slightly, and thus leakage was reported to be less than for AH 26 with gutta-percha over a period of 12 months [4].

GuttaFlow 2 Fast (Coltène/Whaledent, Altstätten, Switzerland), is an advanced next-generation product of GuttaFlow using gutta-percha powder with particle size of less than 30 nm. It is available in dual barrel syringes with mixing tips and capsules. GuttaFlow Bioseal has been introduced with the natural repair mechanism of regeneration by forming hydroxyapatite crystals. This is also available as an automix syringe.

Nanoseal Plus Sealer

Researchers from Universiti Sains Malaysia developed the first endodontic sealer based on nanotechnology, which actively seals tiny gaps. It is made of calcium phosphate hydroxyapatite nanoparticles ranging from 40 to 60 nm. Thus, Nano Seal Plus has a similar structure to the tooth. These particles can penetrate the dentinal tubules and enter accessory canals to ensure that all the spaces are effectively sealed. The sealer is biocompatible, has antibacterial effect, has apical healing ability, provides a good hermetic apical seal, is inexpensive, and prevents leakage by increasing adhesive strength.

Bioceramics: iRoot SP/Endosequence Sealer (Brasseler, Savannah, GA, USA)

The properties associated with bioceramics, such as being nontoxic, are very advantageous to dentistry. They can be classified [16–18] as bioinert, bioactive, or biodegradable. Bioinert materials do not interact with biological systems. Bioactive materials are durable tissues that can undergo interfacial interactions with surrounding tissue. Biodegradable materials eventually replace or are incorporated into tissue.

Numerous bioceramics are currently in use in dentistry. Alumina and zirconia are among the bioinert ceramics used for prosthetic devices. Calcium silicates such as MTA and BioAggregate (DiaDent, Burnaby, BC, Canada) have been used in dentistry as root repair materials and for apical retrofills.

Bioceramics are biocompatible, are nontoxic, do not shrink, and are chemically stable within the biological environment. Most importantly, they do not result in an inflammatory response if an overfill occurs during the obturation process. This is of prime importance in endodontics. A further advantage of the material is its ability to form hydroxyapatite and to create a bond between dentin and the appropriate filling materials.

EndoSequence BC Sealer (Brasseler) makes use of all the above-mentioned advantages associated with bioceramics. It is a nontoxic hydraulic calcium silicate cement for use as an endodontic sealer. This is also known as iRoot SP (injectable root canal sealer) (Innovative BioCeramix, Vancouver, BC, Canada) [16, 19, 20]. The major inorganic constituents include tricalcium silicate, dicalcium silicate, calcium phosphates, colloidal silica, and calcium hydroxide. It also contains zirconium oxide as a radiopacifier and a water free-vehicle that thickens the paste system. It is available as a premixed paste in a syringe with intraoral tips to deliver the paste inside the root canals [21, 22], thus improving convenience and delivery. The introduction of a premixed sealer eliminates the potential for heterogeneous consistency during mixing.

Endosequence BC sealer does not set until it is water activated and hence uses the moisture present in the dentinal tubules after the last irrigation to initiate the setting process, speed up the hydration reaction, and thereby reduce the overall setting time. When the sealer is placed in the root canal, the material absorbs water from the dentin tubules, causing a hydration reaction of the dicalcium silicate and tricalcium silicate. Calcium phosphate reacts with calcium hydroxide at the same time to precipitate hydroxyapatite and water. This water continues to be used for the hydration of the calcium silicates and leads to the formation of a composite network of gel-like calcium silicate hydrate, which mixes with the hydroxyapatite bioceramics and forms a hermetic seal inside the root canal. The pH during the setting process is very alkaline (pH 12.9), which increases its bactericidal properties.

A study on bioceramic sealer showed that even if the sealer extrudes out of the canal, the patient might not experience any pain as compared to other conventional sealers, because the sealer hardens to form hydroxyapatite, which is osseoconductive [23]. This hydroxyapatite has the ability to expand and harden inside the canal, which helps to create a perfect seal with the walls.

Conventional retreatment techniques can be used to remove this sealer when it is used in combination with gutta-percha, but Hess and colleagues [24] observed in retreatment cases that removal of bioceramic sealer using solvent and a rotary instrument and reaching the correct working length was not easy, and patency was gained in only 20% of their experimental samples.

According to Ghoneim and colleagues [25], bioceramic-based sealer is a promising sealer in terms of increasing *in vitro* resistance to the fracture of endodontically treated roots, particularly when accompanied with ActiV GP cones. Further studies need to be conducted to evaluate the cytotoxicity of EndoSequence BC sealer.

Mineral trioxide aggregate–based sealers

In 1993 Torabinejad introduced MTA, a calcium-based material, in endodontics. This has been vastly recommended for pulp capping, pulpotomy, forming an apical barrier, repairing root perforation, and root canal obturation. In 1999, Holland and colleagues concluded that MTA as a sealer induces closure of the main apical foramen by deposition of cementum in the absence of inflammatory cells (Box 5.1). It produces calcium hydroxide, which is released in solution and produces an interstitial layer that resembles hydroxyapatite structures in simulated body fluids. The moisture (biological fluids) is necessary to initiate the setting reaction and to induce bioactivity resulting in the formation of apatite precipitates

MTA is composed principally of Portland cement with the addition of bismuth trioxide to render it radiopaque. Being an entirely inorganic material, Portland cement undergoes chemical shrinkage following hydration. Moreover, hydration forms calcium silicate hydrate (CSH) gel that adheres to the gutta-percha cone. Its role as a sealer where it adheres well to dentin and obturating material, its cohesive strength, wetting properties, low viscosity, cytotoxicity, and biocompatibility were later compared to other sealers.

The novel sealer based on MTA has efficacious sealing ability. When in contact with a simulated body fluid, the MTA releases calcium ions in solution and encourages the deposition of calcium phosphate crystals. But MTA-based root canal sealers do not fulfill all the criteria described by Grossman. Most experiments are laboratory based or in animal models, which may differ from a clinical scenario.

Currently, MTA sealer formulations include Endo CPM Sealer (EGEO SRL, Buenos Aires, Argentina), MTA Obtura (Angelus Odonto, Londrina, Brazil), ProRoot Endo Sealer (Dentsply Maillefer, Ballaigues, Switzerland), and Fillapex (Angelus Odonto). (Box 5.1)

Pro-Root Endo Sealer (Dentsply Tulsa)

ProRoot Endo Sealer is a calcium silicate–based endodontic sealer used in either lateral warm vertical or carrier-based obturation techniques. The major components are tricalcium silicate and dicalcium silicate, with inclusion of calcium sulfate as setting retardant, bismuth oxide as a radiopacifier, and a small amount of tricalcium aluminate. Tricalcium aluminate is necessary for the initial hydration reaction of the cement. The liquid part consists of viscous aqueous solution of a water-soluble polymer to improve the workability and flow. Its addition does not affect the biocompatibility of the material [26–29] or alter the hydration characteristics of MTA. When placed in the canal, it releases

Box 5.1 Mineral trioxide aggregate as a root canal sealer

Advantages

Compatible and stimulates mineralization
Antimicrobial
Forms hydroxyapatite on the surface and provides a biological seal
Bioactive; i.e., it encourages differentiation and migration of hard tissue–producing cells
Exhibits high adhesiveness to dentin as compared to other conventional sealers
Sealing ability is similar to that of epoxy resin–based sealers
Forms calcium hydroxide that releases calcium ions
Nontoxic and nonmutagenic
Provides effective seal against dentin and cementum and promotes biological repair and regeneration of the periodontal ligament

Disadvantages

Can cause discoloration due to the release of the ferrous ions
Long setting time
Short working time of less than 4 minutes
Inadequate compressive strength
Improper handling characteristics
No known solvent is available

calcium and hydroxyl ions from the set sealer liquid, producing hydroxyapatite, which aids in the formation of a physical bond between sealer and MTA.

Endo CPM Sealer (EGEO SRL)

Endo CPM Sealer was developed in 2004 in an attempt to combine the sealing and physiochemical properties of root canal sealer with the biological characteristics of MTA. The powder consists of fine hydrophilic particles that form a gel in the presence of moisture. The main constituents are tricalcium silicate, tricalcium oxide, and tricalcium aluminate. The liquid part contains saline solution and calcium chloride. Research has shown that addition of calcium chloride to MTA reduces setting time, improves its sealing ability, and facilitates insertion into cavities. The material solidifies and forms a hard sealer in 1 hour. It is manufactured as a white modified Portland cement.

The most significant difference is the presence of large amounts of calcium carbonate, which is intended to increase the release of the calcium ions and improve the adhesion to the dentinal walls with adequate flow and biocompatibility. It has been reported that Endo CPM sealer has an alkaline pH. Addition of the calcium carbonate reduces the pH from 12.5 to 10 after setting. This allows better action of alkaline phosphatase. But CPM sealer showed higher ratio of leakage as compared to AH Plus and Sealapex.

Fillapex (Angelus Odonto)

Fillapex is a recent introduction; it is made of two pastes. The first paste contains MTA-based salicylate resin, bismuth trioxide, and fumed silica. This is versatile for every obturation technique. It delivers easily and exhibits excellent handling characteristics and an improved setting time. The other half of the MTA Fillapex paste contains fumed silica, titanium dioxide, MTA (40%), and base resin. Salicylate resin is tissue friendly and therefore a better choice over epoxy-based resins.

The setting reaction relies upon the salicylate reacting with calcium hydroxide. Because there is no calcium hydroxide in the pastes, MTA within the mixture reacts with water from the dentinal fluid. The two pastes combine in a homogeneous mix to form a rigid but semipermeable structure. It exhibits an alkaline pH, has a good flow rate, has an ideal working time of 35 minutes, is antimicrobial, and has a low film thickness to easily penetrate into the accessory canals.

However, there are some concerns. It is reportedly very soluble and has not met the ANSI/ADA requirements on solubility. The greater solubility can result in higher cytotoxicity as the material continues to leak and irritate the neighboring tissue [30–33].

MTA Obtura (Angelus Odonto)

MTA Obtura was developed by replacing saline with liquid resin as the cure inhibitor. The composition is a mixture of white MTA with a proprietary viscous liquid consisting of Portland cement and bismuth oxide. This sealer demonstrated stable leakage values at 15 and 30 days and good sealing ability. However, at 60 days, the material exhibited a considerable increase in leakage and low flow rate.

Fluoride-doped MTA cements

In fluoride-doped MTA cements, the powder consists of white Portland cement, bismuth oxide, anhydrite, and sodium fluoride (NaF). The liquid component contains alphacaine SP solution. NaF was added as an expansive and retarding agent. This helped in increasing the sealing ability of the sealer due to greater expansion achieved. Fluoride ions can penetrate into the dentin and enhance the mineralization of the dentin.

The setting reaction involves the continuous formation of hydration products that contribute in reducing the microchannels in the sealer. The pH is increased up to 12 and may play a protective role in preventing bacterial recontamination of a filled root canal. It has been shown that the cytotoxicity of MTA-F is decreased and the sealer presents suitable bioactivity to stimulate hydroxyapatite crystal nucleation [34].

Methacrylate resin–based sealers

Methacrylate resin–based sealers (MRBSs) have gained popularity due to their hydrophilic properties, which enable them to wet the canal walls and penetrate dentinal tubules. Their bondability to the radicular dentin and root canal materials is also superior compared to other cements.

Four generations have been introduced. However, the monoblock concept is explained first for better understanding of their setting reaction.

Monoblock concept

The term *monoblock,* meaning a single unit, has been employed in dentistry since the turn of the century. A monoblock obturation system is the unit in which the core material, sealing agent, and the root canal dentin form a single cohesive unit. There are two prerequisites for the monoblock to function as a mechanically homogeneous unit. First, the materials that constitute the monoblock should have the ability to bond strongly and mutually to each other, as well as to the substrate that the monoblock is intended to reinforce. Second, these materials should have a modulus of elasticity that is similar to that of the substrate. Monoblocks in the root canal spaces may be classified as primary, secondary, or tertiary depending on the number of interfaces present between the bonding substrate and the bulk material core. (Figure 5.1)

Primary monoblock

Primary monoblock has a single interface that extends circumferentially between the material and the root canal wall. Hydron MTA is an example. Orthograde obturation with MTA (ProRoot MTA, Dentsply Tulsa) as an apexification material represents a contemporary version of the primary monoblock in attempts to strengthen immature tooth roots. A classic example of primary monoblock would be obturating the root canals with gutta-percha without using the sealer. The lack of sufficient strength and stiffness is the major drawback, and this led to the development of secondary monoblocks.

Secondary monoblock

Conventional sealers do not bond strongly to dentin and gutta-percha; therefore, gutta-percha does not form a monoblock, even with the use of a resin-based sealer. Although glass ionomer cements and resin-modified glass ionomer cements bond to root dentin and have been marketed as root canal sealers, they do not bond to gutta-percha [35, 36]. The combined use of a sealer and a core material introduces additional interfaces into a monoblock during obturations. Secondary monoblocks have two circumferential interfaces, one between the cement and dentin and another between cement and the core material. This is of great importance in restorative and endodontic practice. A classic example is the use of sealer for obturation, wherein one interface is between the gutta-percha point and sealer and the second one is between the sealer and the root canal wall. Examples are Resilon and iRoot SP.

Reinforcing the root canals with bondable filling materials was reintroduced in 2004 as the Resilon/Epiphany system (Epiphany, Pentron Clinical Technologies,

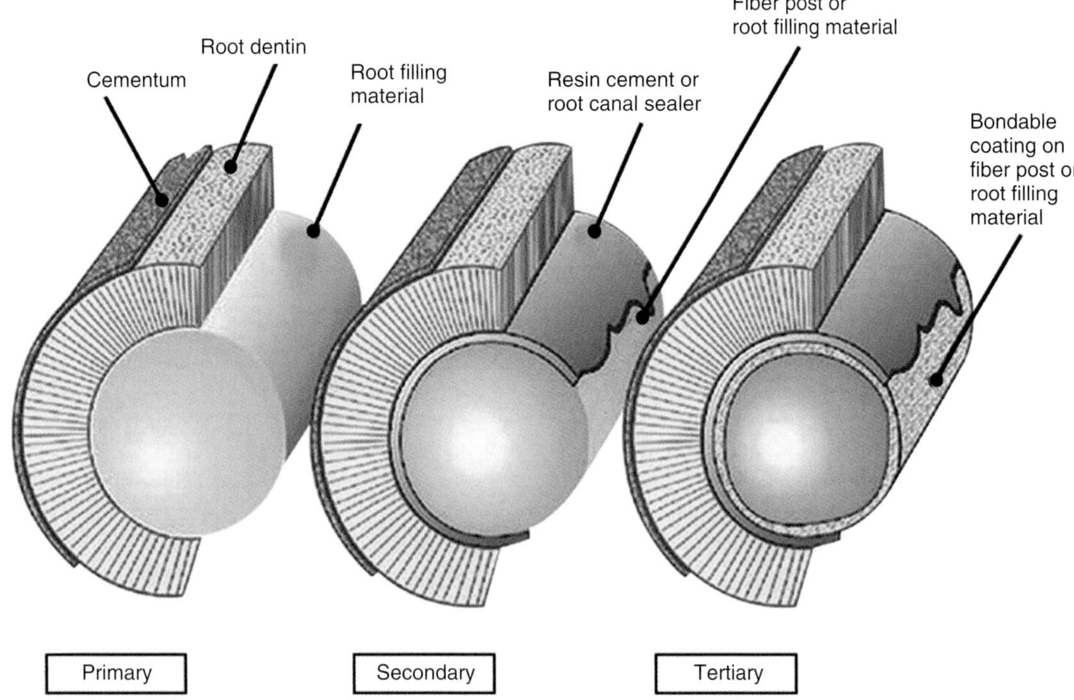

Figure 5.1 The monoblock concept.

Wallingford, CT). The concept was to create a root canal monoblock to achieve a total bond and a total seal of the root canal space, which prevented by the lack of chemical union between the gutta-percha and the resin-based or glass ionomer–based sealer.

Tertiary monoblock

A third circumferential interface is introduced between the bonding substrate and the abutment material by coating the nonbondable gutta-percha with materials that make them bondable to the sealers, thus creating tertiary monoblocks. Because the tertiary interface exists as an external coating on the surface of the gutta-percha, such systems are designed to be used with either a single-cone technique or placement of accessory cones without lateral compaction, to avoid disrupting the external coatings. Fiber posts that contain an external silicate coating or nonpolymerized resin composite for lining root canals that are oval or not perfectly round or wide so that the fiber post can be fitted properly are considered a tertiary monoblock. Examples of tertiary monoblock are ActiveGP and Endorez (Ultradent, South Jordan, UT).

Challenges with monoblocks

Although the idea of creating a mechanically homogeneous unit with root dentin is excellent in theory, accomplishing these ideal monoblocks in the root canal space is challenging, because bonding to dentin is compromised by volumetric changes that occur in resin-based materials during polymerization.

There appears to be no adhesive root canal material that can perfectly obturate the canal space with a tight seal that consists of different interfaces, simultaneously improving the fracture resistance of the tooth. Even when the effect of dentin permeability in endodontically treated teeth is minimal, entrapment of residual moisture within the root canal can result in the permeation of this unbound water through hydrophilic adhesive layers [37, 38]. This can work as stress raisers and promote crack growth and propagation during loading along the interface. The highly unfavorable and complex geometry of the substrate, namely root canal space, also proves to be detrimental to the polymerization of the resin cements or sealers. However, continued research and development is carried out and is likely to result in improvements.

Monoblocks aim at achieving a single unit that would reinforce the tooth structure. However, all the root canal filling materials available today have a modulus of elasticity that is far less as compared to dentin (i.e., 14,000 MPa), which questions the effectiveness of this concept.

First-generation methacrylate resin–based sealers

Hydron (Hydron technologies,Inc. Pompano Beach, FL, USA) is is an example of a primary monoblock used to fill the root canals extensively in the late 1970s. It consists of 2-hydroxy ethyl methacrylate (HEMA). But it was not stiff enough to strengthen the canal surfaces. Though it demonstrated ease of application, antibacterial properties, and adaptability to the canal wall, adverse inflammatory reactions and leakage issues were also observed [39, 40].

Second-generation methacrylate resin–based sealers

Second-generation MRBS materials do not depend on separate dentin conditioning. The generation of an endodontic seal is dependent on the penetration of the hydrophilic sealer into the dentinal tubules and lateral canals following removal of the smear layer. This forms a hybrid layer by creating resin tags with the collagen network [41–43]. Although both the tensile bond strength and apical seal to intraradicular dentin may be improved using a dual-cured self-etching primer/adhesive, there is still a potential problem of rapid polymerization of the adhesive in an environment with reduced oxygen concentration [44, 45].

EndoReZ Sealer (Ultradent Products, South Jordan UT)

EndoReZ was introduced by coating butta-percha cones with a polybutadiene diisocyanate–methacrylate adhesive [45]. The sealer can be used with gutta-percha or with resin-coated gutta-percha, the latter with the objective of forming a monoblock.

It is a two-component system in a double-barrel automix syringe containing the base, which constitutes of diurethane dimethacrylate monomer (UDMA), triethylene glycol dimethacrylate, bismuth compounds, and barium sulfate as fillers, peroxide initiators, and photo initiators. The catalyst also contains diurethane dimethacrylate, triethylene glycol dimethacrylate, bismuth compounds, and some amount of other ingredients as radiopaque fillers. The sealer has hydrophilic qualities and hence can be used in root canals that pose a challenge of moist environment. In this system, no dentin adhesive is employed and an accelerator is used along with the resin-coated gutta-percha cones to provide rapid cure process and also to promote better bonding between the gutta-percha cone and the sealer, which in turn bonds well to the canal wall to establish a complete monoblock seal [46].

This adhesive resin includes a hydrophobic portion that chemically binds with a hydrophobic polyisoprene substrate and a hydrophilic portion that is chemically compatible with a hydrophilic dentinal wall. With the use of this adhesive resin coating, a strong chemical union may be achieved between the gutta-percha and the MRBS. This type of resin-coated cone is recommended for use with the EndoReZ system (explained later). However, it is still unrealistic to expect a mechanically homogeneous unit with the root canal with the EndoRez system, because the bulk of the material inside the root canal still consists of thermoplastic gutta-percha, an elastomeric polymer that flows when stressed.

Third-generation methacrylate resin–based sealers

As the resin era improved, a third generation of self-etching sealers was introduced, which contained self-etching primer along with dual-cured resin sealer for root canal obturation procedures. This introduces the concept of incorporating the smear layer in the sealer–dentin interface.

Fibrefill Resin Sealer (Pentron Clinical Technologies)

Fibrefill is a radiopaque dual-cured methacrylate resin sealer based on urethane dimethacrylate (UDMA) used in combination with a self-curing, self-etching primer system (Fibrefill Primer A and B). This system consists of fiber-reinforced obturators. The apical part of the obturator is gutta-percha, and the coronal two-thirds consists of a resin and a glass fiber post for adhesive bonding. Studies have shown the Fibrefill root canal sealer possesses good sealing ability and adhesive properties to the radicular dentin. MTAD is recommended as the final rinse to enhance the bond strength of the material.

Epiphany (Pentron Clinical Technologies)

Epiphany is a third generation dual-cure resin-based sealer (Figure 5.2). This system uses a self-etching primer and comprises a Resilon cone. Resilon (Resilon Research LLC, Madison, CT) is a dimthacrylate-containing, polyaprolactone-based thermoplastic root-filling material that contains bioactive glass, bismuth oxychloride, and barium sulfate [47].

The sealer is a dual-cure sealer composed of urethane dimethacrylate (UDMA), poly dimethacrylate (PEGDMA), ethoxylated bisphenol A dimethacrylate (EBPADMA), bisphenol A glycidyl methacrylate (BIS-GMA), barium borosilicate, barium sulfate (BaSO4), bismuth oxychloride, calcium hydroxide, photo initiators, and a resinuous solvent (thinning resin). The thinning resin increases the bond strength of the Epiphany sealer to dentin walls when followed by photoactivation. The Epiphany sealer, being dual cure, takes about 45 minutes to completely self-cure in the canal, and hence presents ease of handling. It can be light cured to achieve a hard coronal seal immediately to prevent any contamination issues. Epiphany primer is a self-etch primer, which contains sulfonic acid–terminated functional monomer, HEMA, water, and polymerization initiator. The Primer is applied to the dentin walls of the root canals that are to be filled with Resilon obturating material. The preparation of the dentin through these chemical agents may prevent shrinkage of the resin filling away from the dentin wall and aid in sealing the roots with the Resilon material.

The self-etching primers are further reduced from a two-bottle system to a single-bottle system. In the single-bottle self-etching primer, the functional acidic monomers, solvents, water that is necessary for ionization of the acidic monomers, and self-cured catalysts are incorporated into one component in the single bottle.

The premise behind the material is the formation of a monoblock, that is, the primer forms a hybrid layer with dentin, which bonds to sealer and then bonds to the Resilon core. This results in low apical leakage and good resistance to bacterial infiltration (Figure 5.3). The ability of Resilon to bond to methacrylate-based root canal sealers has been questioned. Unpolymerized resin was found to be available between the core material and the resin sealer. This led to the conclusion that the amount of dimethacrylate in the thermoplastic composite might not be optimum for chemical coupling. Hence, although the sealer had low viscosity, keeping all the above factors in mind, the sealing ability of thin films inside the canal remained questionable [48, 49].

RealSeal (SybronEndo, Orange, CA, USA)

By combining self-etching adhesives and methacrylate resin–based sealers with Resilon, the manufacturer introduced a new era in root canal obturation (4,49,50). Resilon/Epiphany sealer was then introduced again as RealSeal by adding a thinning solvent ethoxylated bisphenol-A-dimethacrylate to adjust the viscosity but did not include photoactivation. However, addition of

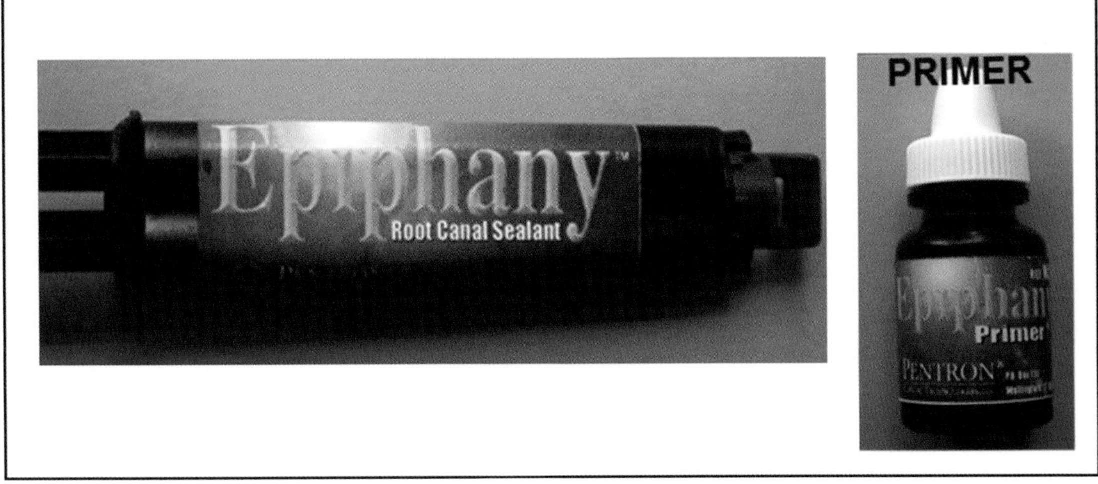

Figure 5.2 Epiphany root canal primer and sealant.

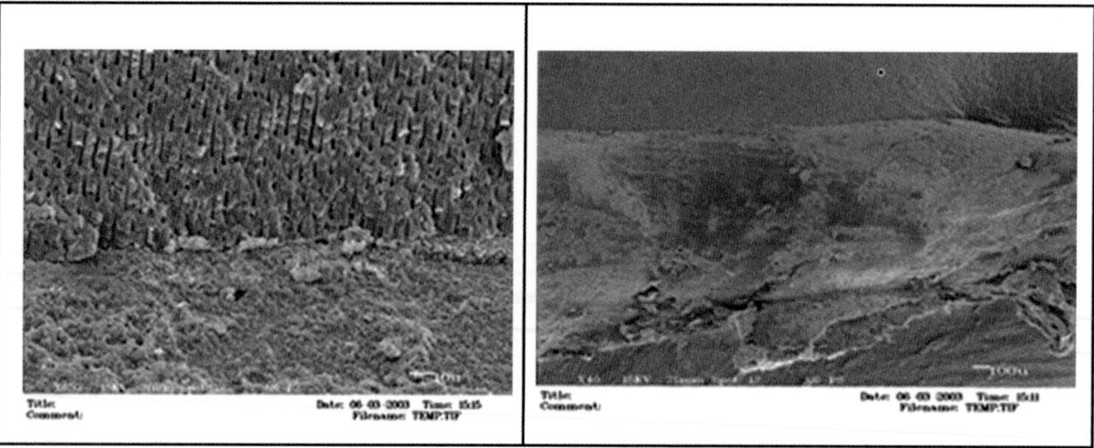

Figure 5.3 Scanning electron microscope images of Resilon Epiphany System. (Image courtesy of Dr. Mohan Sakri.)

the thinning solvent to the sealer without photoactivation did not increase adhesion to dentin [50].

Fourth-generation methacrylate resin–based sealers

Fourth-generation MRBSs are functionally similar and comparable to self-adhesive resin luting composites in that they have further eliminated the separate etching/bonding step [51]. Dentin adhesive primers are now incorporated into the resin-based sealer/composite to render them self-adhesive to dentin substrates. The combination of an etchant, a primer, and a sealer into an all-in-one self-etching, self-adhesive sealer is advantageous in that it reduces the application time as well as errors that might occur during each bonding step. Therefore, in theory, the bonding mechanism of self-adhesive sealers is similar to self-adhesive resin materials. These materials are relatively new, and detailed information and research is limited.

MetaSEAL (Parkell)

MetaSEAL is the first commercially available fourth-generation self-adhesive dual-cured sealer [52, 53]. The inclusion of an acidic resin monomer, 4-methacryloyl oxyethyl trimellitate anhydride (4-META), makes the sealer self-etching and hydrophilic, and it promotes monomer diffusion into the underlying intact dentin to produce a hybrid layer after polymerization. It is recommended for use exclusively with cold-compaction or single-cone techniques. The sealer purportedly bonds to thermoplastic root-filling materials as well as radicular dentin via the creation of hybrid layers in both substrates. MetaSEAL is also marketed as Hybrid Bond SEAL (Sun Medical Co Ltd, Shiga, Japan) in Japan and had been reported to produce similar or slightly inferior sealing properties to conventional nonbonding epoxy resin–based sealers [54, 55].

RealSeal SE and RealSeal 1(SybronEndo)

RealSeal SE is the simplified dual-cured version of RealSeal and uses a polymerizable methacrylate carboxylic acid anhydride (i.e., 4-META) as the acidic resin monomer leading to the elimination of the separate etching/bonding step [56, 57]. The acidic resin monomers in the self-etching primer are incorporated in the RealSeal SE sealer, thus making the technique an all-in-one step. The sealer is claimed to bond to both the Resilon core and radicular dentin via hybrid layers in both substrates, leading to a monoblock unit.

It may be used with Resilon cones or pellets by using cold lateral or warm vertical techniques or with RealSeal 1, a carrier-based Resilon obturator system [58]. This combines adhesive bonding technology with a carrier product and provides benefits of an efficient obturation technique combined with optimal leakage resistance (explained later).

Problems associated with resin-based sealers

Bonding within a deep and narrow root canal is a challenge due to the complex geometry of the root canal. The resin penetrates into the dentinal tubules, whereas the filler particles remain at the interface. This can result in low bond strength. In addition, penetration with a curing light is limited in a root canal system. Proper and uniform application of the adhesive and primer is critical, but it is difficult to achieve this in the apical third of the canal. Polymerization shrinkage is inherent to methacrylate resin–based sealers, which tend to produce debonding at the resin–dentin interface.

Modern root canal filling core materials

Gutta-percha

Since its introduction in 1914 by Callahan, gutta-percha is the standard material of choice as a solid core-filling material for root canal filling (Box 5.2). It is a *trans*-isomer of polyisoprene and exists in two crystalline forms (alpha and beta) with differing properties. The use of alpha phase gutta-percha has increased as thermoplastic techniques have become more popular. Gutta-percha cones consist of approximately 20% gutta-percha, 65% zinc oxide, 10% radiopacifiers, and 5% plasticizers. Alpha phase gutta-percha is brittle at room temperature and is runny, tacky, and sticky (low viscosity), whereas beta phase gutta-percha is stable and flexible at room temperature and is solid and compactible (high viscosity). Beta phase gutta-percha is available as standardized and nonstandardized points.

Although gutta-percha has many desirable properties, such as chemical stability, biocompatibility, nonporosity, radiopacity, and the ability to be manipulated and removed, it does not always bond to the internal tooth structure, resulting in the absence of a hermetic seal [59] (Box 5.2). This produces a poor barrier to bacteria microleakage. Many attempts have been made to resolve the problem through variations in obturation techniques such as vertical and lateral condensation, the use of reverse-fill or touch and heat systems. These methods have reduced microleakage to a certain degree but not completely.

The disadvantages of gutta-percha in endodontic therapy have led to the development of a new material known as the Resilon/Epiphany (R/E) system.

Resilon (Pentron Clinical Technologies)

Resilon is a core obturation material alternative to gutta-percha and requires a sealer to complete obturation of the canal system. Resilon, a synthetic resin-based polycaprolactone polymer, is used with Ephiphany, (Pentron Clinical Technologies), a resin sealer, in an attempt to form an adhesive bond at the interface of the synthetic polymer-based core material, the canal wall, and the sealer. These have gutta-percha–like handling properties and the ability to bond to the sealer, which in turn bonds to dentin within the root canal. This eliminates the probability of microleakage between the core material–sealer interface and the sealer–dentin interface. In 2003, Resilon Research introduced Resilon obturating points and Epiphany sealer into the commercial market. SybronEndo licensed the material as RealSeal. The system consists of Epiphany primer, Epiphany sealer, and Resilon core material (Box 5.3).

Based on polymers of polyester, *Resilon* Material contains bioactive glass and radiopaque fillers. It is a high-performance industrial polyurethane adapted for endodontic use and resembles gutta-percha in color, texture, radiopacity, and handling properties. It consists of a resin core material, available in conventional/standardized cones or pellets, and a resin sealer. The filler content within Resilon is approximately 65% by weight. It is obturated with RealSeal sealer, formerly known as Epiphany, which incorporates self-etching primers.

Resilon is nontoxic, nonmutagenic, and biocompatible. The manufacturer claims that this system creates a monoblock effect with the canal wall. Such a monoblock eliminates the gaps associated with the core material and sealer, resists shrinkage, and strengthens the root [60–62]. Because the Resilon/Epiphany root filling material is a composite resin-based system, it does not have a deleterious effect on the subsequent resin-bonding procedures often used for coronal restorations.

Any obturation technique may be used with the Resilon system, although it works effectively with vertical and lateral condensation techniques. The Resilon points melt at a lower temperature than gutta-percha: about 70°C to 80°C. Research on apical seal of Resilon-based systems has shown that irrespective of the technique used for obturation—lateral condensation or vertical compaction using thermoplasticized materials—the Resilon-based systems have shown less apical leakage as compared to gutta-percha points used with various sealer combinations or gutta-percha thermoplasticized systems. Advantages of Resilon are:

Box 5.2 Characteristics of gutta-percha

Advantages

Biocompatibility
Flexibility of technique
Easily removed
Thermoplastic

Disadvantages

Does not provide a good hermetic seal
Cannot bond to dentin
Potential for voids
Shrinks upon cooling

Box 5.3 Composition of resilon system

Resilon Primer

The primer is a self-etching system that is cured by the sealer.
The primer penetrates all the dentinal tubules.
Ingredients: Sulfonic acid terminated functional monomer, HEMA, Water, Polymerization initiator

Resilon Sealer

The sealer bonds to the primer, thereby eliminating potential for microleakage.
Organic part: BisGMA, ethoxylated BisGMA, UDMA, hydrophilic difunctional methacrylates
Inorganic part: calcium hydroxide, barium sulfate, barium glass, silica, bismuth oxychloride

Resilon Core Material(Obturator)

The Resilon obturator is a thermoplastic polyester that bonds to the surface of the sealer, which in turn bonds to the primer that has hybridized with the tubular
surfaces
Organic component: thermoplastic synthetic polymer-polycaprolactone
Inorganic component: bioactive glass, bismuth oxychloride, barium sulfate

Thinning Resin

Most systems include a thinning resin, which may be added to thin the sealer to the desired viscosity

BisGMA- bisphenol A-glycidyl methacrylate, UDMA- Urethane dimethacrylate

- Decreased incidence of root fracture
- Better radiopacity than gutta-percha
- Dual cure capabilities for immediate coronal seal
- Less irritation than epoxy or ZOE sealers

Coated cones

Coated gutta-percha is also available to inhibit leakage between the solid core and sealer. Currently, alternatives to Resilon available on the market consist of resin-coated gutta-percha cones (EndoRez cones). A bond is formed when the resin sealer contacts the resin-coated gutta-percha cone. Resilon is also available as a terminus on a fiber obturator that allows one to obturate the canal and place a fiber post simultaneously with a methacrylate sealer. Another example is coating gutta-percha cones with glass ionomer. This system is called Active GP Plus (Brasseler USA).

Obturation with gutta-percha

Several obturation techniques are available for root canal treatment (Table 5.2). The choice depends on the canal anatomy and the unique objectives of treatment in each case. Lateral condensation and warm vertical condensation of gutta-percha are techniques that have stood the test of time. Newer methods include the use of injectable, thermoplasticized gutta-percha systems; carriers coated with an alpha-phase gutta-percha; cold, flowable obturation materials that combine

Table 5.2 Techniques for obturating root canal systems.

Obturation with gutta-percha		
Technique	**Explanation**	**Available Systems**
Lateral condensation	A master cone corresponding to the final instrumentation size and length of the canal is coated with sealer, inserted into the canal, laterally compacted with spreaders, and filled with additional accessory cones.	
Warm vertical condensation	A master cone corresponding to the final instrumentation size and length of the canal is fitted, coated with sealer, heated, and compacted vertically with pluggers.	
Continuous wave obturating technique (CWOT)	Continuous wave is essentially a variation of warm vertical compaction (downpacking) of core material and sealer in the apical portion of the root canal using commercially available heating devices and then backfilling the remaining portion of the root canal with thermoplasticized core material using injection devices.	*Downpacking Devices*: System B (SybronEndo, Orange, CA) and Elements Obturation Unit (SybronEndo, Orange, CA) *Backfilling devices*: Obtura (Obtura Spartan, Earth City, MO), Elements Obturation Unit (SybronEndo)
Warm lateral	A master cone corresponding to the final instrumentation size of the canal is coated with sealer, inserted into the canal, heated with a warm spreader, laterally compacted with spreaders, and filled with additional accessory cones. Some devices use vibration in addition to the warm spreader.	
Injection techniques	A preheated, thermoplasticized, injectable core material is injected directly into the root canal. A master cone is not used, but sealer is placed in the canal before injection.	Obtura (Obtura Spartan, Earth City, MO), or Ultrafil (Coltene Whaledent) or Calamus (Dentsply Tulsa Dental Specialties)
	Cold, flowable matrix that is triturated and consists of gutta-percha added to a resin sealer. The technique involves injecting the material into the canal and placing a single master cone.	GuttaFlow (Coltene Whaledent)
Thermomechanical	A cone coated with sealer is placed in the root canal and engaged with a rotary instrument that frictionally warms, plasticizes, and compacts it into the root canal.	
Carrier-Based	*Carrier-Based Thermoplasticized:* Warm gutta-percha, on a plastic carrier, is delivered directly into the canal as a root canal filling	ThermaFil (Dentsply Tulsa Dental Specialties), Realseal 1 (Sybron), Densfil (Dentsply Maillefer, Tulsa, OK)
	Carrier-Based Sectional: A sized and fitted section of gutta-percha with sealer is inserted into the apical 4 mm of the root canal. The remaining portion of the root canal is filled with injectable, thermoplasticized gutta-percha using an injection gun.	SimpliFill (Discus Dental)

gutta-percha and sealer in one product; and glass ionomer embedded in gutta-percha cones.

Temperature-controlled devices for delivering gutta-percha

The DownPak Cordless device (EI, a Hu-Friedy Company, Chicago, IL), System B, and Touch 'n Heat (SybronEndo) are devices available as alternatives to applying heat with a flame-heated instrument because they permit temperature control (Figure 5.4).

Downpak (Hu-Freidy)

An alternative to cold lateral compaction is ultrasonics and, more recently, a combination of vibration and heat using the DownPak Obturation Device. Lateral condensation can be employed by alternating heat after the placement of each accessory gutta-percha cone; heat can be transferred to the canal to soften the cones for better condensation and homogeneity of both the sealer and the gutta-percha. It is used in Europe under the name EndoTwinn.

The Downpak, introduced in 2007, is cordlessand has a multifunctional endodontic heating and vibrating spreader device; it can be used for both vertical and lateral obturation. It uses a combination of controlled heat application and sonic vibrations to plasticize the gutta-percha. While the temperature can be graduated and controlled in intensity during the procedure, it also allows the vibrations to be turned off when required. This allows Downpak to be used with different materials like gutta-percha, Resilon and hybrid resin filling materials having variable softening temperatures, making it a versatile system.

The heat-carrying tips are designed in nickel–titanium and Ultrasoft stainless steel for use in tapered root canals. The technique involves adapting a master cone in the same manner as with lateral compaction. A master gutta-percha cone that reaches to the working end is selected. This is followed by selecting an appropriate spreader of the system, reaching 2.0 mm short of the working length. The system is activated and heated in the temperature cum vibration mode for 2 seconds and subsequently inserted till it reaches the predetermined binding point. A spreader is then used to condense the filling material. This is followed by the insertion of accessory cones, and the procedure is repeated till the spreader can insert for no more than 2.0 mm into the canal.

The heat-carrying tips are designed in nickel–titanium and Ultrasoft stainless steel for use in tapered root canals.

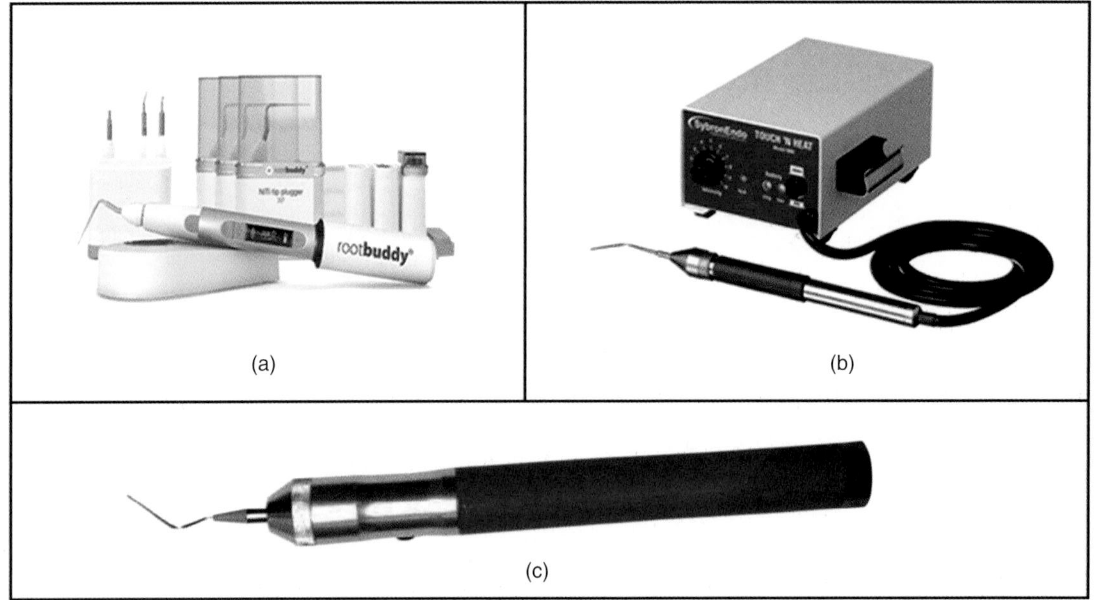

Figure 5.4 *a*, Downpak Obturation System (now marketed as Rootbuddy) (Nikinc Dental, Eindhoven, Netherlands). *b*, Touch 'N Heat System (SybronEndo, Orange, CA, USA). *c*, Endotec II (Medidenta International Inc.).

The combined use of heat and vibration by this system has been proven to provide denser, more compact fillings than heat alone. The system is no longer under Hu-Freidy and is now directed under Nikinc Dental with the name *Root Buddy.*

Endotec II (Medidenta International, Woodside, NY, USA)

Developed by Dr. Harvard Martin, this is a battery-powered, heat-controlled spreader/plugger used for warm lateral compaction of gutta-percha. It combines the simplicity and accurate length control of the lateral compaction technique with the clinical advantages of warm vertical compaction to attain superior obturations where the gutta-percha is made to coalesce and fuse into a dense, homogeneous mass with better adaptability to the root canal [63]. Investigators have found that warm lateral compaction with the Endotec II increased the weight of the gutta-percha mass when compared with traditional cold lateral compaction The Endotec II thermal endodontic condenser reportedly can be used with any curved canal preparation technique and provides calibrated heating with a 3D fill [64].

The instrument consists of a cordless battery-operated handpiece with a heat depressor button for a precise temperature control and with a quick-change top that is used to deliver heat and to thermo-soften the gutta-percha using a specially designed and shaped instrument tip. These tips contain a microheating element. The tips are autoclavable and can be angulated to adjust to any access.

Once the master cone is placed, the Endotec tip is fitted and canal length is marked to 2 to 4 mm short of the apex. The tip is then heat activated outside the canal for 3 to 4 seconds and inserted to the marked length in a circumferential rotation manner for 5 to 8 seconds and removed cold while laterally spreading on withdrawal. The procedure is repeated till the entire canal is completely filled [65].

Touch 'n Heat system (Sybron Endo)

The Touch 'n Heat system was designed by Dr. Herbert Schilder and provides an excellent source of heat for searing off excess gutta-percha during any obturation technique. The Touch 'n Heat eliminates the need for open flame in the operatory, resulting in added safety and controlled heat delivery to the working site. It has the added advantages of adjustable heat intensity and single touch activation, and it allows multiple tip styles to be accommodated. Studies have shown Touch 'n Heat to produce lesser voids in the root filling than other temperature-control devices, such as System B [66].

System B Heat Source (Sybron Endo)

System B is a new generation of portable obturation devices. This cordless obturation system permits fill and pack units for use with any warm vertical technique. System B uses a continuous wave compaction technique, which is a variation of warm vertical compaction. Tapered stainless steel pluggers are used with the System B for this technique. The gutta-percha cones mimic the tapered preparation, permitting application of greater hydraulic force during compaction. After fitting the master cone, a plugger is sized to fit within 5 to 7 mm of the canal length.

The System B unit is set to 200°C in touch mode. The plugger is inserted into the canal to remove the excess coronal material. Compaction is done by placing the cold plugger against the gutta-percha in the canal orifice. Firm pressure is applied, along with heat. The plugger is moved rapidly (for 1 to 2 seconds) to within 3 mm of the binding point. The heat is inactivated while firm pressure is being maintained on the plugger for 5 to 10 seconds. After the gutta-percha has cooled, the plugger is removed. In ovoid canals when the canal configuration may prevent the generation of hydraulic forces, an accessory cone can be placed alongside the master cone before compaction. Filling the remaining space left by the plugger can be accomplished with a thermoplastic-injection technique or by fitting an accessory cone into the space with sealer, heating it, and compacting it with short applications of heat and vertical pressure [67].

Injection techniques for gutta-percha

Obtura (Obtura Spartan, Earth City, MO, USA)

The Obtura II system consists of a hand-held "gun" with a chamber into which pellets of gutta-percha are loaded, along with silver needles of varying gauges of 20, 23, and 25, used to deliver the thermoplasticized material to the canal. This allows control of the viscosity of the gutta-percha through a control on the chamber temperature. A hybrid filling technique is recommended by filling the canal to approximately 4 to 5 mm from the apex, using the lateral compaction technique before gradually filling the coronal portion with thermoplasticized gutta-percha [68]. The needle backs out of the canal as it is filled, and pluggers may be then used to compact the gutta-percha. This compaction should continue until the gutta-percha cools and solidifies.

The Obtura III Max is an update that offers better tactile sensing and ergonomics. It has a redesigned handpiece and a unit that thermoplastisizes gutta-percha. The unit takes up less counter space than Obtura (Figure 5.5).

Calamus 3D Obturation system (Dentsply, Tulsa Dental Speciality)

This system uses a method of warm vertical condensation for filling the root canal. Ever since Schilder introduced the vertical condensation technique more than 40 years ago there have been various advancements in the warm gutta-percha methods, and these advancements help in filling the accessory canals. This quest has led to the development of the Calamus 3D obturation system, which progressively and continuously carries more of the gutta-percha along the master cone, starting from the coronal portion of the canal to the apical foramen.

The Calamus Dual 3D Obturation System consists of the Calamus Pack handpiece for downpacking and the Flow handpiece for backpacking (Figure 5.6). The Calamus Pack handpiece is the heat source that, in conjunction with an appropriately sized Electric Heat Plugger, is used to thermosoften and condense gutta-percha during the downpacking phase of obturation. There are three variably sized EHPs, and they are selected based on the apical size, taper, and curvature of the finished preparation.

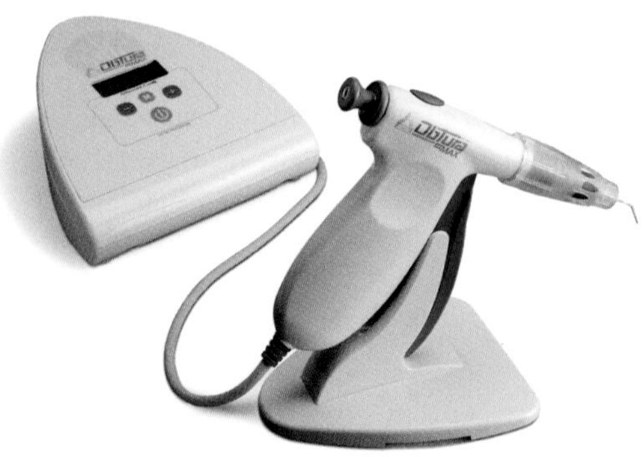

Figure 5.5 Obtura III (Obtura Spartan).

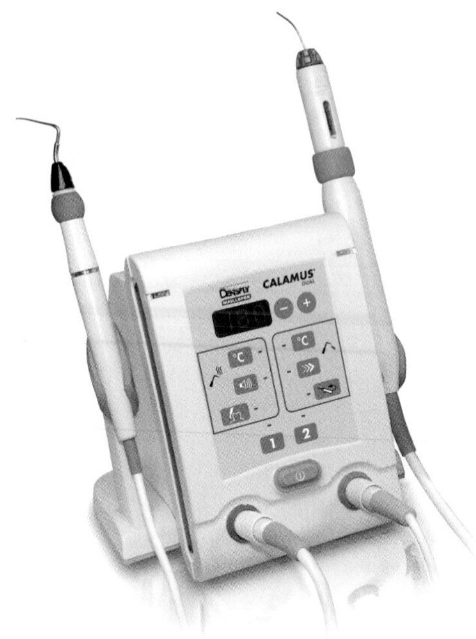

Figure 5.6 Calamus Obturation System (Dentsply) with two hand pieces for downpacking and backpacking.

The Calamus Flow handpiece is used with a gutta-percha cartridge and integrated cannula to dispense warm gutta-percha into the preparation during the backpacking phase of obturation. The cartridges are available in 20- and 23-gauge sizes. The Calamus Dual 3D Obturation System provides a bending tool that may be used to place a smooth curvature on the cannula. The choice of gutta-percha cannula depends on the desired consistency and whether or not the gutta-percha will be condensed. The temperature of the thermoplasticized gutta-percha as it is extruded through the needle tip ranges from 38°C to 44°C. The gutta-percha remains able to flow for 45 to 60 seconds, depending on the viscosity.

The downpacking phase consists of selecting the appropriate Electric Heat Plugger, which is used to sear off the gutta-percha at the orifice of the canal after selecting the master cone. The working end of the plugger is used to vertically condense the warm gutta-percha for 5 seconds, which serves in filling the root canal multidimensionally. This is termed the *wave of condensation*. This wave of condensation provides a piston effect on the sealer and produces proper hydraulics, which helps in compacting the gutta-percha laterally as well as vertically. The plugger is then deactivated, is allowed to cool, and is removed. Then the second wave of condensation is carried out. Three or four heating cycles are required depending on the length of the canal to place the Electric Heat Plugger within 5 mm of the apex.

The backpacking phase involves the back filling or reverse filling of the gutta-percha in the remaining coronal portion of the root canal. The thermosoftened gutta-percha cartridge is placed into the canal with the help of the warm cannula and dispensed on the downpacked gutta-percha. The Calamus handpiece is activated and 2 to 3 mm of gutta-percha is dispensed into the apical portion of the canal. The handpiece helps in the backout from the canal. The backfilling technique is continued till the entire canal has been filled [69].

The Elements Obturation Unit (Sybron Endo)

The Elements system combines a System B device and a gutta-percha extruder in a motorized handpiece to make obturation efficient, predictable, and accurate (Figures 5.7 and 5.8). From downpack to backfill, the Elements Obturation Unit puts the continuous wave of condensation technique into one simple-to-operate device that takes up only one third of the space of two separate machines. The extruder tips are sized 20-, 23-, and 25-gauge and are prebent.

System B forms the right portion of the system, with functions preset for temperature and duration. The tip temperature is continuously maintained and displayed, and the system has a time-out feature that prevents overheating. Extruder forms the left portion of the system, which is a handpiece for gutta-percha delivery. It consists of a precise temperature control in a motorized handpiece that eliminates hand fatigue and precludes voids. Both the handpieces have a silicon booting that serves as an insulator to avoid heat conduction to the clinician's hands during its operation [70].

GuttaFlow Obturation System (Coltène/Whaledent, Altstätten, Switzerland)

The GuttaFlow was introduced in pursuit of complete 3D sealing of root canal walls. It uses silicone polymer technology consisting of finely ground gutta-percha (Roekoseal) and nanosilver (Inside Dentistry). This is a cold fluid obturation system that combines polydimethylsiloxane sealer (explained earlier), powdered gutta-percha with a particle size of less than 30 μm, and nanosilver particles (Figures 5.9 and 5.10). The manufacturer claims GuttaFlow does not shrink, but it expands minimally (0.2%) to seal the root canals, is and it is thixotrophic, which decreases the viscosity under pressure and allows it to flow in the lateral canals. GuttaFlow has very promising properties because of its insolubility, biocompatibility, post-setting expansion, great fluidity, and ability for providing a thin film of sealer, and hence greater adhesion with the dentinal wall [7] and the gutta- percha master cone [13]. GuttaFlow consists of nanosilver in its composition. Nanosilver is metallic silver that is distributed uniformly on the surface of the filling. The nanosilver particles found in GuttaFlow provide better protection against reinfection, are highly compatible, and prevent any corrosion or discoloration [14].

The apical preparation should be as small as possible to prevent extrusion. The viscosity diminishes under pressure, enabling flow into the smallest canals. GuttaFlow can be applied directly into the canal. After thorough debridement and cleaning and shaping of the root canals with copious amount of irrigation, the canals are dried and the master cone is selected. The GuttaFlow is dispensed in capsule from, which can be mixed in a triturator. The canal tip is placed on the capsule, which is fitted on the dispensing gun. It is always better to dispense some amount of the mixed GuttaFlow onto the pad to confirm the color is pink, the sign of a complete mix. The obturation begins by applying a small amount of GuttaFlow into the root canal with the help of a master cone or master apical file or by directly dispensing the GuttaFlow into the canal with the help of canal tip. The master cone is then coated with additional GuttaFlow and inserted to the working length. The GuttaFlow dispenser is used to backfill the root of the canal and is seared off at the orifice of the canal. The working time is 15 minutes, and GuttaFlow sets in 25 to 30 minutes [71, 72].

Ultrafil System (Hygienic-Coltene-Whaledent, Akron, OH, USA)

The Ultrafil system is based on the technique of low-temperature (70°C) injection of thermoplasticized gutta-percha. The cannula that contains gutta-percha is preheated and inserted into the root canal with an injection syringe. The system comes with a portable heating unit and sets regardless of the temperature or moisture. It has low solubility as well.

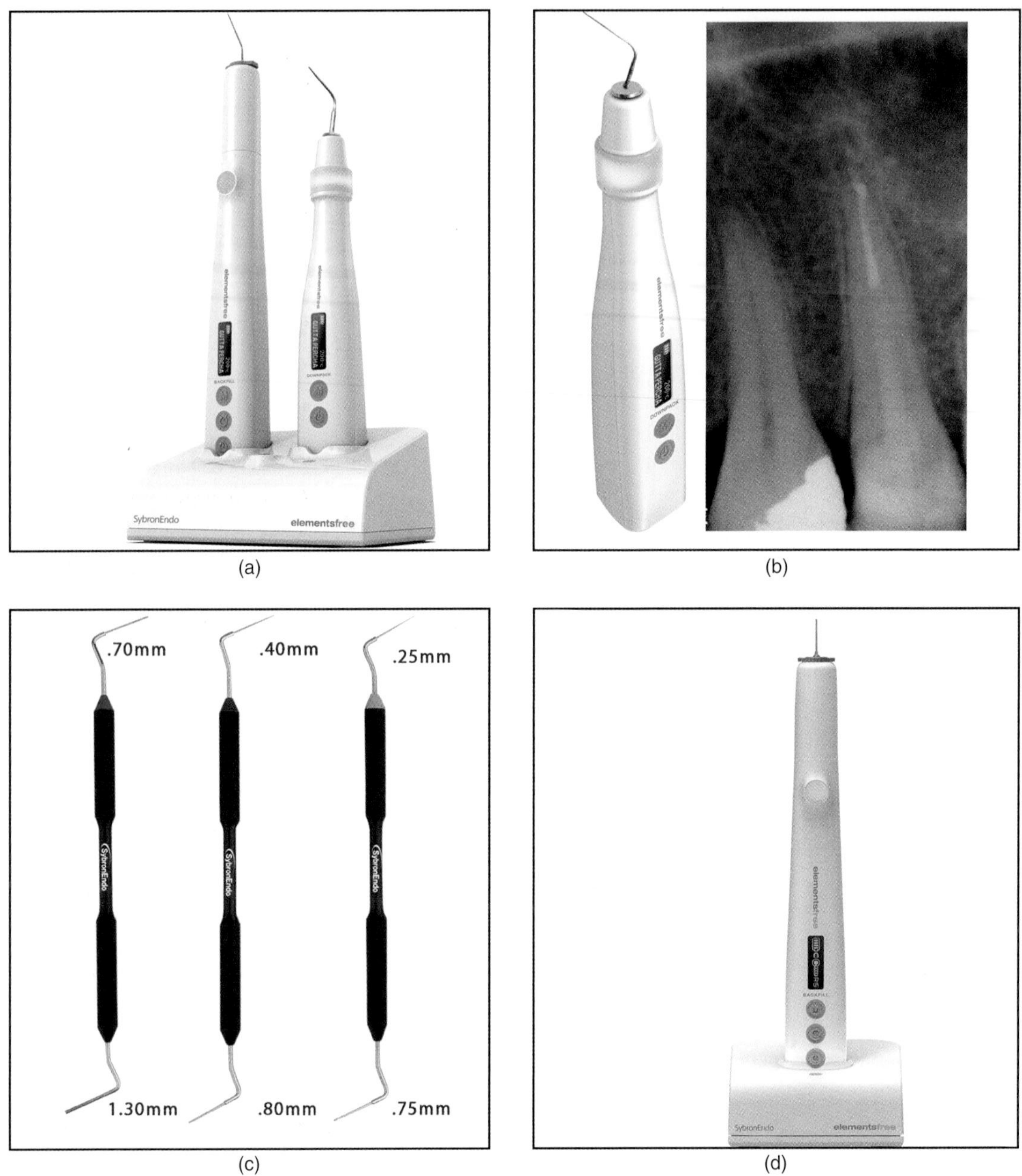

Figure 5.7 *a*, Elements Free Obturation System. *b*, Downpack with the Downpack Unit. *c*, Buchanan hand pluggers with one end stainless steel and the other end nickel titanium. *d*, Backfill unit.

Carrier-based obturation (CBO)

An endodontic obturator is a plastic rod with an attached handle (which in combination is known as a carrier), that has either gutta-percha or Resilon attached to it. Carrier-based obturation is one of the most popular techniques of root canal filling worldwide. This simple and effective procedure significantly reduces dentists' working time while ensuring high-quality obturation, especially in narrow root canals and anatomically complex canals.

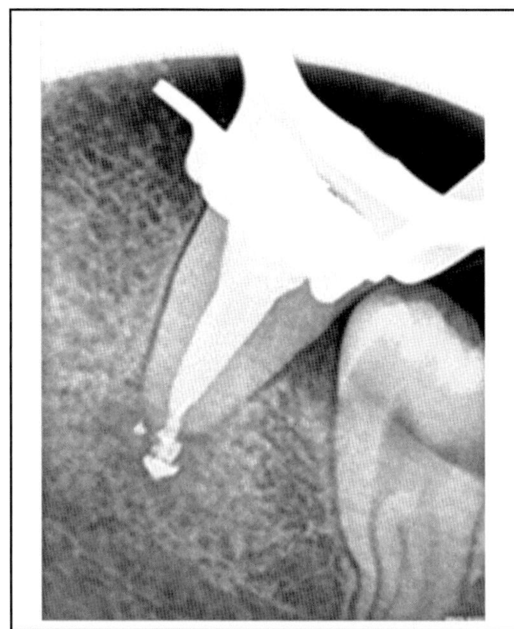

Figure 5.8 Case treated using Elements Obturation Unit. (Image courtesy of Dr. Shilpa V. Shettigar.)

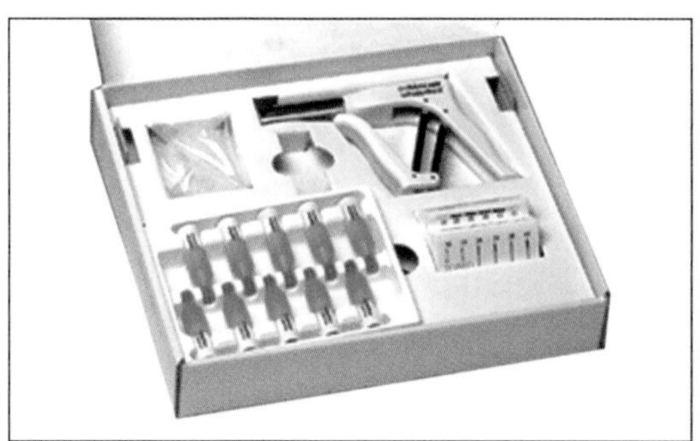

Figure 5.9 Gutta flow system including capsules, ISO-sized canal tips, and dispenser. (Image courtesy of Dr. Ruchika Roongta.)

Carrier-based obturation was first described in 1978 and involved the coating of endodontic files with thermoplasticized gutta-percha, with the carrier remaining in the canal as an integral part of the obturating material. Carriers for core-based techniques can be fabricated using different materials. Thermafil small obturators (up to size 40) (Dentsply Tulsa Dental, Tulsa, OK, USA) are made of Vectra, which is a liquid crystal polymer, and larger sizes are made of polysulfone, whereas GuttaCore carriers (Dentsply Tulsa Dental) are made of cross-linked gutta-percha. These materials are coated with alpha-phase gutta-percha.

Thermafil (Dentsply Tulsa Dental, Tulsa, OK, USA)

Thermafil was first introduced in the United States with a metal carrier coated with gutta-percha. The current version uses specialized plastic carriers coated with gutta-percha, which are thermoplasticized in a special oven before they are inserted into the canal (Figure 5.11). They are known as Thermafil Plus. Both the old and the new system have been found to be biocompatible.

SimpliFill (Discus Dental, Culver City, CA, USA)

The SimpliFill device is a cold carrier-based obturation system that features a removable carrier, leaving nothing in the canal except for the obturation material. Only the apical portion of the carrier has a coating of gutta-percha or Resilon. This technique may be used with the conventional sealers or the resin-based sealers. The carrier has an apical plug attached with 5 mm of gutta-percha. With the plug at the corrected working length, the handle is quickly rotated counterclockwise a minimum of four complete turns. The coronal space can then be filled with gutta-percha.

Other systems

Successfil (Coltene-Whaledent) uses gutta-percha in a syringe. Carriers may be either titanium or radiopaque plastic. This technique offers flexibility with regard to shape and the amount of gutta-percha extruded onto the carrier.

The *JS Quick-Fill* (JS Manufacturing) is an obturation system with alpha-phase gutta-percha on a specially designed titanium carrier.

The *Microseal* endodontic obturation system (Sybron Endo) associates a master gutta-percha cone with thermoplasticized gutta-percha, which is inserted into the root canal with a compactor.

Other examples of carrier-based obturation systems currently available are ProSystem GT Obturators (Dentsply), Soft Core (Axis Dental, Coppell, TX, USA), and Densfil (Dentsply).

Limitations of carrier-based obturation

The combination of thermoplasticized gutta-percha and a plastic carrier acting as a compactor inserted close to working length seems to minimize the presence of

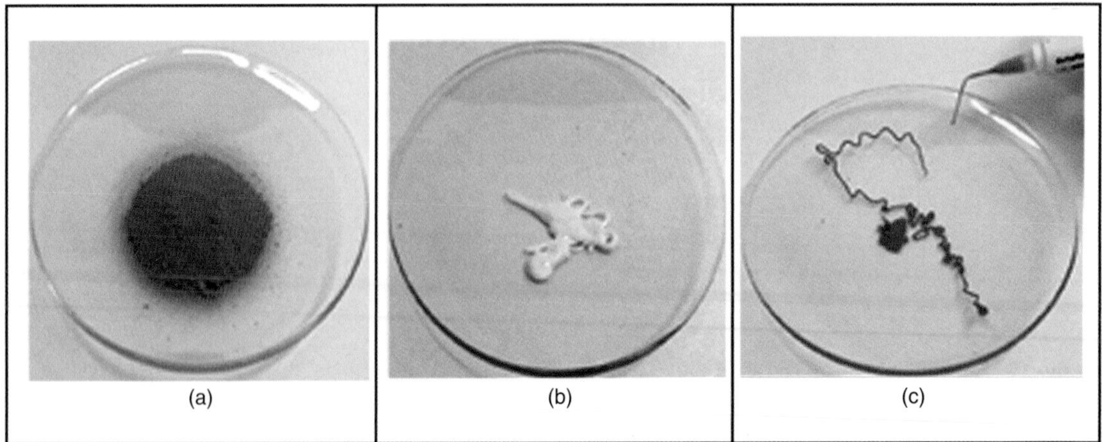

Figure 5.10 *a,* GuttaFlow powder. *b,* GuttaFlow sealer. *c,* Mixed Gutta Flow powder and sealer. (Image courtesy of Dr. Ruchika Roongta.)

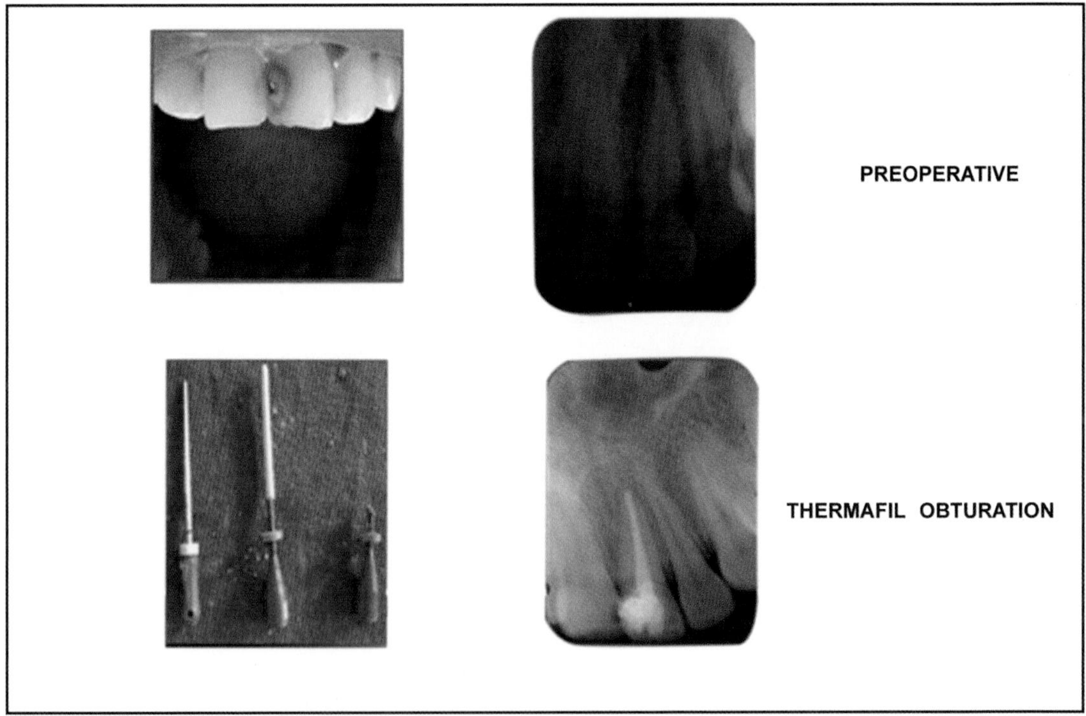

Figure 5.11 Thermafil obturation.

voids when compared to lateral compaction. One of the critiques of any carrier-based obturation technique is the risk of extruding sealer and gutta-percha from the apical foramen, although there are conflicting results in the literature.

A potential disadvantage of a carrier-based root-filling system is denudation of the core with stripping of the gutta-percha coating [73]. Stripping of gutta-percha from the carrier might happen during the insertion of the carriers into the root canal space, particularly in narrow or severely curved canals. This would result in voids and inadequate filling of the root canal space [74]. Studies have shown that the most common cause of stripping of the gutta-percha coating are twisting the carrier during insertion into the root canal space [75, 76]. Adhesion between the carrier and gutta-percha coating is an important aspect in the choice of a core-based obturation system and would help avoid stripping of the gutta-percha coating, creating a root canal filling with fewer voids.

Another potential disadvantage of currently available carrier-based obturation systems is that the volume of gutta-percha is not uniformly distributed around the carrier. This might cause stripping of the gutta-percha from the carrier material when the obturator is inserted into the root canal space, leading to possible voids [73]. The frictional forces present between the gutta-percha and the root canal walls can create an extrusion effect, whereby the filling material is retained at the orifice of the canal [77].

There are a number of myths surrounding the use of carrier-based obturation. Some researchers believe that application of obturators causes periodontal tissue damage, manifested by postoperative sensitivity. This can occur due to the extrusion of the air from the root canal space into the periapical tissues during insertion of the obturator. Such sensitivity resolves spontaneously, without subsequent development of any complications. In addition, some clinicians believe that it is hard to remove obturators from the canal for retreatment, but literature suggests that removing an obturator filling from a canal takes even less time than retreatment of a canal filled with gutta-percha [78, 79]. Dentists also find it difficult to prepare a post space when a carrier-based technique has been used.

GuttaCore System (Dentsply Tulsa Dental Specialties)

The main concern of dentists using carrier-based systems is the presence of the plastic carrier in them. The GuttaCore system demonstrates a new application in the concept of carrier-based gutta-percha. The obturator carriers are not made from plastic, but from a gutta-percha elastomer with intermolecular cross links (cross-linked gutta-percha). Thus, the obturator is made entirely of gutta-percha in two different forms and does not have the polysulfone carrier. It has an internal core of cross-linked gutta-percha, which means the outer surface of the cross-linked gutta-percha will have alpha gutta-percha. This gives a sandwich of gutta-percha (Figure 5.12).

This accounts for not only rapid and high-quality three-dimensional root canal obturation but also for an easy post space preparation and root filling removal, in case retreatment is required. The carrier can be removed from the root canal just as easily as gutta-percha can, since it also is gutta-percha. The same instruments

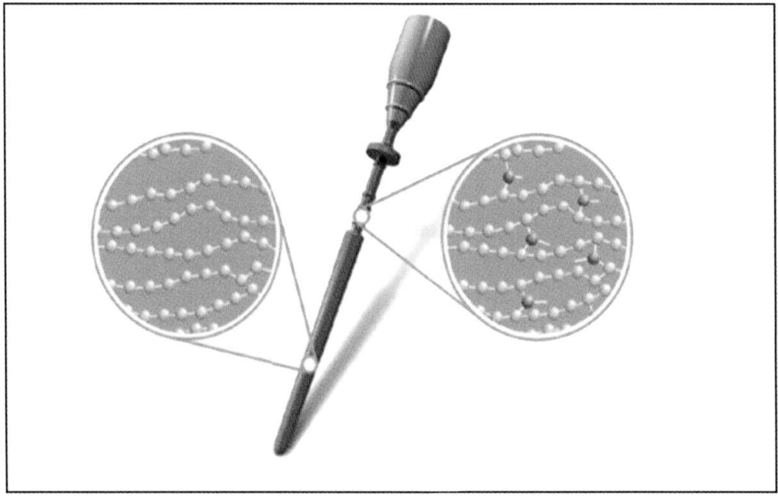

Figure 5.12 GuttaCore obturator structure. (Image courtesy of Dentsply MEA.)

used in lateral or vertical condensation techniques may be used.

Technique

The root canal must be properly shaped and disinfected. It is recommended that when using the GuttaCore system, the root canal must be widened to at least size 20/.06 or 25/.04. Select the right GuttaCore obturator diameter. If .06 or larger instruments were used to prepare the root canal, then select an obturator of the same size as the final nickel–titanium file. If .04 instruments were employed, then select an obturator one size smaller. Under no circumstances should any gutta-percha be cut off from the obturator, because this can damage the carrier.

Gauging the root canal is a very important stage. This can be done with a verifier that is passively inserted to the working length of the root canal. If the verifier does not passively fit to working length, it can be used as a finishing file for apical enlargement.

A thin layer of sealer is then applied to the coronal or, in case of long root canals, the coronal and middle thirds of the canal. The working length is set on the oburator, after which it is placed into a holder of one of the ThermaPrep 2 (Dentsply Tulsa Dental Specialties) oven's heating elements. Unlike obturators with a plastic carrier, a minimum heating level of 20°C to 25°C is required, regardless of the obturator size with the GuttaCore system. The distinguishing characteristics of the ThermaPrep 2 oven are rapid three-dimensional heating of obturators while maintaining the properties of the gutta-percha carrier, as well as the option of having both heating elements operating simultaneously.

The obturator is inserted into the root canal to the working length slowly, without rotation. The heated gutta-percha can be condensed with a plugger in the coronal part of the root canal. This generates additional hydrodynamic pressure, enabling the gutta-percha to fill the ramifications of the main canal. The carrier can then be cut off at the orifice using a regular round bur.

Adhesive obturation

With the development of the new material, Resilon, a number of manufacturers have introduced newer Resilon-based obturation systems.

Epiphany System (Pentron Clinical Technologies)

Epiphany is available as standardized points or pellets to be used with conventional thermoplasticized gutta-percha systems. The Epiphany sealer is recommended to be used with the Epiphany self-etch primer.

RealSeal/RealSeal SE (SybronEndo)

RealSeal points are identical to Resilon obturating points composed of polyester polymers, methacrylate resins, bioactive glass, and radiopaque fillers. The points look, feel, and handle clinically almost identically to gutta-percha. The material can be re-treated with gutta-percha solvents. RealSeal sealer contains UDMA, PEGDMA, EBPADMA and BisGMA resins, silane-treated barium borosilicate glasses, barium sulfate, silica, calcium hydroxide, bismuth oxychloride with amines, peroxide, photo initiator, stabilizers, and pigment, as described earlier. RealSeal Primer is an acidic monomer solution in water.

The RealSeal system is quite similar to the Epiphany system: It includes standardized and nonstandardized points and pellets. The system is available in two variants: the RealSeal system and the RealSeal Self-Etch (SE) system. The Self-Etch system eliminates the priming step. The RealSeal Hi Flow pellets available with the RealSeal system are used with the Elements obturation unit. The reduction of coronal microleakage occurs as a function of RealSeal's ability to be bonded to the canal wall through the creation of a hybrid layer. This requires the removal of the smear layer by rinsing with EDTA. This opens the tubules, and the dentin wall is then covered with the self-etching primer. A hybrid layer is created on top of this with the placement of the sealer. This bonding helps to decrease the amount of bacteria that might be able to migrate in a coronal-to-apical direction. The root canals are then obturated with either a lateral or vertical condensation technique. RealSeal can be compacted, and can also be used in an Obtura gun as injectable filling material.

Carrier-based adhesive obturation

RealSeal One (SybronEndo)

Real Seal One is carrier-based bonded obturating material containing a radiopaque core of polysulfone coated with RealSeal. Like the original RealSeal obturation system, RealSeal One uses Resilon as the filling material. It coats the outside of the core and is thermoplasticized by a proprietary oven. The current carrier-based obturation systems use gutta-percha. Due to the nature of gutta-percha, it cannot be injection molded. Rather, it must be applied to the carrier by dipping. This process can lead to an uneven distribution of gutta-percha on the carrier. When these carriers encounter a constriction in the canal, the gutta-percha coating can be stripped off rather easily, as explained earlier.

On the other hand, the RealSeal One obturator is formed and covered with Resilon using injection molding, making a consistent covering of the core. The compatibility of the resin-based Resilon and the resin core material allows the adhesion of the Resilon to the core. Therefore, when the obturator encounters a constriction in the canal, only the surface portion of the Resilon is stripped away. A thin layer of Resilon still remains adhered to the carrier, which is sufficient to the allow adhesion of the resin-based sealer to the core.

For post space preparation and re-treatment purposes, the removal of the Resilon filling material and the core of the RealSeal One obturators is relatively easy to accomplish. For re-treatment, solvent will soften both the Resilon and the obturator core in just a few minutes.

Because The RS One is one injection-molded unit, the core is always centered in the obturating point. This helps the placement with the core centered and an even layer of RealSeal available around it to bond to the sealer. Only methacrylate-based sealer can be used with this. All other sealers are contraindicated. RealSeal One is recommended for use with RealSeal SE self-etching dual cure resin primer. Since Resilon is hydrophilic, a slightly moist canal is required for optimal bond strength. This provides the same benefit as RealSeal and Resilon, with the potential for reduced microleakage, and a monoblock bonded obturation of the root canal.

Resinate (Obtura Spartan)

The Resinate system is similar to the Epiphany system in that it includes standardized and nonstandardized points and pellets. The sealer is delivered from an automix syringe. The Resinate pellets are designed to be used with the Obtura thermoplasticized obturation system.

Structural obturators: fiber resin post obturation systems

In 2001, Pentron Clinical Technologies introduced the first obturator, FibreFill, with a precisely-sized gutta-percha cone on the end of its highly successful resin fiber post, allowing the simultaneous placement of the obturator and a post. In 2005, Heraeus Kulzer introduced a similar system, InnoEndo, that used Resilon instead of gutta-percha as the obturation material.

Both systems make use of an adhesive bonding agent, a light-curable $Ca(OH)_2$-based resin sealer and a fiber post with an apical terminus of Resilon. A primer included in the system is a self-etching two-bottle liquid that allows the sealer to chemically bond to the canal dentin. The primer is a self-curing adhesive. The root canal sealer is a radiopaque dual-cure resin sealer that contains UDMA, PEGDMA, HDDMA, and BISGMA resins with silane-treated barium borosilcate glasses, barium sulfate, and calcium hydroxide together with polymerization initiators. The material is supplied in a two-barrel automix syringe.

These systems offer several advantages to the clinician. Research has shown that they provide a bonded resin apical and coronal seal, which is superior to gutta-percha, and AH-26 placed either laterally or as a warm vertical compaction [80–82]. The obturator and sealer strengthen the root against fracture [83] and help in the retention of the core. Because the obturators are placed passively, it eliminates any possibility of root strain, which could result in root fracture. The sealers are biocompatible, noninflammatory, and nonmutagenic [84].

The InnoEndo system contains drill-less posts (the same size and taper as .04 files), which eliminates the need to remove additional structure from the root, shortening the length of the procedure and safeguarding the root against fracture. The bond of the post to the radicular dentin is maximized, because there is no opportunity for obturation material to be burnished into the walls of the dentin that would minimize bonding sites [85].

Fiberfill offers a parallel-sided fiber post with either a 5- or 8-mm gutta-percha terminal portion or a tapered obturator with Resilon terminus. The taper obturator has a continuous taper and is available in either .02 or .04 tapers with a 12-mm Resilon terminus. This permits retreatment of the canal should it become necessary. The gutta-percha comes in lengths of 5 mm or 8 mm.

The diameter of the post includes sizes 30, 40, 50, 60, 70, and 80.

The Next endodontic obturating system was introduced initially, followed by the InnoEndo endodontic obturating system. The system uses a two-bottle bonding system followed by the use of either an InnoEndo obturator (for straight single canals) or the tapered obturator designed with a resin fiber carrier (for posterior teeth) bonded using a dual-cured root canal sealant. The advantage is that the system provides a post and core in a single appointment.

After the cleaning and shaping procedures are completed, an appropriate-sized obturator is selected according to the diameter of the canal. The yellow Peeso-reamer (available in the kit) is inserted, which is either set at 5 mm or 8 mm from the apical terminus, followed by the introduction of the blue Peeso-reamer to a similar depth. The canal is then finally rinsed, irrigated, and dried. This is followed by the application of primer. The primer is applied to the depth made by the Peeso-reamer. The sealer is then introduced into the canal. The obturator is gently placed to the working length so that it allows excess sealer to be coronally expressed. The Fiberfill RCS is then cured to stabilize the coronal portion. This is followed by resin core buildup over the obturator, and the material is light cured.

SmartSeal (Prosmart-DRFP Ltd., Stamford, UK)

Materials used in dentistry can be classified as bio-inert (passive), bioactive, and bioresponsive or smart materials based on their interactions with the environment. Smart materials can be defined as designed materials that have one or more properties that can be significantly changed in a controlled fashion by external stimuli, such as stress, temperature, moisture, pH, and electric or magnetic fields [86]. These materials are also referred to as *responsive materials*.

SmartSeal is a root canal obturating system based on polymer technology. Its principle is based on the hydrophilic nature of the obturating points, which can absorb surrounding moisture and expand, resulting in filling of voids and spaces. This is known as ProSmart outside the United Kingdom. This is considered to exhibit smart behavior and incorporates developments in hydrophilic polymer plastics. SmartSeal is a two-part system consisting of Propoint and Smart paste/Smart paste Bio.

Propoint

Propoint is also known as C Point. The C Point system (EndoTechnologies, LLC, Shrewsbury, MA, USA) is a point-and-paste root canal filling technique that consists of premade hydrophilic endodontic points and an accompanying sealer. It consists of two parts. The inner core of C Point is a mix of two proprietary nylon polymers: Trogamid T and Trogamid CX. This provides the point with the flexibility to allow it to easily pass around any curves in the canal space, while being rigid enough to pass easily to length in narrower canals.

The outer polymer layer is a cross-linked copolymer of acrylonitrile and vinylpyrrolidone, which has been polymerized and cross-linked using allyl methacrylate and a thermal initiator. This hydrophilic hydrogel layer allows the point to swell laterally by absorbing residual water from the instrumented canal space and from naturally occurring intraradicular moisture. It does not swell axially, so there is no length change, and radial swelling stops once a seal is created. This lateral expansion of C Point is dependent on the extent to which the hydrophilic polymer is prestressed (i.e., contact with a canal wall reduces the rate or extent of polymer expansion) [87]. The points can expand up to around 17% and will still give the same x-ray appearance as with conventional root-filling materials [88]. The expansion is minuscule and is claimed by the manufacturer to be within the reported tensile strength of dentin. The expansion occurs within the first 4 hours after placing the point into the canal. This allows the sealer and the polymer to penetrate into the dentinal tubules and produce a seal that is highly impermeable to bacterial microleakage.

The clinical steps include selection of a Propoint that matches the last file used to prepare the canal. It is tried, inserted into the canal up to the working length, and confirmed by the use of radiographs. Then the premixed sealer is introduced into the canal using syringe tips. The Propoint is then introduced into the canal, with the help of tweezers, using slow, uniform pressure. Care should be taken that the sealer is applied evenly on the canal walls and that the Propoint is trimmed at the canal orifice using a high-speed handpiece with a diamond bur and ultimately restored using any conventional material [88, 89].

Smartpaste

Smartpaste is a resin-based sealer containing an active polymer that swells to fill any voids or cavities in the root canal. The degree of swelling is controlled by the amount of active polymer used. The polymer can also swell at a later date to fill any voids that might develop.

Smartpaste Bio is a resin-based sealant with the addition of bioceramics. The manufacturer claims that this gives the sealer exceptional dimensional stability and makes it nonresorbable inside the root canal. Smartpaste Bio produces calcium hydroxide and hydroxyapatite as byproducts of the setting reaction, making the material antibacterial and biocompatible. The setting time is delayed (4–10 hours), thus, allowing the Propoint to hydrate and swell to fill any voids. The sealant is delivered in a premixed syringe and does not require mixing, so it can be applied directly into the canal using an intracanal tip, minimizing wastage of material. The cement absorbs water from within the canal, and once set Smartpaste Bio produces a radiopaque biocompatible cement.

Activ GP Precision Obturation System (single cone technique) (Endosequence and Brasseler USA)

Activ GP is the second tertiary monoblock material that uses conventional gutta-percha cones that are surface coated with glass ionomer fillers using a proprietary technique [1]. The first is EndoREZ, already explained earlier. Both systems require the use of either a single-cone technique or a technique that involves the passive placement of accessory cones without lateral compaction (harpooning technique), to avoid the disruption of these external coatings.

The Activ GP Precision Obturation System uses glass ionomer technology, extending the working time of the glass ionomer sealer by modifying its particle size to the nanoparticle level (Figure 5.13). The gutta-percha cones are coated with glass ionomer particles at a thickness of 2 μm. By coating the cones, a stiffer gutta-percha cone is achieved that transforms it into a gutta-percha core/cone, enabling the latter to function as both the tapered filling cone and as its own carrier core, thus avoiding the need for a separate interior carrier of plastic or metal [90]. This also allows it to be bonded to the root dentin via a glass ionomer sealer [91]. Because this system is new, limited information is available.

The cones are available in ISO sizes 15 to 60 in either a .04 or .06 taper in traditional-style cones. The sealer is provided in a liquid–powder formulation with a working time of 12 minutes. Heated downpack techniques are not advised because heat accelerates the setting of the sealer. The Activ GP system cones are available in two designs: the traditional design and the newer enhanced version Activ GP Plus. The Activ GP Plus has calibration rings for easy depth measurement and a unique barrel

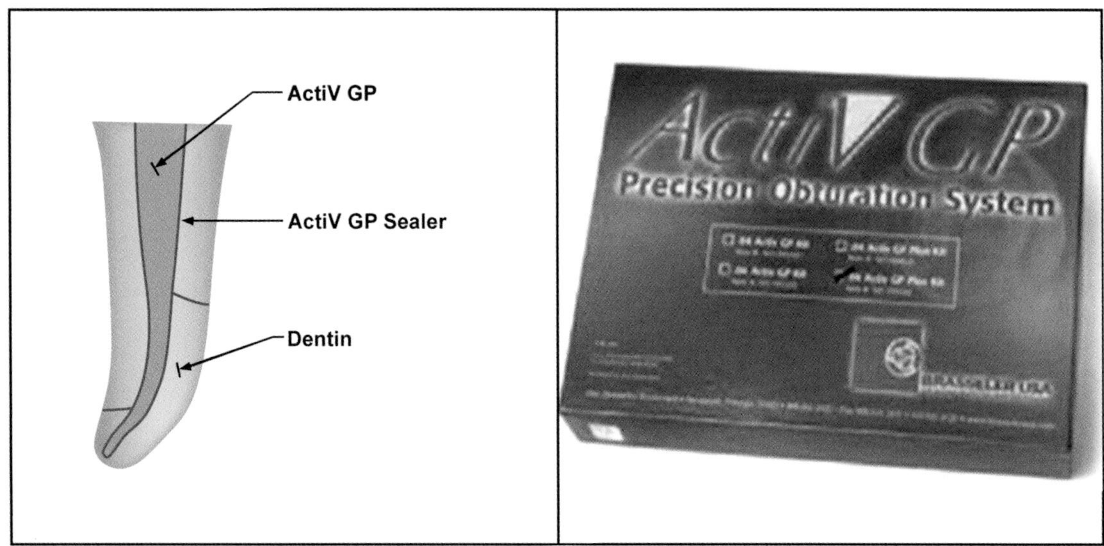

Figure 5.13 ActiV GP.

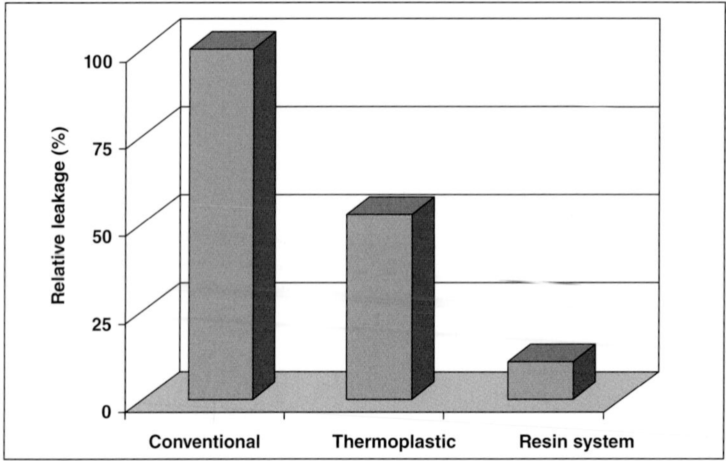

Figure 5.14 Relative leakage behavior of endodontic obturation techniques. (From Von Fraunofer JA. Dental materials at a glance. Oxford: Wiley-Blackwell; 2009).

handle for easier insertion into the canal when used with a transporter. The Activ GP cones are verified by laser measurement to match the preparation made by .04 or .06 tapered EndoSequence file system.

The clinical steps comprise completion of the preparation followed by verification of the fit of the Activ GP cone. Sodium hypochlorite can be used as the final irrigant. A file is coated with the Activ GP sealer and is applied on the canal walls. The Activ GP cone is also coated with the sealer and slowly inserted into the canal to the working length. This allows the excess sealer to extrude coronally, if present. After the Activ GP cone has been seated, the GP is seared off at the orifice and the coronal 2 mm of GP is removed and filled with GP sealer on top. Both the sealer and the Activ GP cone provide a dense radiopaque fill.

The cones can be bent up to 180 degrees and are matched in size to the preparations created by the files. Matching of the primary cone to the preparation is very important with any single-cone technique, because the accurate fit of the cone to the preparation minimizes the amount of sealer used, as well as minimizing any potential shrinkage. However, studies have demonstrated that because it is a single-cone technique, coronal leakage of the Activ GP system was probably due to the increase in the volume of the glass ionomer cement sealer [92]. Therefore, it is also unlikely that the use of the Activ GP system will improve the fracture resistance of endodontically treated teeth.

Conclusion

The art and science of endodontic therapy has changed drastically with the introduction of evidence-based protocols (Figure 5.14). Although gutta-percha and the traditional sealers might not meet all the criteria for an ideal root canal filling material, they have withstood the test of time. The obturation material selected, whether a traditional or a more modern one, must be consistent with the principles of clinical practice, namely, to provide the best treatment for patients. A seal of the root canal system is desirable and essential for the success of the treatment, but modern materials and methods available for obturation do not always achieve this physical and biological goal. The clinician must make the appropriate use of the selected material and method. The advent of new devices and techniques are revolutionizing the science of endodontics and making root filling procedures more predictable.

References

1 Koch K, Brave D. A new endodontic obturation technique, http://www.dentistrytoday.com/endodontics/1104.

2 al-Khatib ZZ, Baum RH, Morse DR, Yesilsoy C, Bhambhani S, Furst ML. The antimicrobial effect of various endodontic sealers. *Oral Surg Oral Med Oral Pathol Oral Radiol Endod* 1990; 70:784.

3 Peters LB, Wesselink PR, Moorer WR. The fate and role of bacteria left in root dentinal tubules. *Int Endod J* 1995; 28:95.

4 Kontakiotis EG, Tzanetakis GN, Loizides AL. A 12-month longitudinal *in vitro* leakage study on a new silicon-based root canal filling material (Gutta-Flow). *Oral Surg Oral Med Oral Pathol Oral Radiol Endod* 2007; 103: 854–859.

5 Willershausen I, Callaway A, Briseño B, Willershausen B. *In vitro* analysis of the cytotoxicity and the antimicrobial effect of four endodontic sealers. *Head Face Med* 2011; 7: 15.

6 Saleh IM, Ruyter IE, Haapasalo M, Ørstavik D. Survival of *Enterococcus faecalis* in infected dentinal tubules after root canal filling with different root canal sealers *in vitro*. *Int Endod J* 2004; 37: 193–198.

7 Upadhyay V, Upadhyay M, Panday RK, Chturvedi TP, Bajpai U. A SEM evaluation of dentinal adaptation of root canal obturation with GuttaFlow and conventional obturating material. *Indian J Dent Res* 2011; 22: 1–6.

8 Buonocore MG. A simple method of increasing the adhesion of acrylic filling materials to enamel surfaces. *J Dent Res* 1955 Dec; 34(6): 849–853.

9 Schäfer E, Zandbiglari T. Solubility of root-canal sealers in water and artificial saliva. *Int Endod J* 2003; 36: 660–669.

10 Bouillaguet S, Shaw L, Barthelemy J, Krejci I, Wataha JC. Long-term sealing ability of pulp canal sealer, AH-Plus, GuttaFlow and epiphany. *Int Endod J* 2008; 41: 219–226.

11 Roggendorf M. Wurzelkanalfüllmaterialien up-to-date Klassische und moderne Wurzelkanalsealer im Vergleich. Bayerisches Zahnärzteblatt. 2004 (Sept); 32–34.

12 Bouillaguet S, Wataha JC, Tay FR, Brackett MG, Lockwood PE. Initial *in vitro* biological response to contemporary endodontic sealers. *J. Endod* 2006; 32: 989–992.

13 Coltene Group. ROEKO GuttaFlow® 2 / ROEKO GuttaFlow® 2 FAST: Root Canal Obturation. https://www.coltene.com/products-coltenewhaledent/endodontics/root-canal-obturation/roeko-guttaflowR-2-roeko-guttaflowR-2-fast/

14 De Deus G, Brandão MC, Fidel RA, Fidel SR. The sealing ability of GuttaFlow in oval-shaped canals: an *ex vivo* study using a polymicrobial leakage model. *Int Endod J* 2007; 40: 794–799.

15 Nakashima K, Terata R. Effect of pH modified EDTA solution to the properties of dentin. *J Endod* 2005; 31: 47–49.

16 Best SM, Porter AE, Thian ES, Huang J. Bioceramics: past, present and for the future. *J Eur Ceram Soc* 2008; 28: 1319–1327.

17 Dubok VA. Bioceramics – yesterday, today, tomorrow. *Powder Metallurgy Metal Ceram* 2000; 39: 7–8.

18 Hench L. Bioceramics: from concept to clinic. *J Am Ceram Soc* 1991; 74(7): 1487–510.

19 Richardson IG. The calcium silicate hydrates. *Cem Concr Res* 2008; 38: 137–158.

20 Koch K, Brave DG. A new day has dawned: The increased use of bioceramics in endodontics. *Dental Town*. 2009 (April): 39–43.

21 Yang Q, Lu D. Premix biological hydraulic cement paste composition and using the same. United States Patent Application 2,008,029,909, 2008.

22 Xu HH, Carey LE, Simon CG Jr,, Takagi S, Chow LC. Premixed calcium phosphate cements: Synthesis, physical properties, and cell cytotoxicity. *Dent Mater* 2007; 23: 433–441.

23 Kossev D, Stefanov V. Ceramics-based sealers as new alternative to currently used endodontic sealers. *Roots*. 2009; 1: 42–48.

24 Hess D, Solomon E, Spears R, He J. Retreatability of a bioceramic root canal sealing material. *J Endod* 2011; 37: 1–3.

25 Ghoneim AG, Lutfy RA, Sabet NE, Fayyad DM. Resistance to fracture of roots obturated with novel canal-filling systems. *J Endod* 2011; 37: 1590–1592.

26 Camilleri J, Montesin FE, Brady K, Sweeney R, Curtis RV, Ford TR. The constitution of mineral trioxide aggregate. *Dent Mater* 2005; 21: 297–303.

27 Camilleri J. The physical properties of accelerated Portland cement for endodontic use. *Int Endod J* 2008; 41: 151–157.

28 Camilleri J. Characterization and chemical activity of the Portland cement and two experimental cements with potential for use in dentistry. *Int Endod J* 2008; 41: 791–799.

29 Camilleri J. Modification of MTA. Physical and mechanical properties. *Int Endod J* 2008; 41: 843–849.

30 Borges RP, Sousa-Neto MD, Versiani MA, Rached-Júnior FA, D-Deus G, Miranda CE, et al. Changes in the surface of four calcium silicate-containing endodontic materials and an epoxy resin-based sealer after a solubility test. *Int Endod J* 2012; 45: 419–428.

31 Faria-Junior NB, Tanomaru-Filho M, Berbert FL, Guerreiro-Tanomaru JM. Antibiofilm activity, pH and solubility of endodontic sealers. *Int Endod J* 2013; 46(8): 755–762.

32 Silva EJ, Rosa TP, Herrera DR, Duque TM, Jacinto RC, Gomes BP, et al. Evaluation of cytotoxicity and physicochemical properties of calcium silicate–based endodontic sealer MTA Fillapex. *J Endod* 2013; 39: 274–277.

33 Silva EJ, Santos CC, Zaia AA. Long-term cytotoxic effects of contemporary root canal sealers. *J Appl Oral Sci* 2013; 21: 43–47.

34 Salles LP, Gomes-Cornélio AL, Guimarães FC, Herrera BS, Bao SN, Rossa-Junior C, et al. Mineral trioxide aggregate-based endodontic sealer stimulates hydroxyapatite nucleation in human osteoblastlike cell culture. *J Endod* 2012; 38: 971–976.

35 Koch K, Min PS, Stewart GG. Comparison of apical leakage between Ketac Endo sealer and Grossman sealer. *Oral Surg Oral Med Oral Pathol* 1994; 78: 784–787.

36 Saunders WP, Saunders EM, Herd D, Stephens E. The use of glass ionomer as a root canal sealer: a pilot study. *Int Endod J* 1992; 25: 238–244.

37 Fogel HM, Marshall FJ, Pashley DH. Effects of distance from the pulp and thickness on the hydraulic conductance of human radicular dentin. *J Dent Res* 1988; 67: 1381–1385.

38 King NM, Hiraishi N, Yiu CK, Pashley EL, Loushine RJ, Rueggeberg FA, et al. Effect of resin hydrophilicity on water-vapour permeability of dental adhesive films. *Eur J Oral Sci* 2005; 113: 436–442.

39 Langeland K, Olsson B, Pascon EA. Biological evaluation of Hydron. *J Endod* 1981; 7: 196–204.

40 Rhome BH, Solomon EA, Rabinowitz JL. Isotopic evaluation of the sealing properties of lateral condensation, vertical condensation, and Hydron. *J Endod* 1981; 7: 458–461.

41 Hammad M, Qualtrough A, Silikas N. Extended setting shrinkage behavior of endodontic sealers. *J Endod* 2008; 34: 90–93.

42 Tay FR, Loushine RJ, Monticelli F, et al. Effectiveness of resin-coated gutta-percha cones and a dual-cured, hydrophilic methacrylate resin-based sealer in obturating root canals. *J Endod* 2005; 31: 659–664.

43 Bergmans L, Moisiadis P, De Munck J, Van Meerbeek B, Lambrechts P. Effect of polymerization shrinkage on the sealing capacity of resin fillers for endodontic use. *J Adhes Dent* 2005; 7: 321–329.

44 Doyle MD, Loushine RJ, Agee KA, Gillespie WT, Weller RN, Pashley DH, et al. Improving the performance of EndoRez root canal sealer with a dual-cured two-step self-etch adhesive. I. Adhesive strength to dentin. *J Endod* 2006; 32: 766–770.

45 Gillespie WT, Loushine RJ, Weller RN, Mazzoni A, Doyle MD, Waller JL, et al. Improving the performance of EndoREZ root canal sealer with a dual-cured two-step self-etch adhesive. II. Apical and coronal seal. *J Endod* 2006; 32: 771–775.

46 Jensen SD, Fisher DJ. Method for filling and sealing a root canal. United States Patent & Trademark Office. Patent number 6,811,400, November 2, 2004.

47 Jainaen A, Palamara JE, Messer HH. Push-out bond strengths of the dentine-sealer interface with and without a main cone. *Int Endod J* 2007; 40: 882–890.

48 Baroudi K, Saleh AM, Silikas N, Watts DC. Shrinkage behaviour of flowable resin composites related to conversion and filler-fraction. *J Dent* 2007; 35: 651–655.

49 Jia WT, Trope M, Alpert B. Dental filling material. United States Patent & Trademark Office. Patent number 7,211,136, May 1, 2007.

50 Rached-Junior FJ, Souza-Gabriel AE, Alfredo E, Miranda CE, Silva-Sousa YT, Sousa-Neto MD. Bond strength of Epiphany sealer prepared with resinous solvent. *J Endod* 2009; 35: 251–255.

51 Radovic I, Monticelli F, Goracci C, Vulicevic ZR, Ferrari M. Self-adhesive resin cements: a literature review. *J Adhes Dent* 2008; 10: 251–258.

52 Lawson MS, Loushine B, Mai S, Weller RN, Pashley DH, Tay FR, et al. Resistance of a 4-META-containing, methacrylate-based sealer to dislocation in root canals. *J Endod* 2008; 34: 833–837.

53 Pinna L, Brackett MG, Lockwood PE, Huffman BP, Mai S, Cotti E, et al. In vitro cytotoxicity evaluation of a self-adhesive, methacrylate resin–based root canal sealer. *J Endod* 2008; 34: 1085–108.

54 Belli S, Ozcan E, Derinbay O, Eldeniz AU. A comparative evaluation of sealing ability of a new, self-etching, dual-curable sealer: hybrid root seal (MetaSEAL). *Oral Surg Oral Med Oral Pathol Oral Radiol Endod* 2008; 106: 45–52.

55 Onay EO, Ungor M, Unver S, Ari H, Belli S. An *in vitro* evaluation of the apical sealing ability of new polymeric endodontic filling systems. *Oral Surg Oral Med Oral Pathol Oral Radiol Endod* 2009; 108: 49–54.

56 Babb BR, Loushine RJ, Bryan TE, Ames JM, Causey MS, Kim J, et al. Bonding of self adhesive (self-etching) root canal sealers to radicular dentin. *J Endod* 2009; 35: 578–582.

57 Mai S, Kim YK, Hiraishi N, Ling J, Pashley DH, Tay FR. Evaluation of the true self-etching potential of a fourth generation self-adhesive methacrylate resin-based sealer. *J Endod* 2009; 35: 870–874.

58 Duggan D, Arnold RR, Teixeira FB, Caplan DJ, Tawil P. Periapical inflammation and bacterial penetration after coronal inoculation of dog roots filled with RealSeal 1 or Thermafil. *J Endod* 2009; 35: 852–857.

59 Saunders WP, Saunders EM. Assessment of leakage in the restored pulp chamber of endodontically treated multirooted teeth. *Int Endod J* 1990; 23(1): 28–33.

60 Fransen JN, He J, Glickman GN, Rios A, Shulman JD, Honeyman A. Comparative assessment of ActiV GP/Glass ionomer sealer, Resilon-Epiphany and gutta-percha/AH PLUS obturation: a bacterial leakage study. *J Endod* 2008; 34(6): 725–727.

61 Sagsen B, Er O, Kahraman Y, Orucoglu H. Evaluation of microleakage of roots filled with different techniques with a computerized fluid filtration technique. *J Endod* 2006; 32(12): 1168–1170.

62 Sahli-Canalda C, Jimeno-Berastegui E, Aguade-Brau E. Apical sealing using two thermoplasticized gutta-percha techniques compared with lateral condensation. *J Endod* 1997; 23(10): 636–638.

63 Liewehr FR, Kulild JC, Primack PD. Improved density of gutta-percha after warm lateral condensation. *J Endod* 1993; 19: 489–491.

64 Castelli WA, Caffesse RG, Pameijer CH, Diaz-Perez R, Farquhar J. Periodontium response to a root canal condensing device (Endotec). *Oral Surg Oral Med Oral Pathol* 1991; 71: 333–337.

65 Caicedo R, Clark SJ. Modern perspectives in root canal obturation. *Dent C E Dig* 2007; 4: 1–12.

66 Silver GK, Love RM, Purton DG. Comparison of two vertical condensation obturation techniques: Touch n Heat modified and System B. *Int Endod J* 1999; 32(4): 287–295.

67 Johnson BT, Bond MS. Leakage associated with single or multiple increment backfill with the Obtura II gutta-percha system. *J Endod* 1999; 5: 613–614.

68 QED Endo. Obtura III Max. http://www.qedendo.co.uk/acatalog/Obtura_III_Max.html.

69 Ruddle CJ. Filling root canal systems: the calamus 3D obturation technique. *Dent Today* April 1, 2010. http://www.dentistrytoday.com/endodontics/2611-filling-root-canal-systems-the-calamus-3-d-obturation-technique

70 Kerr Dental. Elements product brochure. https://www.kerrdental.com/kerr-endodontics/elements-free-cordless-continuous-wave-obturation-system

71 GuttaFlow for the permanent obturation of root canals: a technique review. *Inside Dentistry*. 2006 Jan/Feb;2(1). https://www.dentalaegis.com/id/2006/02/guttaflow-for-the-permanent-obturation-of-root-canals-a-technique-review

72 Coltene. Roeko GuttaFlow 2 / Roeko GuttaFlow 2 FAST Root Canal Obturation. https://www.coltene.com/products-coltenewhaledent/endodontics/root-canal-obturation/roeko-guttaflowR-2-roeko-guttaflowR-2-fast/

73 Rapisarda E, Bonaccorso A, Tripi TR. Evaluation of two root canal preparation and obturation methods: the McSpadden method and the use of ProFile–Thermafil. *Minerva Stomatol* 1999; 48(1–2): 29–38.

74 Weller RN, Kimbrough WF, Anderson RW. A comparison of thermoplastic obturation techniques: adaptation to the canal walls. *J Endod* 1997; 23(11): 703–706.

75 Levitan ME, Himel VT, Luckey JB. The effect of insertion rates on fill length and adaptation of a thermoplasticized gutta-percha technique. *J Endod* 2003; 29(8): 505–508.

76 DuLac KA, Nielsen CJ, Tomazic TJ, Ferrillo Jr, PJ, Hatton JF, Comparison of the obturation of lateral canals by six techniques. *J Endod* 1999; 25(5): 376–380.

77 Bertacci A, Baroni C, Breschi L, Venturi M, Prati C. The influence of smear layer in lateral channels filling. *Clin Oral Investig* 2007; 11(4): 353–359.

78 Frajlich SR, Goldberg F, Massone EJ, Cantarini C, Artaza LP. Comparative study of retreatment of Thermafil and lateral condensation endodontic fillings. *Int Endod J* 1998; 31(5): 354–357.

79 Royzenblat A, Goodell GG. Comparison of removal times of Thermafil plastic obturators using ProFile rotary instruments at different rotational speeds in moderately curved canals. *J Endod* 2007; 33(3): 256–258.

80 Shipper G, Trope M. *In vitro* microbial leakage of endodontically treated teeth using new and standard obturation techniques. *J Endod* 2004; 30(3): 154–158.

81 Platt J, Duke S, Moore K, *et al.* An *in vitro* evaluation of a novel endodontic obturation system. University of Indiana Dental School. Unpublished study.

82 Kim S, Chang P, Iqbal M; University of Pennsylvania School of Dental Medicine. A comparison of coronal and apical dye leakage with two obturation systems. Abstract submitted to American Association of Endodontists meeting, 2002.

83 Ferrari M. University of Sienna. Fracture strength of endodontically treated monoradicular teeth with a new endodontic obturating system (Fibrefill): an *in vitro* study. Unpublished study.

84 Thongthammachat S, Platt JA, Katona TR, Hovijitra S, Moore BK. Fracture resistance and fracture resistance after fatigue loading of 4 different post and cores in endodontically treated teeth. *Compend Contin Educ Dent* 2006; 27(7): 340–346.

85 Serafino C, Gallina G, Cumbo E, Ferrari M. Surface debris of canal walls after post space preparation in endodontically treated teeth: a scanning electron microscopic study. *Oral Surg Oral Med Oral Pathol Oral Radiol Endod* 2004; 97(3): 381–387.

86 Wikipedia. Smart material. http://en.wikipedia.org/wiki/Smartmaterial.

87 Highgate DJ, Lloyd JA. Expandable/contractable composition for surgical or dental use. US patent no. 7,210,935, 2007.

88 Smartseal DRFP Limited. How It Works. 2012, http://www.smart-seal.co.uk/how-it-works.

89 Pathivada L, Munagala KK, Dang AB. Smartseal: a new age obturation. *Ann Dent Spec* 2013; 1(1): 13–15.

90 Koch K, Brave D. Integral gutta percha core/cone obturation technique. *United States Patent* 7,021,936, 2006.

91 Hiraishi N, Loushine RJ, Vano M, Chieffi N, Weller RN, Ferrari M, *et al.* Is an oxygen inhibited layer required for bonding of resin-coated gutta-percha to a methacrylate-based root canal sealer? *J Endod* 2006; 32: 429–433.

92 Monticelli F, Sword J, Martin RL, Schuster GS, Weller RN, Ferrari M, et al. Sealing properties of two contemporary single-cone obturation systems. *Int Endod J* 2007; 40(5): 374–385.

Questions

1 The rationale for obturation of the root canal system states that

i. The seal at the apex is more important than the seal in the coronal part of the canal.

ii. The primary aims of obturation are to prevent reinfection of the root canal and entomb any residual microorganisms.

iii. A root canal filling material should be, among other properties, bacteriostatic, sterilizable, and radiopaque.

a. All are true.

b. Both ii and iii are true.

c. Both i and ii are true.

d. All are false.

2 Which of these has not been used as a sealer?
A Zinc oxide eugenol
B Calcium hydroxide
C Calcium silicate
D Amalgam

3 Root canal sealer is necessary
A To seal the space between the dentinal wall and the obturating core interface
B To provide a hermetic seal
C For all techniques
D Both a and c

4 Alpha-phase gutta-percha is
A Not flowable
B Pliable
C Able to flow under pressure
D Both b and c

5 Temperature control during warm condensation techniques can be achieved using the device
A DownPak
B System B
C Endotec II
D All of the above

6 Plastic injection techniques have the potential for significant overfilling of the canal.
A True
B False

7 The carrier-based technique
A Can enable movement of gutta-percha into lateral and accessory canals.
B Can be used with or without heat depending upon the specific product used.
C Both a and b are true.
D Both a and b are false.

8 GuttaFlow is a
A Cold flowable technique
B Injection-based technique
C Carrier-based system
D Both a and b

9 Monoblock can be achieved with
A Gutta-percha
B Resilon
C Both a and b
D Neither a nor b

CHAPTER 6

Treatment planning of pulpless teeth

Faysal Succaria[1] and Sami M. Chogle[2]

[1] *Private practice, Dubai, UAE*

[2] *Boston University, Henry M. Goldman School of Dental Medicine, Boston, Massachusetts, USA*

When planning restoration of pulpless teeth, it is important to take into account structural differences that exist between them and vital teeth. Weakening is initially because of the loss of tooth structure to dental caries. This weakening continues with consecutive restorative procedures. Finally, more tissue loss results from endodontic access and canal shaping. The result is a structure that exhibits lower resistance to fracture [1]. Thus, much of the planning is to ensure maximumal structural integrity and, as a result, longevity.

The main mechanism of fracture is attributed to cuspal flexure [2–6]. Although some dentists believe in the brittle theory of dentin associated with decreased water content and collagen fiber changes [7], contradictory evidence [8] suggests that no changes occur in dentin brittleness. Tooth position in the arch has an effect on amount and directions of loads subjected to it (Figure 6.1). That, in addition to different root anatomy, necessitates some differentiation in approaches to treatment planning for anterior and posterior teeth.

Treatment options

Treatment options for pulpless teeth can vary from a simple composite resin restoration up to full-coverage restoration. In certain cases, it is necessary to use a post, whereas in others, adding a post can have negative consequences. Treatment options are influenced by many factors such as amount of tooth structure loss and position of the tooth in the arch.

Studies have shown that endodontically treated posterior teeth are prone to fracture at higher rates than vital teeth [9]. A 20-year retrospective study on posterior teeth restored with silver amalgam without cuspal coverage had up to 73% failure for premolars [9]. Another in vivo study followed patients with endodontically treated molars restored without cuspal coverage. The result showed that after 5 years the survival rate was a mere 36% [10].

Off-axis loading in anterior teeth has been shown to cause more structural damage than axial loading [11]. This fact, in addition to the relatively narrower dimensions of anterior teeth, makes tissue conservation paramount. In cases with a conservative access cavity and minimal tooth loss, a composite resin restoration can suffice. Crowns are only necessary in cases where there is extensive tooth loss or need for esthetic enhancement. A post can be used in case the remaining tooth structure is not sufficient for crown retention. However, residual tooth thickness height and position are necessary so the tooth can resist fracture. Treatment options are summarized in Table 6.1.

Ferrule

Ferrule is defined as a ring or a cap that is placed around a structure to strengthen it against fracture. In dentistry, Eissman and Radke [12] introduced the term *ferrule,* although the concept was described earlier. The ferrule effect has been studied extensively in the literature, showing positive impact on strength of restored endodontically treated teeth [13]. Rosen in 1961 described the "hugging action," which strengthens the crown–tooth complex. The ferrule effect is a function of ferrule height, thickness, and continuity.

Current Therapy in Endodontics, First Edition. Edited by Priyanka Jain.
© 2016 John Wiley & Sons, Inc. Published 2016 by John Wiley & Sons, Inc.

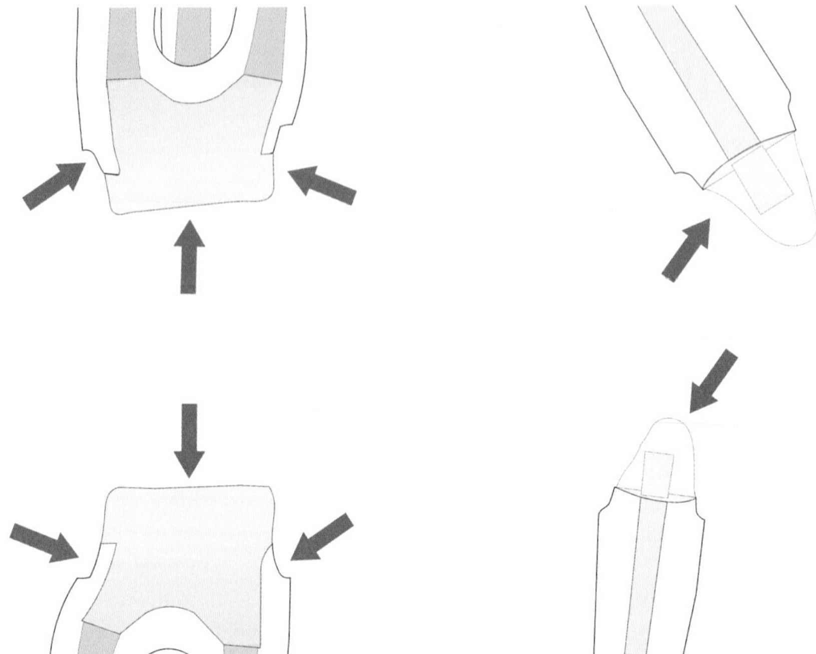

Figure 6.1 Force vectors on anterior and posterior teeth. Anterior teeth undergo off-axis loading, and posterior teeth undergo axial and some off-axis loading.

Table 6.1 Restorative treatment plans for anterior and posterior teeth.

Location	Amount of tissue loss	Recommended restoration type
Posterior teeth	Moderate to severe tooth loss	Cuspal coverage (crown)
	Moderate tooth loss	Cuspal coverage (onlay)
	Extremely minimal amount of tooth loss limited to access opening	Noncuspal coverage
Anterior teeth	Moderate to severe tooth loss	Post and crown
	Moderate tooth loss	Either composite resin restoration or ceramic partial or full coverage depending on esthetic need
	Minimal amount of tooth loss limited to access opening	Composite resin restoration

The effect of height has also been studied. A height of 1 mm doubled the fracture resistance when compared with teeth with no ferrule [14]. Some authors suggest at least 2 mm [15, 16], whereas 3 mm of vertical height is recommended others [17] (Figure 6.2).

Although there is some consensus on ferrule height, there are contradictory results on width (thickness). Some studies suggest a positive effect on fracture resistance [18, 19], but others did not find a significant effect [20]. There is not enough evidence to lead to exact clinical recommendations on width. Nevertheless, maximumal conservation of the axial thickness is advised.

Theoretically it is more advantageous to have a 360-degree ferrule [21]; however, this is not always the case clinically. A number of studies explored the effect of decreased number of walls on fracture resistance. One study showed that four walls of remaining tooth structure exhibited significantly higher fracture strength than three [11].

Both in vivo and in vitro studies have demonstrated that the amount of remaining tooth structure, and in return the ferrule, has more impact on strength than other factors such as post and core system or luting agent used [13, 22, 23]. Advantages of the ferrule include decreased incidence of root and post fracture, decreased post dislodgement, and decreased leakage and failure of the cement seal.

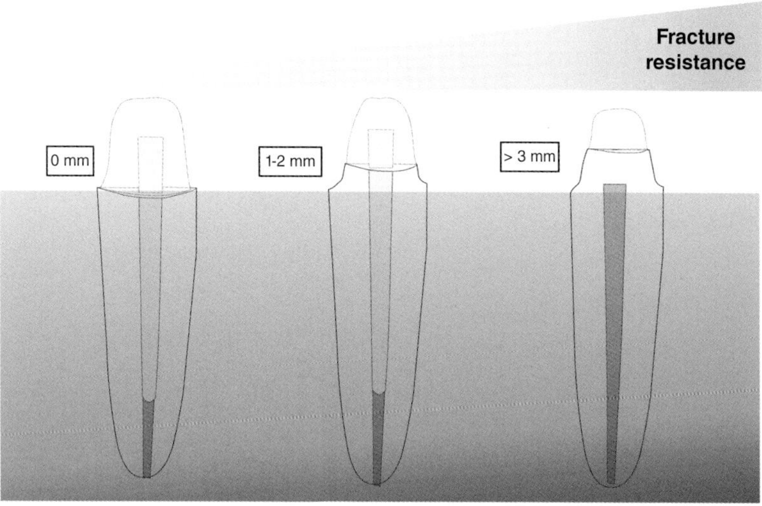

Figure 6.2 Fracture resistance.

Treatment options in cases of insufficient ferrule

Crown lengthening

Crown lengthening is a surgical procedure designed to increase the extent of supragingival tooth structure by apically positioning the gingival margin, removing supporting bone, or both [24]. Indications can be functional or esthetic or both. Although crown-lengthening surgery can be used across the dentition, it has certain limitations. Short roots can be a limiting factor because the surgery increases the crown-to-root ratio. Other anatomical limitations such as molar furcation and minimal keratinized tissue can limit the extent of surgery. Tapering roots present an esthetic limitation anteriorly due to interdental triangular spaces appearing after healing. Lastly, in the esthetic zone, crown lengthening increases the crown-to-root ratio (Figure 6.3). In vitro studies [25, 26] tested crown-lengthened extracted teeth for fracture resistance. The results showed that after simulated crown lengthening, the resistance to fracture had decreased. Therefore, benefits of exposing more of the root should be weighed against the possibility of weakening.

Orthodontic extrusion

Extrusion of roots is accomplished by applying vertical traction forces. With moderate force, the root pulls the periodontium along, and the gingiva migrates with the tooth coronally. This result would be counterproductive for exposing the coronal parts of the root. To achieve extrusion without tissue migration, stronger traction is needed. After the necessary extrusion is accomplished, it is advised to provide long-term retention to limit relapse [27]. Limitations of extrusion are short teeth, shallow furcation, and unfavorable root anatomy for multirooted teeth. When compared with surgical crown lengthening, the crown-to-root ratio is not increased as much as is shown in Figure 6.3. Thus, studies have established higher fracture resistance of this technique [26, 27].

Esthetic considerations in deeply discolored pulpless teeth

Endodontic therapy should not only focus on biological and functional aspects, but it should also take esthetic considerations into account. To reduce the risk of posttreatment tooth discoloration, all materials should be applied carefully. Especially in the esthetic zone, tooth discoloration can have a negative impact on appearance. Discoloration can be caused by pulpal hemorrhage, remnants of pulpal tissue, endodontic obturating materials, intracanal medicaments, or restorative materials [28]. Endodontic materials such as mineral trioxide aggregate (MTA)

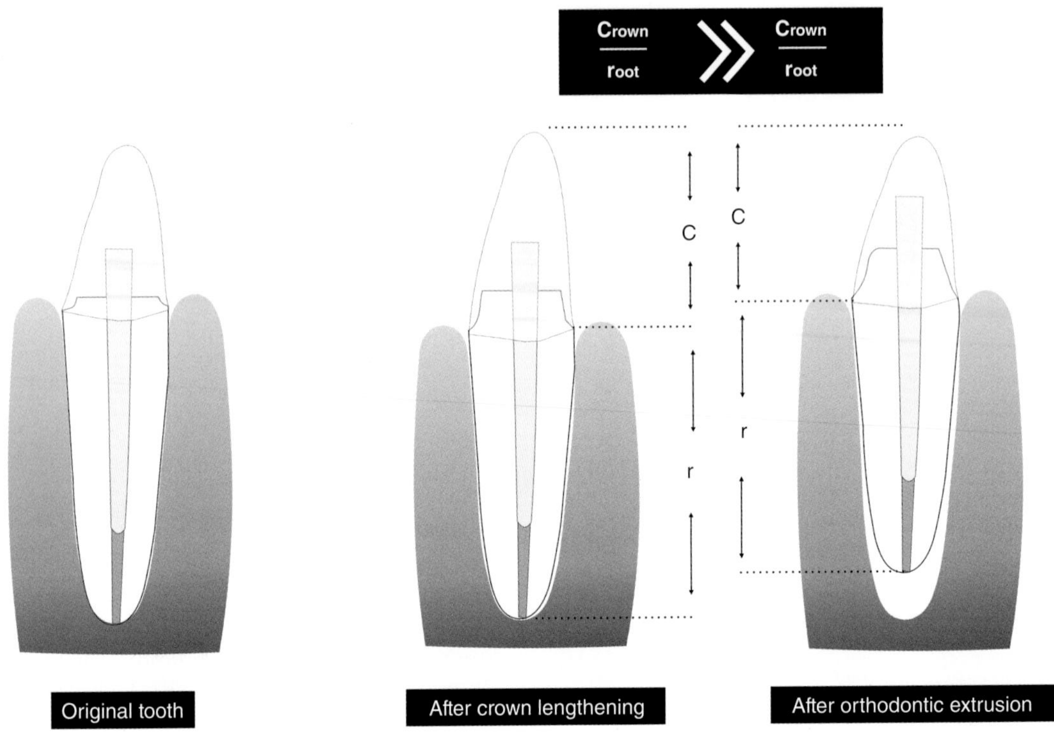

Figure 6.3 Crown-to-root ratio changes after crown lengthening and orthodontic extrusion. The ratio is more favorable with orthodontic extrusion.

and bioceramics can contribute to discoloration as well.

Causes of discoloration

Discoloration from pulpal hemorrhage is often a consequence of trauma to the tooth. The resulting extravasation from the coronal blood vessels into the dentinal tubules leads to release of iron from the red blood cells. In the presence of hydrogen sulfide from microbial origin, iron sulfide is formed, giving the tooth a grayish to blackish hue. The tooth may also show discoloration due to pulpal remnants in the chamber from inadequate pulpotomy or pulpectomy. The onset and degree of discoloration usually depends on the interval between pulpal hemorrhage and/or necrosis and the start of endodontic therapy. The longer this interval, the greater the degree of discoloration and the greater the difficulty in regaining normal color through bleaching [29].

Endodontic obturating materials are probably the most common cause of single-tooth discoloration. Presence of gutta-percha and sealer in the pulpal chamber on completion of treatment often results in dark discoloration. Sealers, whether zinc oxide–eugenol (ZOE) based or resins, are the main offenders, which themselves discolor [30] and can cause progressive coronal discoloration with time [31]. However, gutta-percha contains staining pigments as well that can pigment the tooth. Therefore, especially in anterior teeth, obturation should end at or below the buccal cementoenamel junction to prevent coronal discoloration. The prognosis of bleaching in such discoloration cases depends on the composition of the obturating materials. Sealers with metallic components do not bleach well and can even regress with time.

Phenolic and iodoform-based medicaments have the potential to cause internal discoloration as well [32]. Such intracanal medications when in direct contact with dentin for long periods could allow penetration and oxidization. Fortunately, these types of discoloration are readily and permanently corrected by bleaching, although iodoform-induced discolorations tend to be more severe.

Coronal restorations are generally either metallic or composite. Silver amalgam has been the worst offender, giving the dentin a dark gray or even blackish hue. Such discoloration is difficult to correct with bleaching and is unsatisfactory [33, 34]. In fact, Goldstein and Feinman [35] believe that discoloration from silver amalgam is a contraindication to bleaching, which might necessitate restoration with full-coverage crowns. Zerbinati and Pirero [36] recommend that teeth pigmented by amalgam require prosthetic treatment. Discoloration can also occur from metal posts and pins or thinner tooth structure, yielding a metallic hue due to the increased translucency. In such cases, replacement with resin–composite restorations may suffice.

With composite resin restorations, microleakage is more of a concern regarding discoloration that allows other pigmenting chemicals to penetrate and discolor dentin. The composite itself can also discolor with time. Replacement with a proper sealed composite resin restoration may suffice. If required, internal bleaching provides good results for the dentin before replacing the restoration.

A number of new formulations of MTA, such as white and gray MTA (ProRoot Dentsply, York, PA), MTA Plus, Neo MTA Plus (Avalon Biomed Inc, Bradenton, FL), and bioceramics such as EndoSequence root repair material putty and paste (Brasseler, Savannah, GA), and Biodentine (Septodont, France), have been introduced. These materials are being used coronally in cases of cervical or furcal perforations, revascularization, and pulp-capping procedures with acceptable results. However, most studies have reported that all forms of MTA tested have shown a light yellow to dark brown coronal discoloration [37–40] and can undermine an otherwise successful procedure. Although the discoloration is not as severe as with the use of ZOE-based sealers [41], it might be enough to present a significant clinical complication in esthetic zones [42]. The reason seems to be the bismuth oxide content in combination with irrigant fluids used [43, 44], and these teeth are not responsive to bleaching with the material in place [45]. It is crucial to place these materials below the cementoenamel junction whenever possible to avoid coronal discoloration. In situations that necessitate the coronal use of such materials, full-coverage restoration is suggested.

Another option suggested in pulp-capping procedures may be to remove the material after confirming a dentinal bridge formation under the MTA and then possibly internal bleaching [45, 46]. In such cases, pulp vitality may be concern, and a follow-up visit may be needed to demonstrate pulp vitality and the absence of signs and symptoms.

Management of discolored pulpless teeth

Internal bleaching

Internal bleaching is particularly effective in endodontically treated anterior teeth that discolored due to long-standing necrosis or residual sealer that had disintegrated internally (Figure 6.4). This method was initially described in the 1960s using hydrogen peroxide and sodium perborate [47]. Later, sodium perborate with water came into use.

Internal bleaching relies primarily on oxidizing gels that release nascent oxygen. These can be in the form of hydrogen peroxide, carbamide peroxide, or sodium perborate. The gel is placed into the pulpal chamber after carefully cleaning and sealing the canal with a suitable base such as glass ionomer cement [47–51].

Caution must be exercised to avert leakage of the gel through cementum to alveolar bone, causing external resorption. The literature recommends staying within

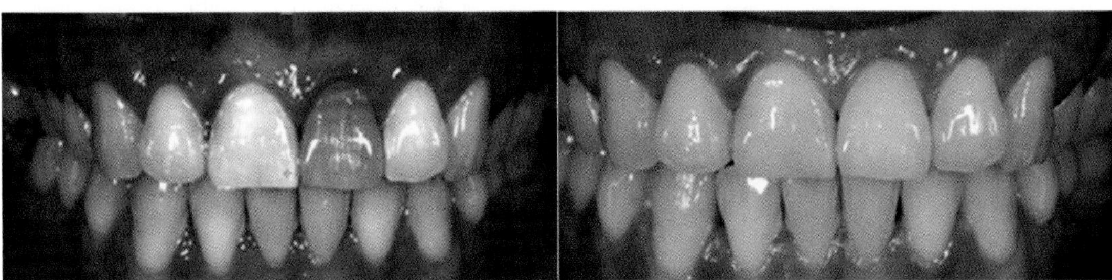

Figure 6.4 *Left,* Preoperative tooth #9 showing severe discoloration. *Right,* After internal bleaching.

1 mm of the cementoenamel junction, ensuring the base is well adapted [49, 51, 52], and using sodium perborate instead of hydrogen peroxide.

This method is the most conservative and is indicated for discolored teeth with minimal restorations and/or need for reconstruction. If this method fails, ceramic coverage is indicated.

Partial and full-coverage restorations

Generalized discoloration, generalized discoloration accompanied by a failing restoration, or loss of sound tooth structure necessitate a treatment modality that will improve esthetics and extend longevity. Depending on severity, treatment can range from minimal-preparation veneers up to full-coverage crowns. This masking ability is a function of the type of ceramic material used [53], thickness [53, 54], and cement used [55] (Figure 6.5).

Masking ability of all-ceramic materials

Lithium disilicate and zirconia-based restorations constitute the two main all-ceramic materials currently used. The dental technician can use the appropriate core and veneering material to attain the desired final shade [56].

It is the dentist's responsibility to provide the technician with dental photographs and stump shade estimation so the technician can make an accurate decision on the type of ceramic to be used [57].

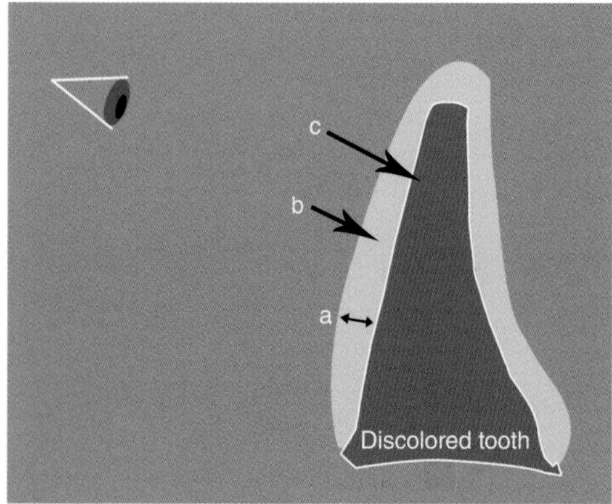

Figure 6.5 Masking ability is a function of ceramic thickness (a), ceramic type (b), and cement opacity (c).

Effect of thickness

Thicker ceramic restorations can mask underlying discoloration better. Thus, in those cases, more preparation is required to create more room for ceramic [57, 58].

Effect of cement

Early cements came with specific shades and opacities. At present, resin cements are supplied with a wide range of shades and opacities. In cases where restorations are being bonded to severely discolored teeth, it is advised to use cements with higher opacity [58].

Posts

Posts serve as retaining structures for core buildups and ultimately the final restoration. The earliest form of post was cast metal, but since then, various other designs and materials have become available.

Some controversy exists pertaining to the strengthening effect of posts on teeth. While some clinicians believe that posts strengthen teeth, studies have shown that posts do not have a positive effect on strength [57–62]. Moreover, some studies suggest that in the presence of enough sound tooth structure, the process of creating post space and the presence of the post can decrease the strength of the tooth [63–65]. Hence, clinicians should avoid using posts when other anatomic features are available to retain the core. Molars might not require posts because a core can usually be retained by the pulpal chamber and canals.

When a post is necessary, it is recommended to be placed in a distal canal in mandibular molars and in the palatal canal in maxillary molars, because the other canals usually tend to be thinner and more curved. In bicuspids with more than one canal, the straighter canal should be used. Multiple posts are seldom indicated. Posts may be prefabricated (metal, carbon fiber, glass fiber, quartz fiber, or zirconia) or custom made.

Factors influencing post design

Root length

The length and shape of the remaining root determine the length of the post. It has been demonstrated that the greater the post length, the better the retention and stress distribution. Post retention is directly proportional to its length. Because the most common causes of post failure is post dislodgment [66], it is important to maximize the length of the post without disturbing the apical seal. 3 to 5 mm of apical gutta-percha has been shown to maintain the apical seal [62, 67]. It is not always possible to use a long post, especially when the remaining root is short or curved. In such cases, the benefit of added length has to be weighed against possible perforation or weakening of the apical seal.

When the root length is short, the clinician must decide whether to use a longer post or maintain the recommended apical seal and use a parallel-sided threaded post. Lack of sufficient length is not only detrimental to retention; data on shorter posts was associated with higher root fractures [60, 68].

Post width (diameter)

Preserving tooth structure, reducing the chances of perforation, and permitting the restored tooth to resist fractures are criteria in selecting the post width. There have been different approaches regarding the selection of post diameter. One approach suggests the post width should not be greater than one third of the root width at its narrowest dimension, whereas another proposes that the post should be surrounded by a minimum of 1 mm of sound dentin.

Conversely to post length, an increase in diameter is not beneficial to retention [68]. Furthermore, increasing post diameter is undesirable and can lead to higher failure rates associated with root fractures. This is because the resistance to fracture is directly related to the thickness of remaining dentin, especially in the buccolingual direction [69].

The post diameter should be as small as possible while providing the necessary rigidity; it is always important to leave as much tooth structure as possible in all phases of treatment. Hence in prefabricated post systems, the narrowest possible post that will fit the canal space should be used. In custom cast posts and cores, minimal flaring to remove undercuts is recommended to preserve as much tooth structure as possible.

Post design

Posts are available in several designs: parallel, tapered, or a combination of both. Parallel posts can provide more retention. However, tapered posts, especially custom-made posts and cores, do not require more intracanal preparation and so are more conservative to tooth structure. Another difference is stress distribution. With tapered posts, stress is concentrated at the cervical area, whereas with parallel posts, the stress is at the apex.

The surface topography can be smooth, serrated passive, or self-threading. Retention is higher for serrated posts. However, it is not recommended to use the self-threaded type because it engages in dentin and can lead to increased undesirable stresses within the root.

Prefabricated posts versus custom posts-and-cores

Canal configuration, esthetics, chairside time, and strength are factors that dictate the type of system to be used. It has been suggested that if a canal requires extensive preparation, a well-adapted cast post and core restoration is more indicated. An example is mandibul anterior teeth with narrow canals. The opposite is true for molars. In molars, the existing walls will interfere with the path of insertion of the post. Removing the interferences would further weaken the tooth. Thus, a prefabricated post is recommended.

Nonmetallic tooth-colored prefabricated posts offer an esthetic advantage over metal posts and carbon fiber posts. Although some techniques exist to apply opaque ceramic to cast metal cores or to use yellow gold, nonmetallic posts with composite cores offer more flexibility with stump shade. The clear advantage of prefabricated posts is with the number of visits and chairside time. Whereas cast post and cores require two appointments, prefabricated posts can be completed in one visit. An additional obvious advantage to the patient is that the canal is sealed without the possibility of leakage between the two appointments.

When comparing fracture resistance, evidence suggests that in general, teeth restored with cast posts-and-cores exhibited higher fracture resistance than fiber posts and metal prefabricated posts. This refutes earlier claims that flexure of posts increases resistance to fractures.

Post materials

When restoring teeth with posts, it is important to carefully choose the material to be used. Historically, all posts were metal based. Alloys ranged from chrome–cobalt to semiprecious silver-based to precious gold-based alloys. Silver- and gold-based alloys offer easier adjustment. In addition, yellow gold alloys offer a warmer nongray stump shade that can be used with all-ceramic crowns.

In the 1990s, earlier carbon fiber posts were introduced. The initial products were black. The color of these posts gave them no advantage over metal post. Furthermore, they were radiolucent and difficult to remove from inside the canal. Later modifications added a coating to make them more esthetic. With the increased use of all-ceramic restorations comes a greater demand for tooth-colored posts and cores. Several systems were introduced over the years including zirconia, glass fiber, and quartz fiber posts.

Zirconia posts are made of fine-grained, dense tetragonal zirconium polycrystals (TZP). These posts are rigid, with a modulus of elasticity higher than stainless steel. The main disadvantages of using zirconia posts is that if fractures happen, the posts are not retrievable, and that bonding of the core to the post can also be a problem with the zirconium posts.

Glass and quartz fiber posts are less rigid than zirconia and offer similar modulus of elasticity to dentin. It makes them a good substitute for carbon fiber posts. They bond easily to composite cores and are easy to handle (Figure 6.6). Nevertheless, compared to metal posts, retrievability is still an issue.

Nonmetallic posts (tooth-colored posts)

Cementation of posts

Cementation relies on both the cement's physical properties and the techniques used. Cement should have high tensile and compressive strength, bond to dentin, have low solubility in oral fluids, and be easy to handle. As for the technique, regardless of the system used, it is recommended to have maximal spread of cement on the post surface with the least voids. Numerous cement types are available for post and core cementation. These cements differ in mechanical properties, clinical handling, and indication.

Zinc phosphate is one of the earliest cements used in dentistry. It possesses favorable physical properties, is inexpensive, is easy to use, and remains an excellent choice for post cementation. Glass ionomer has adequate physical properties; however, it is a slow-setting material that requires many hours to achieve adequate strength and has high initial solubility in oral fluids. Resin-modified glass ionomer cement, as originally formulated, had significant delayed expansion that could lead to root fracture. The current generation of resin ionomer cement has overcome this setback.

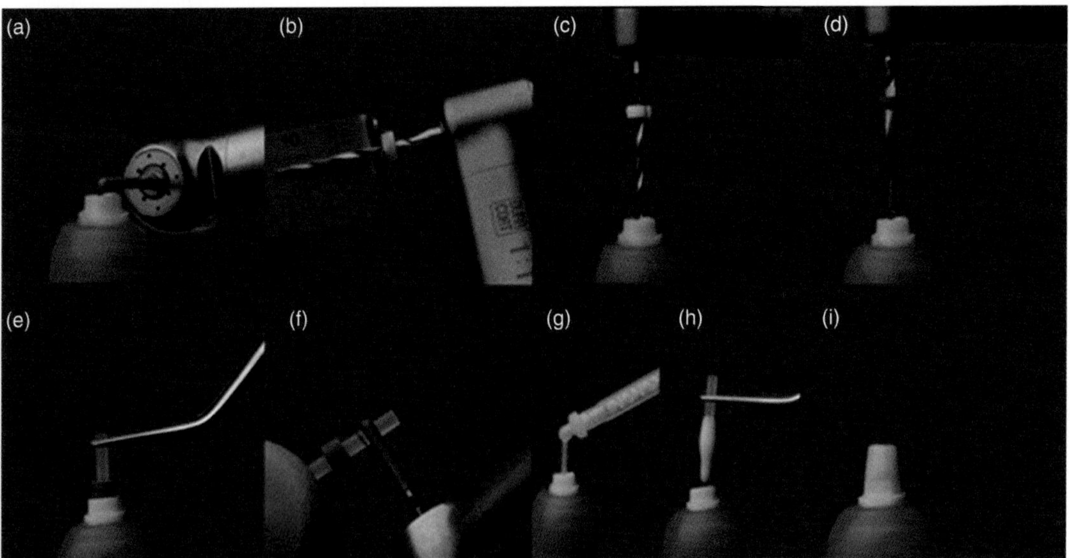

Figure 6.6 Technique for manufacturing a direct fiber-reinforced composite post and composite core. *a,* Initial preparation. *b,* Measuring the required length of the final post. *c,* Using the initial drill to clear the endodontic filing material. *d,* Based on the size of the canal, the final drill is used. *e,* The fiber-reinforced composite post is tried in, making sure it is completely seating. *f,* The excess length of post is sectioned. *g* and *h,* Dual-polymerizing resin cement is applied both into the canal *(g)* and onto the post *(h)*. *i,* Incremental buildup and final preparation of composite.

Table 6.2 Dental cements.

Cement	Advantages	Disadvantages	Indications
Zinc phosphate	Inexpensive Long working time Rapid initial set	Can snap set if the mixing protocol is not followed Mechanical bond only	Metal posts
Glass ionomer	Can bond to dentin Easy to mix and apply	Soluble in oral fluids Prolonged final set	Metal posts
Resin-modified glass ionomer	Can bond to dentin Easy to mix and apply	Earlier formulations were prone to expansion, leading to root fracture	Metal posts Nonmetal posts
Resin cement	Bonds to tooth and to silanated glass fiber posts Controlled set (dual polymerizing)	Relatively expensive	Metal posts Nonmetal posts

There is greater interest now in the use of resin cement to bond posts. These cements offer an immediate set and promise higher retention through bonding. Because eugenol interferes with the setting of resin cements, some caution must be exercised in the use of resin cements in conjunction with ZOE-containing sealers. Controversially, others found no decrease in bond strength of posts in similar conditions (Table 6.2).

Surface treatment

To achieve optimal luting and bonding results, the dentin surface should be carefully cleaned of remnants of endodontic sealer and gutta-percha. Retained remnants can decrease the effectiveness of cement irrespective of type of sealer and choice of cement. The post surface should also undergo treatment. For cast post and cores, sandblasting with 50-μm aluminum oxide particles increases micro roughness and increases the effectiveness of the cement. For glass fiber posts, the surface should be cleaned with ethyl alcohol if a post was tried in. Silane should be then applied to improve bond strength between the resin cement and the post.

Cement application

For zinc phosphate, glass ionomer, and resin-modified glass ionomer cements, apply the cement to the post and inside the canal using a lentulo spiral. This procedure limits air voids and as a result increases bond strength. For resin cements, apply cement to the post and inside the canal using thin cement-mixing tips designed for this purpose. The use of lentulo spirals is not recommended because it can cause undesirably rapid set of some resin cements.

Conclusion

Success is a function of the structural integrity of the tooth-restoration system. Hence it is paramount to preserve coronal and radicular dentin. Posts are only required when it is necessary to retain a core buildup. The choice of post system is not as integral as planning restorations based on principles of hard tissue conservation.

References

1 Aquilino SA, Caplan DJ. Relationship between crown placement and the survival of endodontically treated teeth. *J Prosthet Dent* 2002; 87(3): 256–263.

2 Tidmarsh BG. Restoration of endodontically treated posterior teeth. *J Endod* 1976; 2(12): 374–375.

3 Larson TD, Douglas WH, Geistfeld RE. Effect of prepared cavities on the strength of teeth. *Oper Dent* 1981; 6(1): 2–5.

4 Panitvisai P, Messer HH. Cuspal deflection in molars in relation to endodontic and restorative procedures. *J Endod* 1995; 21(2): 57–61.

5 Bianchi E Silva AA, Ghiggi PC, Mota EG, Borges GA, Burnett LH Jr, Spohr AM. Influence of restorative techniques on fracture load of endodontically treated premolars. *Stomatologija* 2013; 15(4): 123–128.

6 Scotti N, Rota R, Scansetti M, Paolino DS, Chiandussi G, Pasqualini D, Berutti E. Influence of adhesive techniques on fracture resistance of endodontically treated premolars with various residual wall thicknesses. *J Prosthet Dent* 2013; 110(5): 376–382.

7 Pontius O, Nathanson D, Giordano R, Schilder H, Hutter JW. Survival rate and fracture strength of incisors restored with different post and core systems and endodontically treated incisors without coronoradicular reinforcement. *J Endod* 2002; 28(10): 710–715.

8 Sedgley CM, Messer HH. Are endodontically treated teeth more brittle? *J Endod* 1992; 18(7): 332–335.
9 Hansen EK, Asmussen E, Christiansen NC. *In vivo* fractures of endodontically treated posterior teeth restored with amalgam. *Endod Dent Traumatol* 1990; 6(2): 49–55.
10 Nagasiri R. Chitmongkolsuk S. Long-term survival of endodontically treated molars without crown coverage: a retrospective cohort study. *J Prosthet Dent* 2005; 93(2): 164–170.
11 Arunpraditkul S, Saengsanon S, Pakviwat W. Fracture resistance of endodontically treated teeth: three walls versus four walls of remaining coronal tooth structure. *J Prosthodont* 2009; 18(1): 49–53.
12 Eissmann HF, Radke RA. Postendodontic Restoration. In: Cohen S, Burns RC, editors. *Pathways of the pulp*. St. Louis: CV Mosby Co; 1987.
13 Santos-Filho PC, Veríssimo C, Soares PV, Saltarelo RC, Soares CJ, Marcondes Martins LR. Influence of ferrule, post system, and length on biomechanical behavior of endodontically treated anterior teeth. *J Endod* 2014; 40(1): 119–123.
14 Sorensen JA, Engelman MJ. Ferrule design and fracture resistance of endodontically treated teeth. *J Prosthet Dent* 1990; 63(5): 529–536.
15 Assif D, Bitenski A, Pilo R, Oren E. Effect of post design on resistance to fracture of endodontically treated teeth with complete crowns. *J Prosthet Dent* 1993; 69(1): 36–40.
16 Trabert KC, Cooney JP. The endodontically treated tooth. Restorative concepts and techniques. *Dent Clin North Am* 1984; 28(4): 923–951.
17 Pereira JR, de Ornelas F, Conti PC, do Valle AL. Effect of a crown ferrule on the fracture resistance of endodontically treated teeth restored with prefabricated posts. *J Prosthet Dent* 2006; 95(1): 50–54.
18 Mattison GD. Photoelastic stress analysis of cast-gold endodontic posts. *J Prosthet Dent* 1982; 48(4): 407–411.
19 Trabert KC, Caput AA, Abou-Rass M. Tooth fracture—a comparison of endodontic and restorative treatments. *J Endod* 1978; 4(11): 341–345.
20 Al-Wahadni A, Gutteridge DL. An *in vitro* investigation into the effects of retained coronal dentine on the strength of a tooth restored with a cemented post and partial core restoration. *Int Endod J* 2002; 35(11): 913–918.
21 Morgano SM, Brackett SE. Foundation restorations in fixed prosthodontics: current knowledge and future needs. *J Prosthet Dent* 1999; 82(6): 643–657.
22 Creugers NH, Mentink AG, Fokkinga WA, Kreulen CM. 5-year follow-up of a prospective clinical study on various types of core restorations. *Int J Prosthodont* 2005; 18(1): 34–39.
23 Ichim I, Kuzmanovic DV, Love RM. A finite element analysis of ferrule design on restoration resistance and distribution of stress within a root. *Int Endod J* 2006; 39(6): 443–452.
24 The glossary of prosthodontic terms. *J Prosthet Dent*, 2005. 94(1): 10–92.
25 Meng QF, Chen LJ, Meng J, Chen YM, Smales RJ, Yip KH. Fracture resistance after simulated crown lengthening and forced tooth eruption of endodontically-treated teeth restored with a fiber post-and-core system. *Am J Dent* 2009; 22(3): 147–150.
26 Gegauff AG. Effect of crown lengthening and ferrule placement on static load failure of cemented cast post-cores and crowns. *J Prosthet Dent* 2000; 84(2): 169–179.
27 Bach N, Baylard JF, Voyer R. Orthodontic extrusion: periodontal considerations and applications. *J Can Dent Assoc* 2004; 70(11): 775–780.
28 Zimmerli B, Jeger F, Lussi A. Bleaching of nonvital teeth. A clinically relevant literature review. *Schweiz Monatsschr Zahnmed* 2010; 120(4): 306–320.
29 Brown G. Factors influencing successful bleaching of the discolored root-filled tooth. *Oral Surg Oral Med Oral Pathol* 1965; 20: 238–244.
30 Davis MC, Walton RE, Rivera EM. Sealer distribution in coronal dentin. *J Endod* 2002; 28(6): 464–466.
31 Parsons JR, Walton RE, Ricks-Williamson L. *In vitro* longitudinal assessment of coronal discoloration from endodontic sealers. *J Endod* 2001; 27(11): 699–702.
32 Kim ST, Abbott PV, McGinley P. The effects of Ledermix paste on discoloration of mature teeth. *Int Endod J* 2000; 33(3): 227–232.
33 Frank AL. Bleaching of vital and non-vital teeth. In Cohen S., Burns R.C. eds. *Pathways of the pulp*. 2nd ed. St. Louis: C.V. Mosby; 1980. pp. 568–575.
34 Goldstein RE, Feinman RA. Bleaching of vital and non-vital teeth. In Cohen S., Burns R.C. eds. *Pathways of the pulp*. 4th ed. St. Louis. C.V. Mosby; 1994. pp. 593–598.
35 Zerbinati A, Pirero M. Il trattamento delle alterazioni cromatiche dei denti. *Il Dentista Moderno*. 1984; 7:969.
36 Kohli MR, Yamaguchi M, Setzer FC, Karabucak B. Spectrophotometric analysis of coronal tooth discoloration induced by various bioceramic cements and other endodontic materials. *J Endod* 2015; 41(11):1862–1866.
37 Camilleri J. Staining potential of Neo MTA Plus, MTA Plus, and Biodentine used for pulpotomy procedures. *J Endod* 2015; 41(7): 1139–1145.
38 Felman D, Parashos P. Coronal tooth discoloration and white mineral trioxide aggregate. *J Endod* 2013; 39(4): 484–487.
39 Ioannidis K, Mistakidis I, Beltes P, Karagiannis V. Spectrophotometric analysis of coronal discolouration induced by grey and white MTA. *Int Endod J* 2013; 46(2): 137–144.
40 Ioannidis K, Mistakidis I, Beltes P, Karagiannis V. Spectrophotometric analysis of crown discoloration induced by MTA- and ZnOE-based sealers. *J Appl Oral Sci* 2013; 21(2): 138–144.
41 Subay RK, Ilhan B, Ulukapi H. Mineral trioxide aggregate as a pulpotomy agent in immature teeth: long-term case report. *Eur J Dent* 2013; 7(1): 133–138.

42 Marciano MA, Duarte MA, Camilleri J. Dental discoloration caused by bismuth oxide in MTA in the presence of sodium hypochlorite. *Clin Oral Investig* 2015; 19(9): 2201–2209.
43 Berger T, Baratz AZ, Gutmann JL. *In vitro* investigations into the etiology of mineral trioxide tooth staining. *J Conserv Dent* 2014; 17(6): 526–530.
44 Jang JH, Kang M, Ahn S, Kim S, Kim W, Kim Y, Kim E. Tooth discoloration after the use of new pozzolan cement (Endocem) and mineral trioxide aggregate and the effects of internal bleaching. *J Endod* 2013; 39(12): 1598–1602.
45 Belobrov I, Parashos P. Treatment of tooth discoloration after the use of white mineral trioxide aggregate. *J Endod* 2011; 37(7): 1017–1020.
46 Nutting EB, Poe GS. Chemical bleaching of discolored endodontically treated teeth. *Dent Clin North Am* 1967 Nov: 655–662.
47 Fisher NL, Radford JR. Internal bleaching of discoloured teeth. *Dent Update* 1990; 17(3): 110–111, 113–114.
48 Friedman S, Internal bleaching: long-term outcomes and complications. *J Am Dent Assoc* 1997; 128 Suppl: 51S–55S.
49 Abbott P, Heah SY. Internal bleaching of teeth: an analysis of 255 teeth. *Aust Dent J* 2009; 54(4): 326–333.
50 Attin T, Paqué F, Ajam F, Lennon AM. Review of the current status of tooth whitening with the walking bleach technique. *Int Endod J* 2003; 36(5): 313–329.
51 Lee GP[1], Lee MY, Lum SO, Poh RS, Lim KC. Extraradicular diffusion of hydrogen peroxide and pH changes associated with intracoronal bleaching of discoloured teeth using different bleaching agents. *Int Endod J* 2004; 37(7): 500–506.
52 Antonson SA, Anusavice KJ. Contrast ratio of veneering and core ceramics as a function of thickness. *Int J Prosthodont* 2001; 14(4): 316–320.
53 Claus H. The structure and microstructure of dental porcelain in relationship to the firing conditions. *Int J Prosthodont* 1989; 2(4): 376–384.
54 Chang J, Da Silva JD, Sakai M, Kristiansen J, Ishikawa-Nagai S. The optical effect of composite luting cement on all ceramic crowns. *J Dent* 2009; 37(12): 937–943.
55 Holloway JA, Miller RB. The effect of core translucency on the aesthetics of all-ceramic restorations. *Pract Periodontics Aesthet Dent* 1997; 9(5): 567–574; quiz 576.
56 Shokry TE, Shen C, Elhosary MM, Elkhodary AM. Effect of core and veneer thicknesses on the color parameters of two all-ceramic systems. *J Prosthet Dent* 2006; 95(2): 124–129.
57 Turgut S, Bagis B. Effect of resin cement and ceramic thickness on final color of laminate veneers: an *in vitro* study. *J Prosthet Dent* 2013; 109(3): 179–186.
58 Morgano SM, Hashem AF, Fotoohi K, Rose L. A nationwide survey of contemporary philosophies and techniques of restoring endodontically treated teeth. *J Prosthet Dent* 1994; 72(3): 259–267.
59 Sorensen JA, Martinoff JT. Clinically significant factors in dowel design. *J Prosthet Dent* 1984; 52(1): 28–35.
60 Sorensen JA. Preservation of tooth structure. *J Calif Dent Assoc* 1988; 16(11): 15–22.
61 Morgano SM. Restoration of pulpless teeth: application of traditional principles in present and future contexts. *J Prosthet Dent* 1996; 75(4): 375–380.
62 Sidoli GE, King PA, Setchell DJ. An *in vitro* evaluation of a carbon fiber–based post and core system. *J Prosthet Dent* 1997; 78(1): 5–9.
63 Guzy GE, Nicholls JI. *In vitro* comparison of intact endodontically treated teeth with and without endo-post reinforcement. *J Prosthet Dent* 1979; 42(1): 39–44.
64 Trope M, Maltz DO, Tronstad L. Resistance to fracture of restored endodontically treated teeth. *Endod Dent Traumatol* 1985; 1(3): 108–111.
65 Goodacre CJ, Spolnik KJ. The prosthodontic management of endodontically treated teeth: a literature review. Part I. Success and failure data, treatment concepts. *J Prosthodont* 1994; 3(4): 243–250.
66 Goodacre CJ, Spolnik KJ. The prosthodontic management of endodontically treated teeth: a literature review. Part II. Maintaining the apical seal. *J Prosthodont* 1995; 4(1): 51–53.
67 Cohen S, Blanco L, Berman L. Vertical root fractures: clinical and radiographic diagnosis. *J Am Dent Assoc* 2003; 134(4): 434–441.
68 Kurer HG, Combe EC, Grant AA. Factors influencing the retention of dowels. *J Prosthet Dent* 1977; 38(5): 515–525.
69 Tjan AH, Whang SB. Resistance to root fracture of dowel channels with various thicknesses of buccal dentin walls. *J Prosthet Dent* 1985; 53(4): 496–500.

Questions

1 For post and core fabrication in multirooted teeth
 A It is essential to make posts for each canal.
 B Posts should be made in the larger canal irrespective of the canal length.
 C Both statements are false.
 D Both statements are true.

2 Which of the following cement are not preferred for cementing posts?
 A Zinc oxide eugenol
 B Zinc phosphate
 C Resin modified glass ionomer
 D Resin cements

3 Ferrule effect means
 A Tooth preparation must extend 2 mm beyond the cervical margin of the tooth.
 B Treatment provides marginal and tooth integration.
 C Both statements are true.
 D Both statements are false.

4 The length of the post in cast posts should be
 A Equal to the root length
 B Equal to the height of the anatomic crown

C 1 mm short of apical seal
D None of the above

5 Regarding the restoration of endodontically treated teeth, all of the following are generally believed to be true except
A A post weakens the tooth.
B All post designs are predisposed to leakage.
C A minimum of 4 mm of gutta-percha is needed to preserve the apical seal.
D Threaded screw posts are preferred over parallel-sided or tapered posts.

6 Post and core is indicated for
A A vital tooth with proximal caries
B A badly damaged endodontically treated tooth
C A badly damaged vital tooth
D A tooth with fractured incisal third

7 Why is it important to retain as much coronal dentin as possible when preparing a post for a crown?
A To resist crown rotation
B To resist post rotation
C To provide a ferrule effect
D All of the above

8 The cast post should be sandblasted by the lab before it is returned for fitting.
A True
B False

9 Tapered posts are less retentive than parallel-sided posts.
A True
B False

10 When cementing a post
A Cement should be placed on the post only.
B Cement should be placed in the canal only.
C Cement should be applied on the post and in to the canal.
D The crown must be cemented immediately with the same mix of cement.

CHAPTER 7

Dental traumatic injuries

Zuhair Al Khatib[1] and Edward Besner[2]

[1] *Formerly, Head of Endodontic Department, Dental Center, Dubai Health Authority, Dubai, UAE*

[2] *Formerly, Associate Professor, Department of Endodontics, Georgetown University School of Dentistry, Washington, DC, USA*

The history of treating dental trauma goes back to 1965, when the guidelines were first developed [1]. Dentoalveolar traumatic injury is one of the most commonly encountered dental emergencies; it occurs quite often in preschool- and school-age children and in young adults. Dental trauma can result in fractured, displaced, or lost teeth, which can have functional or esthetic effects on the individual. It can affect or involve the dental pulp (directly or indirectly), and it can cause extensive damage to the surrounding tissues. This chapter talks about various traumatic dental injuries and their current protocols of management. Root resorption is also described.

Traumatic dental injury (TDI) may be defined as an injury that results from an external force and that involves the teeth, the alveolar portion of the maxilla or mandible, and the adjacent soft tissues [2, 3]. It is imperative to rule out any neurological involvement or any other systemic injuries. Primary dentition is more affected during the period when the child's motor coordination is developing. Most injuries to permanent teeth occur secondary to falls, violence, and sports. The extent of injury can be related to the direction of force against the teeth, which can affect soft tissue as well as hard tissue (Figure 7.1). Object speed, size, and shape also plays a role in how much damage occurs to the teeth and surrounding supporting structure. A sharp object can cause more soft tissue damage than a larger blunt object such as football or fist punch during a fight or an elbow hit during basketball game. Children with an overjet exceeding 4 mm and with incompetent lips and a mouth-breathing habit are more prone to such injuries.

Preventive measures are essential during sports activities such as mouth guards, helmets. Occlusal relationship is a risk factor for traumatic injuries. The best measure for preventing dental and oral injuries is education on both how to avoid them and what to do if an injury occurs, which should include students, teachers, and parents.

General considerations

When faced with a traumatic injury, the biggest challenge for the clinician is to calm the patient and the parents in their panic and confused state. The dental practitioner should be able to reassure them and guide them on what to do if they call the dental office over the phone. A study by Porritt and colleagues investigates how a variety of biopsychosocial variables contribute to parents' adjustments to their children's dentoalveolar trauma [4].

It is critical to obtain standardized data from the patient or accompanying person [5]. This should include a complete history of when, where, and how the injury occurred, including the time elapsed between the incident and the patient's presence in the dental office. If the injury happened on dirty ground, antitetanus shots should be considered. Check for any previous dental injury, and obtain a medical history for allergies or any serious illness. This will have an impact on the outcome and prognosis of the treatment and even on the treatment plan. The type of occlusion and any disturbances in the bite should be determined at this stage.

Current Therapy in Endodontics, First Edition. Edited by Priyanka Jain.
© 2016 John Wiley & Sons, Inc. Published 2016 by John Wiley & Sons, Inc.

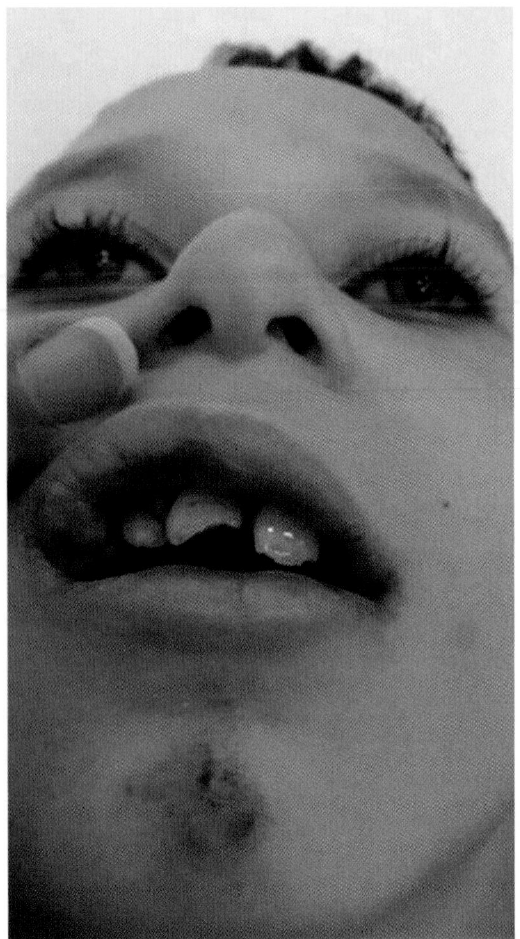

Figure 7.1 Dental trauma involving soft and hard tissues; the trauma was due to fall on the ground during school games.

Additional information, including if the patient vomited or lost conscious, had bleeding from the nose or ears after the injury, was in a state of confusion, or had blurred vision can help the treating dentist in deciding whether or not to pursue medical consultation [6].

Instructions to the patient or guardian calling from the site of the injury should include specific information relating to the type of injury. Tell the parent or patient to stay calm and try not to panic. If the tooth has displaced (moved from original position in the socket) but is still in the socket, the patient should rush to the dentist. If the tooth crown is fractured, the patient should find the fractured piece and bring it along. If the tooth is knocked out (avulsed), the patient should try to find it. The patient should hold the tooth from its crown and either put it back in its socket and bite gently on it or else store it in a glass of cold milk and bring it immediately to the dentist.

A proper diagnosis, treatment planning, and follow-up are critical to ensure a favorable outcome. Recommended guidelines by the International Association of Dental Traumatology (IADT) should assist the dentist and other healthcare professionals in making an informed decision. The primary goal is to delineate an approach for the immediate and urgent care of traumatic dental injuries. The patient's compliance contributes greatly to the outcome of the treatment and to better healing.

Trauma cases need long-term follow-up and evaluation at intervals for at least five years. This is significant for a long-term effective outcome.

Clinical examination

Check for any fractures of the bone or the dentoalveolar complex, any abnormal tooth mobility or tooth displacement, and any tenderness to touch and/or percussion. The adjacent soft tissue should also be examined for any lacerations. A pulp sensibility test, usually at the time of trauma, will give negative results.

Radiographic examination

Radiographs are essential for detecting root fractures, intrusions, extent of root development, periapical damage, degree of tooth displacement, position of unerupted teeth, fractures of the mandible or maxilla, the presence of tooth fragments, and foreign bodies in soft tissue. They also provide information about the patient's age and anticipated tooth maturation. Although some radiographs show negative findings at the initial appointment, they are important as baseline comparisons with subsequent radiographs.

Intraoral views are usually sufficient in assessing most dentoalveolar injuries. Several projections and angulations are routinely recommended, but the clinician should decide which radiographs are required for the patient. Recommended views are periapical view with 90-degree horizontal angle with central beam through the tooth in question, occlusal view, periapical view with lateral angulations from mesial or distal aspects, and soft tissue radiographs in case of soft tissue lacerations. Current imaging modalities like cone-beam computed tomography (CBCT) are not essential but can help in diagnosis and can give specific information about the traumatized teeth [7, 8]. They provide enhanced visualization, particularly in cases of root fractures and lateral luxation.

Initial treatment

Once the diagnosis is established and the local anesthetic is given, the tooth should be examined. If any contamination is visible, the tooth surface should be cleaned with saline and chlorhexidine 0.1%. Suture any lacerations, if required. Fractured tooth structure should be restored using composite resin. In cases of displacement or root or bone fracture, use digital pressure to replace the tooth in its normal position before splinting. Radiographs should be taken to confirm the accuracy of the repositioned tooth.

A short-term, flexible, nonrigid splint is recommended for tooth and bone fractures and for luxated or avulsed teeth. In cases of root fractures in the middle and cervical third of the tooth and alveolar fractures, rigid splinting is recommended. Splinting maintains the repositioned tooth in its correct position and provides patient comfort and improved function. A flexible splint for 2 weeks is generally used for subluxation and extrusive luxation. Lateral luxation (flexible splint), root fractures (rigid), and alveolar fractures (rigid), usually require 4 weeks of splinting [9]. In avulsion cases, where the teeth are not present, fixation is obtained by using firm pressure to realign the bone fragments and stabilize the area by suturing the gingival tissues. This is kept in place for 4 weeks.

Every effort should be made to preserve the pulp vitality in cases of immature permanent teeth to ensure continuous root development. Vitality tests (hot, cold, and electric) may be performed to determine the status of the pulp. At the time of injury, these are not very reliable diagnostic tools because they can give a false positive response or no response. Diagnosing necrotic pulp requires additional signs and symptoms. Emerging therapies have been under research and have demonstrated the ability to regenerate vital pulp tissue. This is discussed later in this chapter and in this book. In immature teeth, it is best not to initiate a root canal unless there are signs of necrotic pulp or radiographic changes. In mature permanent teeth that sustain TDIs, pulpal necrosis is amenable to preventive pulpectomy because root development is substantially completed. Root canal treatment can be initiated 7 to 10 days after trauma just before removing the splint.

Use of adjunctive systemic antibiotics

There is not sufficient evidence to support the use of antibiotics for TDIs. Antibiotics should be limited to certain cases of avulsion: if the tooth is contaminated with soil or debris, if there is a soft tissue laceration, or in cases where surgical intervention is needed and is at the discretion of the treating dentist [9–11]. The patient's medical condition or history necessitates the use of antibiotics in some situations. The first choice of antibiotics is usually tetracycline, and the dose should be adjusted according to the patient's age and weight. There is a growing concern amongst healthcare professionals regarding tooth discoloration with tetracycline, especially in children whose teeth are not completely developed or erupted. An alternative is phenoxymethylpenicillin (penicillin V) or amoxicillin.

Patient instructions and follow-up

Both patient and parents should be advised and given instructions regarding the care of injured teeth for optimal healing and prevention of any further injury. Instructions should include consumption of soft diet for one week, avoidance of participation in contact sports, maintenance of good oral hygiene by using a soft tooth brush and rinsing with an antibacterial like chlorhexidine 0.1% twice a day for one week, and keeping pressure off the injured tooth.

The splint should be removed after two to four weeks, depending on the type of TDI. The tooth and the surrounding tissues should be checked for healing. Follow-up radiographs should be taken and compared with initial images. The patient should be recalled for follow-up after 2 weeks, 6 to 8 weeks, 6 months, 1 year, and yearly for 5 years.

A favorable outcome of the TDI is achieved when on follow-up and recall the tooth is asymptomatic, the sensibility test is positive, and radiographs show intact periodontal space, no changes at the periapical tissues, and no signs of root resorption or root canal calcification or obliteration. Immature teeth should show continuous root development.

An unfavorable outcome of the TDI is when there are signs of external and internal root resorption, pulp necrosis, periapical rarefaction, and radiolucency developing along the fracture line of a fractured root. The tooth is in an infrabony position and is ankylosed.

Classification of traumatic injuries

Dental trauma may be classified according to the types of trauma (Box 7.1). The classification has been modified and updated by Andreasen and colleagues [12]. Since then, the IADT [13] and other researchers have put together all data available to develop classifications and treatment modalities of TDIs [14–16]. The management of these injuries is categorized individually for explanatory purposes.

Management of injuries to the periodontal tissues

Concussion

Concussion is defined as an injury to the tooth supporting structures without abnormal loosening or displacement of the tooth. This is the simplest form of trauma that can affect the teeth. There may be bleeding around the gingiva as a result of injury to the tooth supporting structures. Concussed teeth are tender to touch and percussion and slightly mobile due to an inflamed and injured periodontal ligament. Pulp sensibility testing usually gives positive results. Radiographic examination reveals the tooth is in its normal position within the socket. Treatment objectives are to optimize healing of the periodontal ligament and maintain pulp vitality. This is accomplished by relieving the tooth from occlusion and having the patient avoid using the concussed teeth for a week to reduce any pressure, which in turn reduces the stress on the periodontium. Splinting is usually not indicated. The patient should be placed on a soft diet for two weeks. These cases just need monitoring for about one year at three-month intervals. Radiographs should be taken at recall visits. Vitality should be tested as well at recall visits because there is a risk of pulp necrosis mainly with mature teeth [17]. In immature teeth, due to continuous root development, the risk of pulpal necrosis is much less.

Subluxation

Subluxation is defined as a modest injury to the teeth that affects the supporting structure of the affected tooth with abnormal loosening but without tooth displacement. Diagnostic signs and treatment are similar to those for concussion injury except for managing the mobility of the traumatized tooth. Sensibility testing at the time of the trauma is negative, indicating a transient pulpal damage that is usually reversible. Primary teeth

Box 7.1 Classification of Traumatic Dental Injuries

Injuries to the Periodontal Tissues

Concussion
Luxation
- Subluxation
- Extrusion
- Lateral luxation
- Intrusion

Injuries to the Hard Dental Tissues and the Pulp

Avulsion
Infarction
Enamel fracture
Enamel–dentin fracture
Enamel–dentin–pulp fracture
Crown–root fracture
- Uncomplicated
- Complicated

Root fracture
Alveolar bone fracture

do not require treatment for minor mobility. The prognosis is usually favorable, and the affected tooth returns to its normal condition within two weeks. Follow-up treatment is recommended at one week and six to eight weeks.

Mobile permanent teeth may need to be stabilized and occlusal interferences relieved. A flexible splint may be placed for two weeks if the patient feels pain and discomfort. Mature permanent teeth with closed apices may undergo pulpal necrosis due to associated injuries to the blood vessels at the apex. Therefore, until a definitive pulpal diagnosis is reached, monitoring and testing the affected teeth is important at one week, six to eight weeks, and one year.

Extrusion or extrusive luxation

Extrusion is defined as a partial displacement of the tooth axially from its socket (Figure 7.2A). In such cases the periodontal ligament is usually torn and the tooth appears to be elongated or protruding and mobile (Figure 7.2B). The bony socket usually stays intact. Radiographs reveal an increase in the periodontal space at the apical level. The tooth is tender to touch and percussion, with little or no response to a sensibility test. This is dependent on the degree of displacement of the tooth and its stage of development.

In primary immature teeth, treatment depends on the degree of displacement, occlusal interference, and time to exfoliation. If the injury is not severe (less than 3 mm of extrusion) the tooth may be repositioned or allowed to spontaneously align. In immature teeth, revascularization has a high occurrence rate. Positive reading of the pulp tester is a good indication of revascularization. But when the injury is severe or the tooth is nearing exfoliation or the patient is uncooperative, extraction should be considered as the treatment of choice.

In a permanent mature tooth with a closed root apex, there is increased risk of pulpal necrosis and periapical rarefaction. The tooth crown might discolor. Active repositioning of the tooth with digital pressure into its anatomically correct position should be initiated as soon as possible. Steady and firm finger pressure should be applied in an apical direction to displace the clot formed between the floor of the socket and the tooth apex. Stabilize the tooth for two weeks using a flexible splint. If the tooth is displaced greater than 5 mm and pulp necrosis is anticipated, the pulp should be extirpated within 48 hours and the canal filled with calcium hydroxide, followed by final obturation after three months. Treatment follow-up is two weeks when the splint is removed, and recall visits are scheduled at four weeks, eight weeks, six months, and one year (Figure 7.2C). Patient instructions and follow-ups are essential for good long-term prognosis.

Lateral luxation

Lateral luxation is defined as displacement of the tooth in a direction other than axial, usually in palatal/lingual, labial, or lateral direction (Figure 7.3A). This is accompanied by damage to the periodontal ligament, with fracture of the supporting alveolar bone (Figure 7.3B). The tooth is not mobile and is locked into the new position, giving a metallic sound, resembling an ankylosed tooth, during percussion. The tooth usually is not tender to touch, and pulp sensibility testing yields negative results. In immature teeth, pulpal revascularization usually occurs. Radiographic findings show an increase in the periodontal ligament space, rupture of the periodontal ligament, and displacement of the apex toward or through the labial bone plate. This is most evident on an occlusal radiograph.

Treatment in *mature teeth* consists of repositioning the tooth using firm and gentle digital pressure. Forceps may be used to disengage the tooth from its bony locked position and then repositioned. Such injuries are always accompanied by a dentoalveolar fracture component. The alveolar bone is also repositioned into its correct position to maintain alveolar integrity. The tooth may be stabilized with a flexible splint for four weeks. Pulp condition needs to be monitored. If pulpal necrosis is anticipated or if the tooth is displaced more than 5 mm, pulp should be extirpated within 48 hours to prevent root resorption. Follow-up is every two weeks while the splint is in place and then six to eight weeks, six months, and annually up to five years.

In *primary immature teeth,* continuous development of the root can be confirmed by radiographs indicating revascularization. The teeth may be allowed to passively reposition if this does not interfere with occlusion. If interferences are present, the tooth should be repositioned and splinted to the adjacent teeth for one to two weeks to allow healing. Such teeth have an increased risk of developing pulp necrosis compared to teeth that are left to spontaneously reposition. Follow-up is at two to three weeks and clinical observation and radiographs at six to eight weeks and one year. If there are no signs

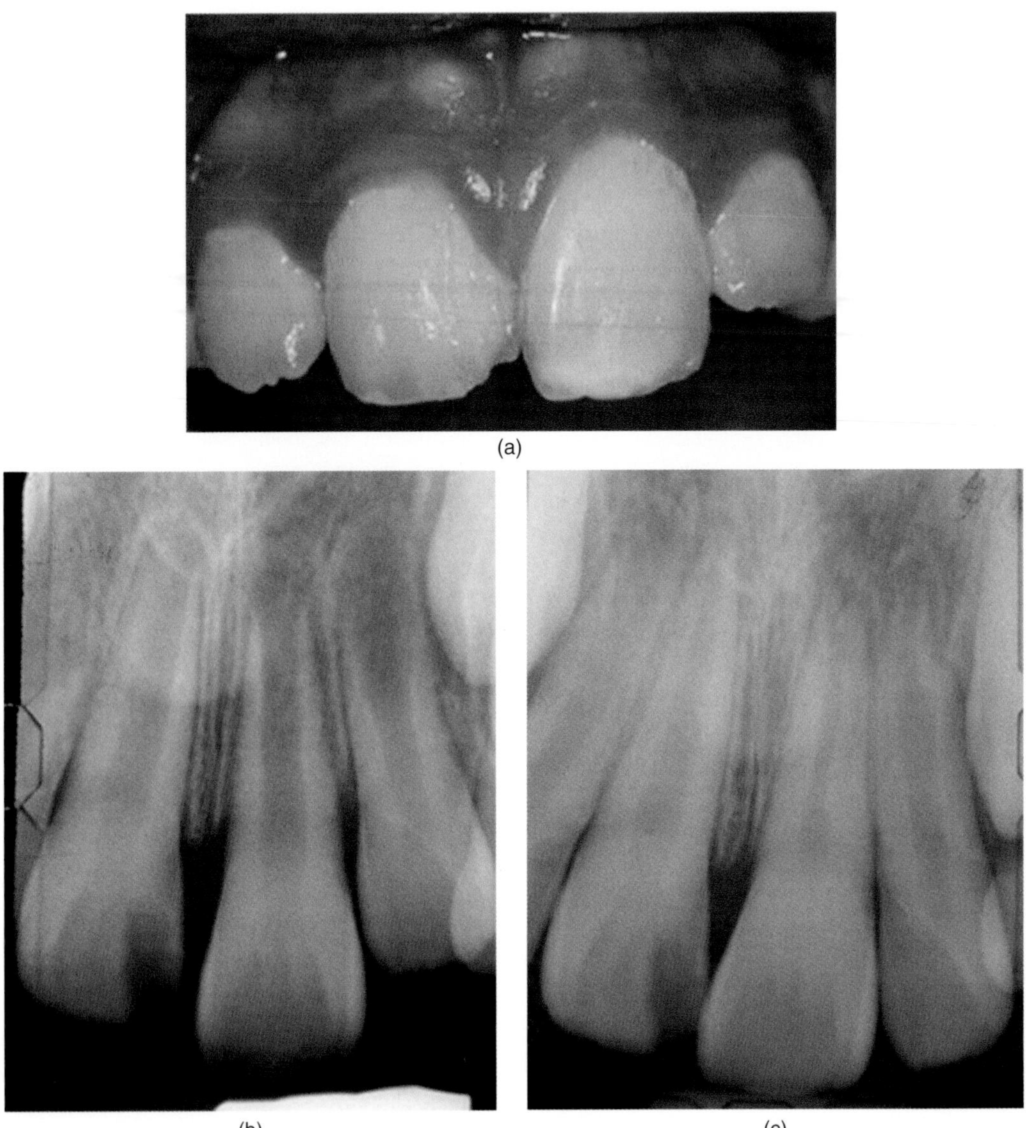

Figure 7.2 Extrusion. *A,* Extrusion of the upper left central incisor of a 9-year-old boy. *B,* A radiograph showing an open apex and chipped crown of upper right central tooth. *C,* Two years after trauma with apical closure and pulp canal calcification. Apical maturation and resorption of upper left lateral incisor.

of root development after three months, root canal therapy should be initiated using nonsetting calcium hydroxide to create an apical seal.

Intrusion or intrusive luxation

Intrusion is defined as the apical displacement of the tooth into the alveolar bone (Figure 7.4). This is due to trauma along the long axis of the tooth. In severe injuries, the tooth becomes intruded and locked in the alveolar bone, causing compression of the periodontal ligament and fracture of the alveolar socket. The intruded tooth is immobile, and on percussion it gives a high metallic sound. Clinically, the tooth appears to be short or even missing. the sensibility test yields negative

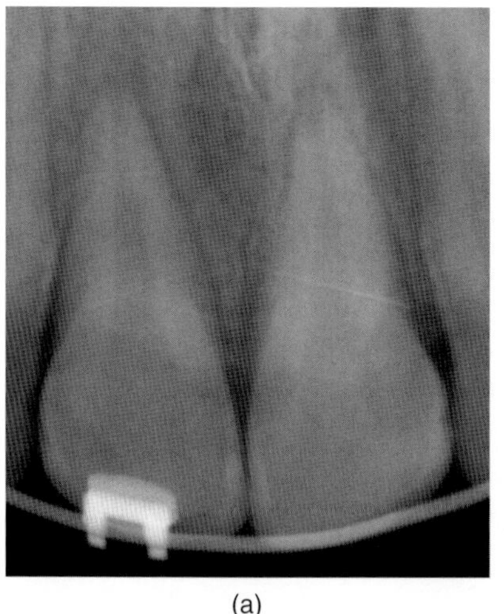

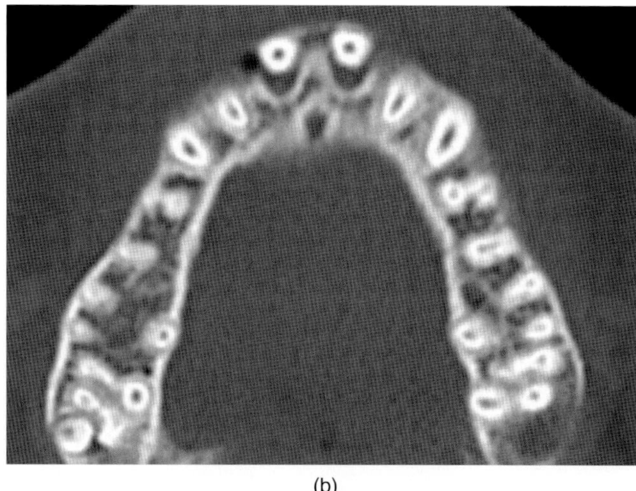

(a) (b)

Figure 7.3 Palatal luxation. *A,* Patient under orthodontic treatment due to trauma to teeth displaced labially. *B,* CBCT showing labial bone fracture with displacement of upper central incisors.

results. The tooth apex is usually displaced labially toward or through the labial bone plate when the affected tooth is of a primary dentition. In permanent teeth the displacement is into the alveolar bone. The position of the primary tooth in relationship to the developing permanent may be determined by a lateral radiograph.

Radiographic findings reveal that the tooth is displaced apically and the periodontal ligament space is not continuous or may be absent from all of the root. The cementoenamel junction is also located more apically in the intruded tooth in comparison to its adjacent tooth. There are three treatment modalities recommended to reposition the intruded tooth.

If the intrusion is less than 3 mm, allow for spontaneous eruption in case of immature teeth with incomplete root formation, and monitor the self-eruption over 6 weeks. If there is no movement within a few weeks, initiate an orthodontic repositioning procedure. In mature, fully developed roots, spontaneous eruption is less likely to occur. Intervention may be essential to prevent ankylosis. In either event, initiate orthodontic forced eruption or surgical repositioning if the tooth does not erupt spontaneously.

If the intrusion is between 3 and 7 mm, orthodontic repositioning should be performed over a few weeks to allow the periapical tissues to heal. The pulling force should be very minimal to help healing of the periodontal ligament and alveolar bone over time. Teeth should be splinted with a soft splint to allow physiologic tooth movement up to 4 weeks. This will stop the tooth from reintruding in the alveolar bone once again.

If the intrusion is more than 7 mm, surgical repositioning may be necessary. The pulp is likely to become necrotic in teeth with complete root formation. Root canal therapy should be initiated with calcium hydroxide 2 to 3 weeks after surgery. The tooth is then stabilized with a flexible splint for 4 to 8 weeks.

Management of injuries to the hard dental tissues and pulp

Avulsion

Avulsion is defined as the complete displacement of a tooth out of its socket. Exfoliated, avulsed, or knocked-out teeth are synonyms for the most serious and critical situation that can happen to adolescents. In young people, most avulsions occur during contact sports like football, basketball, handball, rugby, and boxing. Fights among students at school and assaults can be contributing causes as well. Slipping in bathrooms or other wet floors, car accidents, and bicycling are contributing factors and are common among elderly persons and adolescents. Avulsion of permanent teeth is observed in 0.5% to 3% of all dental injuries [12].

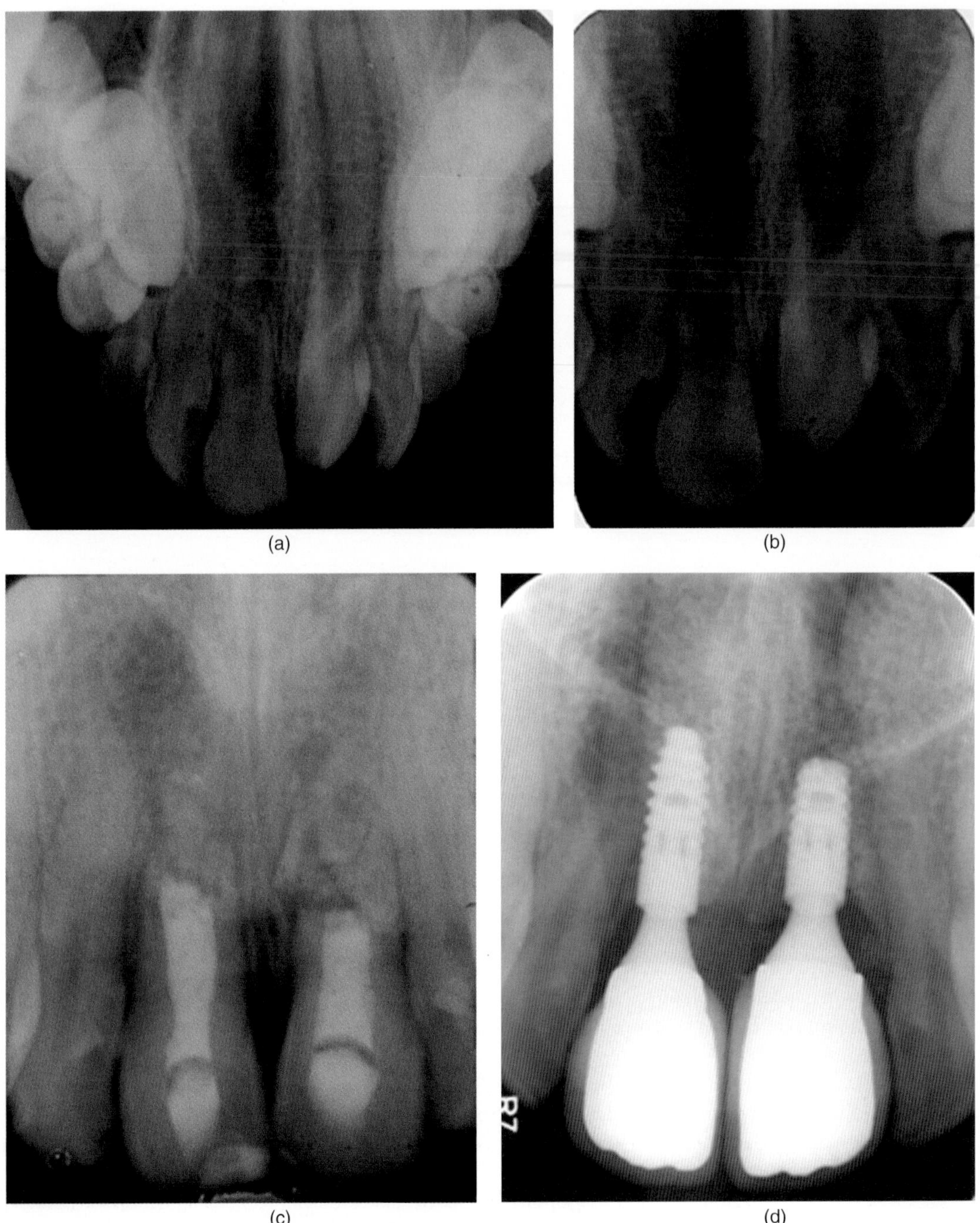

Figure 7.4 Intrusion (upper left lateral incisor). *A*, Occlusal radiograph. *B*, Periapical radiograph. *C*, Tooth erupted and MTA placed in both the central incisors; secondary midroot fracture. (D) Eleven years later, implant was placed.

The most important element for the treating dentist in dealing with traumatic injuries is the awareness of different modalities of treatment for both immature and mature teeth. Avulsion injuries may be accompanied by fracture of the alveolus. Radiographs are necessary to rule out intrusion if the avulsed tooth is not found.

The viability of the periodontal cells depends on the length of time the tooth was out of the mouth, the storage medium used before reaching the dentist, and the stage of development of the tooth. All these influence the treatment planning and prognosis. Immediate treatment is essential for better prognosis. Long-term prognosis also depends on the viable cells of the periodontal ligaments and the extent of damage to the cementum and pulpal tissues. Inflammatory resorption, replacement resorption, and ankylosis are the most significant and common complications after replantation of the avulsed teeth.

Instructions can be given to the parent or guardian or patient over the phone about what they can do at the site of the accident until they reach the dentist's office. The best first aid is to wash the tooth under running cold water for a few seconds, if possible, and immediately replant the tooth in its socket at the site of the accident by holding the tooth by its crown part and let the patient bite on a piece of gauze. Another option is to place the tooth in a storage medium, the most readily available and suitable being cold milk. Alternatively, place the tooth inside the mouth between the teeth and the cheek (buccal vestibule), and tell the patient to be careful not to swallow it. The most detrimental to the cells of the periodontal ligament is if the avulsed tooth is stored in a dry place before it is reimplanted. This affects the vitality of the periodontal cells, which in turn can cause resorption and prevent reattachment.

Success of replantation was initially thought to depend mainly on shorter extraalveolar time. However, researchers have demonstrated that storage medium is one of the most important factors in determining the prognosis of avulsed teeth. A storage medium may be defined as a physiological solution that closely replicates the oral environment with adequate osmolality, pH, and nutritional metabolites and thus create the best possible conditions for storage to help preserve the vitality of periodontal ligament cells following avulsion [18]. The ideal storage medium should maintain the vitality of the periodontal fibroblast cells to help them proliferate to reattach to the alveolar bone and root surface [19–21) and simulate the biological conditions of periodontal ligament cells, such as osmolality of 320 mOsm/kg and pH of 7.2 [22–27].

Types of storage media

Types of storage media, with their characteristics and efficacy, are shown in Table 7.1.

Hank's Balanced Salt Solution

Hank's balanced salt solution (HBSS) (Biological Industries, Beit Haemek, Israel) is a pH balanced solution having an osmolality of 320 mOsm/kg and pH of 7.2 [19, 28]. The main ingredients are 8 g/L sodium chloride, 0.4 g/L of D-glucose (dextrose), 0.4 g/L potassium chloride, 0.35 g/L sodium bicarbonate, 0.09 g/L sodium phosphate, 0.14 g/L potassium phosphate, 0.14 g/L calcium chloride, 0.1 g/L magnesium chloride, and 0.1 g/L magnesium sulfate [19, 26, 27]. These constituents can sustain and reconstitute the depleted cellular components of the periodontal ligament cells. This solution is the best available storage medium according to Krasner [27] and Ashkenazi and colleagues [19] because of its composition of glucose and calcium and magnesium ions, which can preserve periodontal ligament cells for up to 24 hours at 4°C. This solution does not require refrigeration and can be kept on the shelf for two years.

Hank's balanced salt solution is commercially available as Save-A-Tooth (Save-A-Tooth, Inc., Pottstown, PA, USA). Save-A-Tooth showed inferior results as compared to the original product. This could be due to the fact that HBBS is prepared for immediate use for better performance. However, it is not readily available at the accident site, thus making it a bit impractical for use.

Culture medium

Eagle's minimal essential medium consists of 4 ml of L-glutamine, 10^5 IU/L of penicillin, 100 µg/mL of streptomycin, 10 µg/mL of nystatin, and calf serum (10% v/v) [22]. It can maintain the viability of cells and clonogenic capacity for up to 8 hours of storage at 4°C [19].

Eagle's medium supplemented with growth factor has the same contents as Eagle's minimal essential medium. In addition, growth factors of 15% fetal calf serum and antibiotic solution consisting of 100 UI/mL penicillin, 50 µg/mL gentamicin, and 0.3 µg/mL amphotericin B (Fungizone) are added to the solution. According to Ashkenazi and colleagues [21], this is the second best medium after Hank's balanced salt solution in

Table 7.1 Different types of storage media.

Storage Medium	Characteristics	Efficacy
Hank's balanced salt solution	Neutral pH, osmolality, nutrients	++
Viaspan	Neutral pH, osmolality, favors cell growth	++
Minimal essential medium	Nutrients, antimicrobial, growth factors	++
Saline	Neutral pH, osmolality	–
Water	Bacterial contamination, hypotonic, nonphysiological pH, osmolality	– –
Saliva	Bacterial contamination, hypotonic, nonphysiological pH, osmolality	– –
Propolis and green tea	Antiinflammatory, antibacterial, antioxidant	++
Milk	Isotonic, neutral pH, osmolality, nutrients, growth factors, high availability	++
Patient's own serum	Neutral pH, osmolality, essential metabolites	+
Gatorade	Low pH, hypertonic	–
Probiotic lens solution	pH and osmolality not established, basic nutrients	+
Egg white	Low bacterial contamination, nutrients, water	+
Contact lens solution	Antibacterial, preservatives	–

++= Excellent, + = Good, – = poor, – – = Very poor

preserving the viability, mitogenicity, and clonogenic capacity after 24 hours at room temperature of 24°C, which make this medium a better cell preserver than Eagle's medium without growth factor supplement.

ViaSpan

ViaSpan (Belzer VW-CSS, Du Pont Pharmaceuticals, Wilmington, DE, USA) is a new storage medium used for transporting organs. It has been very effective for storing avulsed teeth as well [19, 20]. It has osmolality of 320 mOsm and pH of 7.4 at room temperature, which is ideal for cell growth [19–21]. It also contains adenosine, which is necessary for cell division. It is considered close to an ideal medium, but it has to be refrigerated, is not readily available, and is expensive, thus making it difficult to use [20].

Egg white

Egg white has a pH of 8.6 to 9.3 and an osmolality of 251 to 298 mOsm/kg. Khademi and colleagues compared milk and egg white as solutions for storing avulsed teeth, and the results have shown that teeth stored in egg white for 6 to 10 hours had a better incidence of repair than those stored in milk for the same amount of time [29]. This result was similar to that obtained by Sousa and colleagues, who demonstrated that milk and egg white had similar properties concerning the organization of collagen fibers and the number of cells, which makes egg white a perfect storing media [30].

Milk and milk formulas

Cow's milk has favorable properties for acting as a storage medium for avulsed teeth. It is an isotonic liquid with a neutral pH of 6.5 to 6.7 and physiological osmolality of 273 mOsm/kg. Krasner stated that milk can maintain the viability of human cellular periodontal ligament [27]. The American Association of Endodontists (AAE) indicates milk as a transport solution for avulsed teeth [22, 27, 28, 31]. Milk is significantly better than other solutions because it is easy to obtain, has low or no bacterial content, and contains essential nutrients such as amino acids, carbohydrates, and vitamins [22, 27, 31–35]. It is important that it be used in the first 20 minutes after avulsion [34]. Milk only prevents cell death and does not help in mitosis. Blomlöf and colleagues recommended milk as an excellent medium for 6 hours when it was cold and fresh [24]. Gamsen and colleagues demonstrated that milk is able to maintain the osmotic pressure for periodontal ligament cells but it does not have the ability to restore viability of the already depleted or degenerated cells [33]. Cooler temperatures reduce cell swelling, increase cell viability, and improve the cell recovery. Cold milk maintains cell function for almost twice as long as milk at room temperature.

Long shelf-life milk is an effective storage medium. Pearson and colleagues compared the efficiency of several milk substitutes, which included reconstituted powdered milk, evaporated milk, and baby formulas like Similac or Enfamil, as compared to whole milk [32].

Their findings revealed that Enfamil does not require special storage, has a shelf-life of 18 months, and is a more effective storage medium than pasteurized or whole milk for at least 4 hours [32]. There is no significant difference between regular pasteurized milk and long shelf-life milk; the only advantage of long-life milk is that it does not require refrigeration [35]. Regular pasteurized milk has a shorter shelf life and requires refrigeration, which makes it less readily available at the site of accident. Harkacz and colleagues suggested that milk with lower fat content may be more appropriate than milk with higher fat content [36].

Tap water

Tap water has been shown to be the least desirable storage medium. It causes rapid cellular lysis of the periodontal ligament cells, and it has bacterial contamination, low osmotic pressure (is hypotonic), and nonphysiological pH and osmolality [19, 20, 22–24].

Saliva/buccal vestibule

The buccal vestibule can be used for a short time due to its availability. It has nonphysiological pH and osmolality of 60 to 70 mOsm/kg. Other unfavorable characteristics are high bacterial content and hypotonicity. Storage for more than 2 to 3 hours will result in membrane damage of the cells. However, it is preferred to use saliva rather than keep the tooth in a dry environment when no other storage medium is available.

Gatorade

Gatorade is a sports drink used for rehydration. It is not very suitable for use as a storage medium due to its low acidic pH and hypertonicity, making it impossible for the cell to grow. It can only serve as a short-term storage medium if no other option is available because it preserves more cells than tap water.

Contact lens solution

Contact lens solution contains a fatty acid monoester and a cationic antimicrobial component. It is worse than saline [37]. The presence of preservatives in its formula is harmful to the cells of the periodontal ligament. Contact lens solutions are not generally recommended [38].

Propolis

Propolis is a natural substance produced by honeybees with antiinflammatory, antioxidant, antimicrobial, and tissue-regenerative properties [28]. It has approximately 50 constituents, primarily resins and vegetable balsams 50%, waxes 30%, essential oils 10%, and pollen 5%. Mori and colleagues found that this can be a promising transport medium [39]. The antibacterial and antiinflammatory actions inhibit prostaglandin synthesis, thus promoting healing of the epithelial tissues. Propolis also contains iron and zinc, which are important for collagen synthesis, and bioflavonoids, which help in the contention of hemorrhage of the periodontal ligament tissue. The major drawback is that it is not readily available to the public.

Saline solution

Normal saline provides physiological pH and osmolality of 280 mOsm/kg, which is compatible with the cells of the PDL. However, it lacks essential nutrients needed for cell metabolism, such as magnesium, calcium, and glucose [22, 27]. It has been suggested to use this as an interim storage medium for 2 hours [22, 31].

Recommendation

Although HBSS, ViaSpan, and Eagle's medium have great potential to maintain the PDL cells in a viable state after avulsion, the practicalities of using these solutions, the cost, and the lack of ready availability to the general public make them less than ideal. Milk remains the most convenient, cheapest, and most readily available solution in most situations while also being capable of keeping PDL cells alive. Hence, milk remains the storage medium of choice for avulsed teeth that cannot be replanted immediately or very soon after the avulsion because its pH and osmolality remain within the acceptable biological range.

Current developments in storage media

Antibiotic solution

Limited tooth storage in a cell-compatible medium prior to replantation has been researched and studied. Antibiotic solution has proven antiresorptive properties, thus promoting healing. It also promotes fibroblasts and connective tissue attachment, thereby enhancing regeneration of PDL cells.

Emdogain

Emdogain (Straumann Holding AG, Basel, Switzerland) is an enamel matrix protein shown to promote periodontal cell proliferation. It is composed of a number of proteins that self-assemble to create a matrix. The dominant protein in this matrix is amelogenin, which has been remarkably well conserved throughout evolution and is functionally consistent in many species. Therefore, although the matrix proteins in Emdogain are of porcine origin, they are considered "self" when encountered by the human body. Ashkenazi and Shaked found that it diminishes the percentage of fibroblasts of the periodontal ligament and is capable of forming colonies, which lowers the ability of the fibroblasts to repopulate the radicular surface after tooth avulsion [40]. It can delay, but not stop, the development of replacement resorption and by itself is not efficient in the regeneration of injured periodontal tissues of the avulsed tooth [40, 41].

Alendronate

Alendronate is a third-generation bisphosphonate currently used to inhibit pathologic osteoclast-mediated resorption of hard tissue. Studies have demonstrated that soaking avulsed teeth in alendronate results in significantly less loss in root mass due to resorption, as compared to other storage media.

Fluoride

Pre-replantation treatment of the root surface with fluoride helps eliminate inflammatory root resorption and increases the resistance of the root to replacement root resorption through the formation of fluorapatite on the root surface. This is done in cases when root cells cannot be resurrected by rehydrating in HBBS or milk. Results for this are proved only in in vitro studies [42].

Treatment of avulsed teeth

The guidelines for the treatment of avulsed permanent teeth vary, but the ideal treatment for an avulsed tooth is immediate replantation (Figures 7.5 and 7.6) [15, 43]. However, it cannot always be carried out immediately.

The treatment decision and long-term prognosis of avulsed teeth is related to the maturity of the root apex (open or closed) and the condition of the PDL cells. The condition of PDL cells depends on the storage medium and the time the tooth has been out of the mouth [44–48]. After a dry time of 60 minutes or more, all PDL cells are nonviable [15, 43]. In patients with a prolonged extraoral time, when replantation is being considered, the tooth should be maintained in a suitable medium until it is replanted by a dentist [49, 50]. Replanted teeth must be monitored carefully, and clinical and radiographic findings should be recorded because in children and adolescents, ankylosis is commonly associated with infraposition of the replanted tooth.

There are no guideline for the replantation of primary teeth due to the potential of subsequent damage to the developing permanent tooth. However, replantation of a permanent tooth should be preferably done at the site of trauma.

Avulsed immature teeth (open apex): new treatment regimen and rationale

Tooth is replanted before arrival (immediate replantation)

Immediate replantation has the best long-term prognosis. In such cases, the revascularization rate is high, causing growth continuation of the root apex until it closes completely. The less developed the root at the time of injury, the greater the potential for revascularization. Leave the tooth in place. Ensure that the examination of traumatized teeth and initial treatment mentioned at the beginning of this chapter are performed. Stabilize the teeth with a flexible physiologic splint for two weeks. Prescribe an antibiotic. Avoid root canal treatment unless there is clinical or radiographic evidence of pulp necrosis. In the case of pulp necrosis, the pulp should be extirpated and calcium hydroxide placed immediately, to stimulate apexification and halt the inflammatory response. Patient instructions and follow-up should be followed as mentioned at the beginning of this chapter.

Preserving the periodontal ligament attachment (teeth with less than 60 minutes outside the mouth): enhancing revascularization with the use of topical antibiotics

The decision and management differs for immature and mature teeth. Because the patient's age is not a clear indication of a tooth's maturity, the clinician should rely upon the apical closure as an indication for the stage of development. An immature tooth (open apex) can establish revascularization, but a mature tooth cannot.

If immediate replantation is not possible, the avulsed tooth is transported to the dentist's office in an appropriate storage medium. Detrimental effects occur to the

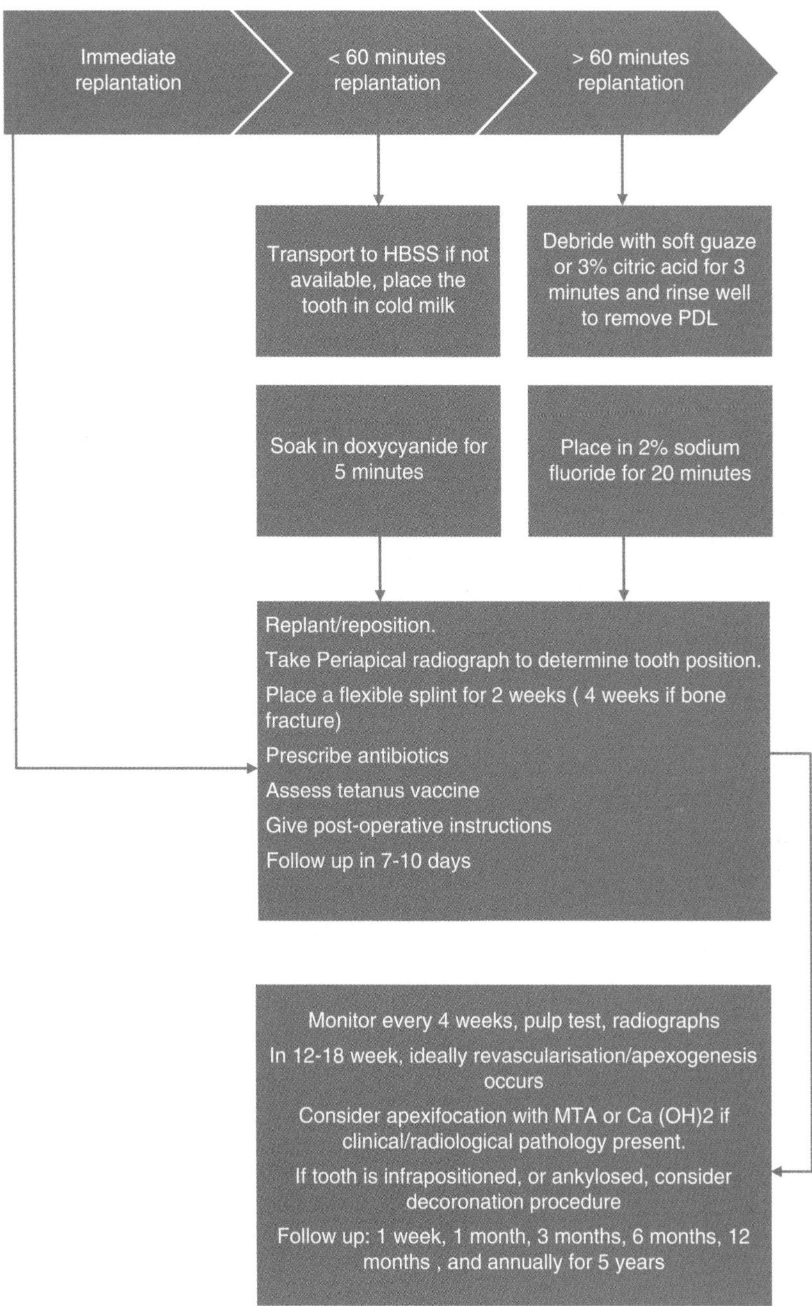

Figure 7.5 Treatment of avulsed immature teeth.

periodontal ligament cells especially if the tooth has been kept dry. Upon the patient's arrival, assess the extraalveolar time and storage medium, because the risk of ankylosis increases significantly with an extraoral dry time of more than 15 minutes. In such a situation, replantation is questionable because the increased risk of ankylosis can have an unaesthetic result. Such teeth, if replanted, should be monitored closely.

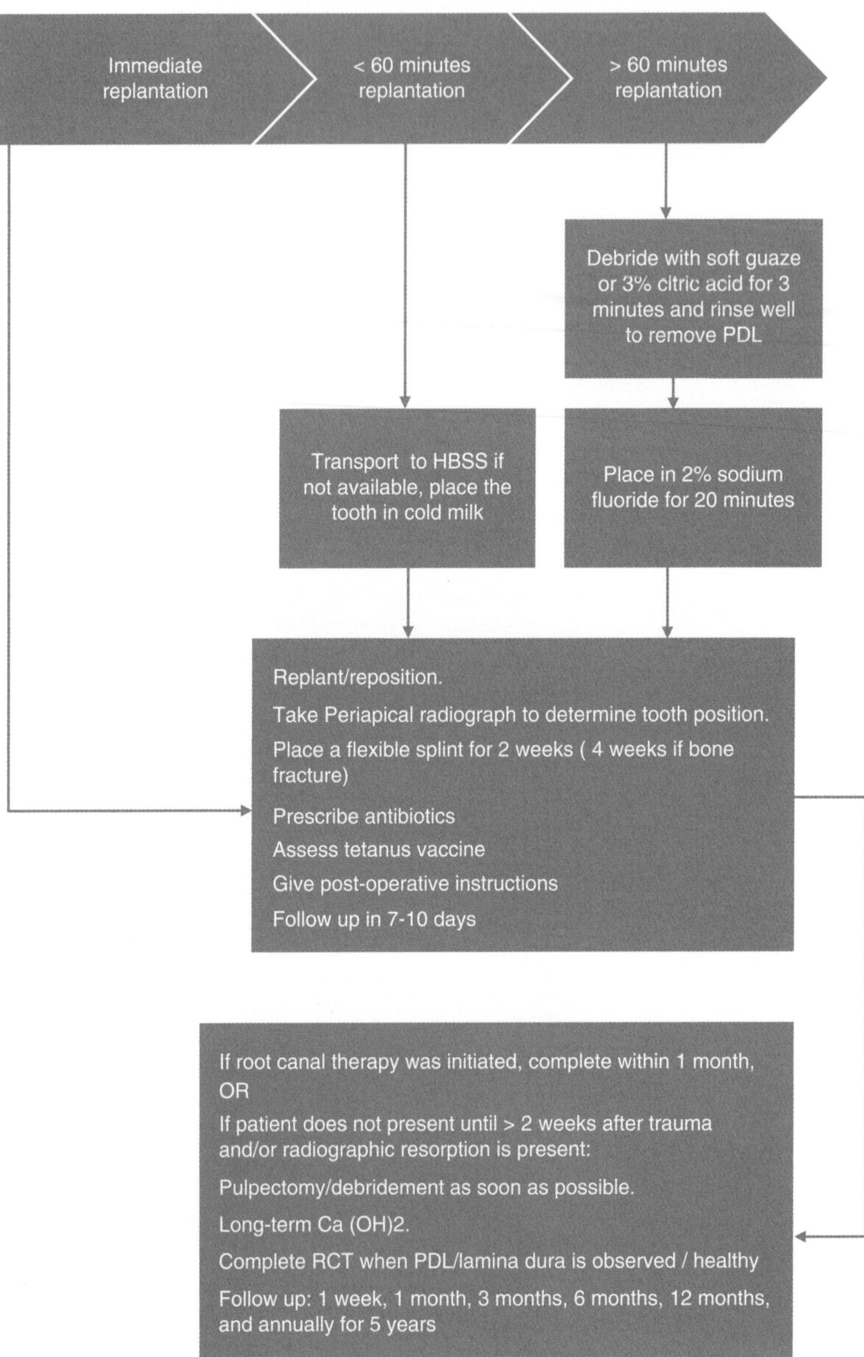

Figure 7.6 Treatment of avulsed mature teeth.

Clean the root surface with saline solution without touching the coronal part. Flush the socket with saline. Soak the tooth in minocycline or 1% doxycycline solution (1 mg doxycycline solution in 20 mL saline or 50-mg doxycycline capsule in 1000 mL saline) for 5 minutes [47, 51, 52]. Cvek and colleagues [47] found that topical application of doxycycline increased the probability of complete pulp revascularization and decreased the probability of microorganisms in the pulpal lumen. The risk of inflammatory root resorption was also decreased. Ritter and colleagues concluded that minocycline facilitates pulp revascularization in immature teeth after replantation [53].

Replant the tooth slowly and gently with firm digital pressure without exerting any force. If resistance is met, check for any bony fractures. Verify the position of the tooth in the socket clinically and radiographically. Prescribe systemic antibiotic. Do not initiate endodontic treatment unless there are signs of pulpal necrosis or radiographic changes. If root canal therapy has to be initiated, it should be performed just before the splint is removed to minimize any pressure. Calcium hydroxide can be used as intracanal medicament for up to one month, followed by root canal filling with a biocompatible material. Bryso and colleagues demonstrated that roots treated with Ledermix Paste roots had statistically significantly more healing and less resorption than the roots treated with calcium hydroxide [54].

Patient instructions and follow-up are the same. Recall visits should be at two weeks (when the splint is removed), four weeks, eight weeks, six months, and one year and annually thereafter. If the tooth exhibits symptoms, mobility, or ankylosis, surgical treatment should be considered.

Teeth with more than 60 minutes outside the mouth

Delayed replantation has a poor long-term prognosis. The periodontal ligament will be necrotic and not expected to heal. Osseous replacement resorption or ankylosis is likely to occur [48, 55]. There is controversy regarding whether such teeth should not be replanted. Recent guidelines recommend replantation, though, to maintain the alveolar bone contour esthetically and psychologically. Ankylosis is often associated with infraposition of the replanted tooth. Decoronation may be necessary when the degree of infraposition increases more than 1 mm [56, 57]. Despite an extended extraalveolar dry storage time, teeth with delayed replantation might be retained in a stable and functional position in the dental arch. In patients for whom growth has not ceased, the replanted tooth can maintain the periodontium and the surrounding bone for a few years until other replacement options, such as implant, can be considered.

Treatment of these cases starts with the removal of attached periodontal ligament from the root surface, using gentle scrubbing with gauze or 3% citric acid for 3 minutes [52, 58] followed by soaking the tooth in 2% sodium fluoride for 20 minutes. Selvig stated that fluoroapatite makes the tooth more resistant to ankylosis than hydroxyapatite [59]. This procedure makes the root surface more resistant to osteoclastic activity, thus reducing the possibility of resorption and ankylosis. After replanting the tooth, splint the tooth in place for four weeks.

Root canal therapy is usually performed extraorally by irrigating the canal and placing an apical plug of about 4 mm thick, using mineral trioxide aggregate (MTA) (ProRoot Endo Sealer, Dentsply Maillefer, Ballaigues, Switzerland) [60–63] or TotalFill BC RRM Putty (Peter Brasseler Holdings, Savannah, GA, USA) [64, 65]. Ghoneim and colleagues [65] concluded that bioceramic root canal filling can strengthen the residual root and increase the *in vitro* fracture resistance of endodontically treated teeth. This is a very significant finding, particularly for the long-term retention of an immature tooth that has thin root canal walls and is susceptible to fracture if any future trauma happens.

Avulsed Mature Permanent Teeth (Closed Apex)

Mature teeth with immediate replantation

The treatment for a mature tooth does not differ from that for an immature avulsed tooth when it is replanted immediately. Follow the same steps and monitor the outcome clinically and radiographically. Initiate root canal therapy 7 to 10 days after replantation and just before removing the splint. The chance of revascularization is minimal in a mature avulsed tooth. Place non-setting calcium hydroxide for one month until the root canal is permanently filled. This can help in reducing any further non-favorable outcome. Fill the canal with biocompatible filling material and follow up the case.

Mature teeth with less than 60 minutes outside the mouth

An avulsed tooth that has been kept outside the mouth will have some necrotic periodontal ligament cells (Figure 7.7). If the avulsed tooth is left dry, wash the root surface with saline and soak it in an appropriate medium, such as HBBS. Treat the surrounding tissues, if they are lacerated. Flush the alveolar socket with a stream of saline to get rid of any coagulum. Replant the tooth back in its socket with gentle pressure, without exerting any force [66]. Osseous inflammatory resorption (ankylosis) is one of the unfavorable potential outcomes [55]. Patient instructions and follow-up are essential, and intervention is done at the first sign of inflammation.

Mature teeth with more than 60 minutes outside the mouth

Extraoral time longer than 60 minutes has a poor long-term prognosis (Figure 7.8). The goal of delayed replantation is to promote alveolar bone growth to encapsulate the replanted tooth and to maintain the integrity of the alveolar bony socket (Figure 7.9). Treatment starts with cleaning the root surface with gentle scrubbing. Soak the tooth in 3% citric acid for 3 minutes. Rinse it with saline and immerse it in 2% sodium fluoride solution for 20 minutes. Root canal therapy can be performed prior to replantation. Otherwise, root canal therapy can be performed two weeks after replantation and the splint can be removed that day.

An unfavorable outcome is ankylosis or inflammatory root resorption without osseous replacement, which will eventually lead to tooth loss (Figure 7.10). If the infrabony position is more than 1 mm, decoronation may be necessary [56, 57]. Lin and colleagues and Malmgren agreed that decoronation of ankylosed young permanent incisors resulted in a decrease in the buccopalatal dimension with time [67, 68]. It did not prevent additional alveolar growth that occurs with age in a developing child and thus may help maintain the alveolar bone ridge width, height, and continuity and assist in future rehabilitation with less-invasive ridge-augmentation procedures required for implant placement. Currently, there is an emphasis on the

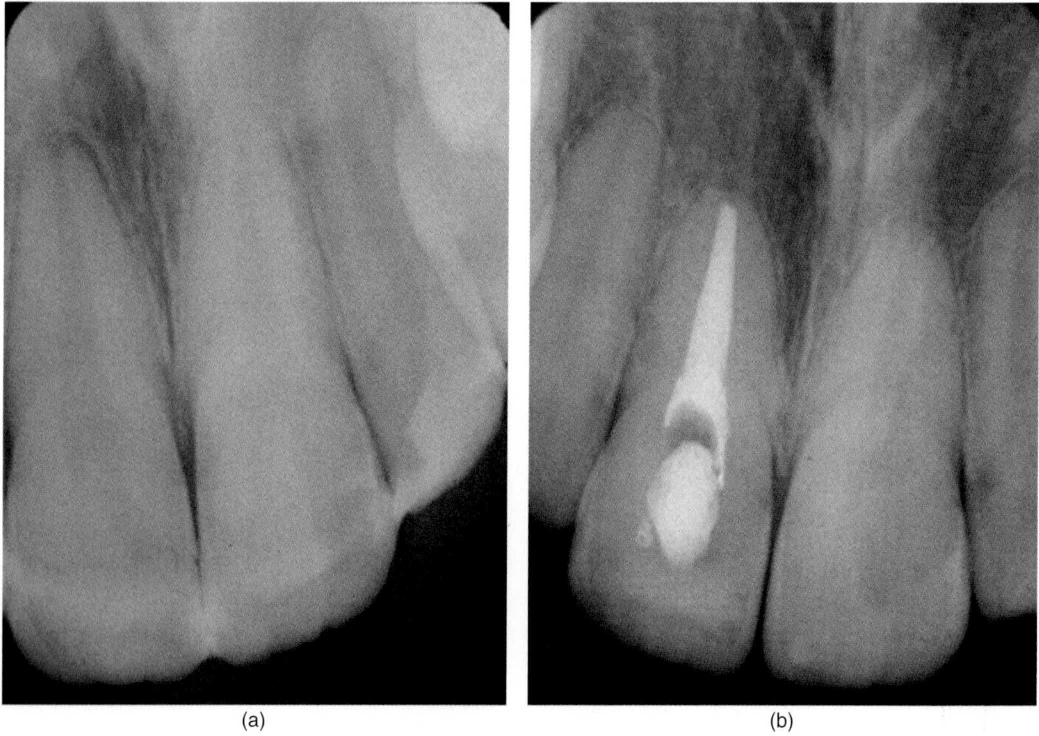

(a) (b)

Figure 7.7 Avulsion with extraoral time less than 60 minutes. *A*, Upper right central incisor replanted. *B*, Follow-up after 4 years.

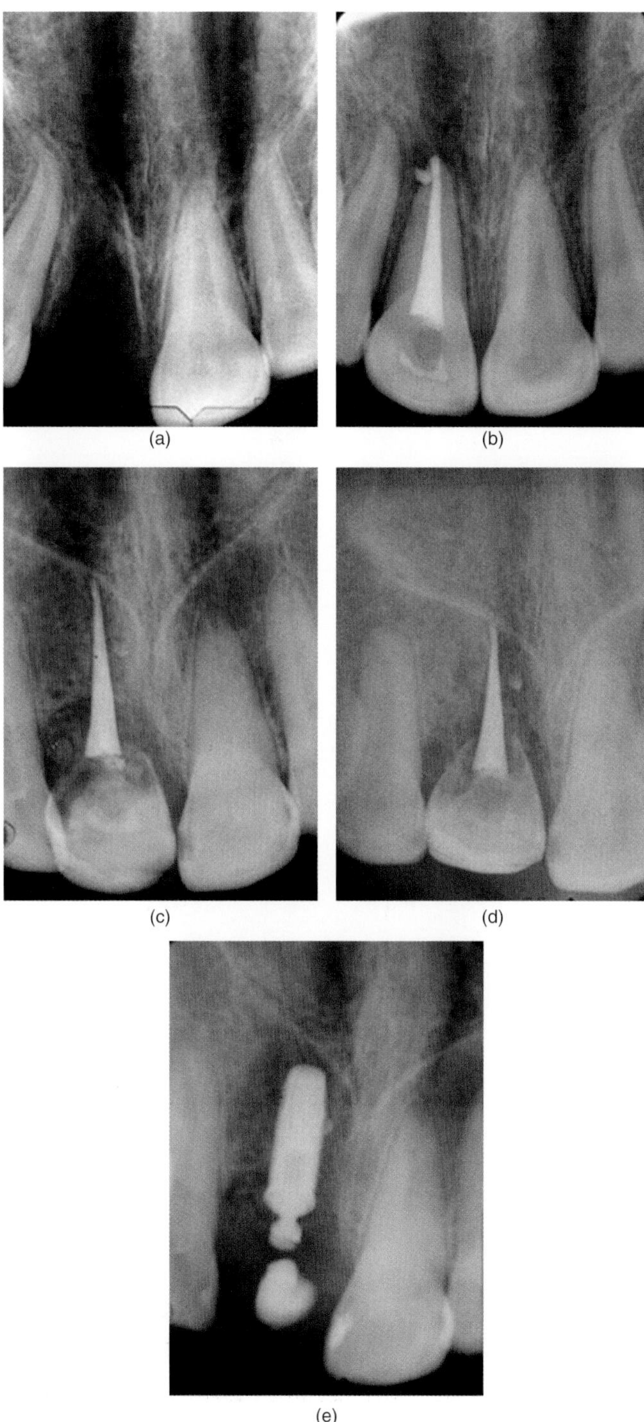

Figure 7.8 *A,* Avulsion with extraoral time of two hours. *B,* Three months after replantation. *C,* Inflammatory root resorption noticed after two and a half years. Left central canal obliterated. *D,* Five and half years later, with the tooth still holding its position in the alveolar bone, with the gutta-percha filling and free gingiva. *E,* Tooth removed and implant placed without bone augmentation.

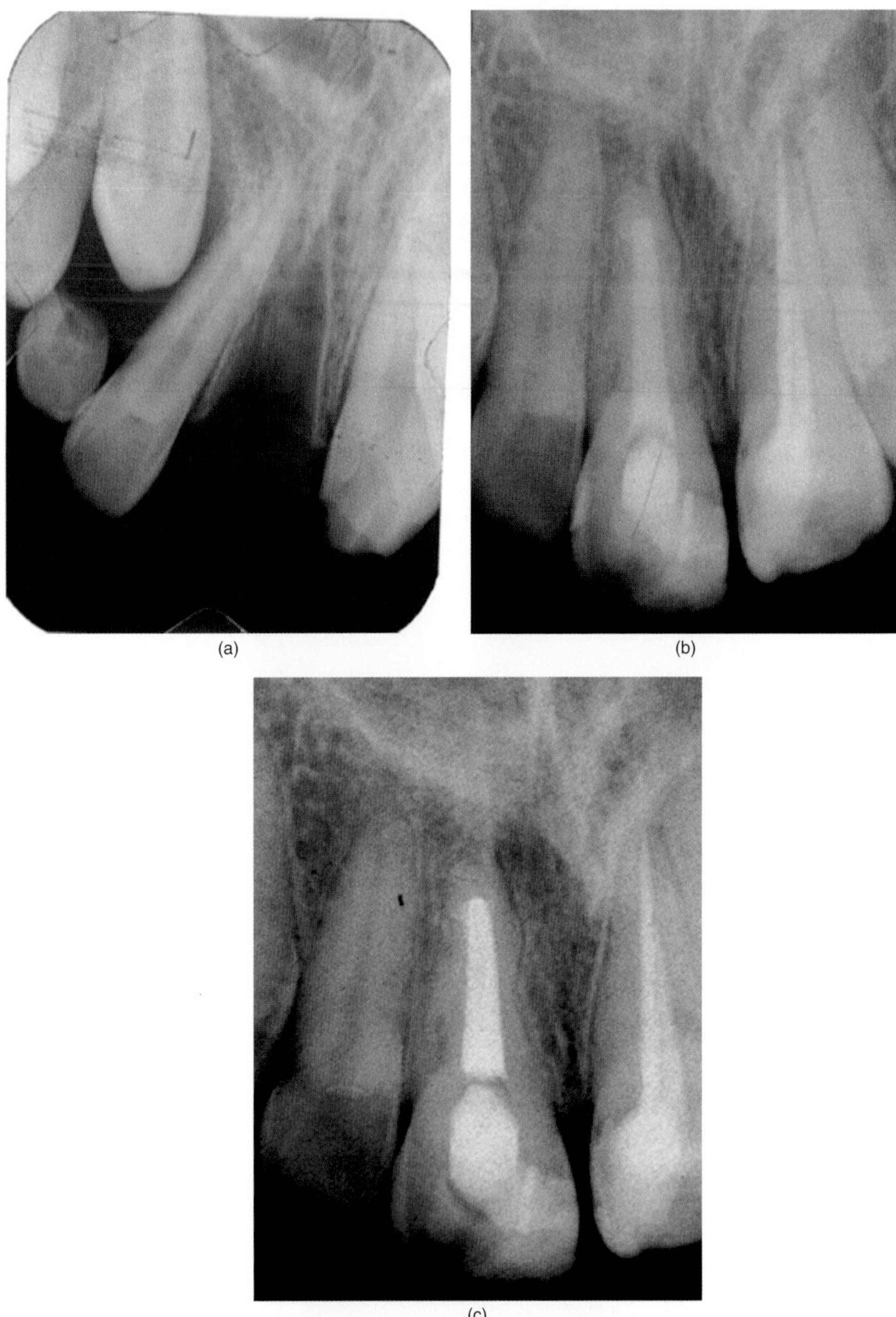

Figure 7.9 Avulsion with extraoral time more than 60 minutes. *A,* Upper right central incisor kept dry for four hours. *B,* Mesial and distal resorption after five years. *C,* Nine years after trauma.

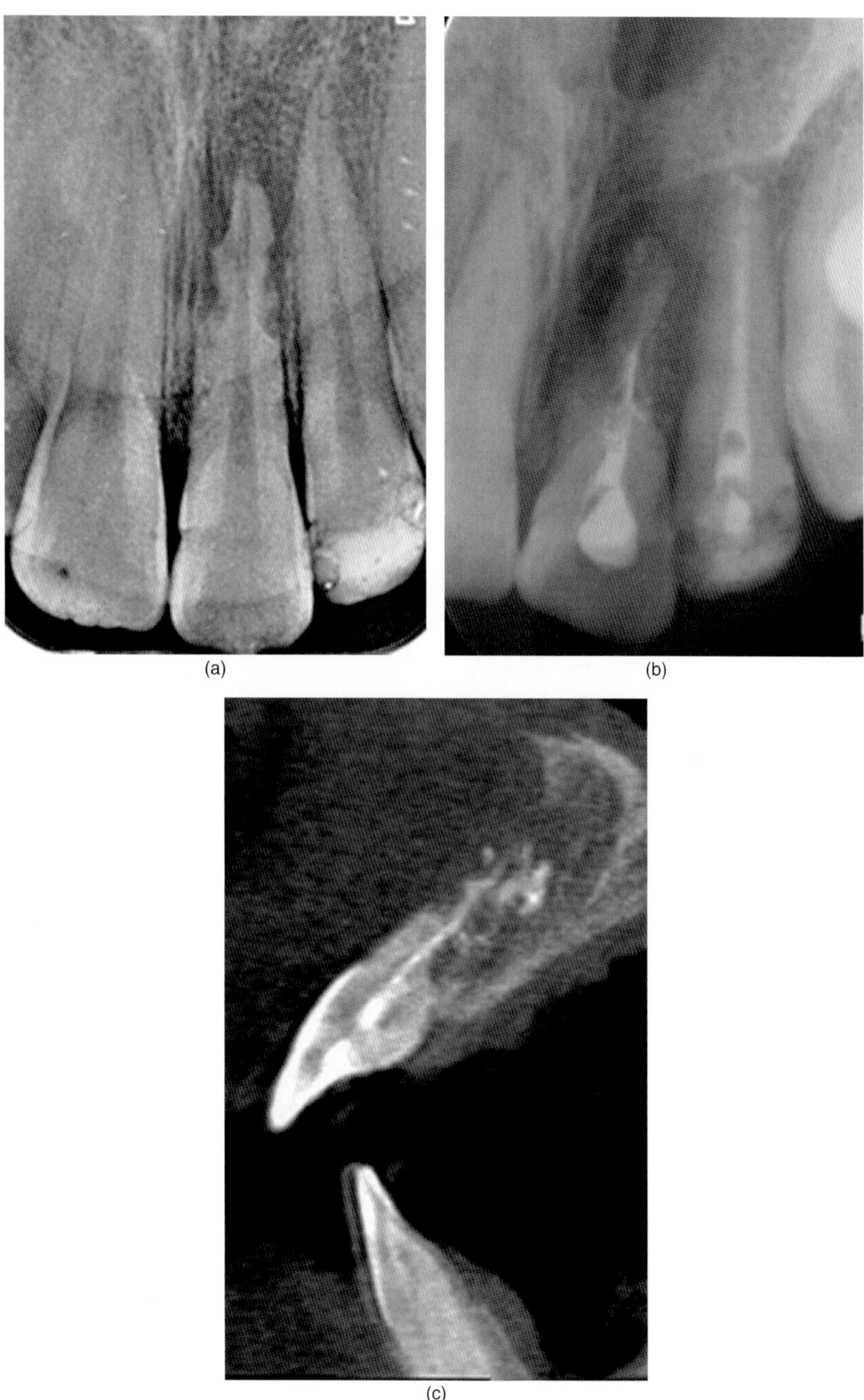

Figure 7.10 *A,* Inflammatory root resorption. *B,* Two years after avulsion and replantation. *C,* CBCT image showing that most of the root is resorbed.

regenerative procedures in managing avulsed teeth with pulpal necrosis.

Pulp revascularization

Regeneration in immature permanent teeth that have necrotic but uninfected pulps following trauma helps to reduce the risk of fracture. Regenerative endodontic procedures can be defined as biologically based procedures designed to predictably replace damaged, diseased, or missing structures, including dentin and root structures as well as cells of the pulp–dentin complex, with live viable tissues, preferably of the same origin, that restore the normal physiologic functions of the pulp–dentin complex [69]. These include direct pulp capping, revascularization, apexogenesis, apexification, stem cell therapy, and tissue engineering [69]. Most therapies use the host's own vascular cells for these procedures, but stem cell therapies are also currently under research and development. (Figure 7.11).

Bioactive substances like Emdogain, an enamel matrix derivative substance, is currently under research for facilitating regeneration of the periodontal ligament

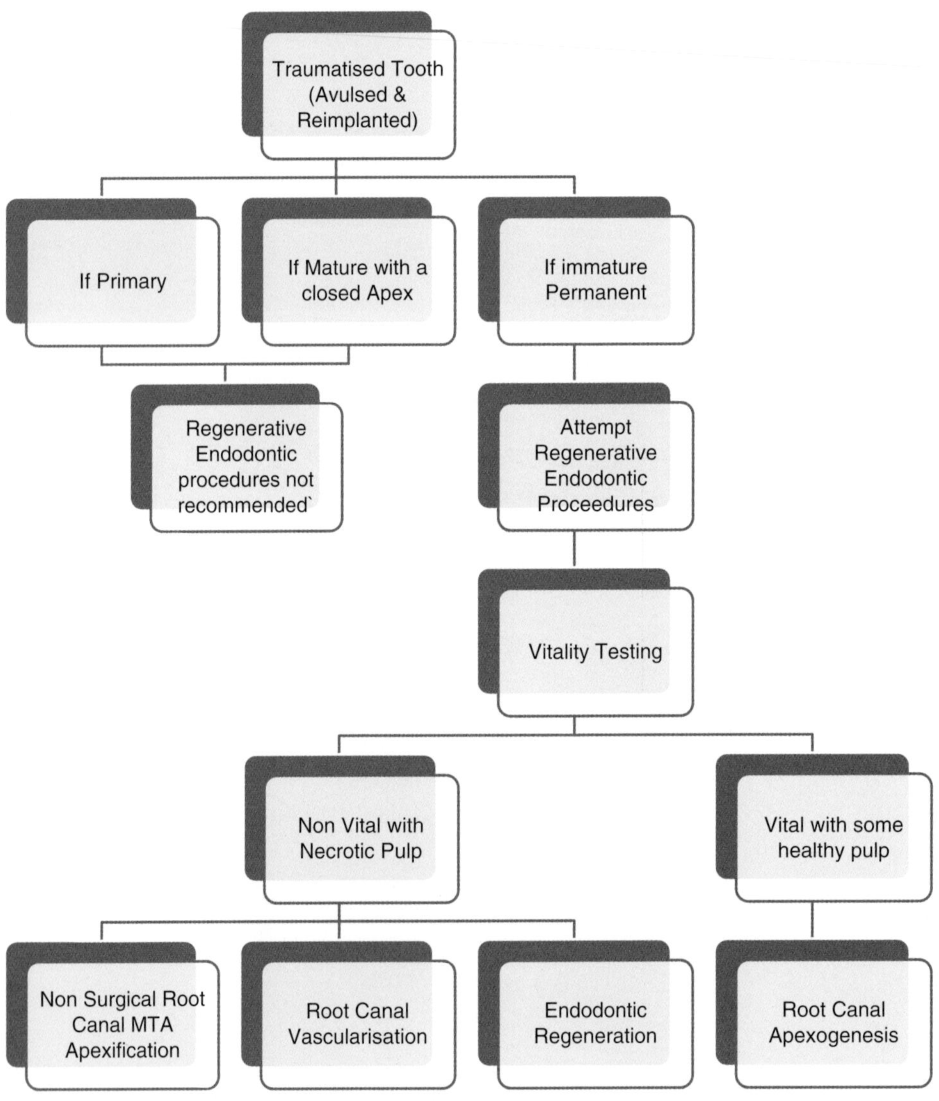

Figure 7.11 When to perform regenerative procedures.

and inhibiting the development of replacement and inflammatory root resorption. It is still in the early stages of evaluation for use. Researchers argue that coating the root surface of avulsed teeth with Emdogain could promote migration, proliferation, and differentiation of periodontal ligament fibroblasts. The topic is dealt in detail in Chapter 11.

Enamel infraction (crack)

Infarction is defined as an incomplete fracture of the enamel without loss of the tooth structure. This is the simplest form of trauma that can occur. Tiny craze lines in the enamel can be seen visually or with transillumination. A periapical radiograph should be taken to rule out any root fractures. A sensibility test may give a negative reading initially, indicating transient pulpal damage. Treatment is aimed at maintaining the structural integrity of the tooth. It can range from plain observation to placement of composite resin, depending on the extent and the aesthetics. No follow-up is needed for these cases [14].

Enamel fracture

Enamel fracture is confined to tooth crown enamel and is visible clinically with rough enamel surface. Regardless of its simplicity, treatment procedure should be followed with pulp testing, mobility, and radiographs. If a tooth fragment is available, it can be replaced after smoothing sharp enamel edges and bonding the fragment to the tooth using composite resin [14]. Follow-up is scheduled for 6 to 8 weeks and then one year.

Enamel–dentin fracture without involvement of the pulp (uncomplicated crown fracture)

Enamel–dentin fracture involves only enamel and or enamel–dentin structure without the involvement of the pulp. This is clinically detectable. Lips, tongue, and gingiva should also be examined for embedded tooth fragments and debris. Pulp sensibility testing is essential to monitor pulpal changes. Initial testing may be negative, indicating transient pulpal damage. Soft tissue radiographs should also be taken, especially when the patient presents with soft tissue lacerations, because sometimes the tooth fragment is embedded in one of the lips (Figure 7.12).

Treatment objectives are to maintain pulp vitality and restore normal esthetics and function. For small fractures, rough edges may be smoothed. For larger fractures, lost tooth structure may be restored with calcium hydroxide (if the fracture is close to the pulp), glass ionomer cement, and composite. The prognosis of uncomplicated crown fractures depends primarily upon the extent of dentin exposed. Follow-up clinically and radiographically at 6 to 8 weeks and one year [14, 70].

Enamel–dentin fracture involving the pulp (complicated crown fracture)

A complicated crown fracture is defined as an enamel–dentin fracture with pulp exposure. As with the uncomplicated tooth fracture, the lips, tongue, and gingiva should be examined for tooth fragments and debris. The routine radiographs should include soft tissue

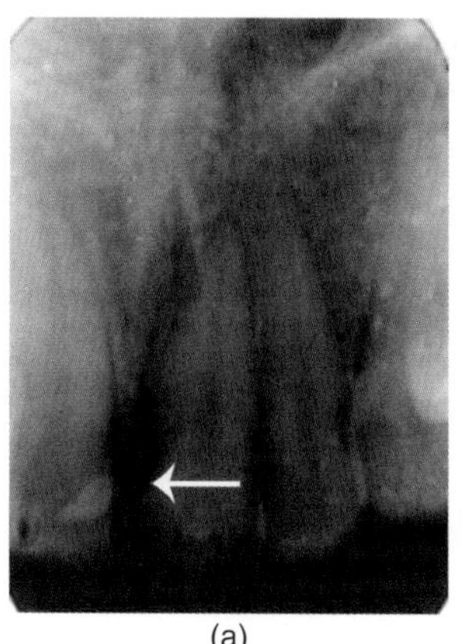
(a)

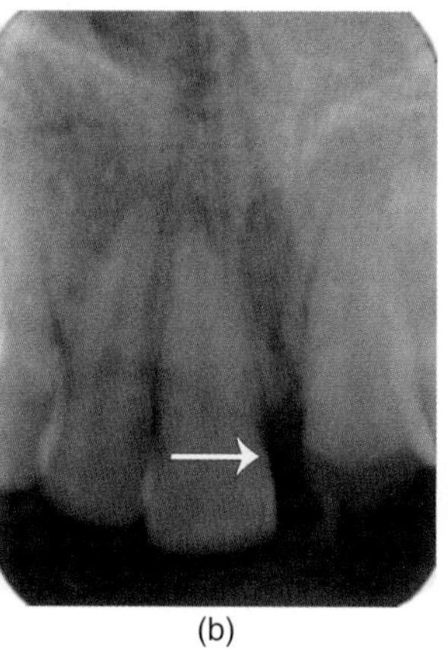
(b)

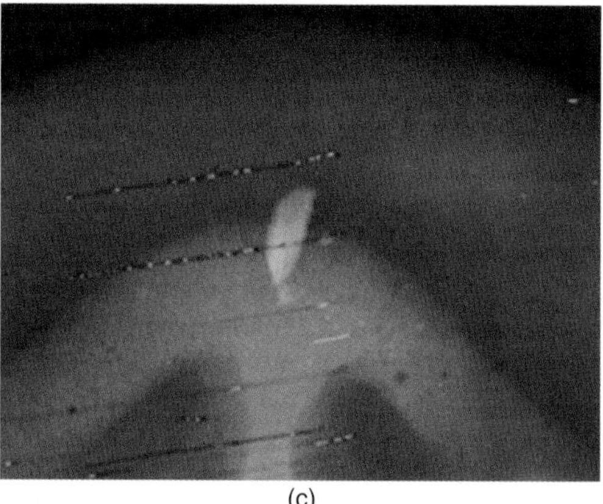
(c)

Figure 7.12 Enamel dentin fracture. *A*, Arrow indicates fractured crown fragment. *B*, Arrow indicates the displacement of the fragment. *C*, Soft tissue radiograph of the upper lip showing the fractured fragment.

radiograph in addition to periapical and occlusal radiographs. A sensibility test is not indicated because pulpal exposure and involvement is evident clinically by sight.

For primary teeth, pulpal treatment options are pulpotomy, pulpectomy, or extraction, but it is advantageous to preserve the pulp's vitality. In permanent teeth, pulp treatment options are direct pulp capping or partial pulpotomy with calcium hydroxide or MTA or pulpectomy, depending on the extent of the exposure and the time elapsed since injury [71]. The tooth should be isolated and decontaminated with chlorhexidine. The tooth is then restored with composite resin [14]. These procedures will maintain the viability of pulpal tissue cells, thus helping in continuous root maturation in immature teeth. Mature teeth will maintain their viability to prevent any further pulp complications. Follow-up is in 6 to 8 weeks and one year.

Crown–root fracture without pulp involvement

This type of crown–root fracture is a result of an enamel, dentin, and cementum fracture with or without exposing the pulp. A mobile coronal fragment attached to the gingiva with or without a pulp exposure is clinically evident. The fracture line extends palatally below the gingival margin or sometimes even below the bone crest, making the fracture line invisible. Anteriorly, the fractured coronal portion extends in an incisal direction, resulting in pain upon occlusion. In the posterior region the fracture is usually confined to the buccal cusps. Root fractures can only be diagnosed radiographically.

Radiographic findings reveal a radiolucent oblique area usually perpendicular to the central radiographic beam. If definitive treatment cannot be performed at the initial visit, the emergency treatment should be carried out to reposition the coronal fragment and temporarily splint it to the adjacent teeth with composite for up to four weeks to reduce the patient's discomfort.

Treatment modalities depending on the position of the fractured fragment (according to DiAngelis and colleagues [14]) include fragment removal only, fragment removal and gingivoplasty and/or osteoplasty, orthodontic extrusion, surgical extrusion, decoronation, or extraction.

Fragment removal only

If the fractured fragment is at the level of the free gingiva, it is removed. Dentin is protected and the tooth is restored with composite resin. Long-term prognosis is not assured.

Fragment removal and gingivoplasty and/or osteoplasty

If the fracture is subgingival—it is at the level of or under the bone crest—surgical exposure of the fractured surface by gingival apical repositioning or osteoplasty should be performed to convert the fracture to a supragingival level. This should be limited to the palatal aspect so as not to compromise the aesthetics. Root canal therapy is carried out before the crown-lengthening procedure.

Orthodontic extrusion

Orthodontic extrusion of the apical fragment to expose the subgingival fracture site is used if pulp vitality needs to be preserved in cases of uncomplicated crown–root fractures (Figure 7.13). Upon removal of the separated fragment, root canal therapy should be performed. Using the space of the canal, a temporary post is cemented. This is attached with orthodontic brackets to the neighboring teeth to permit extrusion of the tooth along its long axis. If there is sufficient tooth structure, the orthodontic bracket may be placed on the labial surface of the injured tooth. Once the desired length and results achieved, stabilize to prevent prolapse of the tooth. Casted post and crown can be placed later. This procedure is time consuming and causes discomfort for elderly patients.

Surgical extrusion

Surgical extrusion is performed when there is complete root development and the apical fragment is long enough to retain a post and crown. Once the fractured segment is removed, surgically reposition the tooth coronally, using forceps, to its new position with minimal luxation. Stabilize with a flexible splint. A rotation of the tooth to 90 or 180 degrees can offer a better position for periodontal ligament healing. As the fracture site becomes exposed labially, more periodontal ligament can be saved [72]. There is a risk of root resorption with this procedure and marginal breakdown of the periodontium.

Decoronation

Decoronation is indicated in young patients as an alternative to extraction when the above-mentioned options

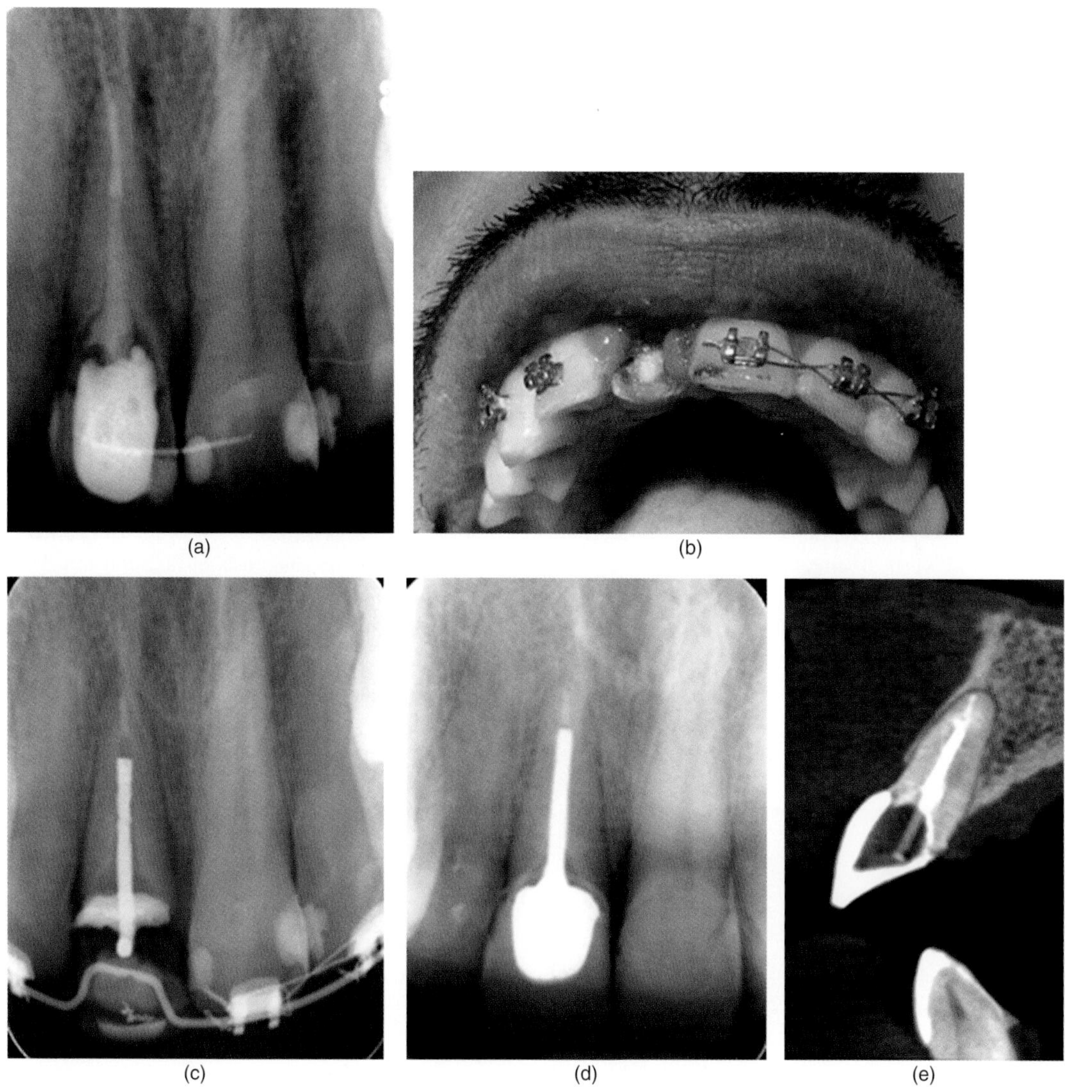

Figure 7.13 *A,* Cervical crown root fracture as presented with the wire splint. *B,* After removing the fractured part and preparing for orthodontic extrusion. *C,* Placing a hook wire in the root canal, with orthodontic wire labially on the adjacent teeth and force erupting over two months. *D,* Cast post and crown placed after four months. *E,* CBCT image showing the cemented crown in position.

cannot be carried out and implant is the treatment of choice in the future. Submerging the root will maintain the alveolar bone contour and prevent alveolar bone resorption.

Extraction

The prognosis of teeth with crown–root fractures depends on the location of the fracture and the extent of enamel, dentin, cementum, and pulp involvement. Fractures extending significantly below the gingival margin might not be restorable. The splint is removed at 4 weeks. Patient instructions should be the same. Follow-up is at 6 to 8 weeks and one year. For patient assurance, it can be every 3 months.

Crown–root fracture with pulp involvement

A crown–root fracture involving enamel, dentin, and cementum with pulp exposure can affect immature and even mature teeth. Every attempt should be made to ensure root development in immature teeth and prevent resorption in mature teeth. Treatment modalities are the same as described for crown–root fracture without pulp exposure, excluding the first point of fragment removal only, which is not applicable here. Patient instructions and follow-up should be the same.

Root Fracture

A root fracture is restricted to the root of the tooth and involves cementum, dentin, and pulp. It can result in a vertical or transverse root fracture. It is uncommon, occurring in less than 3% of dental injuries [73]. The direction and location of the fracture determine the long-term prognosis of the tooth. Because the crown of the tooth is often intact, diagnosis of a root fracture can only be made radiographically and can require multiple radiographic exposures at different horizontal and vertical angulations to arrive at an accurate diagnosis. Root fractures in primary teeth may be obscured by superposition of an erupting tooth.

The more cervical the position of the fracture, the worse the prognosis. The apical fragment usually remains in its original position while the coronal fragment is displaced. If a transverse fracture is close to the root apex, the success rate is considered high (Figure 7.14). However, the closer the fracture is to the vicinity of the gingival line and the more vertical it is, the poorer the long-term success rate. Immature teeth with vital pulp rarely sustain root fracture [73]. Severity of root fracture and its location along the root depends on the speed and direction of the object. Depending on the distance of displacement between the coronal and apical segment, the neurovascular supply can be severed at the fracture line and the periodontal ligament separation.

Transverse root fracture can be categorized as three types according to the location of the fracture line: apical one third (Figure 7.15), middle one third, or coronal one third (Figure 7.16). Diagnosing such cases is easy; it resembles diagnosis of luxation injuries. The coronal segment may be mobile and tender to touch or percussion. If the coronal part is displaced, the teeth will be disturbed on occlusion. Radiographs are an essential diagnostic tool and should include a periapical bisecting exposure for locating a root fracture in the cervical

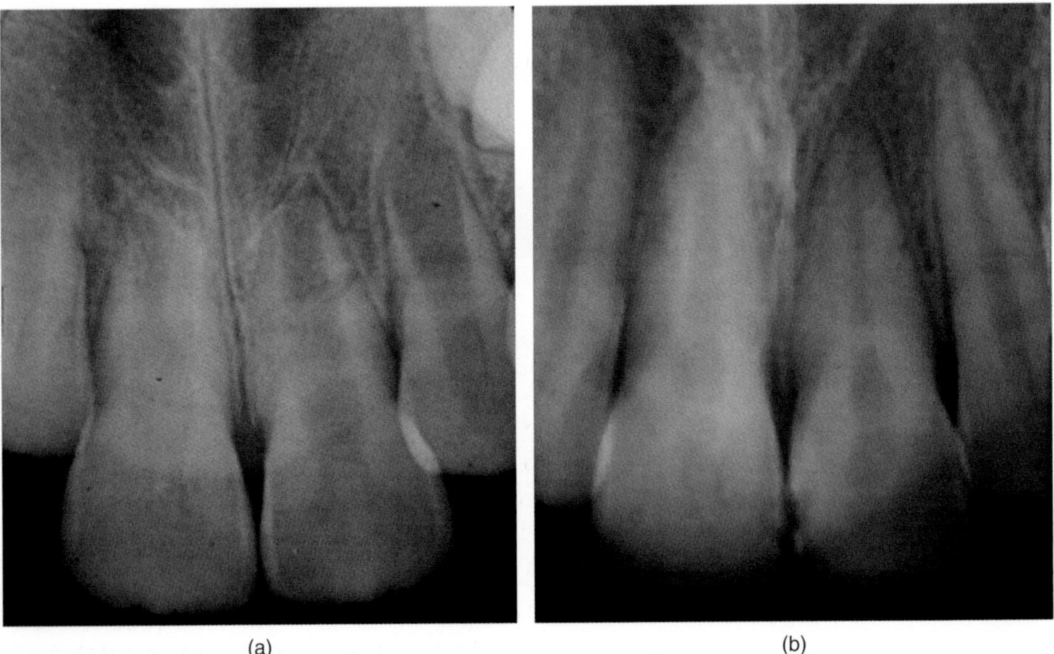

(a) (b)

Figure 7.14 *A,* Middle root fracture of an immature tooth without displacement. *B,* Five years after the injury without treatment, all anterior teeth matured and the fracture line healed with hard tissue.

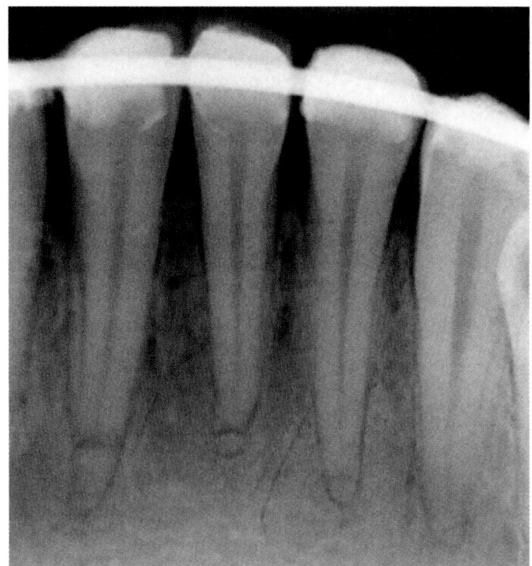

Figure 7.15 Apical third root fracture of lower anterior teeth.

third of the root and occlusal exposure for locating root fractures in the apical and middle third. A permanent tooth with root fracture and positive pulp sensitivity may be repositioned and stabilized with a flexible splint for 4 weeks to permit pulpal healing and hard tissue repair of the fracture. If the root fracture is near the cervical area, stabilization may be required for a longer period, up to 4 months.

The tooth is splinted for four months if the fracture is in the in the cervical third. Apical and middle one third transverse root fracture treatments are almost the same. If coronal fragments are mobile, reposition and stabilize the fragment with flexible splinting of composite resin and wire or orthodontic appliances for 4 weeks

Do not initiate endodontic treatment unless there is an indication to do so. If root canal treatment has to be carried out, the root canal should be instrumented to the fracture line only and filled with nonsetting calcium hydroxide for up 3 months to initiate a fracture line stop and prevent resorption. Follow-up is 6 to 8 weeksand then every 3 months for 1 year (Figure 7.17). Patient instructions are the same as for other root fractures.

Treatment of coronal one third root fractures is the most troublesome and technically sensitive. It has a poor long-term prognosis because of the proximity of the fracture line to the gingival sulcus. The tooth is splinted for 4 months if the fracture is in the in the cervical third. Maintaining excellent oral hygiene is absolutely critical. Poor oral hygiene can cause gingival inflammation and apical migration of the base of the gingival crevice, leading to exposure of the fracture line and its communication with the oral cavity, thus resulting in the loss of the coronal segment.

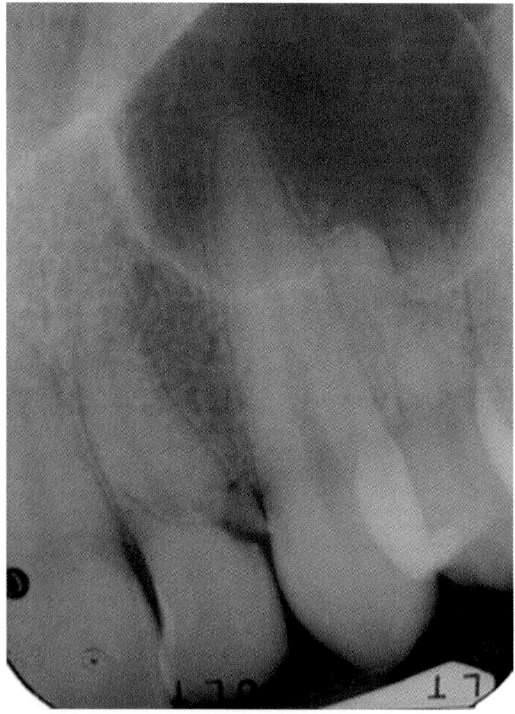

Figure 7.16 Multiple fractures of the cervical margin of a lateral incisor.

Fracture line healing patterns

Different healing modalities after root fracture have been described in the literature by several authors [74–77] radiographically and histologically. Four more commonly described are healing with hard tissue formation, healing with fibrous connective tissue formation, healing with bone and connective tissue formation, and granulation tissue formation.

Healing with hard tissue formation

In this type of a healing pattern, the fracture line is visible radiographically (Figure 18A). According to Andreasen [77], healing can be diagnosed from the radiographs after follow-up. If the root canal anatomy

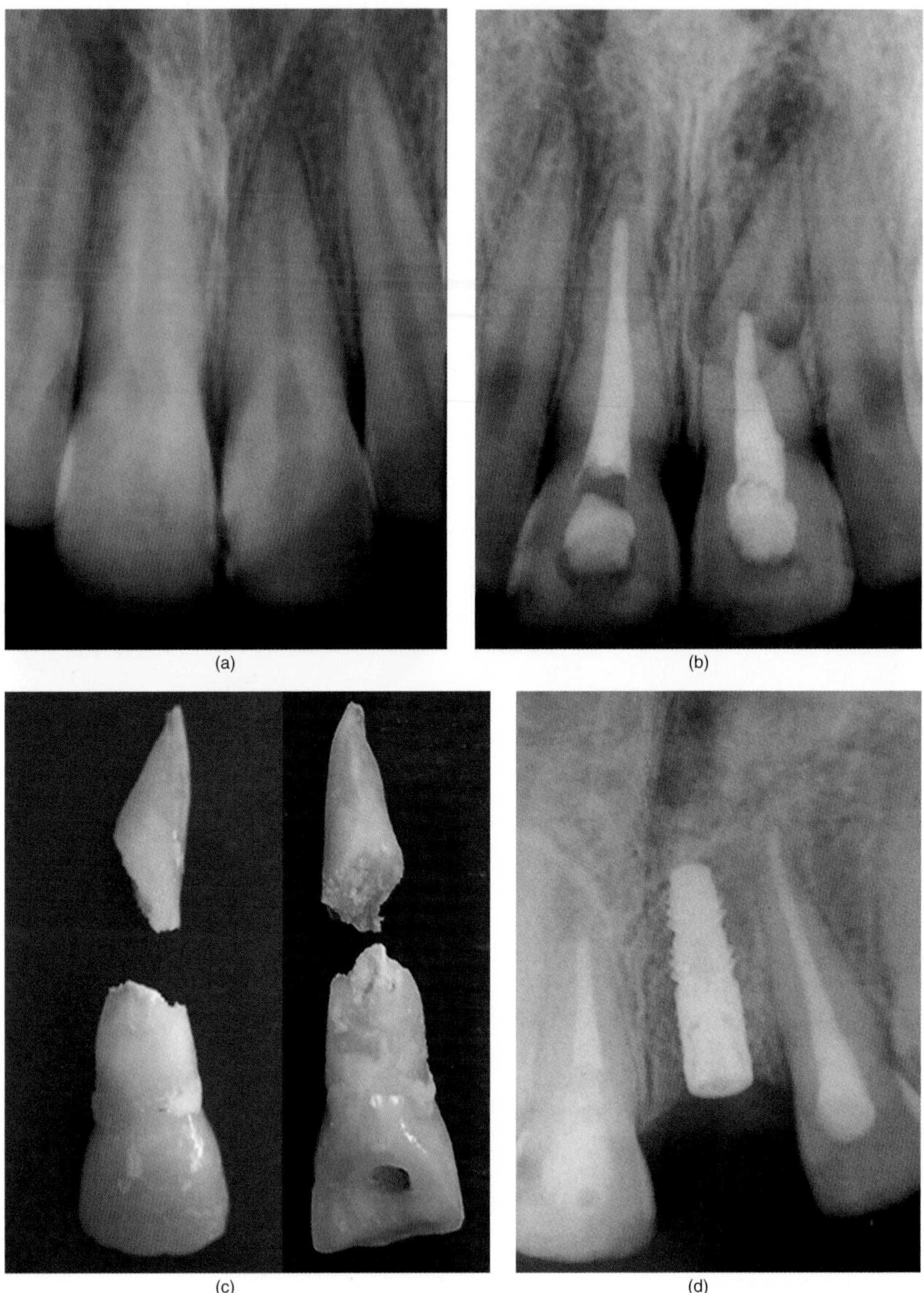

Figure 7.17 *A,* Middle root fracture without displacement of the fractured segments. *B,* Four years with displacement of the apical segment endodontic therapy has been performed. *C,* Nine years after trauma, extracted tooth showing the two separated fragments. *D,* Implant placed after extraction.

of the coronal fragment remains unchanged, healing is usually by hard tissue formation.

Healing with fibrous connective tissue formation

In this type of a healing pattern, there is an ingrowth of connective tissue between the two fragments. The fragments are displaced radiographically and have rounded fractured edges, and the coronal root canal becomes obliterated with time.

Healing with bone and connective tissue formation

The apical and coronal fractured segments are separated, and radiographically a bony ridge can be seen in the fracture line (Figure 7.18B).

Granulation tissue formation

No signs of healing or obvious radiolucency can be seen radiographically of the fracture line due to the inflammation and necrosis of the coronal segment. If the coronal segment has been treated endodontically, healing may be with connective tissue formation with a good long-term prognosis [75].

Alveolar Bone Fracture

Alveolar bone fracture is common in situations when there is trauma to several teeth together causing the alveolar process to fracture. This does not necessarily involve the alveolar socket. On clinical examination, the fractured process will move several teeth at the same time during the mobility test. Neurovascular supply is affected negatively by cutoff. The periodontal ligament is compressed and the root apex is wedged in the buccal bone [14]. The fractured alveolar displacement causes occlusion disturbance, pain, and tenderness to touch and percussion. Tooth root fracture may or may not occur with alveolar fracture.

Treatment consists of reduction and splinting, using firm and gentle digital pressure to replace the alveolar bone and teeth to their original position, in a downward (axial) and backward (buccal) movement to help to release the teeth from the bone. Physiologic splinting for 4 weeks, with radiographs and monitoring over 1 year, is recommended. Endodontic intervention is essential on any sign of periapical rarefaction.

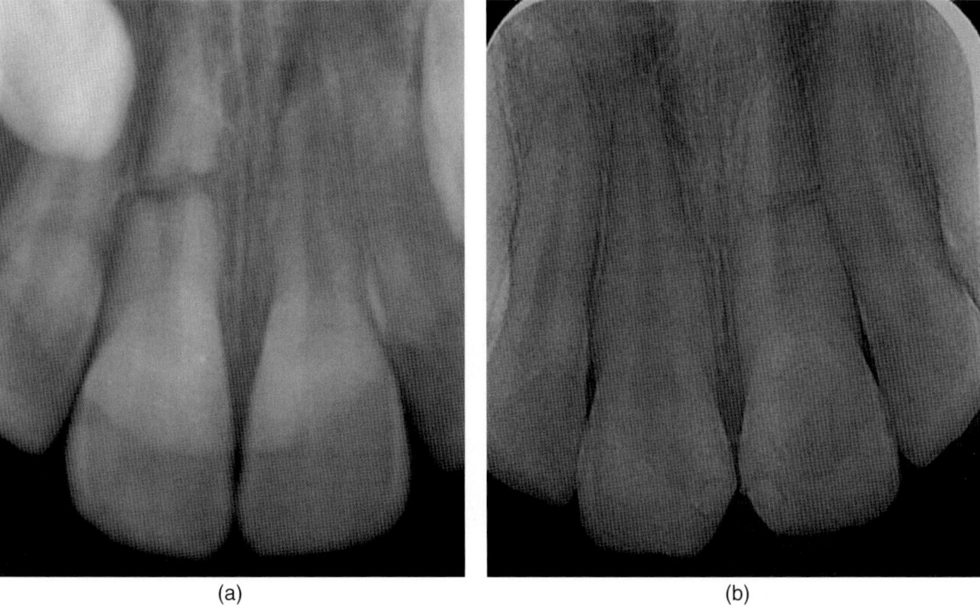

Figure 7.18 *A,* Healing with bone and connective tissue. *B,* Healing with hard tissue and connective tissue without endodontic treatment.

Root Resorption

One of the common sequelae after a traumatic injury is root resorption. Root resorption is either a physiological or pathological process. It can occur when there is damage to the periodontal ligament, cementum, or dentin and may be self-limiting or progressive. The extent of the resorption depends on the surface area that was damaged and the presence of persisting stimulation. If the trauma is self-limiting and the injury to the periodontal ligament is mild, then repair with new cementum to the root will take place [78]. Because pain is so infrequently associated with resorption, routine follow-up is imperative after trauma. The process of root resorption is initiated either outside of the tooth, giving rise to external resorption, or from within the canal, where it is termed internal resorption (Figure 7.19).

Types of Resoprtion

Internal resorption

Internal resorption is the result of osteoclastic activity nourished by a highly vascularized granulation tissue that has replaced normal pulp. It is a progressive

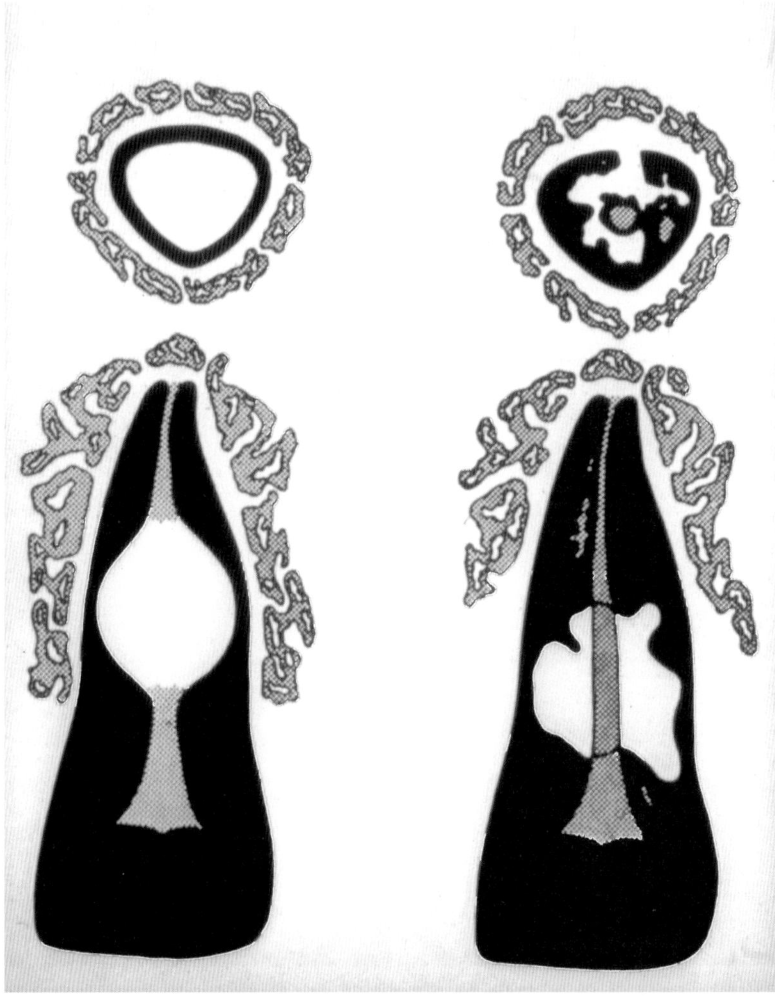

Figure 7.19 Differential diagnosis of internal and external resorption. *A,* Internal resorption. Radiographically, the canal appears interrupted. *B,* External resorption. The canal appears irregular, and a radiolucent area appears overlying the canal.

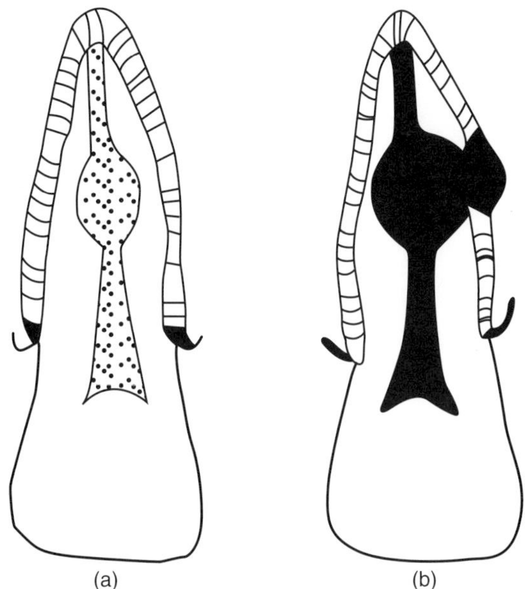

Figure 7.20 Internal resorption. *A,* Resorption that is confined within the root canal. *B,* The resorption has progressed to extend beyond the root, perforating the root.

dissolution of dentin, enamel, and cementum and can be halted only by removing pulp. Internal resorption may be rapid, decimating the tooth in months; in other cases, the process can take years. Because there is no way of predicting the rate of devastation, it is imperative to remove the altered pulp tissue when the pathosis is first discovered [79]. If the resorption process goes on for too long, the root can be perforated (Figure 7.20). The enlarged, unevenly shaped resorption cavities, which extend in all directions, present additional problems in treatment. In these situations, access cavities must be enlarged sufficiently to provide all adequate approach to the irregular metaplastic tissue (Figures 7.21 and 7.22). Internal resorption has been categorized into internal replacement and internal inflammatory resorption [80].

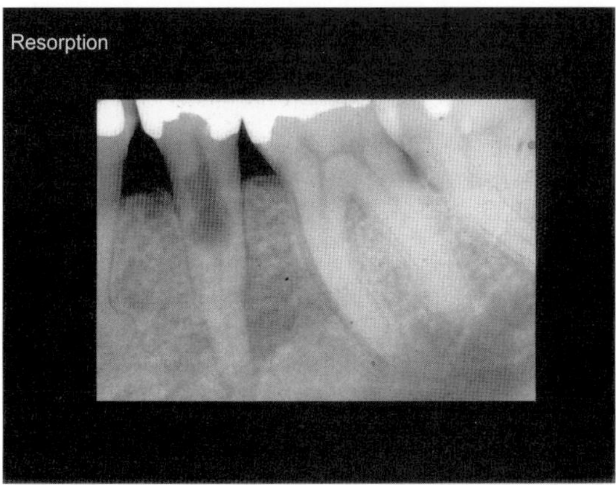

Figure 7.21 Internal resorption with irregular shape can present challenges on treatment.

External resorption

External resorption is another form of root resorption, which is characterized by small excavations in cementum on the root (Figure 7.23). This can be much more complicated to diagnose and treat. Such resorptive process is diagnosed radiographically as an irregular radiolucent area overlying the root canal. The canal outline remains intact (Figure 7.1B). In internal resorption, the outline of the canal is interrupted (Figure 7.19A).

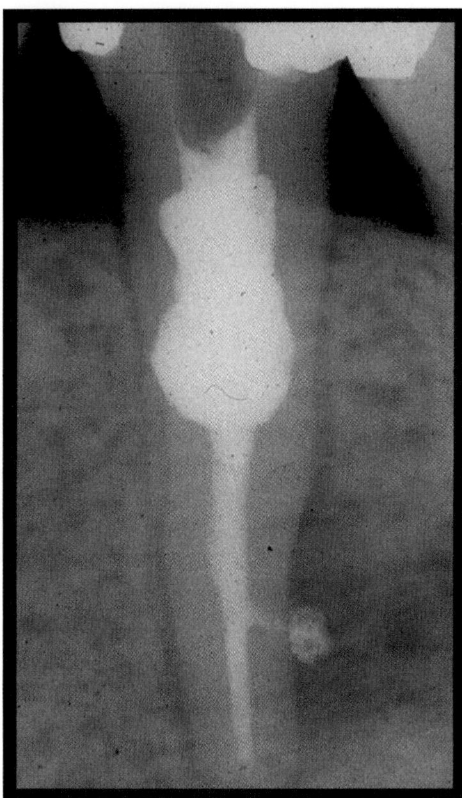

Figure 7.22 Internal resorption after endodontic therapy was performed.

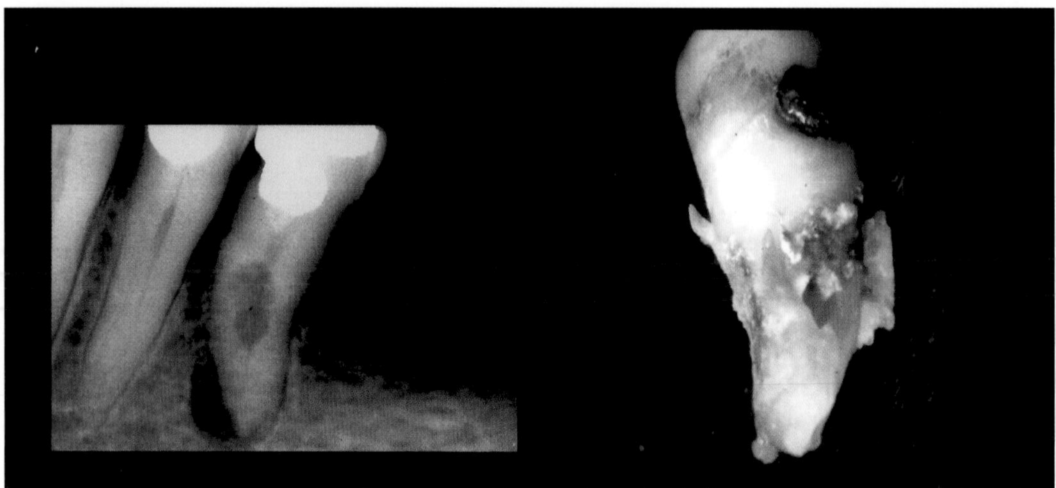

Figure 7.23 The extent of external resorption radiographically usually appears less extensive than it actually is in reality. *A,* Radiograph showing resorption. *B,* Resorption in the extracted tooth.

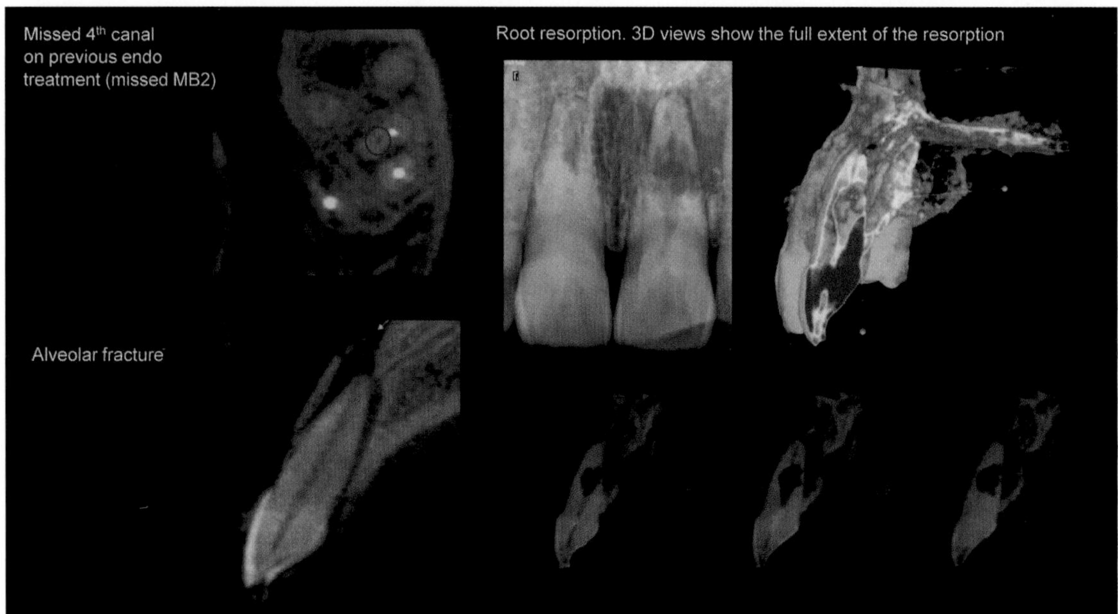

Figure 7.24 Using CBTC scan for diagnosing internal and external resorption.

The use of a cone beam can be helpful in diagnosing internal and external resorption (Figure 7.24). A shift/angle radiograph can also help in differentiating internal versus external resorption. External resorption can be transient or pathologic. Transient resorption can be in the form of surface or pressure resorption (Figure 7.25).

Surface resorption

Surface resorption is a self-limiting superficial process that occurs on the root surface and is followed by spontaneous repair (Figure 7.25A and B). Large areas of denuded root surfaces are subjected to excessive osteoclastic action and subsequent osseous replacement. After some weeks, this resorptive cavity is repaired by

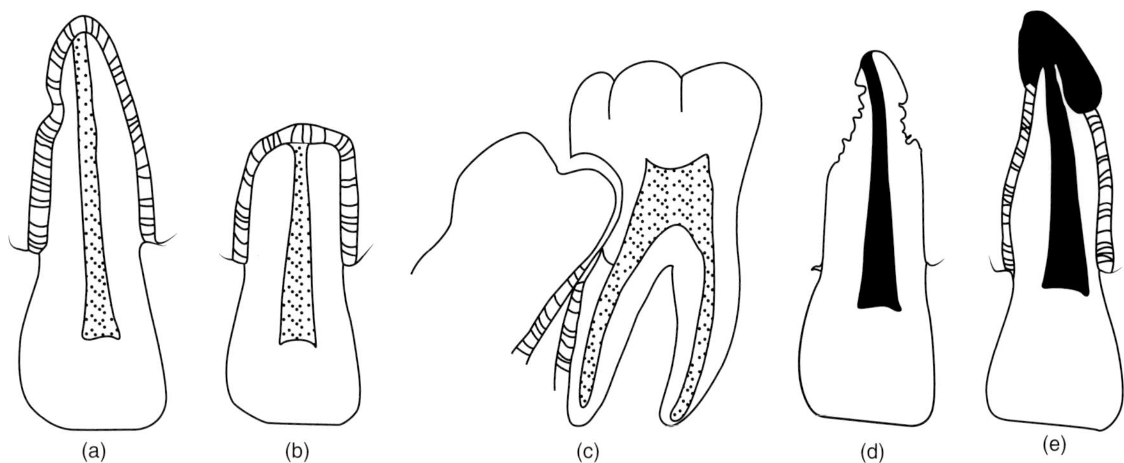

Figure 7.25 External resorption. *A*, Transient resorption. *B*, Surface pressure (orthodontic). *C*, Surface pressure (impaction). *D*, Pathologic resorption (ankylosis). *E*, Pathologic resorption (inflammatory).

new cementum and Sharpey's fibers [80]. Table 7.2 lists the classifications of root resorptions.

Pressure resorption

Pressure resorption is due to erupting or impacted teeth, orthodontic movement, or trauma from occlusion. The resorptive process will discontinue when the pressure is no longer present. No root canal treatment is necessary in surface or pressure resorption [81]. Pathological resorption occurs when there is no periodontal ligament space at the resorptive site. This is where the initial resorption cavity has penetrated cementum and reached the dentinal tubules. This event leads to a continuation of the osteoclastic process and progressive resorption of the root surface, ultimately perforating to the root canal. If the infection in the root canal and the dentinal tubules is eliminated by endodontic therapy, osteoclastic activity will be arrested, and healing with new cementum and Sharpey's fibers will take place (Figure 7.25D and E).

When the periodontal ligament has been extensively damaged, ankylosis will be permanent. This will lead to progressive external inflammatory root resorption. In inflammatory resorption, the root resorption is a direct response to the inflammatory process. Elimination of the inflammation by endodontic therapy is essential in order to abate the process. Periodontal therapy is necessary if the resorption is of periodontal origin.

Invasive cervical root resorption

Invasive cervical root resorption is an aggressive form of external root resorption that is characterized by its cervical location and invasive nature and is progressive (Figure 7.26). Predisposing factors can be intracoronal bleaching, trauma, orthodontic treatment, and periodontal surgery. Nonsurgical treatment of invasive cervical resorption involves the topical application of a 90% aqueous solution of trichloracetic acid to the resorptive tissue, curettage, endodontic treatment where necessary, and restoration with a biocompatible cement. When the cervical resorption communicates with the oral cavity, a surgical approach is necessary.

Access to the resorptive area is key to treatment to this condition. Treatment is aimed at inactivating all resorbing tissue and repairing the resorptive defect by placing a biocompatible nonsoluble cement. A flap is reflected, and the resorptive crater on the root surface is cleaned and repaired with a restorative material.

A good restorative material to use is BC sealer (Brasseler USA, Savannah, GA, USA), which is premixed. It chemically bonds to dentin and is extremely biocompatible, with no shrinkage (Figure 7.27). ProRoot mineral trioxide aggregate (MTA; Dentsply Tulsa Dental Specialties, Tulsa, OK, USA) is another highly biocompatible material with excellent long-term results. A powder component is mixed with water to create a paste. The MTA is placed in the preparation and

Table 7.2 Classification of root resorption.

Type	Differential Diagnosis	Treatment	Prognosis
External Resorption			
Transient			
Surface	Small excavations are separated from bone by periodontal ligament Pulp is responsive	No treatment is necessary	Excellent
Pressure	Pulp is responsive Resorption stops when pressure is discontinued	Correction and discontinuance of pressure No root canal therapy	Excellent when etiologic pressure is discontinued
Pathologic			
Ankylosis (replacement)	There is no periodontal space at the resorptive site Margins of defect are irregular Canal maintains original form	Root canal therapy	Poor
Inflammatory	There is a radiolucency next to the resorption Margin of resorption varies from smooth to ragged but is not comparable to the irregular defects of ankylosis Multiple angulated x-ray films will shift lesion when superimposed over pulp Canal maintains original form Tissue may be fluctuant or a fistula may be present owing to non-responsive pulp	Root canal therapy	Unpredictable
Cervical Invasive Resorption	There is an irregular radiolucency within the tooth, often superimposed over the pulp canal Radiolucency becomes more regular in advanced stage Canal maintains original form Pulp remains responsive	Root canal therapy Debridement of the defect through the coronal access opening with a slow-speed round bur or surgical procedure Filling of the defect with glass ionomer cement	Poor to good depending on the ability to debride the defect and the quality of the filling
Internal Resorption			
Intracanal resorption with no extended perforation	Bulbous enlargement of pulp chamber or canal Responsive pulp during active phase	Root canal therapy	Excellent
Intracanal resorption with extraosseous perforation	Bulbous enlargement exists to or near the oral environment Radiolucency at the site of perforation Pulp is unresponsive Tissue may demonstrate fluctuance or fistula	Root canal therapy Well-condensed filling of the root canal and resorptive defect	Fair to excellent depending on the quality of obliteration of the canal space and resorptive defect
Intracanal resorption with supraosseous perforation	Bulbous enlargement to or near the oral environment Periodontal breakdown extends to perforation Pulp is unresponsive Tissue may demonstrate fluctuance	Root canal therapy and surgical repair	Depends on location, surgical access, and the periodontal defect that will remain

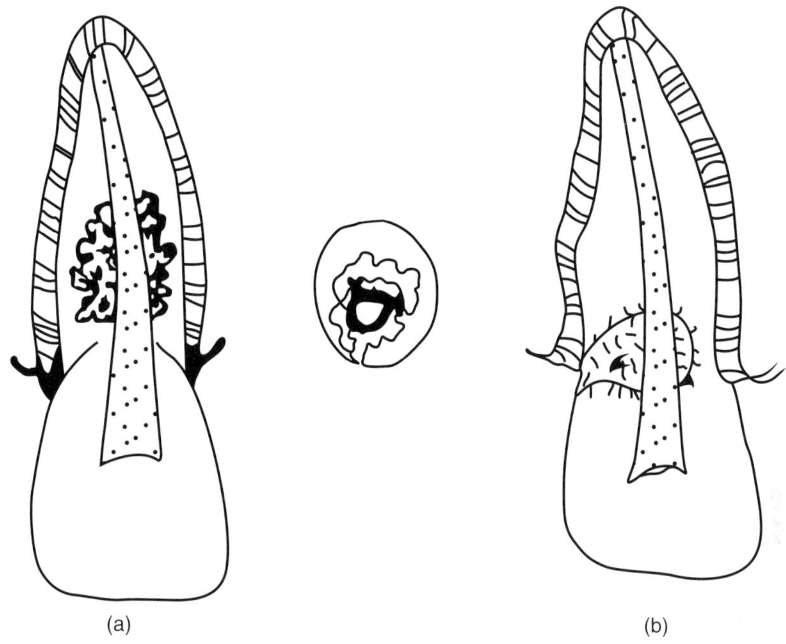

Figure 7.26 Invasive cervical root resorption. *A*, root resorption without penetrating the crest. *B*, Root resorption with penetration of crestal bone.

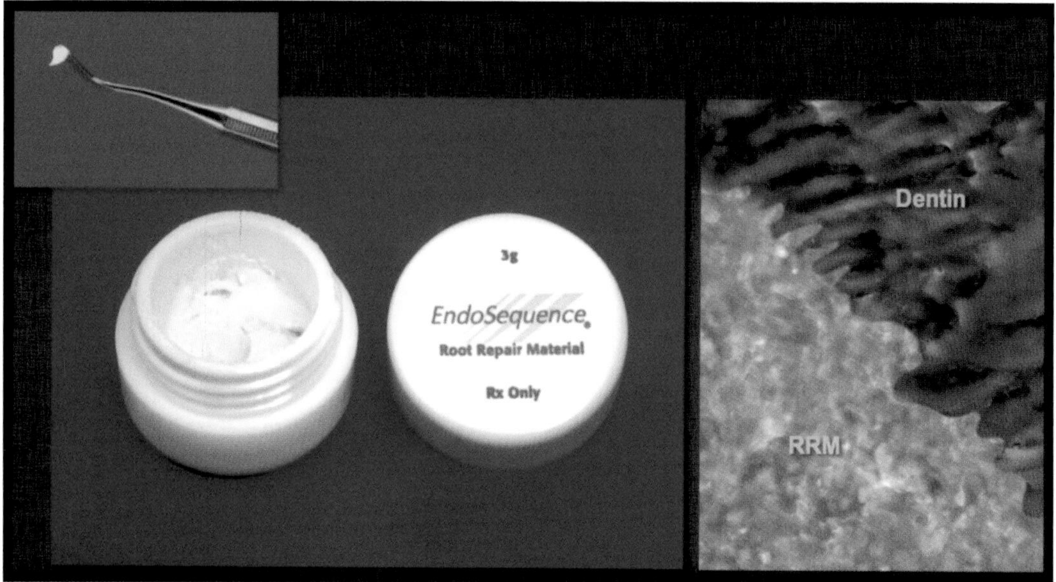

Figure 7.27 EndoSequence bioceramic root repair material to fill a resorption crater.

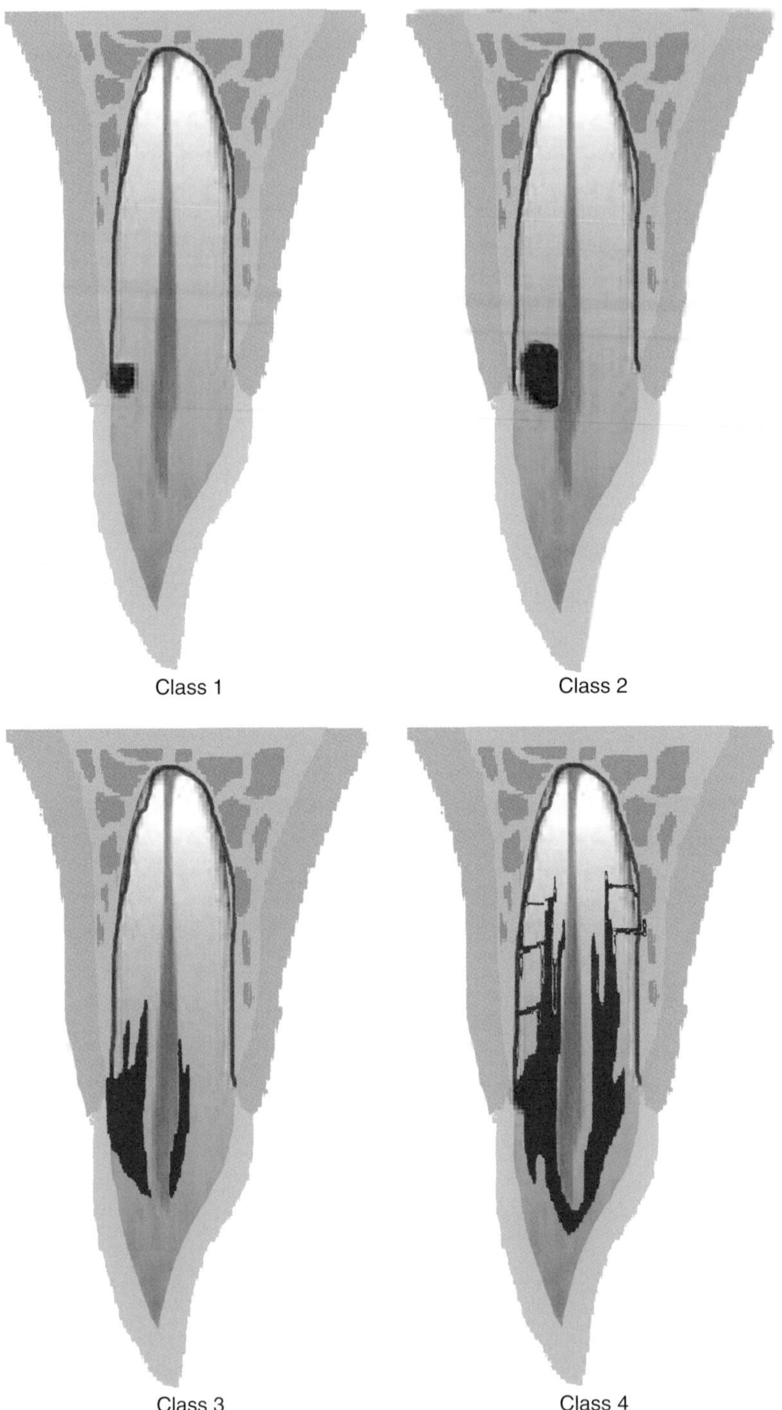

Figure 7.28 Clinical classification of invasive cervical resorption. Class 1: Small invasive resorptive lesion near the cervical area with penetration into dentin. Class 2: Well-defined invasive resorptive lesion that has penetrated close to the coronal pulp chamber. Class 3: Deeper invasion of dentin by resorbing tissue;. Class 4: Large invasive resorptive process extending beyond the coronal third of the root.

compacted. It is then allowed to set and create a seal [82]. Biodentine (Septodont, Saint Maurdes Fossés, France) is a fast-setting calcium silicate–based restorative material with biocompatibility similar to that of MTA. Compared to MTA, Biodentine has a considerably shorter setting time and is easier to handle, making it a material worth considering when repairing resorptive defects [83].

Heithersay [84] classified invasive cervical resorption into four classes: Class I denotes a small invasive resorptive lesion near the cervical area with shallow penetration into dentin. Class 2 denotes a well-defined invasive resorptive lesion that has penetrated close to the coronal pulp chamber but shows little or no extension into the radicular dentin. Class 3 denotes a deeper invasion of dentin by resorbing tissue, not only involving the coronal dentin but also extending into the coronal third of the root. Class 4 denotes a large invasive resorptive process that has extended beyond the coronal third of the root [84] (Figure 7.28).

Classification according to stimulation factors is listed in Box 7.2. Figure 7.29 demonstrates the progression of root resorption. Figure 7.30 demonstrates ankylosis-related root resorption.

Box 7.2 Classification of resorption listed according to stimulation factors

Injury alone: only stimulus for the resorption is the injury itself,; self-limiting

Surface resorption
Replacement resorption

Injury *plus* additional inflammatory stimulus; progressive

Internal inflammatory root resorption
External inflammatory root resorption
Pressure resorption
Invasive cervical resorption

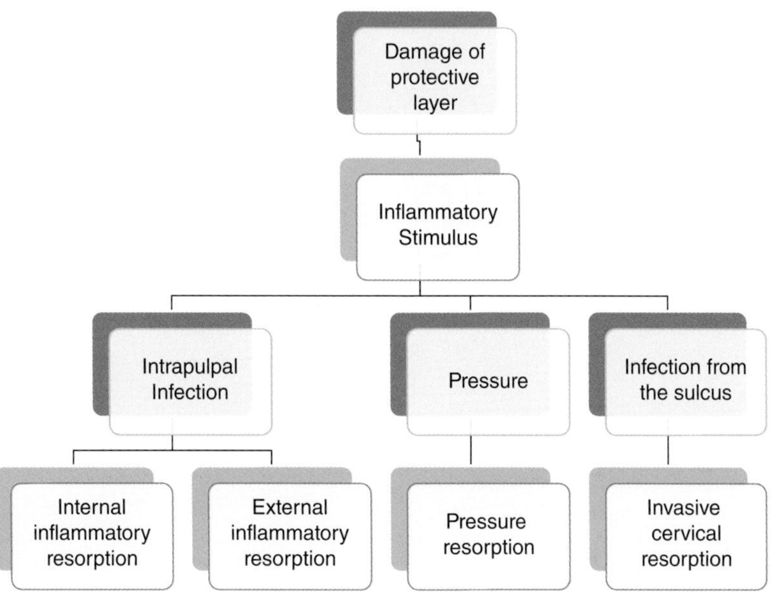

Figure 7.29 Progression of root resorption.

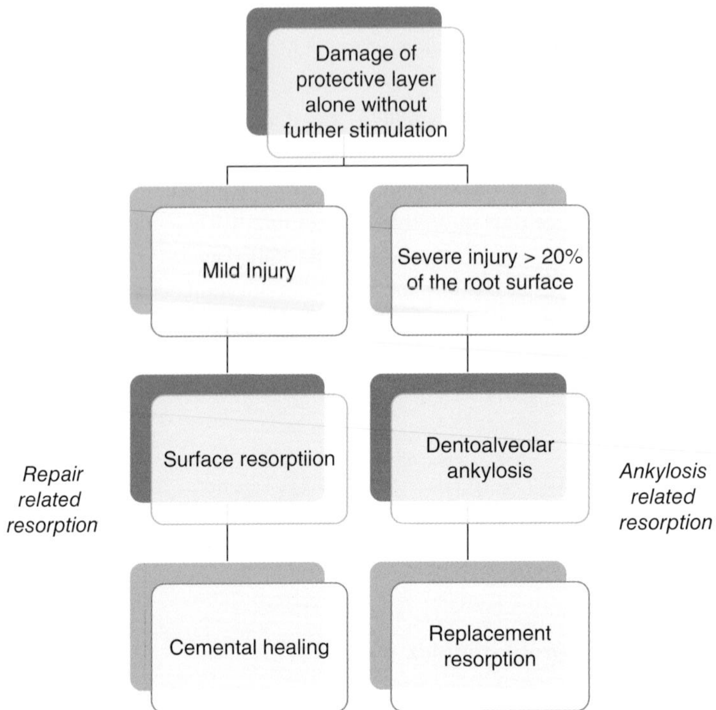

Figure 7.30 Ankylosis related root resorption.

Future

Successful management of dental trauma involves four major areas of consideration: type of trauma, management of changes to the pulp vitality, control of inflammatory periodontal disease, and continuous evaluation and management with restoration of the dentition. Clinicians should always follow current guidelines and evidence-based recommendations. If a revascularization procedure is attempted, care must be taken.

References

1 Andreasen JO, Ahrensburg SS. History of dental trauma. *Dent Traumatol* 2012; 28: 336–344.

2 Gassner R, Tuli T, Hachl O, Moreira R, Ulmer H. Craniomaxillofacial trauma in children: a review of 3,385 cases with 6060 injuries in 10 years. *J Oral Maxillofac Surg* 2004; 62: 399–407.

3 Dale RA. Dentoalveolar trauma. *Emerg Med Clin North Am* 2000; 18: 521–538.

4 Porritt JM, Rodd HD, Baker SR. Parental quality-of-life impacts following children's dento-alveolar trauma. *Dent Traumatol* 2013; 29: 92–98.

5 Andreasen FM, Kahler B. Diagnosis of acute dental trauma: the importance of standardized documentation: a review. *Dent Traumatol* 2015;31(5):340–349.

6 Hofman PA, Nelemans P, Kemerink GJ, Wilmink JT. Value of radiological diagnosis of skull fracture in the management of mild head injury: meta-analysis. *J Neurol Neurosurg Psych* 2000; 68: 416–422.

7 Cohenca N, Simon JH, Roges R, Morag Y, Malfaz JM. Clinical indications for digital imaging in dento-alveolar trauma. Part 1: traumatic injuries. *Dent Traumatol* 2007; 23: 95–104.

8 Cohenca N, Simon JH, Mathur A, Malfaz JM. Clinical indications for digital imaging in dento-alveolar trauma. Part 1: Root Resorption. *Dent Traumatol* 2007; 23: 105–113.

9 Andreasen JO, Andreasen FM, Mejàre I, Cvek M. Healing of 400 intra-alveolar root fractures. 2. Effect of treatment factors such as treatment delay, repositioning, splinting type and period and antibiotics. *Dent Traumatol* 2004; 20: 203–211.

10 Hinckfuss SE, Messer LB. An evidence-based assessment of the clinical guidelines for replanted avulsed teeth. Part II: prescription of systemic antibiotics. *Dent Traumatol* 2009; 25: 158–164.

11 Andreasen JO, Storgaard Jensen S, Sae-Lim V. The role of antibiotics in presenting healing complications after traumatic dental injuries: a literature review. *Endod Topics* 2006; 14: 80–92.

12 Andreasen JO, Andreasen FM, Andersson L. *Textbook and Color Atlas of Traumatic Injuries to the Teeth*, 4th ed. Oxford: Wiley–Blackwell; 2007.

13 International Association of Dental Traumatology. Guidelines for the evaluation and management of traumatic dental injuries. *Dent Traumatol* 2001; 17:1, 49, 97, 145, 193.

14 DiAngelis AJ, Andreasen JO, Ebeleseder KA, Kenny DJ, Trope M, Sigurdsson A, et al. International Association of Dental Traumatology guidelines for the management of traumatic dental injuries: 1. Fractures and luxations of permanent teeth. *Dent Traumatol* 2012; 28: 2–12.

15 Andersson L, Andreasen JO, Day P, Heithersay G, Trope M, DiAngelis AJ, et al. International Association of Dental Traumatology guidelines for the management of traumatic dental injuries: 2. Avulsion of permanent teeth. *Dent Traumatol* 2012; 28: 88–96.

16 Andreasen JO, Bakland LK, Flores MF, Andreasen FM, Andersson L. *Traumatic Dental Injuries: A Manual*. 3rd ed. Chichester, UK: Wiley–Blackwell; 2011.

17 Lauridsen E, Hermann NV, Gerds TA, Ahrensburg SS, Kreiborg S, Andreasen JO. Combination injuries 1. The risk of pulp necrosis in permanent teeth with concussion injuries and concomitant crown fractures. *Dent Traumatol* 2012; 28: 364–370.

18 Ingle JI, Bakland LK, Baumgartner JC. *Ingles's endodontics*. 6th ed. Hamilton, ON: B.C. Decker; 2008.

19 Ashkenazi M, Sarnat H, Keila S. *In vitro* viability, mitogenicity and clonogenic capacity of periodontal ligament cells after storage in six different media. *Dent Traumatol* 1999; 15: 149–156.

20 Ashkenazi M, Marouni M, Sarnat H. *In vitro* viability, mitogenicity and clonogenic capacity of periodontal ligament cells after storage in four media at room temperature. *Dent Traumatol* 2000; 16: 63–70.

21 Ashkenazi M, Marouni M, Sarnat H. *In vitro* viability, mitogenicity and clonogenic capacity of periodontal ligament fibroblasts after storage in four media supplemented with growth factors. *Dent Traumatol* 2001; 17: 27–35.

22 Blomlöf L. Milk and saliva as possible storage media for traumatically exarticulated teeth prior to replantation. *Swed Dent* 1981; 8: 1–26.

23 Lindskog S, Blomlöf L. Influence of osmolality and composition of some storage media on human periodontal ligament cells. *Act Odontol Scan* 1982; 40: 435–441.

24 Blomlöf L, Lindskog S, Andersson L, Hedström K-G, Hammarström L. Storage of experimentally avulsed teeth in milk prior to replantation. *J Dent Res* 1983; 62: 912–916.

25 Lindskog S, Blomlöf L, Hammarström L. Mitoses and microorganisms in the periodontal membrane after storage in milk or saliva. *Scand J Dent Res* 1983; 91: 465–472.

26 Krasner P, Person P. Preserving avulsed teeth for replantation. *J Am Dent Assoc* 1992; 23: 80–88.

27 Krasner P. Tooth avulsion in the school setting. *J Sch Nurs* 1992; 8: 20–26.

28 Özan F, Polat ZA, Er K, Özan Ü, Deger O. Effect of propolis on survival of periodontal ligament cells: new storage media for avulsed teeth. *J Endod* 2007; 33: 570–573.

29 Khademi AA, Atbaee A, Razavi S-M, Shabanian M. Periodontal healing of replanted dog teeth stored in milk and egg albumen. *Dent Traumatol* 2008; 24:510–514.

30 Sousa HA, Alencar AHG, Bruno KF, Batista AC, Carvalho ACP. Microscopic evaluations of the effect of different storage media on the periodontal ligament of surgically extracted human teeth. *Dent Traumatol* 2008; 24: 628–632.

31 Courts FJ, Mueller WA, Tabeling HJ. Milk as an interim storage media for avulsed teeth. *Pediatr Dent* 1983; 5: 183–186.

32 Pearson RM, Liewehr FR, West L, Patton WR, McPherson J, Runner RR. Human periodontal ligament cell viability in milk and milk substitute. *J Endod* 2003; 29: 184–186.

33 Gamson EK, Dusmsha TC, Sydiskis R. The effect of drying time on periodontal ligament cell vitality. *J Endod* 1992; 18: 186–189.

34 Blomlöf L, Otteskog P, Hammarström L. Effect of storage in media with different ion strengths and osmolalities on human periodontal ligament cells. *Scan J Dent Res* 1981; 89: 180–187.

35 Marino TG, West LA, Liewehr FR, Mailhot JM, Buxton TB, Runner RR, McPherson III, JC. Determination of periodontal ligament cell viability in long shelf-life milk. *J Endod* 2000; 26: 699–702.

36 Harkacz OM, Carnes DL, Walker WA III,. Determination of periodontal ligament cell viability in the oral rehydration fluid Gatorade and milks of varying fat content. *J Endod* 1997; 23: 687–690.

37 Chamorro MM, Regan JD, Opperman LA, Kramer PR. Effect of storage media on human periodontal ligament cell apoptosis. *Dent Traumatol* 2008; 24: 11–16.

38 Sigalas E, Regan JD, Kramer PR, Witherspoon DE, Opperman LA. Survival of human periodontal ligament cells in media proposed for transport of avulsed teeth. *Dent Traumatol* 2004; 20: 21–28.

39 Mori GG, Nunes DC, Castilho LR, de Moraes IG, Poi WR. Propolis as storage media for avulsed teeth: microscopic and morphometric analysis in rats. *Dent Traumatol* 2010; 26: 80–85.

40 Ashkenazi M, Shaked I. *In vitro* clonogenic capacity of periodonatal ligament fibroblasts cultured with Emdogain. *Dent Traumatol* 2006; 22: 25–29.

41 Wiegand A, Attin T. Efficacy of enamel matrix derivatives (Emdogain) in treatment of replanted teeth: a systematic review based on animal studies. *Dent Traumatol* 2008; 24: 498-502.

42 Selvig KA, Bjorvatn K, Bogle GC, Wokesjo UME. Effect of stannous fluoride and tetracycline on periodontal repair after delayed tooth replantation in dogs. *Scand J Dent Res* 100:200–203.

43 Kaba AD, Maréchaux SC. A fourteen-year follow-up study of traumatic injuries to the permanent dentition. *ASDC J Dent Child* 1989; 56(6): 417–425.

44 Andreasen JO, Andreasen FM. "Avulsions," in *Textbook and Color Atlas of Traumatic Injuries to the Teeth*, J. O. Andreasen and F. M. Andreasen, Eds., pp. 383–425, Mosby, Munksgard, Copenhagen, Denmark, 1994.

45 Cohenca N, Karni S, Eidlitz D, Nuni E, Moshonov J. New treatment protocols for avulsed teeth. *Refuat Hapeh Vehashinayim*. 2004; 21: 48–53.

46 Ram D Cohenca ON. Therapeutic protocols for avulsed permanent teeth: review and clinical update. *Pediatr Dent* 2004; 26(3): 251–255.

47 Cvek M, Cleaton-Jones P, Austin J, Lownie J, Kling M, Fatti P. Effect of topical application of doxycycline on pulp revascularization and periodontal healing in reimplanted monkey incisors. *Endod Dent Traumatol* 1990; 6(4); 170–176.

48 Andreasen JO, Borum MK, Andreasen FM. Replantation of 400 avulsed permanent incisors. 3. Factors related to root growth. *Endod Dent Traumatol* 1995; 11(2): 69–75, 1995.

49 Barrett EJ, Kenny DJ. Avulsed permanent teeth: a review of the literature and treatment guidelines. *Endod Dent Traumatol* 1997; 13(4): 153–163.

50 Pohl Y, Filippi A, Kirschner H. Results after replantation of avulsed permanent teeth. II. Periodontal healing and the role of physiologic storage and antiresorptive–regenerative therapy. *Dent Traumatol* 2005; 21(2): 93–101.

51 Bryson EC, Levin L, Banchs F, Trope M. Effect of minocycline on healing of replanted dog teeth after extended dry times. *Dent Traumatol* 2003; 19: 90–95.

52 Yanpiset K, Trope M. Pulp revascularization of replanted immature dog teeth after different methods. *Dent Traumatol* 2001; 16: 211–217.

53 Ritter AL, Ritter AV, Murrah V, Sigurdsson A, Trope M. Pulp revascularization of replanted immature dog teeth after treatment with minocycline and doxycycline assessed by laser Doppler flowmetry, radiography, and histology. *Dent Traumatol* 2004; 20: 75–84.

54 Bryson EC, Levin L, Banchs F, Abbott PV, Trope M. Effect of immediate intracanal placement of Ledermix Paste on healing of replanted dog teeth after extended dry times. *Dent Traumatol* 2002; 18: 316–321.

55 Kinirons M, Boyd D, Gregg T. Inflammatory and replacement resorption in reimplanted permanent incisor teeth: A study of the characteristics of 84 teeth. *Endod Dent Traumatol* 1999; 15: 269–272.

56 Andersson L, Malgren B. The problem of dentoalveolar ankyloses and subsequent replacement resorption in the growing patient. *Aust Endod J* 1999; 25: 57–61.

57 Filippi A, Pohl Y, von Arx T. Decoronation of an ankylosed tooth for preservation of alveolar bone prior to implant placement. *Dent Traumatol* 1001; 17: 134–137.

58 Nyman S, Houston F, Sarhed G, Lidhe J, Karring T. Healing following reimplantation of teeth subjected to root planing and citric acid treatment. *J Clin Periodontol* 1985; 12: 294–305.

59 Selvig KA, Zander HA. Chemical analysis and microradiography of cementum and dentin from periodontally diseased human teeth. *J Periodontol* 1962; 33: 303–310.

60 Torabinejad M, Hong CU, Lee SJ, Monsef M, Pitt Ford TR. Investigation of mineral trioxide aggregate for root-end filling in dogs. *J Endod* 1995; 21: 603–608.

61 Torabinejad M, Pitt Ford TR, McKendry DJ, Abedi HR, Miller DA, Kariyawasam SP. Histologic assessment of mineral trioxide aggregate as a root-end filling in monkeys. *J Endod* 1997; 23: 225–228.

62 Torabinejad M, Chivian N. Clinical applications of mineral trioxide aggregate. *J Endod* 1999; 25: 197–205.

63 Camilleri J, Gandolfi MG, Siboni F, Prati C. Dynamic sealing ability of MTA root canal sealer. *Intl Endod J* 2011; 44: 9–20.

64 Lovato KF, Sedgley CM. Antibacterial activity of EndoSequence root repair material and ProRoot MTA against clinical isolates of *Enterococcus faecalis*. *J Endod* 2011; 37: 1542–1546.

65 Ghoneim AG, Lutfy RA, Sabet NE, Fayyad DM. Resistance to fracture of roots obturated with novel canal filling system. *J Endod* 2011 ;37:1590–1592.

66 Ray HA, Trope M. Periapical status of endodontically treated teeth in relation to the technical quality of the root filling and the coronal restoration. *Intl Endod J* 1995; 28: 12–15.

67 Lin S, Schwarz-Arad D, Ashkenazi M. Alveolar bone width preservation after decoronation of ankylosed anterior incisors. *J Endod* 2013; 39: 1542–1544.

68 Malmgren B. Ridge preservation/decoronation. *J Endod* 2013; 3: S67–S72.

69 Murray PE, Garcia-Godoy F, Hargreaves KM. Regenerative endodontics: a review of current status and call for action. *J Endod* 2007; 33: 337–90.

70 Andreasen FM, Norén JG, Andreasen JO, Engelhardtsen S, Lindh-Strömberg U. Long-term survival of crown fragment bonding in the treatment of crown fractures: a multicenter clinical study. *Quintessence Int* 1995; 26: 669–681.

71 Cvek M. A clinical report on partial pulpotomy and capping with calcium hydroxide in permanent incisors with complicated crown fracture. *J Endod* 1978; 4: 232–237.

72 Andreasen JO, Andreasen FM, Bakland LK, Flores MT. Crown–root fracture. *Traumatic Dental Injuries. A Manual.* Oxford: Blackwell/Munksgaard; 2003. pp. 32–33.

73 Zachrisson BU, Jacobsen I. Long-term prognosis of 66 permanent anterior teeth with root fracture. *Scand J Dent Res* 1975; 83: 345–354.

74 Andreasen JO, Hjorting-Hansen E. Intraalveolar root fracture: radiographic and histologic study of 50 cases. *J Oral Surg* 1967; 25: 414–426.

75 Andreasen FM, Andreasen JO, Bayer T. Prognosis of root fractured permanent incisors: prediction of healing modalities. *Endod Dent Traumatol* 1989; 5: 11–22.
76 Heithersay GS, Kahler B. Healing responses following transverse root fracture: a historical review and case reports showing healing with (a) calcified tissue and (b) dense fibrous connective tissue. *Endod Dent Traumatol* 2013; 29: 253–265.
77 Andreasen FM, Kahler B. Pulpal response after acute dental injury in the permanent dentition: clinical implications: a review. *J Endod* 2015; 41: 299–308.
78 Andreasen JO, Andreasen FM. *Essentials of traumatic injures to the teeth.* Copenhagen: Munksguard; 1990. pp. 116–117.
79 Andreasen JO. *Traumatic injuries to the teeth.* Philadelphia: WB Saunders; 1981. p. 23.
80 Tronstad L. Root resportion: etiology, terminology and clinical manifestations. *Endod Dent Traumatol* 1988: 4: 241–252.
81 Frank AL, Simon JHS, Abou-Rass M, Glick DH. Clinical and surgical endodontics concepts in practice. Philadelphia: JB Lippincott; 1983. p. 153.
82 Mente J, Leo M, Panagidis D, Saure D, Pfefferle T. Treatment outcome of mineral trioxide aggregate: repair of root perforations: long term results. *J Endod* 2014; 40: 790–796.
83 Zhou HM, Shen Y, Wang ZJ, Li L, Zheng YF, Häkkinen L, Haapasalo M. *In vitro* cytotoxicity evaluation of a novel rot repair material. *J Endod* 2013; 39: 478–483.
84 Heithrsay GS. Clinical, radiographic, and histopathologic features of invasive cervical resorption. *Quintessence* 1999: 30: 27–37.

Questions

1 Which of the following is the commonest type of injury in the orofacial region?
A Laceration
B Contusion
C Abrasion
D Avulsion

2 In vertical root fractures, chances of success are
A Poor
B Good
C Fair

3 An avulsed tooth must be replanted into the socket
A Within 20 minutes
B Within 10 minutes
C As early as possible
D Within 40 minutes

4 The tooth most commonly involved in a traumatic accident is
A Maxillary lateral incisor
B Maxillary central incisor
C Mandibular central incisor
D Mandibular lateral incisor

5 Chances of rapid root resorption and pulpal necrosis are higher in cases with intrusion of permanent teeth. To prevent this, pulp tissue is extirpated and calcium hydroxide is placed inside the root canal as an interim dressing. This is done
A Within 2 weeks of the injury
B Within 6 weeks of the injury
C Immediately after the injury
D Within 8 weeks of the injury

6 In root fractures, the best prognosis is with
A Coronal third fracture
B Middle third fracture
C Apical third fracture

7 Which is the least-favorable form of repair after root fracture?
A Healing with calcified tissue
B Healing with interposition of connective tissue
C Healing with interposition of bone and connective tissue
D Healing with interposition of granulation tissue

8 Internal resorption may follow
A Trauma
B Root fracture
C Successful root canal filling
D Enamel fracture

9 External root resorption may be attributed to which of the following?
i. Tumors and cysts
ii. Impacted teeth
iii. Excessive mechanical or occlusal forces
iv. Periapical inflammation
a. i and ii
b. ii and iii
c. i, ii, and iii
d. ii, iii, and iv
e. All of the above

10 Cells responsible for root resorption are
A Fibroblasts
B Cementoblasts
C Osteoblasts
D Osteoclasts
E Odontoblasts

CHAPTER 8

Visualization in endodontics

Carla Cabral dos Santos Accioly Lins[1], Diógenes Ferreira Alves[2], and Angelo Barbosa de Resende[3]

[1] *Department of Anatomy, Federal University of Pernambuco, Recife, Brazil*

[2] *Department of Endodontics, University of Pernambuco, Recife, Brazil*

[3] *Faculty of Dentistry, Recife, Brazil*

Endodontics is a specialty that has evolved with the use of new materials and technologies developed by engineering, computer science, and medicine, which has provided more precise treatments and more predictable prognosis in procedures that were performed in the darkness and dependent on the experience and skill of the operator [1]. The optical science through the use of endoscopes, orascopes, magnifying glasses, and microscopes has contributed to the precision of procedures in places deemed inaccessible to human vision, both in conventional and in surgical endodontics [2, 3].

Visualization devices in endodontics

Endoscopes are devices formed by a set of tubular lenses, coupled to a camera, light source, and a display [4]. They are widely used in medicine and were introduced into endodontics in 1979 to diagnose root fractures [5]. The term *endoscopy* is derived from Greek *endon*, "inside," and *skopion*, "to see," hence the meaning "to see inside." Endoscopes may be rigid, semiflexible, or flexible. The flexible endoscope has a coating of Nitinol, and its optical part is 0.9 mm in diameter, allowing a magnification of 20×. In nonsurgical endodontics, a 4-mm lens diameter, an angle of 30 degrees, and 4-cm length rod-lenses are recommended. In surgical endodontics, a lens of 2.7 mm in diameter, 70-degree angle, and 3 cm in length rod-lenses are recommended [3, 6, 7].

Orascopes began to be used in endodontics from 1990 onwards. Orascopes differ from endoscopes by being made of optical fiber (glass or plastic) and are recommended for root canal visualization. They have a diameter of 0.8 mm at the tip, a 0-degree lens, and a working portion that is 15 mm long. Like endoscopes, orascopes also work with a camera, a light source, and a monitor. These devices are used for visualization in conventional and surgical endodontics and are small, lightweight, and very flexible, thus allowing visualization of the treatment field at various angles and distances without losing focus and depth. Before the orascopes can be used, the root canal must have 15 mm of the cervical third prepared with a file #90 and then dried to better capture the image [3, 8, 9].

For decades, magnifying glasses were used by dentists to expand their visual capacity [10]. Although magnifying glasses improve visualization and are easy to use and handle, they have many limitations, including weight, image distortion, small depth of focus, limited and fixed magnification, and need for auxiliary light source. Using a magnifying glass causes eye and muscle fatigue as the view is converged when used for long periods, and it encourages incorrect posture as the professional attempts to improve the focus [11].

Operating microscope

Listed among the great inventions of medicine, the microscope, created in the early seventeenth century, made it possible to study the progress of biology and a new perception of medical science. The invention of the microscope, attributed to Galileo, was the result of an improvement by the Dutch naturalist Antonie

Current Therapy in Endodontics, First Edition. Edited by Priyanka Jain.
© 2016 John Wiley & Sons, Inc. Published 2016 by John Wiley & Sons, Inc.

van Leeuwenhoek in 1674, who used it to observe living organisms. Equipped with only a glass lens, this primitive microscope increased visual perception by 300 times, with reasonable clarity, achieving the observation of bacteria only 1 to 2 μm in diameter. Years later, Robert Hooke improved the primitive microscope of Leeuwenhoek, giving even greater image magnification [12].

From this date, the magnification systems have evolved and increasingly sophisticated optical assemblies continue to be developed. In dentistry, the use of the clinical microscope was first proposed in 1977 by Baumann, a German specialist in the microsurgery of ear [13]. However, only later, when the operating microscope models began to prioritize the posture of the operator, it was greatly spread in endodontics. In 1992, Gary Carr [14] made the first publication in the dental literature featuring some of the various applications of the operating microscope in endodontics, and this study was the basis for several other authors to deepen the research on its use [15–18]. The biggest development, however, took place in early 1998 when the American Dental Association established the obligation of teaching their use in all graduate courses in endodontics in the United States [19].

The operating microscope is considered one of the most significant influences on the growth of the specialty, because its use revolutionized dental clinical practice [14, 20]. The operating microscope introduces more advantages than disadvantages (Box 8.1), and the dental professional benefits from the advantages of magnification, thus obtaining a very bright operative field. This occurs because the coaxial lighting system is on the same axis view. Thus, there is no shade on the displayed area. In addition, lighting systems produce a uniform light with high power and the possibility to intensity adjustment for different clinical situations. To use the magnification, the professional needs to understand two basic optical principles: depth of field (focus) and field of view. The depth of field is defined as the distance between the closest and the farthest points that appear with acceptable sharpness in a certain scene [21]. Field of view is the total area that can be visualized through an optical instrument. The higher the magnification used, the smaller the depth of focus and the lower the visual field obtained.

Key concepts and applications of the operating microscope

The operating microscope is used in endodontic treatment of all teeth, especially in situations where direct visualization of the internal anatomy is limited. It is a working tool that allows excellent illumination of the operative field and magnification of images. Its routine

Box 8.1 Advantages and disadvantages of the operating microscope

Advantages

It has higher magnification.
It has better lighting.
It gives a three-dimensional view of the work area.
It has good ergonomics.
It does not lead to eyestrain.
It provides adequate working distance.
It has a documentation system.

Disadvantages

The equipment takes up a lot of space when it is movable on the floor.
It must be used in a single room when it is fixed on the ceiling or wall.
It is difficult to transport.
At higher magnification, the field of view and focal depth are reduced.
The equipment is expensive, and it requires proper and regular maintenance.
It has a steep learning curve.

use allows a great improvement in the quality and documentation of clinical trials. It consists of the base, the optical head, the light source, the engine, and the light splitter.

The base is the structure that supports the microscope. The base can be attached to the ceiling, wall, floor, or castors, which permits movement of the equipment according to the clinical need.

The optical head comprises the objective lens, the magnification nosepiece, and the binocular, which takes images to the eyes of the operator (Figure 8.1). The lenses are responsible for different magnification (2.5× to 24×), which can magnify an object 3 to 40 times, depending on the model and configuration of the microscope. The binoculars are tilting, and through the height adjustments they allow ergonomic, functional, and comfortable postures, adapting to the needs of the operator.

The focal distance is measured between the objective lens and the object to be focused. The objective lens can be 200, 250, or 300 mm (Figure 8.2), and the choice of lens is related to the operator's structure. The shorter the distance, the more limited will be the exchange of instruments between operator and assistant. Therefore, one should opt for the longest focal length that the height of the operator permits because this distance provides an excellent ergonomic working position with increased biosafety.

The light source is generated by a halogen lamp, light-emitting diode (LED), xenon, or metal halide. The light is directed to the head of the surgical microscope, usually through an optical fiber. Ideally, the light source supports two lamps (one in use and one reserve) and should be easy to replace.

The engine makes it possible to control increases (zoom) and microfocalization with adjustments in the motorized pedal.

The light splitter is a system for capturing images (photo and/or video). It is adapted through the device, allowing the dentist to document the case and also to transmit the image in real time to a monitor, also enabling the incorporation of a second binocular for the assistant.

Uses

The microscope is a valuable auxiliary tool in conventional endodontic techniques, allowing it to be used at various stages of treatment, such as surgery requiring access to root canals, the diagnosis of fractures and cracks, the observation of floor and location of root canals, in treating the perforations in endodontic retreatment, in periradicular surgery, and

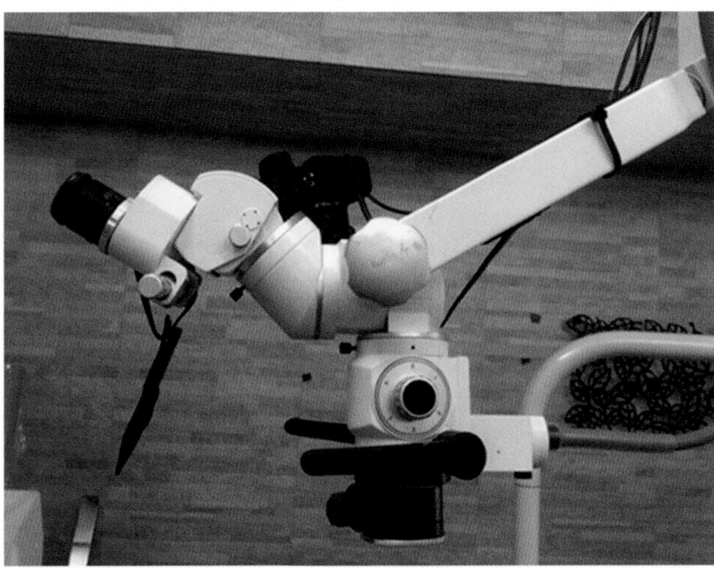

Figure 8.1 Operating microscope showing the binocular, objective, and the nosepiece.

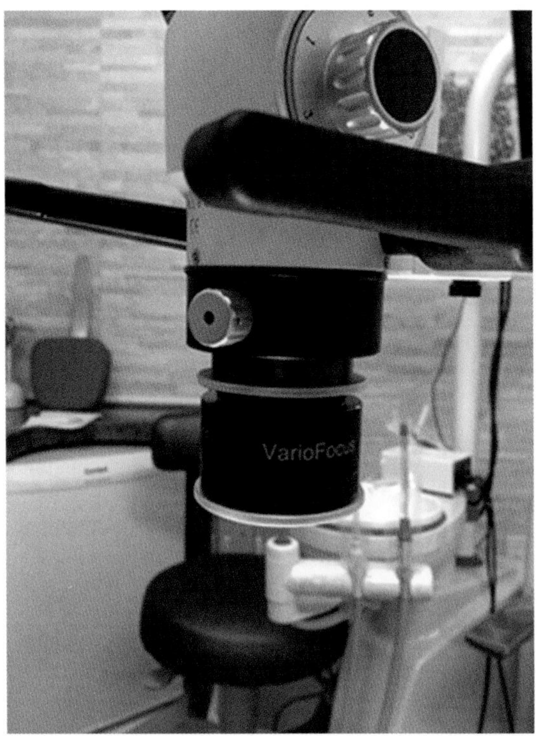

Figure 8.2 Vario Focus da JC-Optik, It Allows focus between 200 and 300 mm.

in removing fractured instruments and intraradicular nuclei [22].

This instrument is very helpful (Figure 8.3) in the diagnosis of root fractures. When the professional suspects a vertical fracture, the diagnosis can be made by observing the inner wall of the root canal, eliminating the need for exploratory surgery to examine the outer surface of the root [1]. To have good visibility, it is important to control the drying of the dentin: if it is too dry, the texture appears as white as chalk, and the fracture is not visible. If the dentin is too moist, reflection of the irrigating fluid can mask the fracture line [23].

Root perforation is a condition that can be caused by reabsorption of internal or external cavities or accidents arising from intraoperative procedures, resulting in communication of the root space with the outer tooth surface [24]. In such a scenario, there is always a doubtful prognosis that could significantly compromise the endodontic treatment. The treatment in the floor of the pulp or in the root canal chamber is performed with

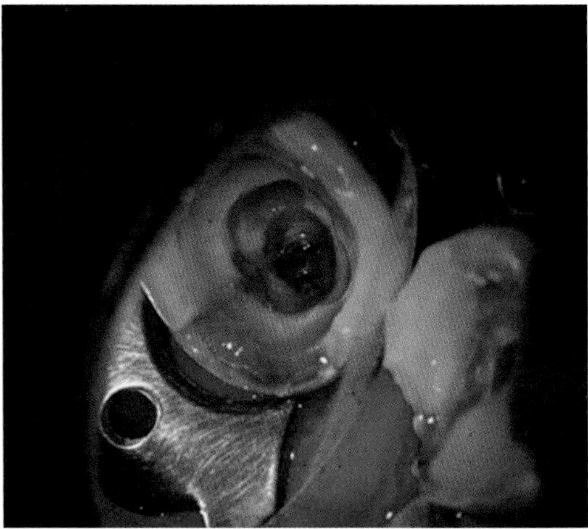

Figure 8.3 Line of coronal fracture located during the access to pulp chamber.

greater success by visualizing through the operating microscope, which allows better magnification and lighting with control of procedures, favoring a better seal [25, 26].

During the cleaning and shaping of the root canal system, overloading the instruments, or bad handling can lead to fracture of files within the channel. In such cases, the operating microscope is very useful because it allows the professional to visualize the fragment within the channel (Figure 8.4), where one can observe the presence of the space between the instrument and the walls of the conduit and the mobile fragment [26, 27]. Thus, the instrument can be removed, minimizing damage to the surrounding dentin [28, 29] and also preventing root perforations, steps, zips, and even root fractures. Among the various techniques for removal, ultrasound used in association with the surgical microscope has a high profile. In these cases, ultrasound is used in thin-gauge nondiamond inserts that penetrate into the root canal and touch only the fractured fragment of the instrument. The vibration transferred to the instrument causes it to release from the walls and be removed by irrigation and aspiration [27, 30].

The operating microscope and ultrasound has been fundamental to the development of conventional endodontics, as well as for paraendodontic microsurgery. The traditional surgical technique has a success rate of below 60%, but the current technique using both microscope and ultrasound yields success rates

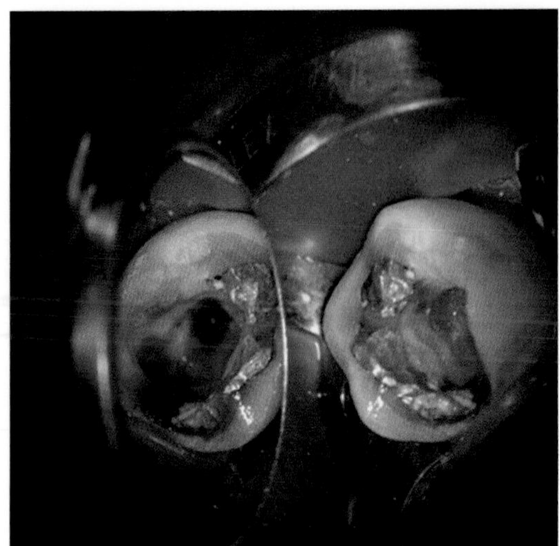

Figure 8.4 Endodontic instrument fractured within root canal.

above 90% [31–33]. This difference in success rates between the techniques makes the use of ultrasound and surgical microscope fundamental and essential in paraendodontic surgical procedures. The coupled use of these devices is especially useful for smaller osteotomies, better visualization of the apical region and its foramina, apicectomy with a cutting angle always perpendicular to the long axis of the tooth, retro repairs with suitable dimensions and inclinations, preparation of an isthmus of the apical or middle third, and in filling cavities [12] (Figure 8.5).

Several explanations for the failure of endodontic treatment have been reported in the literature. Technical failures include apical percolation, root perforations, canals with no sealing, periodontal lesions, incomplete obturations or superobturations, and coronal leakage due to loss of a restoration or recurrent decay [34–36]. In an attempt to eliminate these causes, nonsurgical endodontic treatment is the standard of practice [37]. Within this context, the microscope becomes a great ally for implementing the reintervention, because with the microscope we can observe the remaining filling material still not removed by solvent or by canal instrumentation (Figure 8.6). Thus, when the filling material is completely removed and the walls of the channel are cleaned, many causes of failure can be identified, such as the presence of a vertical fracture, extra channels, or root perforations that may be treated with a higher success rate.

Another aspect of dental practice that has been enhanced by use of the surgical microscope is the documentation. The microscope has a unit that can be adapted to a photo camera, a video camera and a video

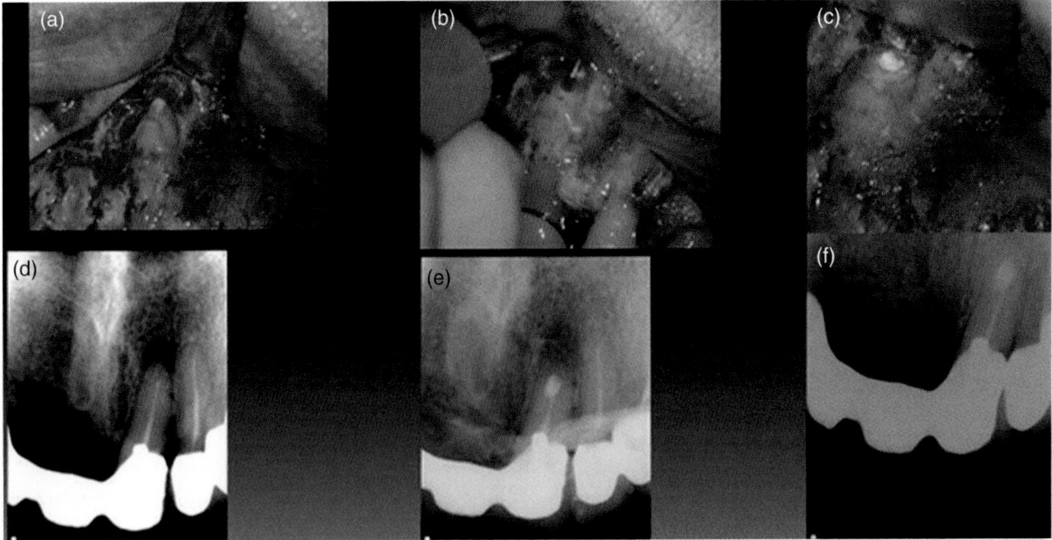

Figure 8.5 Periapical surgery with magnification, allowing the clinician to view: *A,* Gutta-percha cone exhibition. *B,* Apical retropreparation with ultrasonic tip. *C,* Retrograde retrofilling image with MTA. *D,* Initial radiography. *E,* Postoperative radiography. *F,* Radiography of the control after eight months showing the repair process.

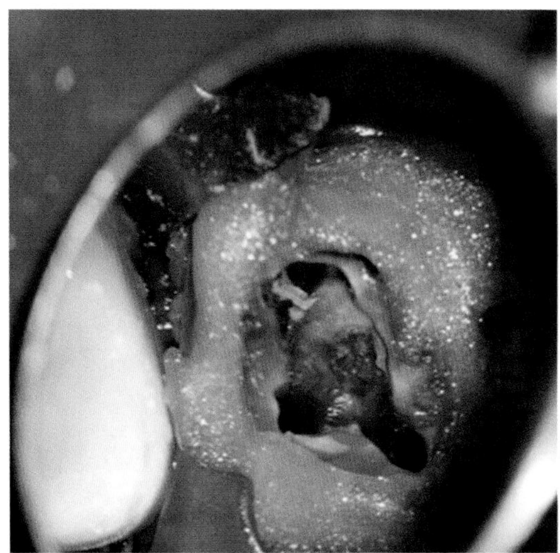

Figure 8.6 View of remaining obturation material during treatment of the root canal system.

printer. The recordings not only help the dentist legally but also can be used to educate patients, who often better understand visual communication [38]. At the end of the treatment, a printed image from the video can be a complement of the final radiograph. It is also possible to scan different images during surgery and then print a single copy. Copies can be used for patient education, legal documentation, insurance, teaching, or exchange between professionals [10, 11].

Resources to locate root canals

Current features and techniques

The surgical microscope has helped endodontists make detailed observations of morphological characteristics of the various dental structures, allowing better results in various stages of endodontic treatment. The bright lighting allows better visualization of the input ports of the root canals [39–43], assists in the removal maneuvers of dentin projections, and facilitates the differentiation of colors between the dentin and the floor of the pulp chamber [44].

In cases with calcifications or obstructions within the root canal, or where the anatomy of the pulp floor was changed, this equipment is very important to the successful treatment of these difficulties. By using the microscope more commonly, more conservative treatments with respect to the internal anatomy of the teeth are now possible, reducing the chance of accidents that can occur during endodontic therapy [45, 46].

To find the root canals, the most useful magnifications are 8× and 12.5×, because with higher magnification, images of the pulpal floor can be distorted, and depth of field can be lost. The operator must control the amount of light so as to be able to discern the variable coloring and texture differences of the dentin [11, 14]. In addition to magnification and illumination, the operator can use the physical and chemical properties of some substances such as sodium hypochlorite and disclosing agents that will serve as a guide to finding atresic canals [47] and increase the chance of detecting additional root canals on the floor of the pulp chamber [48].

The action of sodium hypochlorite on organic matter promotes effervescence, which helps in locating the canal hole [49]. The effervescence time and the amount of irrigating solution influences the ease of locating the canals. It is recommended to leave a minimum amount of pulp in the floor cavity for observation, in order to highlight differences between the coloring dentine present in the pulp cavity and floor [11].

The holes of the canal entrance can also be identified by disclosing agents such as 1% methylene blue [47–49], 1% sodium fluorescein [50, 51] and Sable Seek (Ultradent Products, Inc. South Jordan, Utah, USA) [47]. Sodium fluorescein 1% is an orange eye drop solution that dyes organic structures on the floor of the pulp chamber. A cobalt blue light filter is attached inside or outside the optical head of the operating microscope, and the sodium fluorescein appears as fluorescent green in the canal entrance and blue in the rest of dentin [52].

Modifications to access surgery have been suggested to increase the amount of localized canals, mainly on the upper molars, on which the conventional triangular shape is modified to trapezoidal, rectangular, or rhomboidal using ultrasound and the spherical long-stem insert drills [43]. Stropko's study [53] on the location of the additional canals in the upper molars using the operating microscope revealed the presence of a thin neck, similar to a red or white line, between the first mesiobuccal (MB1) and second mesiobuccal (MB2) canal, except in cases of calcification on this site.

The growing disclosure of additional canals, such as the fourth canal (second mesiobuccal, MB2) in

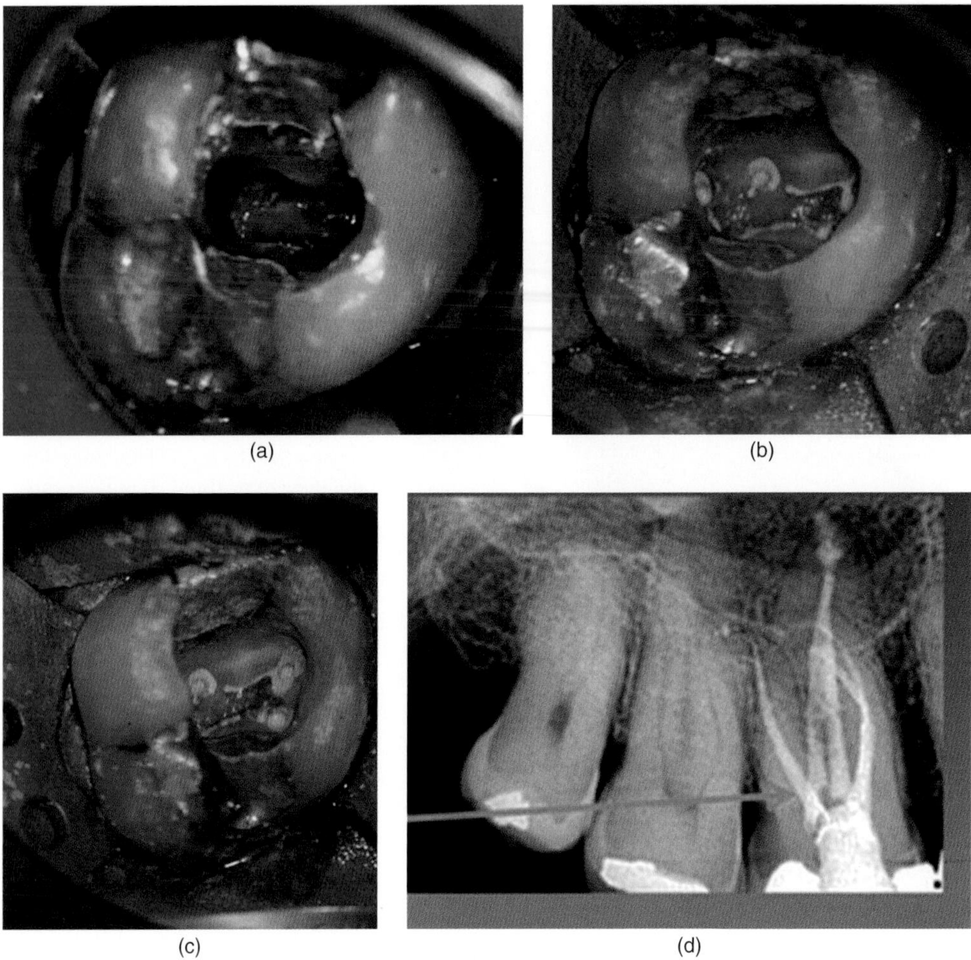

Figure 8.7 *A*, Entrance of five canals after instrumentation. *B* and *C*, Identification of the gutta-percha after obturation. *D*, Final radiograph.

the first and second molars (Figure 8.7) and the fifth canal (mesiomedial) in the mesial root of mandibular molars, have become the most predictable endodontic treatment and with a greater chance of success [51, 54–56]. The most common configuration of the mandibular first molar is the presence of two or three root canals. Martins and Anderson [57] have reported two rare anatomical configurations with six canals in two left molars. Dental surgical microscope and ultrasound probes (Troughing Ultrasonic) were used in the furrows between the mesial and distal canals to successfully locate the middle root canals.

The surgical microscope has caused major changes in endodontics. To use it in the daily routine, it is necessary to promote training courses where professionals can get hands-on experience with this working tool, enabling them to work with the instruments and equipment, seeking to have a new conception of the workplace. Early in training, the microscope can impede the work because the learning curve is long, so training on extracted teeth is highly recommended. However, once the dentist becomes proficient with the microscope, its use gives the dentist a more comfortable and ergonomic working position, reducing fatigue and stress, increasing work efficiency [58].

Conclusion

The technological advances developed over the past few years have allowed endodontists to achieve high levels of excellence, and the visual magnification has become a powerful tool that is providing greater precision in treatment, better quality, and a higher success rate in many cases.

References

1 Feix LM, Boijink D, Ferreira R, Wagner MH, Barletta FB. Operating microscope in endodontics: visual magnification and luminosity. *S Braz Dent J* 2010; 7: 340–348.
2 Ingle JI, Bakland IK. *Endodontics*. Hamilton: BC Decker; 2008.
3 Dhingra A, Nagar N. Recent advances in endodontic visualization: a review. *J Dent Med Sci* 2014; 13: 15–20.
4 Bahcall J, Barss J. Orascope vs. endoscope: a revolution in endodontic visualization. *Dentistry* 2001; 2: 24–27.
5 Detsch S, Cunningham W, Langloss J. Endoscopy as an aid to endodontic diagnosis. *J Endod* 1979; 2: 60–62.
6 Taschieri S, Rosano G, Weinstein T, Del Fabbro M. Endoscopic management of a lateral root lesion. A case report. *Minerva Stomatol* 2008; 57: 587–595.
7 Taschieri S, Rosano G, Francetti L, Agliardi E, Del Fabbro M. A modified technique for using the endoscope in periradicular surgery. A case report. *Minerva Stomatol* 2008; 57: 359–367.
8 Bahcall J, Barss J. Orascopic visualization technique for conventional and surgical endodontics. *Int Endod J* 2003: 36: 441–447.
9 Bahcall J, Barss J. Orascopy: vision for the millennium. *Part II. Dent Today* 1999: 18: 82–85.
10 Rubinstein R. The anatomy of the surgical operating microscope and operating position. *Dent Clin North Am* 1997; 41:391–413.
11 Fregnani E, Hizatugu R. *Endodontics: A contemporay view*. São Paulo: Santos Press, 2012.
12 Hirsch ED Jr., *What Your 5th Grader Needs to Know*. New York: Delta Trade Books; 2006. Anton van Leeuwenhoek, pp. 384–385).
13 Baumann RR. How may the dentist benefit from the operating microscope? *Quintessence Int* 1997; 5: 5–17.
14 Carr GB. Microscopes in endodontics. *J Calif Dent Assoc* 1992; 20: 55–61.
15 Pecora G, Andreana S. Use of dental operating microscope in endodontic surgery. *Oral Surg Oral Med Oral Pathol* 1993; 75: 751–758.
16 Mounce R. Surgical microscopes in endodontics: the quantum leap. *Dent Today* 1993; 12: 88–91.
17 Ruddle CJ. Endodontic perforation repair: using the surgical operating microscope. *Dent Today* 1994; 13: 48– 53.
18 Kim S. Modern endodontic practice: instruments and techniques. *Dent Clin North Am* 2004; 48: 1–9.
19 American Dental Association. *Accreditation Standards for Advanced Specialty Education Programs in Endodontics*. Chicago: American Dental Association; 2013.
20 García Calderín M, Torres Lagares D, Calles Vázquez C, Usón Gargallo J, Gutiérrez Pérez JL. The application of microscope surgery in dentistry. *Med Oral Patol Oral Cir Bucal* 2007; 12: 311–316.
21 Leslie S, Current I, Comton J, Zakia RD. *Basic Photographic Materials and Processes*. Oxford: Focal Press; 2000.
22 Santos Accioly Lins C, de Melo Silva E, de Lima G, Conrado de Menezes S, Coelho Travassos R. Operating microscope in endodontics: a systematic review. *Open J Stomatol* 2013; 3: 1–5.
23 Khayat G. The use of magnification in endodontic therapy: the operating microscope. *Pract Periodontics Aesthet Dent* 1998; 10: 137–144.
24 American Association of Endodontists. *Glossary of endodontic terms*. Chicago: American Association of Endodontists; 2003.
25 Ianes CI, Nica LM, Stratul S, Carligeriu, V. Endodontic retreatment of a mandibular first molar with five root canals: a case report. *Timisoara Med J* 2011; 61: 125–130.
26 Nunes E, Silveira FF, Soares JA, Duarte MA, Soares SM. Treatment of perforating internal root resorption with MTA: a case report. *J Oral Sci* 2012; 54: 127–131.
27 Ward JR, Parashos P, Messer HH. Evaluation of an ultrasonic technique to remove fractured rotary nickel–titanium endodontic instruments from root canals: Clinical cases. *J Endod* 2003; 29: 764–767.
28 Faramarzi F, Fakri H, Javaheri HH. Endodontic treatment of a mandibular first molar with three mesial canals and broken instrument removal. *Aust Endod J* 2010; 36: 39–41.
29 Jadhav GR. Endodontic management of a two rooted, three canaled mandibular canine with a fractured instrument. *J Conserv Dent* 2014; 17: 192–195.
30 Ward JR. The use of an ultrasonic technique to remove a fractured Rotary nickel–titanium instrument from the apical third of a curved root canal. *Aust Endod J* 2003; 29: 25–30.
31 Kim E, Song JS, Jung IY, Lee SJ, Kim S. Prospective clinical study evaluating endodontic microsurgery outcomes for cases with lesions of endodontic origin compared with cases with lesions of combined periodontal–endodontic origin. *J Endod* 2008; 34: 546–51.
32 Setzer FC, Shah SB, Kohli MR, Karabucak B, Kim S. Outcome of endodontic surgery: a meta-analysis of the literature-part 1: Comparison of traditional root-end surgery and endodontic microsurgery. *J Endod* 2010; 36: 1757–1765.
33 Song M, Jung IY, Lee SJ, Lee CY, Kim E. Prognostic factors for clinical outcomes in endodontic microsurgery: a retrospective study. *J Endod* 2011; 37: 927–933.

34 Torabinejad M, Ung B, Kettering JD. *In vitro* bacterial penetration of coronally unsealed endodontically treated teeth. *J Endod* 1990; 16: 566–569.

35 Saunders WP, Saunders EM. Coronal leakage as a cause of failure in root canal therapy: a review. *Endod Dent Traumatol* 1994; 10: 105–108.

36 Sritharan A. Discuss that the coronal seal is more important than the apical seal for endodontic success. *Aust Endod J* 2002; 28: 112–115.

37 Friedman S, Mor C. The success of endodontic therapy: healing and fuctionally. *J Calif Dent Assoc* 2004; 32: 267–274.

38 Koch K. The microscope: its effect on your practice. *Dent Clin North Am* 1997; 41: 619–626.

39 Kottoor J, Velmurugan N, Surendran S. Endodontic management of a maxillary first molar with eight root canal systems evaluated using cone-beam computed tomography scanning: a case report. *J Endod* 2011; 37, 715–719.

40 Karumaran CS, Gunaseelan R, Krithikadatta J. Microscope-aided endodontic treatment of maxillary first premolars with three roots: A case series. *Indian J Dent Res* 2011; 22, 706–708.

41 Kontakiotis EG, Tzanetakis GN. Four canals in the mesial root of a mandibular first molar. A case report under the operating microscope. *Aust Endod J* 2007; 33: 84–88.

42 Karthikeyan K, Mahalaxmi S. New nomenclature for extra canals based on four reported cases of maxillary first molars with six canals. *J Endod* 2010; 36: 1073–1078.

43 Sachdeva GS, Malhotra D, Sachdeva LT, Sharma N, Negi A. Endodontic management of mandibular central incisor fused to a supernumerary tooth associated with a talon cusp: a case report. *Int Endod J* 2012; 45: 590–596.

44 Lababidi EA. Discuss the impact technological advances in equipment and materials have made on the delivery and outcome of endodontic treatment. *Aust Endod J* 2013; 39: 92–97.

45 Selden HS. The role of a dental operating microscope in improved nonsurgical treatment of "calcified" canals. *Oral Surg Oral Med Oral Pathol* 1989; 68: 93–98.

46 Nóbrega LMM, Gadê Neto CR, Carvalho RA, Dameto FR, Maia CADM. *In vitro* evaluation of blockage transposition in the root canal entrance with or without the clinical microscope as assistant. *Cienc Odontol Bras* 2008; 11: 56–63.

47 Nallapati S. Aberrant root canal anatomy: a review. *Sasidar Nallapati PMD* 2007; 2: 50–62.

48 Baldassari-Cruz LA, Lilly JP, Rivera EM. The influence of dental operating microscope in location the mesiolingual canal orifice. *Oral Surg Oral Med Oral Pathol* 2002; 93:190–193.

49 Vertucci FJ. Root canal morphology and its relationship to endodontic procedures. *Endod Topics* 2005; 10: 3–29.

50 Carvalho MC, Zuolo ML. Orifice locating with a microscope. *J Endod* 2000; 26: 532–4.

51 Ryan JL, Bowles WL, Baisden MK, McClanahan SB. Mandibular first molar with six separate canals. *J Endod* 2011; 37: 878–80.

52 Pais ASG, Alves VO, Sigrist MA, Cunha RS, Fontana CE, Bueno CE. Sodium fluorescein and cobalt blue filter coupled to a dental operating microscope to optimise root canal location in maxillary first molars. *J Endod* 2014; 8: 193–198.

53 Stropko JJ. Canal morphology of maxillary molars: clinical observations of canal configurations. *J Endod* 1999; 25: 446–450.

54 Rampado ME, Tjäderhane L, Friedman S, Hamstra SJ. The benefit of the operating microscope for access cavity preparation by undergraduate students. *J Endod* 2004; 30: 863–867.

55 Coutinho-Filho T, La Cerda RS, Gurgel-Filho ED, de Deus GA, Magalhães KM. The influence of the surgical operating microscope in locating the mesiolingual canal orifice: a laboratory analysis. *Braz Oral Res* 2006; 20: 59–63.

56 Görduysus MO, Görduysus M, Friedman S. Operating microscope improves negotiation of second mesiobuccal canals in maxillary molars. *J Endod* 2001; 27: 683–686.

57 Martins JN, Anderson C. Endodontic treatment of the mandibular first molar with six root canals: two case reports and literature review. *J Clin Diagn Res* 2015; 9: 6–8.

58 Marques KCA, Motta Júnior, AG, Fidel RAS, Fidel SR. Clinic adequation of surgical microscope on dental treatment. *Revista Cientific of HCE* 2008; 2: 70–72.

Questions

1 Which of the following equipment is considered the biggest advancement in endodontics?
 A Dental loupe
 B Endoscope
 C Orascope
 D Operating microscope

2 Which of the following statements is false regarding the use of surgical microscope?
 A It facilitates the visualization of cracks and dental fractures.
 B To clearly visualize the dentin, it has to be dry.
 C Its expansion and lighting aids in locating additional canals.

3 The higher the magnification, the smaller the depth of focus.
 A True
 B False

4 Which of these are types of light sources is/are used in surgical microscopes?
 A Halogen lamp
 B LED
 C Xenon
 D All of the above

5 What is the magnification used for endoscopes?
A 5×
B 15×
C 20×
D 25×

6 The operating microscope was first used by
A Ophthalmologists
B Endodontists
C Otologists
D Dermatologists

7 Binoculars of the microscope are available with which of the following tube types?
A Straight
B Inclined
C Inclinable
D All of the above

8 With the operating microscope, use of the mirror
A Remains essential
B Is optional
C Is unnecessary
D None of the above

9 Using the operating microscope has rendered which of the following procedures more reliable:
A Removing a broken instrument
B Repairing a perforation
C Passing a ledge
D All of the above

10 What are the main advantages of the operating microscope in clinical practice?
A Better visualization
B Improved treatment quality
C Ideal treatment ergonomics
D All of the above

CHAPTER 9

Endodontic microsurgery

James D. Johnson[1], Kathleen McNally[2], Scott B. McClanahan[3], and Stephen P. Niemczyk[4]

[1] *Department of Endodontics, School of Dentistry University of Washington, Seattle, Washington, USA*

[2] *Endodontics Department, Naval Postgraduate Dental School Bethesda, Maryland, USA*

[3] *Division of Endodontics, School of Dentistry, University of Minnesota, Minneapolis, Minnesota, USA*

[4] *Advanced Education Program in Endodontics, Harvard School of Dental Medicine, Boston, Massachusetts, USA*

Endodontic microsurgery has become a valuable choice for patients who desire to retain their natural dentition. With new techniques and technology, endodontic microsurgeons can offer their patients a predictable positive outcome for teeth that otherwise would be lost.

Endodontic surgery has experienced many advances in recent years. The use of the dental operating microscope has made surgical procedures, and all endodontic procedures, more precise. Microsurgical instruments, soft tissue management principles and procedures, ultrasonic root end preparations, improved root-end filling materials, guided tissue-regeneration techniques, and improved radiographic three-dimensional imaging with cone beam computed tomography have led to these advances.

Today, endodontic microsurgery relies on techniques and materials from other disciplines in dentistry and medicine, as well as techniques and materials unique in endodontics. Materials and techniques from restorative dentistry and prosthodontics can repair dental structures in surgical and nonsurgical endodontic treatment. Surgical principles from the oral maxillofacial surgeon and the periodontist must also be incorporated into endodontic microsurgery where appropriate. The endodontic microsurgeon of today must be adept at managing and manipulating soft tissues to achieve an esthetic and functional result. With this in mind, it is incumbent upon the endodontic microsurgeon to be an expert in all techniques and materials enhancing microsurgical outcomes. One must be acutely aware of methods and materials to support a state-of-the-art practice that renders predictable results for patients.

Advances in endodontic microsurgery and improved armamentarium

Dental Operating microscope

The dental operating microscope revolutionized endodontic surgery. With increased magnification and illumination, the dental operating microscope allows visualization of the delicate structures in the endodontic surgical field, and it allows precise microinstrumentation needed for successful surgical techniques.

The dental operating microscope is described in detail in another chapter and detailed in references for this chapter [1, 2].

Microinstrumentation

With magnification, smaller instruments can be used. Micro blades, micro mirrors, micropluggers, micro explorers, smaller suture materials, micro curettage instruments, smaller retractors, micro syringes for air and water (Stropko irrigator), micro scissors, Castroviejo needle holders, and ultrasonic instrumentation are required for endodontic microsurgery.

Ultrasonic instrumentation

Ultrasonic piezoelectric units transfer energy to ultrasonic tips that are used to prepare the root end [2]. Dr. Gary Carr designed the first ultrasonic tips that were stainless steel. Ultrasonic tips now come in many sizes and materials, including the Kim Surgical (KiS) tips (Obtura Spartan Endodontics. Algonquin, IL), which are made of zirconium nitride [2]. Ultrasonic tips allow small root-end preparations, which can be made in

Current Therapy in Endodontics, First Edition. Edited by Priyanka Jain.
© 2016 John Wiley & Sons, Inc. Published 2016 by John Wiley & Sons, Inc.

the long axis of the root to a depth of 3 mm. Newer 6- and 9-mm ultrasonic tips are also available for deeper root-end preparations. Ultrasonic tips also come with different angles, so that any canal on any tooth may be prepared for a root-end filling.

Cone beam computed tomography

Cone beam computed tomography (CBCT) has made it possible to view the surgical site in three dimensions and to accurately visualize anatomical structures, including roots, periapical lesions, the inferior alveolar canal, the mental foramen, and the maxillary sinus, to name a few. The microsurgeon now knows exactly what is in the surgical area. This prevents encroachment on neurovascular bundles, lessens the amount of bone that needs to be removed, and provides a better path to the area that will be treated surgically. It is possible to use data from the CBCT images to create a three-dimensional model that is an exact replica of the structures that were imaged on the CBCT.

Figure 9.1 demonstrates a two-dimensional radiographic image that has limitations. Figure 9.2 is a three-dimensional CBCT scan demonstrating the value of a CBCT image that provides information that is necessary for the planned surgical procedure.

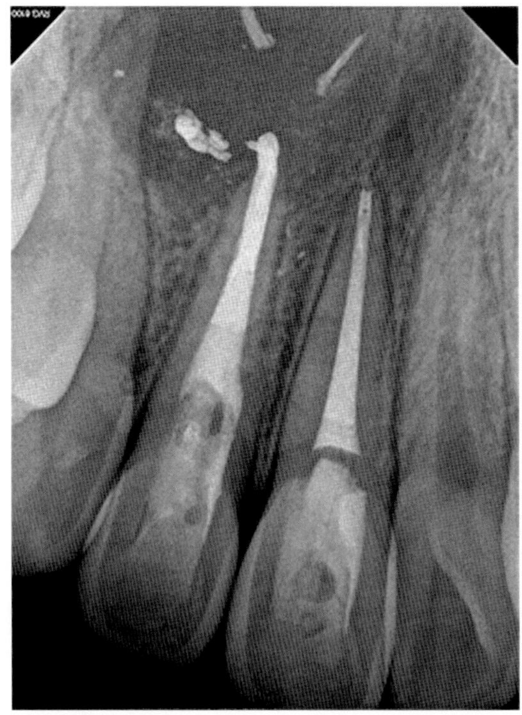

Figure 9.1 Periapical radiograph of a large periapical lesion. The extent of the lesion cannot be determined on a periapical radiograph. (Image courtesy of Dr. Ben Studebaker.)

Root-end filling materials

Root-end filling materials that seal the root-end preparation well and that are extremely biocompatible are now available. These include Super EBA (Harry J. Bosworth Co, Skokie, IL), mineral trioxide aggregate (MTA), and the newer bioceramics. These materials have improved outcomes when compared to older root-end filling materials such as amalgam, or cold burnished gutta-percha.

Guided tissue-regenerative techniques

Guided tissue-regenerative techniques that are used in other areas of medicine and other areas of dentistry, especially periodontics, have made it possible to treat conditions such as through-and-through lesions, periapical defects that communicate with the marginal crestal bone, furcation defects from perforation, and large periapical lesions, and have led to an increase in successful outcomes for these types of cases.

Indications and contraindications for endodontic surgery

Most common indications and contraindications for surgical intervention are listed in Box 9.1 and Box 9.2 [2–5].

Presurgical considerations

Several factors must be considered when planning treatment for endodontic surgery. These include the indications and contraindications previously listed. The endodontic microsurgeon must also consider the patient's medical and dental histories and the overall treatment plan. The overall treatment plan for the patient must be known and planned with all specialists concerned. The patient's motivation to undergo endodontic microsurgery and any degree of apprehension must be taken into account. In esthetic zones, mucoperiosteal flap design is critical and should be considered to prevent gingival recession and possible scarring. Esthetic areas must have soft tissue

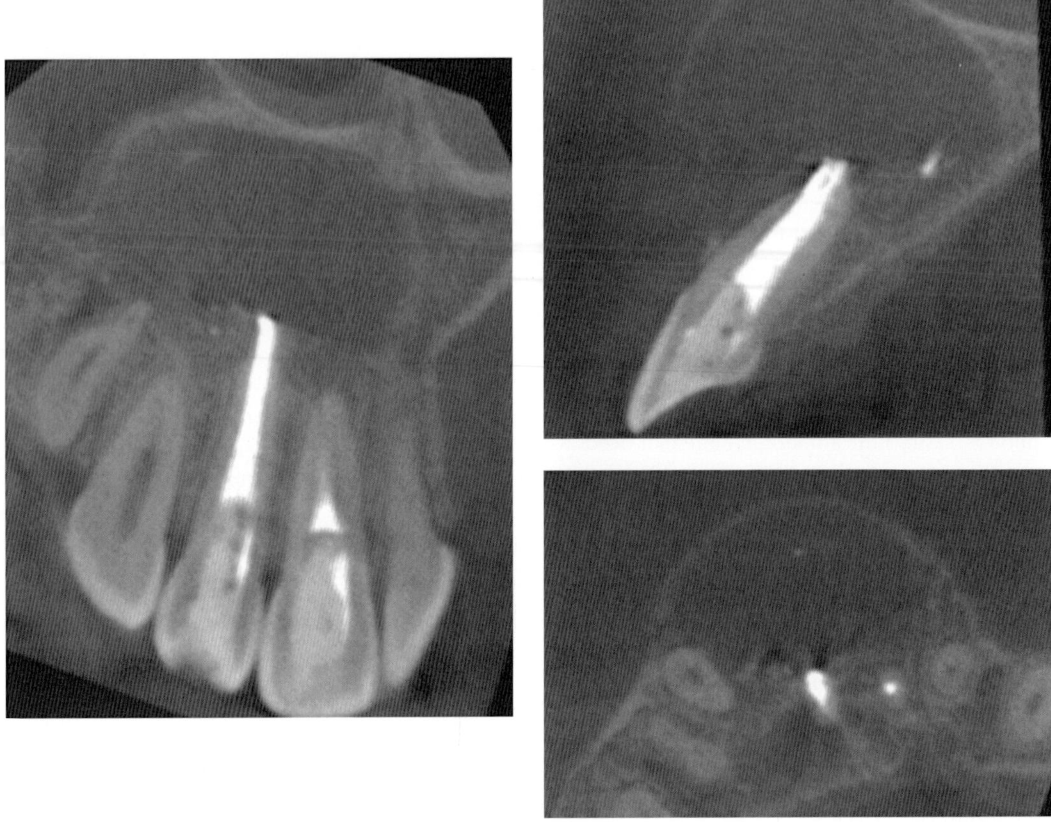

Figure 9.2 In this CBCT image of the large periapical lesions, sealer is evident. The facial–palatal width of the root canal filling is visualized. The bony margins of the lesion are intact on the palatal and nasal floor, but the facial bone is not intact and is expanded. (Image courtesy of Dr. Ben Studebaker.)

management strategies to avoid exposure of crown margins.

Clinical considerations involving the dentition include caries, deficiencies of restorations, cracks, and pulpal vitality of teeth in the surgical area. Soft tissues must be carefully evaluated, and muscle and frenum attachments must be noted. The presence of sinus tracts and preexisting scar tissue are additional factors that can affect the surgical treatment plan and flap design. The patient's periodontal status must be considered. Periodontal probing depths and areas of bleeding on probing must be charted. Areas of gingival recession and width of attached keratinized gingiva must be evaluated. The amount of gingival and periodontal inflammation should be evaluated to determine the need for a dental prophylaxis prior to surgery to reduce inflammation. The amount of bone loss and furcation involvement should be identified because they can influence flap design. Endodontic–periodontal lesions must also be considered in order to determine the sequence of treatment.

Anatomical considerations in treatment planning include height and depth of buccal vestibule, height and depth of the palate, size of the oral cavity, the patient's interocclusal distance, prominence of the mental protuberance, presence of exostoses, and the prominence of the buccal oblique ridge. Root length and the presence, location, and size of periapical lesions are essential in treatment planning and mucoperiosteal flap design. Location of key anatomic structures such as the mental foramen, inferior alveolar canal, and maxillary sinus is critical.

Box 9.1 Indications for endodontic surgical intervention

The following conditions present the most common indications for surgical intervention [1–4]:

Need for surgical drainage
- Fluctuant: releases fluid build-up and provides rapid relief
- Nonfluctuant: releases pressure; may be only blood or serous fluid, but decreases irritants and increases circulation to the area

Pulp canal obliteration and other calcifications

Procedural errors
- Instrument separation
- Nonnegotiable ledging
- Root perforation
- Symptomatic overfilling
- Gross overfills

Anatomic variation
- Root dilacerations
- Apical root fenestration

Biopsy
- Suspicious or nonhealing lesions
- Uncharacteristic signs and symptoms, which require exploratory surgery and biopsy for microscopic evaluation

Corrective surgery
- Repair of resorptive defects
- Root caries
- Root resection
- Hemisection
- Bicuspidization

Replacement surgery
- Intentional replantation (extraction followed by replantation)
- Posttraumatic replantation
- Transplantation of teeth
- Ridge preservation when teeth must be extracted after exploratory surgery reveals an unfavorable prognosis

Box 9.2 Contraindications for endodontic surgery [1–4]

Unidentified cause of treatment failure (identify the cause before surgery)

Medical or systemic complications (may be absolute or relative)
- Blood or bleeding disorders (medical consult, lab work needed)
- Terminal disease
- Uncontrolled diabetes
- Severe heart disease or uncontrolled hypertension
- Immunocompromised state (caution)
- Recent myocardial infarction (within 7–30 days, or longer if unstable angina is present) [5]
- Psychological problems
- Kidney disease requiring dialysis (caution)
- Osteoradionecrosis
- History of bisphosphonate medications

Anatomic factors
- Lack of surgical access
- Root lengths that are too short (precluding root-end resection or making restoration with a post and core inadvisable)
- Severe periodontal disease
- Nonrestorable teeth

Indiscriminate use of surgery: surgery is not indicated if a nonsurgical method presents an equal or better chance of success

The presence of crowns, fixed bridges, posts, and type of post affect treatment planning decisions.

Treatment planning

The medical condition of the patient may or may not affect whether the patient can undergo endodontic microsurgery. Most medical conditions are relative, and most, if well controlled, are not a contraindication to surgery. Consultation with the patient's physician and medical staff is required when dealing with complex medical issues. Monitoring vital signs is important for all patients, and laboratory tests and values may also be required for many medical conditions prior to surgery.

Patients with bleeding disorders, or patients being treated with anticoagulants, should be carefully evaluated and managed. A thorough knowledge and investigation into any possible adverse reactions with local anesthetics and medications the patient may be taking is critical. Patients require premedication with antibiotics for some heart conditions and for some joint replacement conditions. Immunocompromised patients may require antibiotic coverage. It may be necessary to supplement corticosteroid medications in some patients who are taking corticosteroid medications. Many patients require oral sedation or nitrous oxide to reduce anxiety. Other patients require deeper sedation involving intravenous sedation, and still others need to have their endodontic microsurgery procedure in a hospital operating room.

The patient's motivation to save the tooth by means of endodontic surgery can be determined by reviewing their history and discussing their dental goals. Reviewing the patient's medical and dental history is a great opportunity to develop rapport with the patient, which will be an asset during the surgical treatment.

The patient's ability or inability to lie flat or to turn on their side during the endodontic microsurgery may be limited by medical conditions, including arthritis and other conditions. It is beyond the scope of this chapter to outline all of the medical conditions that need to be managed when considering endodontic microsurgery. There are some absolute contraindications for surgery, which were listed above. A medical consultation is always in the best interest of the patient.

The patient's dental history is valuable when formulating an endodontic treatment plan, and the overall dental treatment plan for the patient's dental needs should be understood. This allows the endodontist to know how the specific tooth in question will be restored and used in the restorative plan. The history of the specific tooth or teeth that may require endodontic treatment will give the endodontist the background to know if the tooth should be treated nonsurgically, re-treated nonsurgically, or treated with surgical endodontics. Nonsurgical endodontics has a very high success rate and usually should be the first line of treatment. If initial root canal therapy was not successful, retreatment to correct any deficiencies is indicated prior to surgical intervention, if possible. Nonsurgical retreatment has a very good outcome. Surgical endodontic outcomes with modern techniques is as successful as nonsurgical retreatment, and in some situations is better. Some nonsurgical retreatment involves potential risk, such as removing a large post or requiring removal of additional dentin. These potential risks would make surgical endodontics a better option for these patients.

The extraoral and intraoral examination, pulp sensibility testing, and radiographic examination of periapical images and CBCT images of the patient will further lead the endodontic microsurgeon to a treatment plan.

Clinical considerations

The presence of teeth with nonvital pulps in the surgical field may require nonsurgical endodontics to be performed before surgical endodontics on the tooth in question is completed.

Anatomical structures

Patients who are unable to open their mouth adequately or who have limited movement of the temporomandibular joint (TMJ) may not be good candidates for endodontic surgery. A thick buccal cortical plate with a prominent external oblique ridge may preclude root-end surgery on a mandibular second molar. The same may true for a palatal approach to a maxillary molar palatal root, if there is a shallow palatal vault with thick palatal bone. An extremely shallow facial vestibule can contraindicate root-end surgery, or it can at least be an indication to extend the mucoperiosteal flap in a horizontal direction. Palpation over the root eminences can reveal areas of dehiscence or concavities between roots, thus indicating where vertical incisions may be placed. Care must also be exercised to not place a vertical incision where it could intersect the mental nerve as it exits from the mental foramen. When CBCT imaging and tenderness to palpation over the apex of roots may indicate that the apical ends of roots are outside of the bony housing, root-end surgery should reduce the apical extent of the roots to insure they are within the bony architecture and are not out of the facial cortical bone.

Periodontal considerations

Periodontal probing depths will indicate bone level and dictate a flap design that would allow inspection of the crestal bone in some cases and would detect a periodontal pocket in other cases. Teeth with a poor periodontal prognosis should not be considered for root-end surgery. Teeth with gingival recession, furcation defects, horizontal or vertical bone loss, and endo–perio lesions can affect the decision to treat the tooth with endodontic surgery, and will determine flap design if a tooth will be treated surgically.

Soft tissue considerations

The width of the attached and keratinized gingiva and the periodontal tissue type also influence flap design. The presence of a sinus tract influences the reflection of the mucoperiosteal flap. Muscle attachments and frenums may dictate where vertical releasing incisions are placed. Preexisting scar tissue and exostosis call for careful reflection of the mucogingival flap.

Radiographical considerations

If cracks, vertical root fractures, or cervical resorptive areas are present, an intrasulcular flap may be required to view and examine these areas. The size of the periapical lesion will determine the horizontal component of the mucogingival flap. A large lesion requires a longer horizontal component to the flap as opposed to no lesion or a small periapical lesion. The placement of a vertical incision must be at least one tooth away from the extent of the periapical lesion.

Prosthodontic considerations

Teeth that are not restorable should not be considered for root-end surgery. The presence of crowns in the esthetic zone might lead the endodontic microsurgeon to consider a submarginal flap design or a papilla base incision. The presence of a fixed bridge can influence the location of the incision in the area of the pontic. In some cases, with enough tissue present, the incision can be placed 3 to 4 mm from the pontic so that the flap may be elevated, allowing enough tissue for suturing. In other cases, the incision can be extended to the lingual or palatal side of the pontic and reflected from beneath the pontic as part of the mucoperiosteal flap. The length and type of material of the post in teeth that have been restored with a post must be evaluated, because it can affect the ability to perform root-end preparation.

Presurgical preparations

Before initiating the procedure, the risks and benefits should be explained to the patient. A consent form for endodontic microsurgery should be discussed and signed by the patient. Prior to the procedure, the oral and written postoperative instructions should be given to the patient. Prescriptions for medications should be discussed and provided to the patient.

On the day of the surgery, the patient should be given 400 to 600 mg of ibuprofen to limit the inflammatory response from the surgical procedure. The patient should also rinse for one minute with chlorhexidine mouth rinse. The patient's preoperative vital signs should be recorded. A pulse oximeter should be placed on the patient's finger to monitor their oxygen saturation and heart rate. The patient is then draped with sterile covers or towels, and the endodontic microsurgical team proceeds with their surgical scrub, donning surgical and personal infection-control gear. The patient's lips should be scrubbed with povidone–iodine solution (Betadine) if they are not allergic to iodine.

Anesthesia and hemostasis

Hemostasis during surgical procedures is important to enhance visibility, instrumentation, and placement of root-end filling materials and to maximize the physical properties of the root-end filling materials. Achieving hemostasis starts preoperatively with a thorough examination of the patient's medical history. It is essential to ascertain if the patient is taking any medications that might increase bleeding or if the patient has any bleeding disorders.

Medical conditions that can affect bleeding and clotting include hereditary hemorrhagic telangiectasia, von Willebrand's disease, thrombocytopenic purpura, hemophilia A and B, and lack of some coagulation factors including factors I, II, VII, VIII, IX, X, and XI. Liver disease, including vitamin K deficiency, and alcoholism can increase bleeding. All of these conditions require a medical consultation with a physician [6, 7].

Medications that can increase bleeding including those that alter platelet function are aspirin and other nonsteroidal antiinflammatory drugs (NSAIDs). Other platelet-altering drugs, such as clopidogrel (Plavix), alcohol, and β-lactam antibiotics can effect bleeding. Drugs that alter coagulation include heparin, warfarin (Coumadin), and direct thrombin inhibitors [6, 7].

It is now thought that for relatively minor oral surgical procedures, including root-end surgery, it is better to have the patient who is on anticoagulant therapy, such as aspirin, clopidogrel, or warfarin, to continue these medications rather than risking thromboembolisms. The patient's international normalized ratio (INR) should be monitored on the day of surgery to confirm an acceptable level that is in the range of 1 to 4 [8–12]. Local measures to control bleeding may be used and are usually adequate. Local hemostatic agents are discussed later in this chapter.

Some patients do not consider herbal medications and other dietary supplements to be drugs, but several of these medications can cause bleeding problems. Supplements such as echinacea, gingko biloba, and fish oil can prolong bleeding time. Ginseng can cause hypertension and tachycardia. St. John's wort can prolong the effects of narcotics or anesthetic agents [13–18].

There are two purposes for delivering local anesthetics before surgery. One is the obvious need for anesthesia in the surgical site. The other is for hemostasis due to the epinephrine in local anesthetics.

In general, if the endodontic microsurgeon can use blocks rather than local supraperiosteal infiltrations, a wider area will be anesthetized with fewer injections. Regional blocks can then be supplemented, if needed, with infiltrations. For hemostasis, lidocaine with 1:50,000 epinephrine is infiltrated in the surgical area near root apices, carefully avoiding the skeletal muscle at the depth of the mucobuccal fold. One does not want to activate the β_2-adrenergic receptors in skeletal muscle, which will lead to vasodilation and increased bleeding instead of the desired vasoconstriction. Activation of the α_1-adrenergic receptors in the alveolar mucosa and gingival tissues will lead to the desired vasoconstriction to aid in hemostasis in the surgical field. Lidocaine with 1:50,000 epinephrine has been demonstrated to be an effective means of controlling bleeding during surgical procedures in the oral cavity [19]. The delivery of anesthetic solution should be at a relatively slow rate, perhaps taking one to two minutes to support patient comfort, adequate surgical anesthesia, and effective hemostasis.

A long-acting local anesthetic such as bupivacaine is useful in postoperative pain control by providing anesthesia to the surgical area for 4 to 9 hours [20].

Patient positioning and microscope alignment

Patient positioning is extremely important in endodontic microsurgery. Because the surgeon is required to retract tissues with one hand and use the dominant hand for instrumentation, direct vision through the microscope is necessary, as the microsurgeon does not have a free hand with which to hold a mirror. The exceptions to this rule are surgeries performed on palatal roots, where the palatal flap can be sutured to the other side of the mouth to reflect it, or surgeries on lingual surfaces of mandibular teeth for procedures to repair resorptive defects. On the lingual surface a mirror may be used as a retractor. Different patient positioning schemes have been devised by various authors. One that simplifies patient positioning, microscope alignment, and surgeon position has been developed by Dr. Stephen Niemczyk [21].

The endodontic microsurgeon needs direct visualization through the microscope. The correct positioning of the patient and the microscope allows this to occur. The patient must be positioned in the dental chair so that the long axis of the tooth undergoing the surgical procedure is parallel to the floor. For anterior teeth, the adjustment is to move the patient's head up or down relative to the long axis of the tooth, such that the long axis of the tooth is parallel to the floor. In the case of posterior teeth, the patient should be positioned on their side. This allows direct vision through the microscope and also places the long axis of the tooth parallel to the floor.

The microscope should be aligned so that it is parallel to the long axis of the tooth upon which the procedure is being performed. This is accomplished more easily if the microsurgeon is seated in the 12 o'clock position relative to the patient's head. To clarify, the surgeon is positioned directly behind the patient's head in the middle of the chair as the patient lies in the dental chair. With the long axis of the patient's tooth parallel to the floor, and the long axis of the microscope aligned with the long axis of the tooth, resections and root-end preparations will be at right angles to each other and also the natural influence of gravity will help produce resections that are at right angles to the long axis of the tooth. Once the resection is completed, the root-end preparation will easily be accomplished at a right angle to the root-end resection and in the long axis of the tooth (Figure 9.3).

To prevent neck strain, the patient should be positioned completely on their side, rather than simply turning their neck. This facilitates looking directly down on the tooth at a right angle to the long axis of the tooth. It is absolutely critical that the surgeon be in a comfortable and ergonomically correct position during the crucial phase of the procedure, even if the patient must hold a difficult position for just a short time, in order to obtain the best surgical outcome (Figures 9.4–9.7).

The microscope may be tilted slightly, or the patient may tilt their head up or down once the resection has been completed, so that the resected root end face may be inspected. This inspection will confirm the completion of the resection and identify the location of canals and isthmus, which may be enhanced with methylene blue dye.

With the correct positioning and alignment of the patient, the microscope, and the surgeon, the surgery can be more accurately carried out using the increased magnification and illumination provided by the surgical operating microscope.

Other patient-positioning schemes and microscope alignments have been proposed by Rubinstein [22], by Merino [1], and by Kim [2]. Many of the principles are the same; however, in some of these positions the surgeon is not at the 12 o'clock position of the chair but

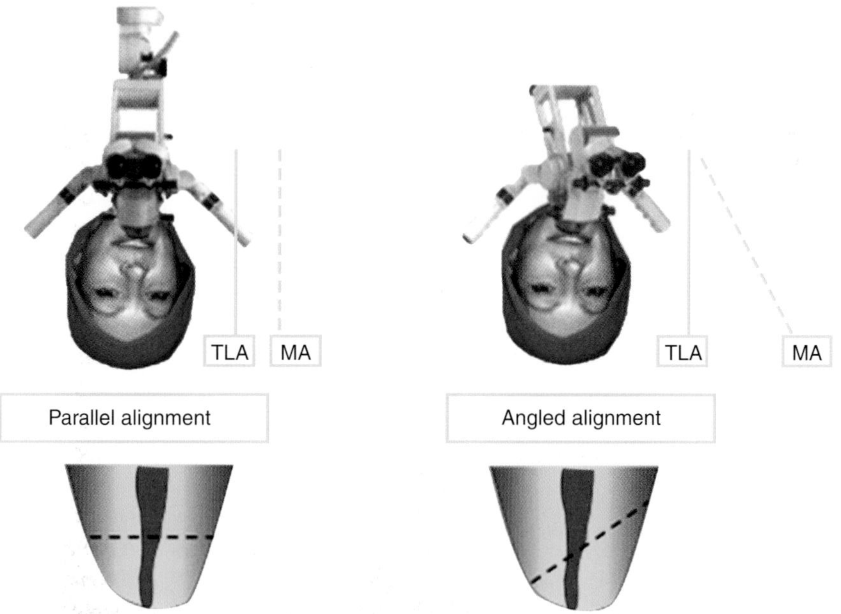

Figure 9.3 The microscope should be positioned so that the long axis of the microscope is parallel to the long axis of the tooth on which the surgical procedure is to be performed. This requires the surgeon to sit at the 12 o'clock position at the head of the dental chair, so that the long axis of the tooth points directly at the surgeon's midsection. This will ensure that the resection cuts are at 90 degrees to the long axis of the tooth. The diagram on the *left* demonstrates a parallel alignment where the microscope axis is parallel to the long axis of the tooth, which leads to a resection of 90 degrees to the long axis of the tooth. The diagram on the *right* demonstrates an angled alignment where the microscope axis does not match the long axis of the tooth, which can result in an angled resection. (from Niemczyk SP. Essentials of endodontic microsurgery. *Dent Clin North Am.* 2010;54:375–399.)

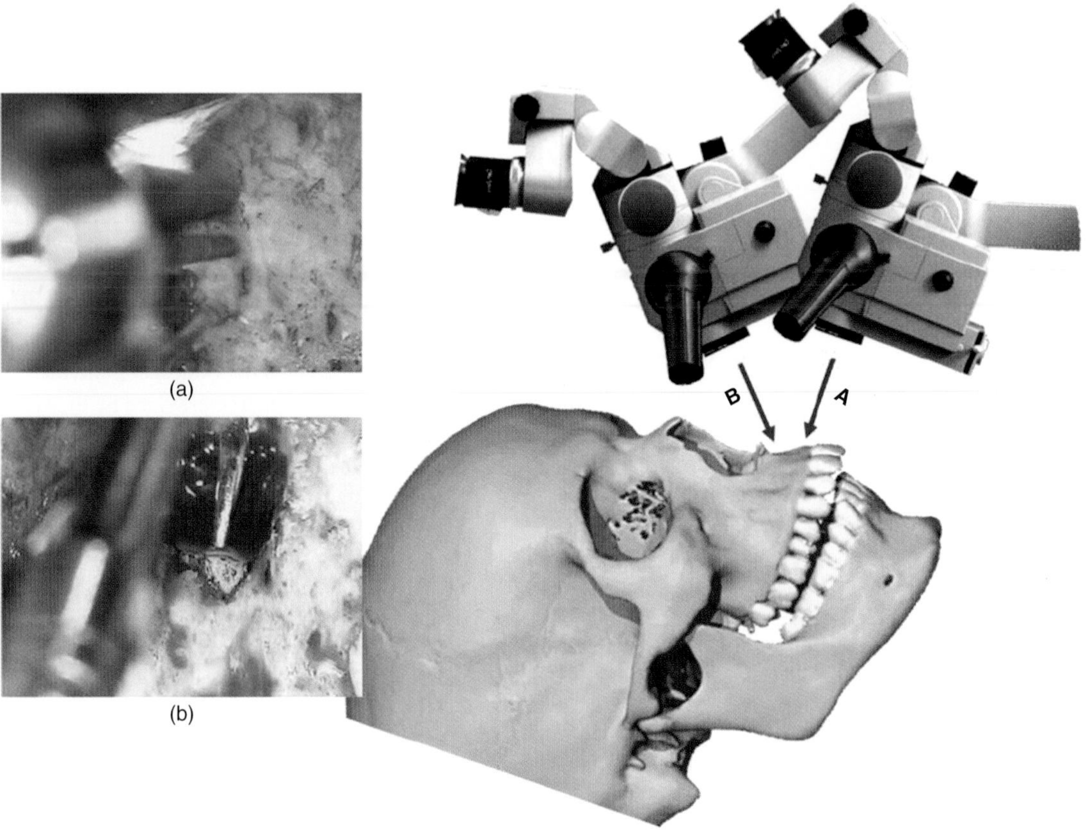

Figure 9.4 Alignment for maxillary anterior teeth. The long axis of the tooth should be parallel to the floor. For ostectomy, curettage, and resection, the microscope can be at a 90-degree angle to the long axis of the root. For root-end preparation, the microscope can be angled to view the resected root end. (from Niemczyk SP. Essentials of endodontic microsurgery. *Dent Clin North Am.* 2010;54:375–399.)

is to the side of the chair. The surgeon is not aligned in the long axis of the tooth in some of these positions. The surgeon in these other schemes needs to be able to move freely between the 10 o'clock and 2 o'clock positions. The patient's position, the microscope's alignment, and the surgeon's position can vary and may be a matter of personal preference of the surgeon and dependent upon certain patient factors.

The use of a surgeon's stool or chair that has arm rests will help support and steady the surgeon's arms and hands to ensure precise movements and lessen fatigue. Memory foam may be customized and fitted to the dental chair to make it more comfortable for the patient, especially when the patient must lie completely on their side during the surgical procedure.

Mucogingival flap designs and soft tissue management

The selection of the most favorable mucoperiosteal flap design affects access during surgery and healing outcomes. The choice of flap design should be based on many factors to ensure maximum access and visibility of the surgical site, favorable hard and soft tissue response, minimal gingival recession, and good healing with little or no morbidity.

The mucogingival flap designs used in endodontic microsurgery include the envelope flap, the intrasulcular flaps (triangular and rectangular), the submarginal flap (Ochsenbein–Luebke), the palatal flap, and the papilla base flap. The semilunar flap design is an outdated design and, for the most part, has no place in

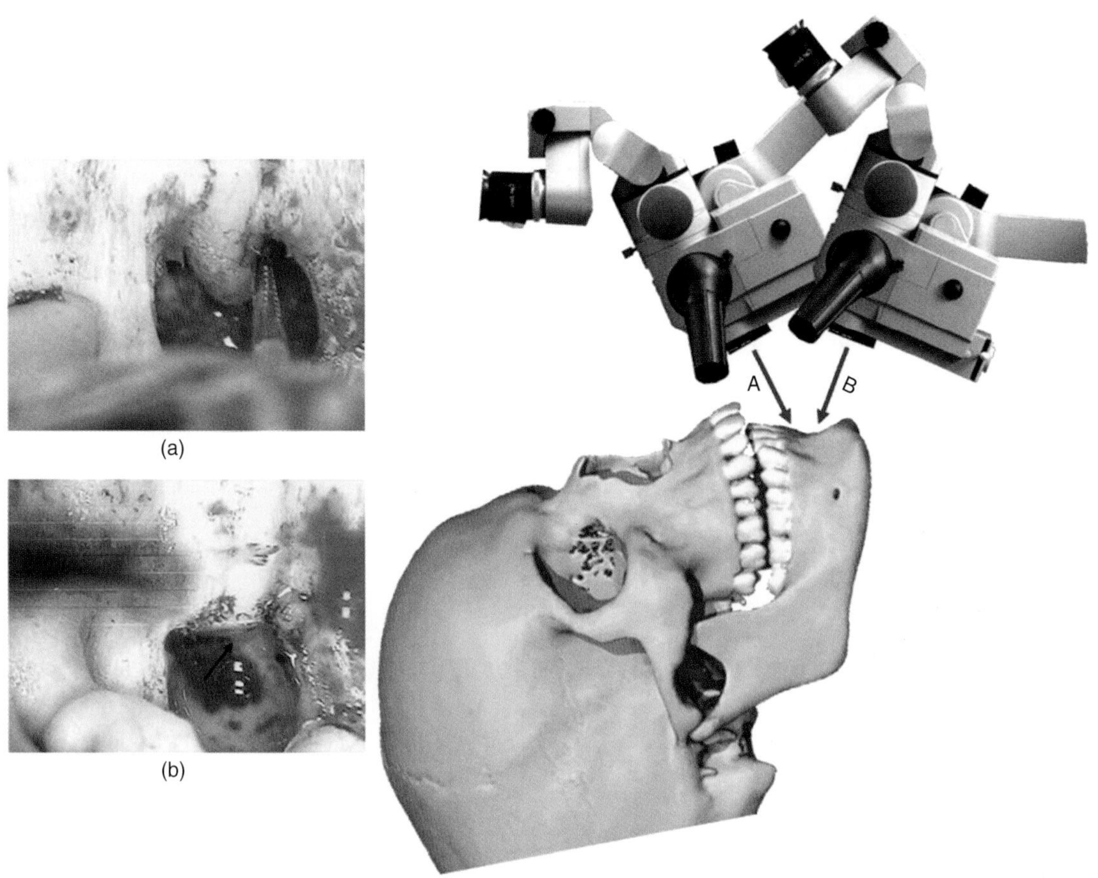

Figure 9.5 Alignment for mandibular anterior teeth. The long axis of the tooth should be parallel to the floor. For ostectomy, curettage, and resection, the microscope can be at a 90-degree angle to the long axis of the root. For root-end preparation, the microscope can be angled to view the resected root end. (from Niemczyk SP. Essentials of endodontic microsurgery. *Dent Clin North Am.* 2010;54:375–399.)

modern endodontic microsurgery. The semilunar flap has many disadvantages and minimal advantages or indications in endodontic microsurgery. Some of the disadvantages include limited access and disruption of blood supply to unflapped tissues, which can result in delayed healing and scarring.

Envelope flap

The envelope flap is an intrasulcular incision without a vertical releasing incision. It is not used for surgery in the apical area. It may be used for repair of cervical defects such as resorption repairs, submarginal caries removal, or other corrective surgery in the cervical areas of teeth or crestal bone areas.

Intrasulcular flaps

There are two types of intrasulcular flaps. The triangular flap design has a horizontal intrasulcular incision and one vertical releasing incision (Figure 9.8) [23]. The rectangular flap design has a horizontal intrasulcular incision with two vertical releasing incisions, one on each end of the horizontal incision (Figure 9.9) [23]. The difference in the triangular and rectangular flap design is that the rectangular flap has two vertical releasing incisions, whereas the triangular flap has only one.

The horizontal incision for the triangular and the rectangular intrasulcular mucogingival flaps is made in the gingival sulcus and extends to the crestal bone, cutting through the gingival attachment and the periodontal

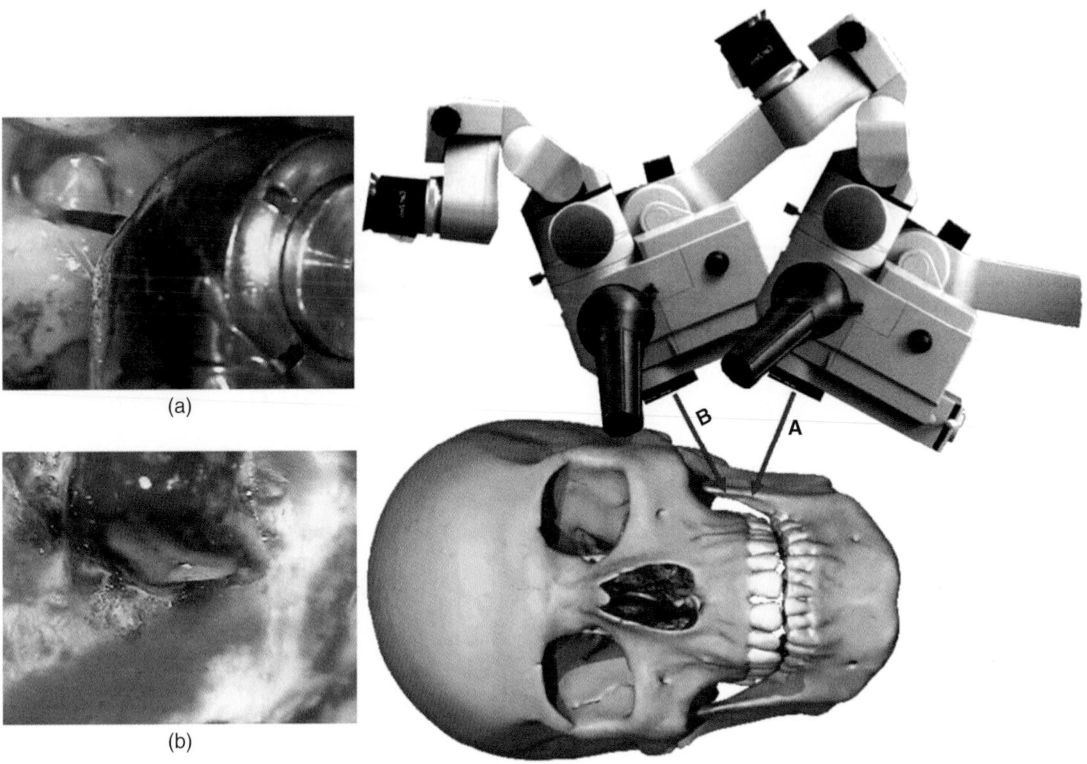

Figure 9.6 Alignment for maxillary posterior teeth. The long axis of the tooth should be parallel to the floor. For ostectomy, curettage, and resection, the microscope can be at a 90-degree angle to the long axis of the root. For root-end preparation, the microscope can be angled to view the resected root end. (from Niemczyk SP. Essentials of endodontic microsurgery. *Dent Clin North Am.* 2010;54:375–399.)

ligament fibers. It includes the dental papilla and frees the entire dental papilla [24].

The vertical incision should be parallel to the supraperiosteal blood vessels, which run in a vertical direction from superior to inferior parallel to the long axis of the tooth roots [3]. Creating an incision with this in mind greatly reduces the number of vessels that will be severed, thus providing better blood supply to the reflected flap. By avoiding the trapezoidal flap design, fewer vessels are severed by the vertical incision, and a better blood supply is maintained to the unflapped tissues (Figure 9.10). The vertical incisions should be over sound bone, avoiding periapical lesions and frenum or muscle attachments [24]. Ideally, the vertical incision should be in the concavities between the bony eminences covering the roots. This follows a plastic surgery principle that states incisions should be placed in shadows or creases to help hide the incision line when the incision is healed.

The vertical incision should start at the line angle of the tooth at the marginal gingiva and should meet the marginal gingiva at a 90-degree angle. This gives the vertical incision a shape similar to a hockey stick, with the blade portion of the hockey stick extending at right angles from the marginal gingiva to the longer vertical portion of the incision, which could be viewed as the handle of the hockey stick. It is critical that this portion of the vertical incision be at right angles to the marginal gingiva to prevent a pointed tip to the flap, which will be difficult to reapproximate and suture and can result in healing with a double papilla. Also, when the incision meets the marginal gingiva in the apical third of the papilla, it reduces the distance for blood profusion to the rest of the papilla. This results in better healing [25, 26]. The vertical portion of the incision can be slightly beveled toward the flap and not extend into the mucobuccal fold. This allows better re-approximation, suturing, and healing (Figure 9.11).

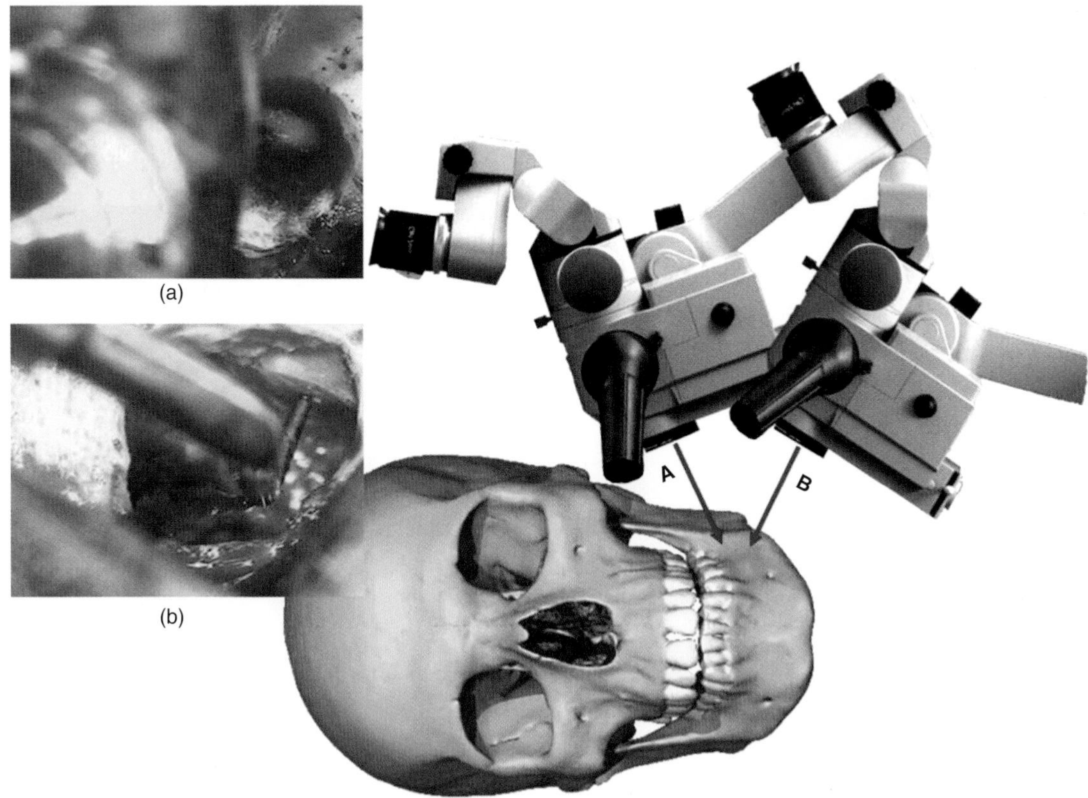

Figure 9.7 Alignment for mandibular posterior teeth. The long axis of the tooth should be parallel to the floor. For ostectomy, curettage, and resection, the microscope can be at a 90-degree angle to the long axis of the root. For root-end preparation, the microscope can be angled to view the resected root end. (from Niemczyk SP. Essentials of endodontic microsurgery. *Dent Clin North Am.* 2010;54:375–399)

The advantages of the intrasulcular incisions include minimal loss of blood supply to flapped tissues and unflapped tissues. Intrasulcular flaps provide a good view of crestal bone, periodontal defects, and vertical root fractures, if present. The triangular flap is easy to extend, if needed. It is relatively easier to reapproximate the triangular and rectangular flaps, and they are easier to suture.

The disadvantages of the intrasulcular flaps are the amount of gingival recession and possible alteration of the gingival papilla.

Submarginal flap

The submarginal flap, or the Ochsenbein–Luebke flap, is a flap design used primarily in the anterior maxilla, particularly where there are full crowns in the area [27]. It is reported to cause less recession around crowns, thus preventing the unesthetic exposure of crown margins.

The flap consists of two vertical releasing incisions and a horizontal incision, which is in the attached keratinized gingiva. There must be a minimum of 3 mm of attached gingiva to perform this procedure. The horizontal incision should be scalloped to match the contour of the gingival margin of the anterior teeth, and it should be beveled toward the flap, so the incision line is more coronal on the exterior surface of the keratinized gingiva and more apical at the alveolar bone surface (Figures 9.12–9.15).

It is extremely important to perform periodontal probing in the area where the flap will be prepared to ensure that there is at least 3 mm of attached keratinized gingiva apical to the probing depths. One method of doing this is with a pocket marking instrument that has one beak inserted into the sulcus and the other beak at a right angle to the tip. When they are closed together, a bleeding point will mark the depth of the sulcus [21]. If

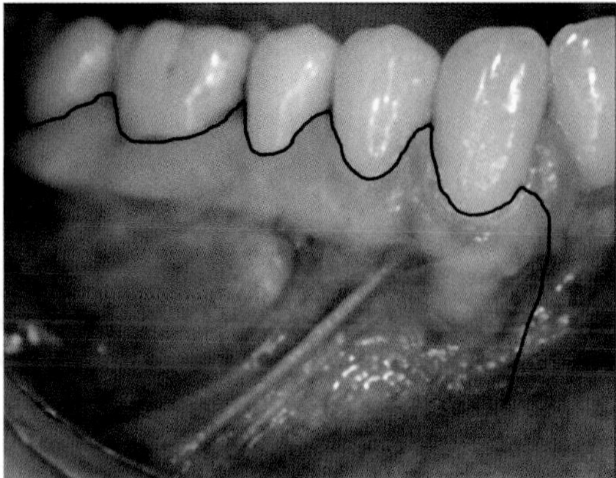

Figure 9.8 Triangular flap design with a sulcular horizontal incision and a vertical releasing incision in the concavity between the canine and the lateral incisor. (Courtesy of Dr. Stephen Niemczyk, adapted from Grandi C, Pacifici L. The ratio in choosing access flap for surgical endodontics: a review. Oral & Implantol. 2009;2(1):37–52. Epub 2009 Dec 10.) [23]

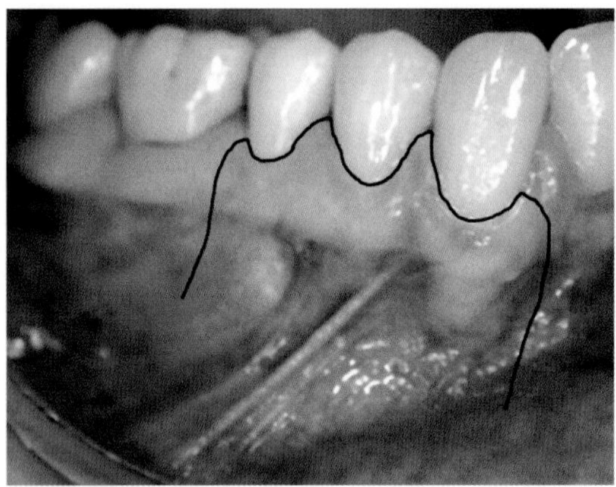

Figure 9.9 Rectangular flap design with two vertical releasing incisions. Both vertical releasing incisions should be in the concavities between the bony eminences over teeth and meet the marginal gingiva at right angles at the junction of the middle and apical third of the interdental papilla. The horizontal incision is in the sulcus. (Courtesy of Dr. Stephen Niemczyk, adapted from Grandi C, Pacifici L. The ratio in choosing access flap for surgical endodontics: a review. Oral & Implantol. 2009;2(1):37–52. Epub 2009 Dec 10.) [23]

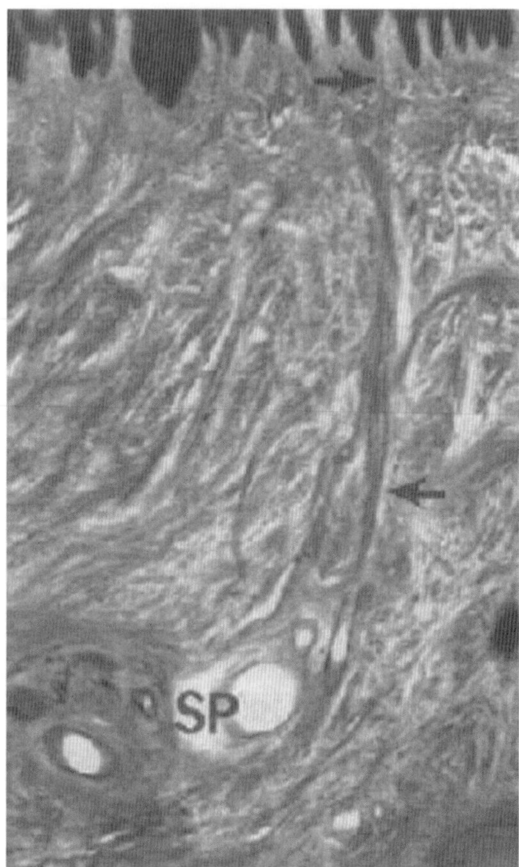

Figure 9.10 Supraperiosteal blood vessels deep in the reticular layer of the lamina propria of attached gingiva. The arrow indicates a vessel passing into the papillary layer to form a capillary plexus next to epithelium. (From Gutmann JL, Harrison JW. *Surgical endodontics*. Boston: Blackwell Scientific Publications; 1991.)

there are periodontal pockets deeper than the attached gingiva, the submarginal flap should not be used, and an intrasulcular flap should be considered.

Once the patient has been anesthetized, a sharp endodontic explorer is used to sound bone through the gingiva to determine the height of the crestal bone. The height of the crestal bone is marked from bleeding points created with the explorer. An indelible pencil or gentian violet stick can be used to delineate this marking as well [21].

The vertical incision should also be beveled toward the flap, just as with the vertical incisions in intrasulcular flaps. The corners where the vertical incision reaches the horizontal incision should be rounded slightly to prevent a sharp tip, which is difficult to reattach and suture (Figure 9.16).

The submarginal flap requires attention when approximating the wound edges. All wounds tend to retract once the tissue is separated due to elastic fibers in connective tissue. Because the submarginal incision

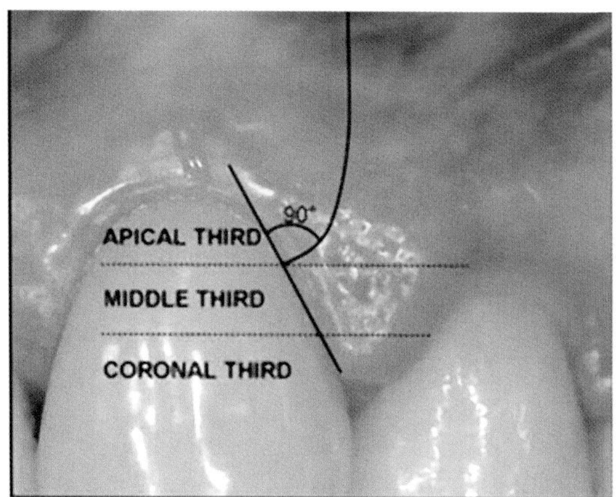

Figure 9.11 The vertical releasing incision starts by visually dividing the interdental papilla into coronal, middle, and apical thirds. At the junction of the middle and apical thirds the vertical releasing incision should begin at the line angle of the tooth and at a 90-degree angle to the marginal gingiva. The vertical releasing incision forms a hockey stick shape, with the horizontal portion of the releasing incision as the blade and the vertical portion of the releasing incision forming the handle of the hockey stick. Placing the incision at the junction of the middle and apical third of the papilla allows short profusion of blood supply to the flap. This ensures a better blood supply to the rest of the papilla. (Courtesy of Dr. Stephen Niemczyk, adapted from Grandi C, Pacifici L. The ratio in choosing access flap for surgical endodontics: a review. Oral & Implantol. 2009;2(1):37–52. Epub 2009 Dec 10.) [23]

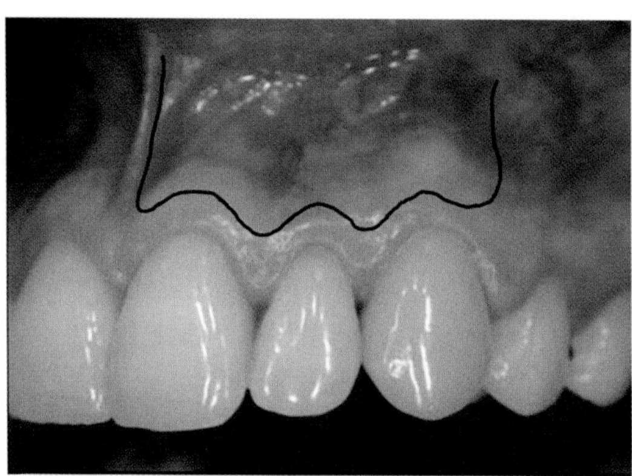

Figure 9.12 The submarginal incision will have a scalloped horizontal portion that will match the marginal gingival contour. It must be placed in the attached keratinized gingiva. There should be at least 3 mm of attached keratinized gingiva present for this incision. (Courtesy of Dr. Stephen Niemczyk, adapted from Grandi C, Pacifici L. The ratio in choosing access flap for surgical endodontics: a review. Oral & Implantol. 2009;2(1):37–52. Epub 2009 Dec 10.) [23]

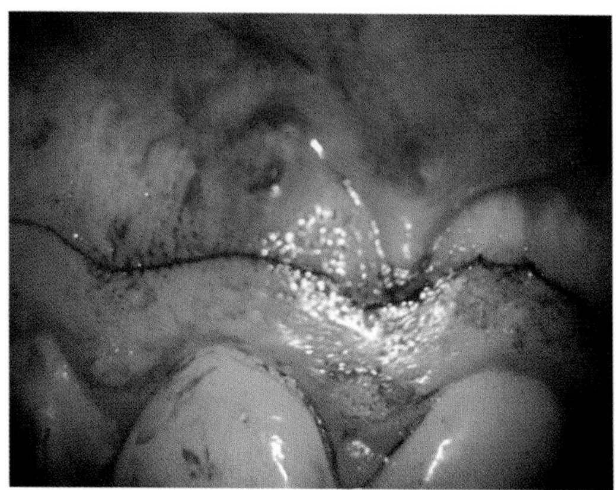

Figure 9.13 Submarginal flap design demonstrating the scalloped incision in the attached keratinized gingiva corresponding to the contour of the marginal gingiva, and the crestal bone. (Image courtesy of Dr. Brandon Yamamura.)

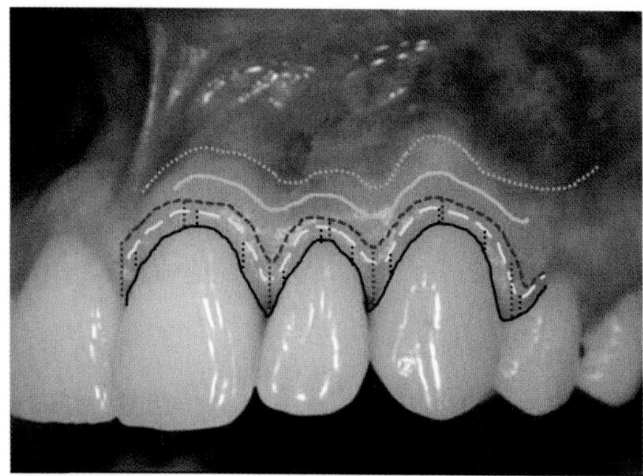

Figure 9.14 Submarginal incision. The dark blue line represents the marginal gingiva. The green line represents the mucogingival junction. The black vertical lines represent the periodontal probing depths. The yellow line represents the depth of the gingival sulcus as determined by periodontal probing. The red line represents the level of the crestal bone as determined by sounding for the crestal bone through the gingiva, which is depicted by the red vertical lines. The turquoise line represents the location of the incision line in the horizontal component of the flap. (Courtesy of Dr. Stephen Niemczyk, adapted from Grandi C, Pacifici L. The ratio in choosing access flap for surgical endodontics: a review. Oral & Implantol. 2009;2(1):37–52. Epub 2009 Dec 10.) [23]

has two edges instead of one, both edges of the incision pull away from each other. To insure closure of the submarginal incision, firm pressure should be applied to approximate the wound edges for 4 to 5 minutes before suturing. As the microsurgeon sutures the submarginal flap, gaps should be identified along the incision line.

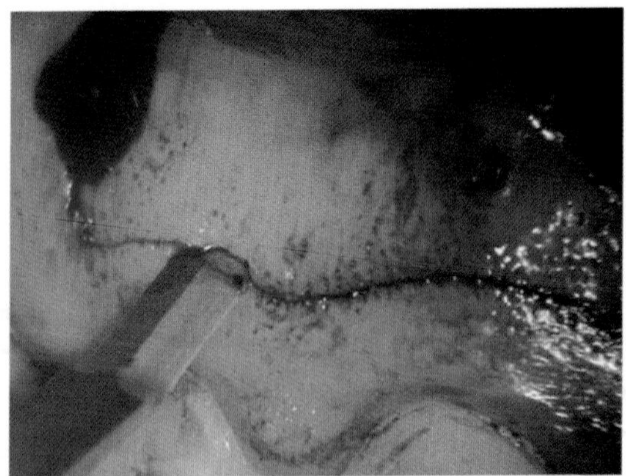

Figure 9.15 Submarginal incision. Note the scalloped incision in the keratinized attached gingiva that corresponds to the contour of the marginal gingiva. Also apparent is the rounded tip where the vertical releasing incision meets the horizontal scalloped incision. The beveling of the horizontal portion of the submarginal flap with a microblade provides the bevel toward the flap, which enhances repositioning and adaption of the flap into its original position and will promote better healing by primary intention. (Image courtesy of Dr. Brandon Yamamura.)

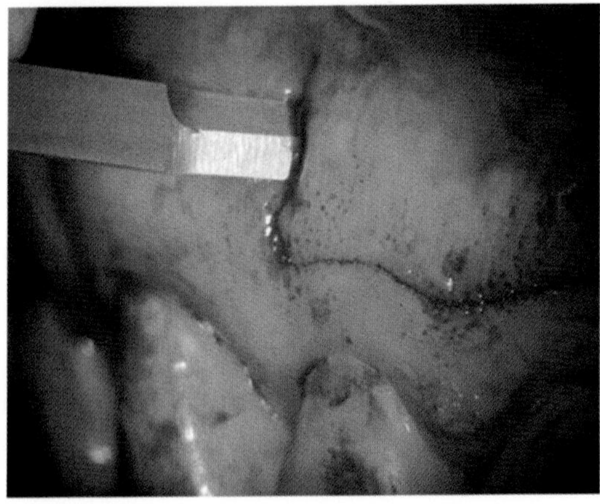

Figure 9.16 Vertical releasing incision of a submarginal incision demonstrating beveling of the incision into the flap, and the rounding off of the flap where the vertical incision meets the horizontal incision to avoid a pointed edge at the corner of the flap. (Image courtesy of Dr. Brandon Yamamura.)

Placing additional sutures appropriately along the incision ensures primary closure with minimal scarring.

Papilla base flap

The papilla base flap was popularized by Velvart [28]. It reportedly results in better surgical outcomes in terms of soft tissue healing, decreased recession, and healthier dental papillae [29, 30].

Although soft tissue outcomes are improved with the papilla base flap design, the procedure is more technique sensitive. It requires two incisions in a split-thickness design, and suturing is more difficult and precise because very small sutures (7–0) are required for closure. However, once the endodontic microsurgeon gains experience in this procedure, it offers excellent results.

The vertical incisions for the papilla base flap is the same as the vertical incisions for the intrasulcular flap. The vertical incision starts at the junction of the middle and apical third of the interdental papilla and meets the marginal gingiva at right angles. It then extends vertically in the concavity between the root eminences. This vertical incision resembles a hockey stick. The vertical portion of the incision should be beveled toward the flap.

The horizontal component of the papilla base flap extends from the vertical incision into the gingival sulcus of each tooth included in the flap and at the apical and middle third junction of the interdental papilla. An incision that arches apically is made that meets the adjacent tooth at right angles to the marginal gingiva at the junction of the apical and middle third of the interdental papilla. The first incision into the papilla should be 1.5 mm in depth and at right angles to the surface of the gingiva. A second incision is made by placing the micro blade to the depth of the first incision and then beveling the second incision apically to reach the crestal bone margin. This second incision produces

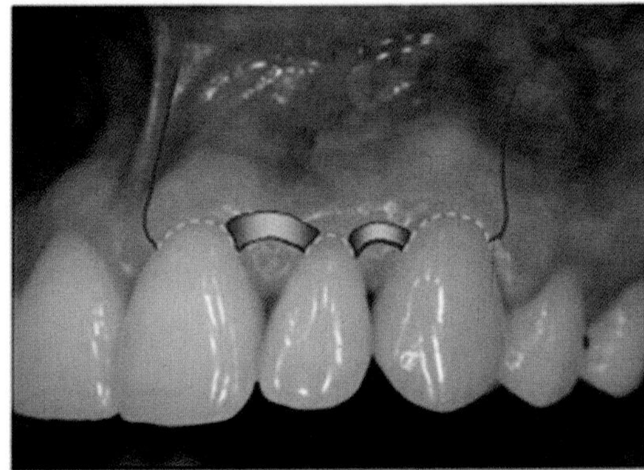

Figure 9.17 Papilla base incision outline with split-thickness incisions of the papillae. (Courtesy of Dr. Stephen Niemczyk, adapted from Grandi C, Pacifici L. The ratio in choosing access flap for surgical endodontics: a review. Oral & Implantol. 2009;2(1):37–52. Epub 2009 Dec 10.) [23]

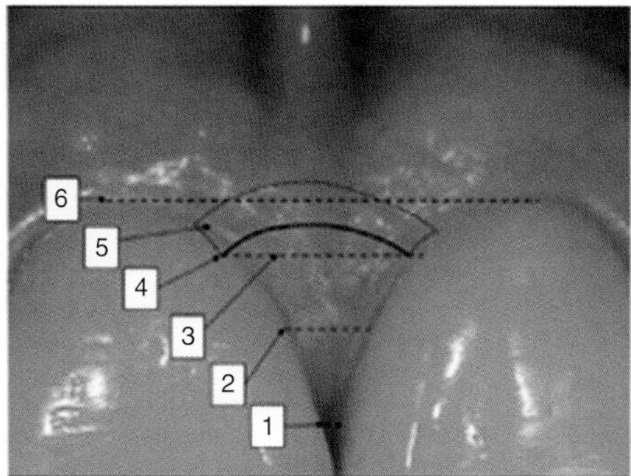

Figure 9.18 Papilla base incision. The interdental papilla is divided into thirds (numbers 1–2, 2–3, 3–6). The initial incision (#4) is 1.5 mm in depth, and it meets the marginal gingiva at the junction of the middle and apical thirds of the papilla. This incision meets the tooth at a right angle to the marginal gingiva, arches apically, and is at a right angle to the surface of the papilla. The second incision (#5) is from the base of the first incision, and it extends to alveolar bone. (Courtesy of Dr. Stephen Niemczyk, adapted from Grandi C, Pacifici L. The ratio in choosing access flap for surgical endodontics: a review. Oral & Implantol. 2009;2(1):37–52. Epub 2009 Dec 10.) [23]

a small split-thickness flap that is beveled to the crest of the alveolar bone. Here onward, the flap is reflected as a full-thickness flap [28–30] (Figures 9.17–9.21).

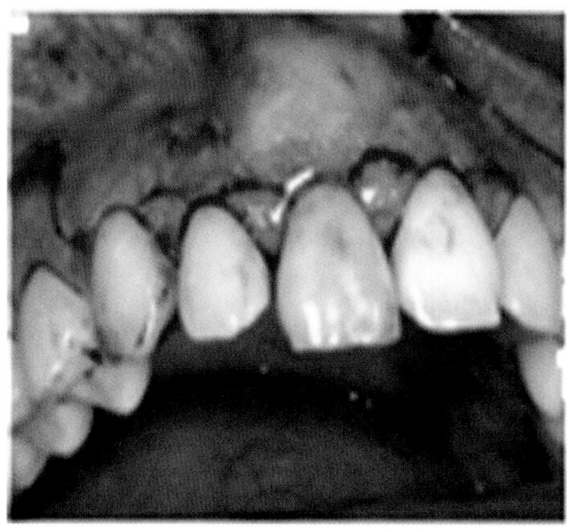

Figure 9.20 Papilla base incision. (Image courtesy of Dr. Susan Roberts.)

Palatal flap

The palatal flap may be used for access to the palatal root of maxillary molars when root-end resection and root-fill procedures are indicated. Palatal flap designs can be either horizontal or triangular. The horizontal portion of the flap consists of an intrasulcular incision. When a vertical incision is required for greater access, as in root-end surgery, the same principles of other vertical

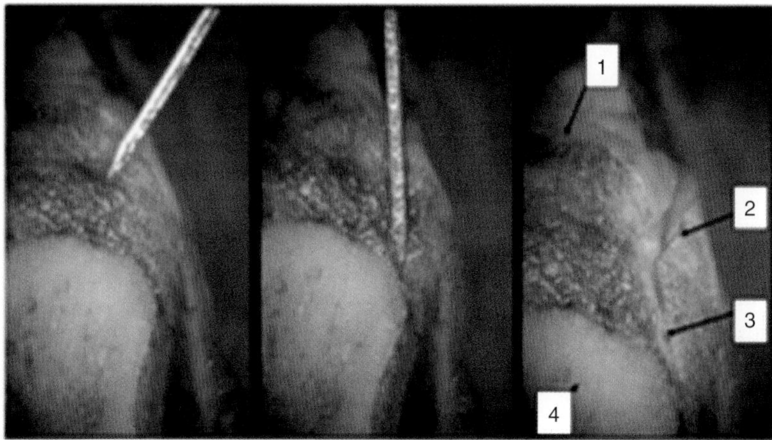

Figure 9.19 Papilla base incision. The image on the left demonstrates the first incision, which is perpendicular to the interdental papilla surface and 1.5 mm in depth. The second incision is depicted in the middle image, and it extends from the base of the first incision to the crest of alveolar bone, creating a split-thickness flap in this area. The image on the right demonstrates the complete incision, with #1 representing the cul of the interdental tissue, #2 the first incision, #3 the second incision to alveolar bone, and #4 the alveolar bone. (Courtesy of Dr. Stephen Niemczyk, adapted from Grandi C, Pacifici L. The ratio in choosing access flap for surgical endodontics: a review. Oral & Implantol. 2009;2(1):37–52. Epub 2009 Dec 10.) [23]

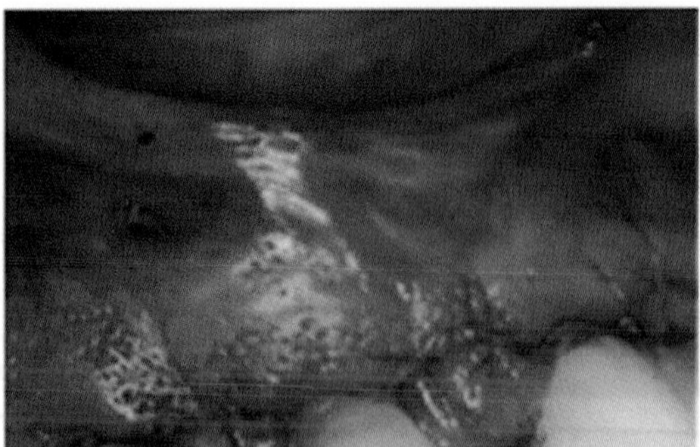

Figure 9.21 Papilla base incision at 3 days. Note the 7–0 suture across the incision line. Good healing is observed for this early postoperative period. (Image courtesy of Dr. Susan Roberts.)

incisions apply. It should meet the tooth at right angles to the marginal gingiva. In the case of palatal flaps, the vertical releasing incision should be at the mesial side of the maxillary first premolar. This will ensure that the incision is in the area of the terminal branches of both the greater palatine vessels and the nasopalatine vessels. By placing the incision at the terminal ends of these vessels, hemorrhage will be reduced in the area, because these vessels are smaller. The vertical releasing incision for a palatal flap should extend to the midline of the palate. If possible, the incision should be placed in the valleys between the palatal rugae. This will be more comfortable for the patient and lead to less scarring. If needed for better access, a mini vertical incision can be placed distal to the second molar. This incision should only be a few millimeters so as to avoid the greater palatine vessels and nerve (Figures 9.22 and 9.23).

Palatal surgery is the one area where direct vision of the surgical field through the microscope is not possible. This challenge can be overcome by suturing the reflected palatal flap to the maxillary teeth on the opposite of the mouth. This reflects the flap out of the field, allowing the surgeon to use a mirror and complete the surgery using indirect vision through the microscope.

If possible, the suture knots for the horizontal portion of the palatal flap should be on the facial gingiva to prevent the patient from feeling them with the tongue. Sutures along the vertical releasing incision are on the palate.

A palatal stent should be fabricated prior to the surgery appointment, and inserted after flap closure to hold the palatal mucosa against the palatal bone to ensure close reapproximation and reduce the chance of hematoma formation (Figure 9.24).

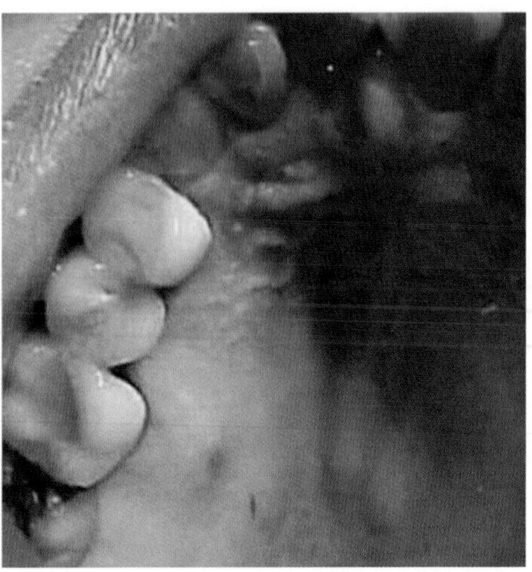

Figure 9.22 Sinus tract on the palate from the palatal root of the maxillary first molar that had been re-treated and did not heal. (Image courtesy of Dr. James Johnson.)

Incisions

Incisions should be made with a firm continuous stroke, rather than small short strokes. The incision line should not be over bony defects, periapical lesions, or frenum attachments, and it should terminate at the line angles of teeth, meeting the marginal gingiva at 90 degrees. They should be in the concavities between bony eminences that cover the roots of teeth. Vertical incisions should not extend into the mucobuccal fold.

Most incisions in endodontic microsurgery should be made with a mini blade #69 or #64. The papilla base incisions should be made with the half radius mini or micro blade #64 (Salvin Dental Specialties, Charlotte, NC) (Figures 9.25–9.27). Incisions for incision and drainage of abscess may be made with a #15 or #15C blade. Some lingual flaps require a #12 blade.

Flap reflection and elevation

Flap reflection and elevation should begin in the vertical releasing incision at the level of the attached keratinized

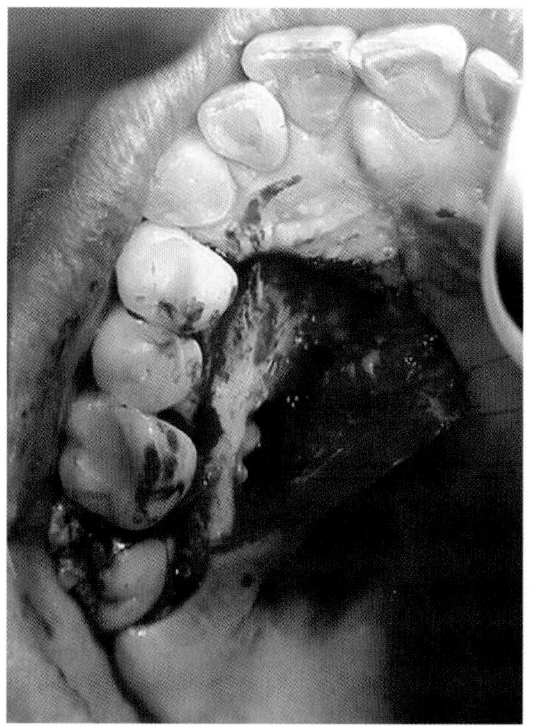

Figure 9.23 Palatal flap reflected, exposing the palatal root apex of the maxillary first molar. The vertical incision meets the marginal gingiva of the maxillary first premolar at right angles and extends to the midline of the palate, staying in the valleys between the rugae. The flap is tied to the teeth on the opposite side of the arch by a wide bracket made by broad loop of the suture rather than a small point. This provides better control of the reflected flap and prevents the suture from pulling out. Suturing the flap to the maxillary teeth on the other side of the arch reflects the flap and allows the surgeon to use indirect vision through the microscope using a mirror. (Image courtesy of Dr. James Johnson.)

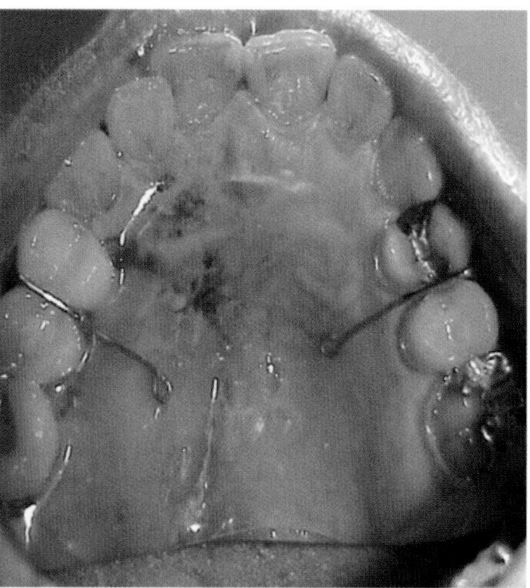

Figure 9.24 Palatal stent in place to adapt the flap to the palatal bone and to prevent hematoma formation between the flap and the palatal bone. (Image courtesy of Dr. James Johnson.)

gingiva and not in the intrasulcular incision. This prevents damage to the root-attached tissues, including the epithelium and connective tissue, and avoids damage to the delicate marginal gingiva [3].

By undermining the mucoperiosteal tissues starting in the vertical releasing incision at the attached keratinized gingival level, the mucoperiosteal tissues are separated from the cortical plate of bone. Left and right Ruddle curettes, as well as sharp periosteal elevators and the Molt #3 instrument, are particularly useful for undermining elevation. As the tissues become separated

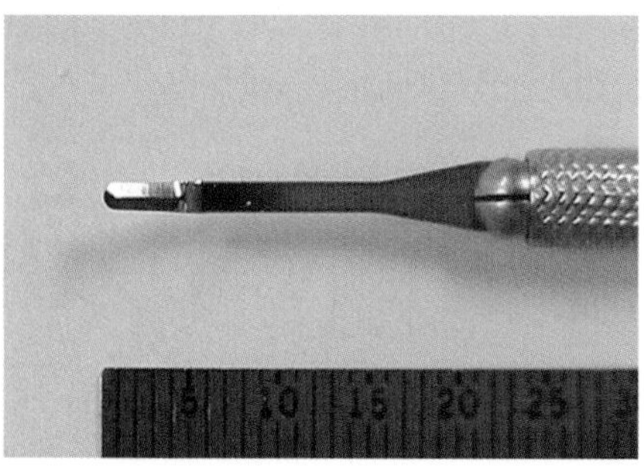

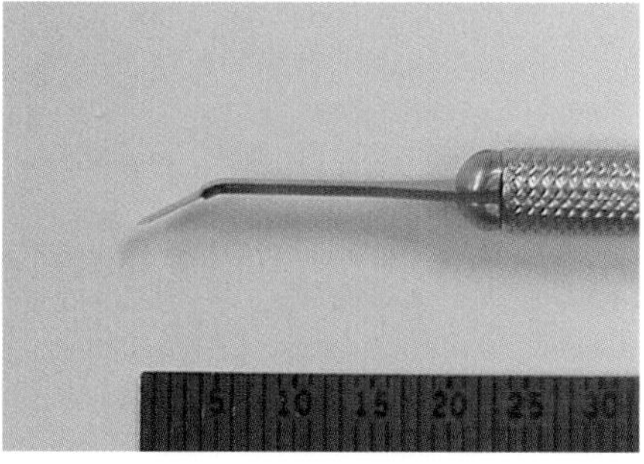

Figure 9.25 Angled microsurgical blades. (Image courtesy of Dr. Scott McClanahan.)

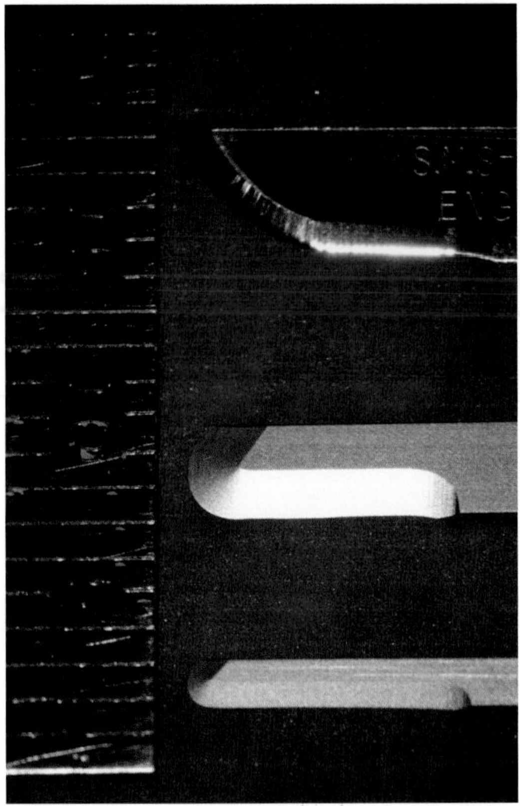

Figure 9.26 From top to bottom, #15 blade, #64 minisurgical blade (half radius), and #64 microsurgical blade (half radius). (Image courtesy of Dr. Stephen Niemczyk.)

from bone, the elevator is directed coronally and the flap is lifted away from crestal bone, in the case of an intrasulcular incision. This undermining elevation allows passive elevation of the supracrestal attached gingiva, marginal gingival, and interdental gingiva [3]. When the gingival tissues are released, elevation continues in an apical direction until there is adequate reflection of the mucoperiosteum to have sufficient access to the periapical areas (Figure 9.28).

Although a clean cortical bone surface is useful for hemostasis and visualization of the surgical area without bleeding, the bleeding tissue tags can help with the reattachment of the flap after the procedure, so they do not all have to be scraped off of the cortical bone.

There are other anatomical considerations when reflecting mucoperiosteal flaps. In the area of the anterior nasal spine, the elevator should be directed in a superior vertical direction, not in a horizontal direction, to prevent possible fracture of this delicate structure.

In the area of the mental foramen, careful reflection is required. As the reflection in the posterior mandible proceeds in an apical direction, the separation of the periosteum from bone is evident. As the mental foramen is reached, the bone drops off into a depression where the mental nerve and accompanying vascular supply becomes visible. Once identified, it can be protected by placing a groove in the bone where a retractor may be placed to protect the neurovascular bundle exiting the mental foramen [3].

If a sinus tract is present and extends from the periapical lesion to the mucogingival surface, the surgeon must use care when reflecting the mucoperiosteal flap. The periosteum around the sinus tract should be elevated so that the sinus tract is the only attachment binding the flap down. Once this is accomplished, tension can be placed so the sinus tract is extended with the flap. The sinus tract is then incised with the micro blade, staying close to the cortical bone. This releases the entire mucoperiosteal flap and provides access to the surgical site. Care must be taken during this procedure to avoid creating a large tear through the flap.

Once the flap is reflected, a groove can be cut with a #6 or #8 round bur in an area apical to where you will perform the ostectomy, avoiding critical structures. This groove should be in a horizontal direction or in a direction to provide the best flap retraction. The retractor is placed in this groove and left there throughout the procedure. This prevents the retractor from impinging on soft tissue, which can cause severe tissue damage and delayed healing (Figure 9.29).

When cortical bone is exposed, it is critical to frequently irrigate with normal saline to ensure the cortical bone and reflected tissue stay moist. The heat from the microscope light can quickly desiccate bone and mucoperiosteal tissues if they are not repeatedly bathed in normal saline solution. Another method for keeping tissues moist is to invert the reflected flap back underneath itself, keeping the surfaces moist.

Ostectomy

An ostectomy is a procedure involving the removal of bone. Dental applications of ostectomy are to specifically remove bone surrounding a tooth in an

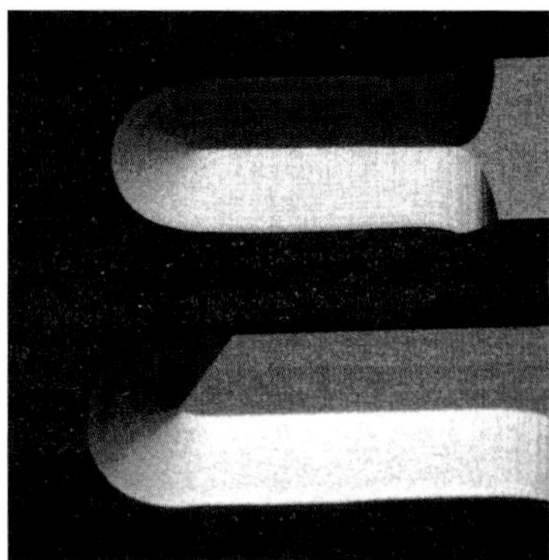

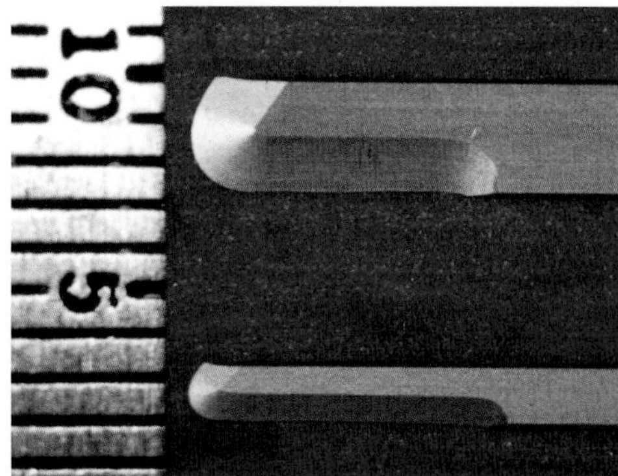

Figure 9.27 Mini and microsurgical blades. They come in half-radius or full-radius designs. The full-radius blade cuts in either direction. The half-radius blade cuts only in one direction. (Images courtesy of Dr. Stephen Niemczyk)

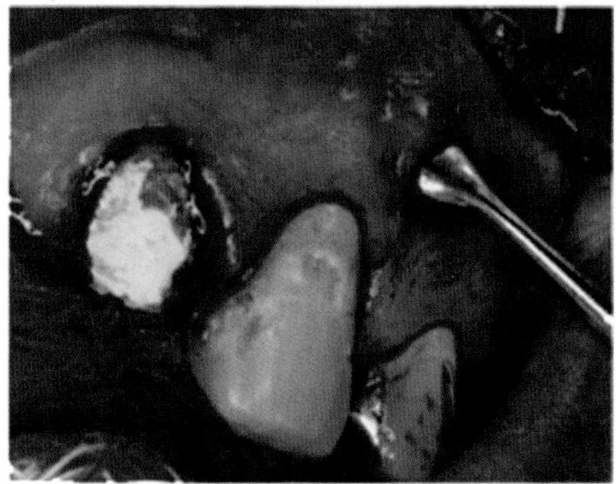

Figure 9.28 Flap elevation should begin in the vertical releasing incision in the attached keratinized gingiva, avoiding placing the elevator on the marginal gingiva. Elevation of the flap should tunnel under the tissue to free the attached gingiva and papilla. Once these tissues are lifted off of the alveolar bone, reflection proceeds in an apical direction. (Image courtesy of Dr. Dwight Moss.)

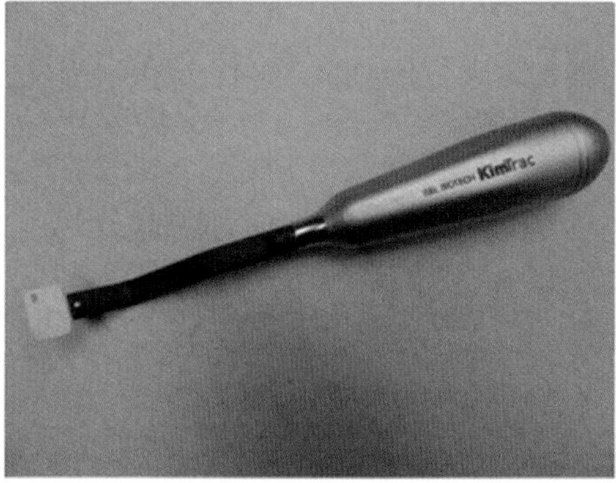

Figure 9.29 KimTrac retractor. (B&L Biotech, Fairfax, VA, USA>). Standard retractors are often too large for endodontic microsurgery, as the operating field is very small. Retractors designed for endodontic microsurgery are available; however, the surgeon might need to customize a retractor.

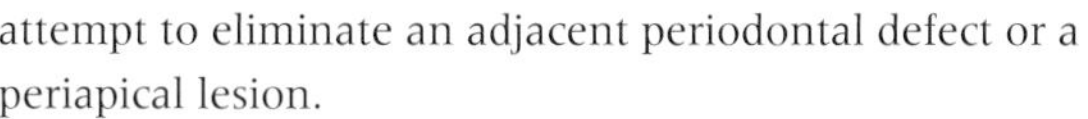

attempt to eliminate an adjacent periodontal defect or a periapical lesion.

Sterile surgical high-speed handpieces with rear exhaust should be used with adequate coolant. This prevents air from entering the surgical site. Sterile saline may be used to keep the bur cooled via separate irrigation. A second option is to have sterile water running through the water lines from a reservoir to the handpiece. It is critical to keep the bone cool while removing bone. Bone that has been anesthetized has a reduced blood supply, which increases its sensitivity to excessive heat that is generated without proper cooling of the bur. Bone should be removed with light pressure utilizing a brush stroke. Larger round burs should

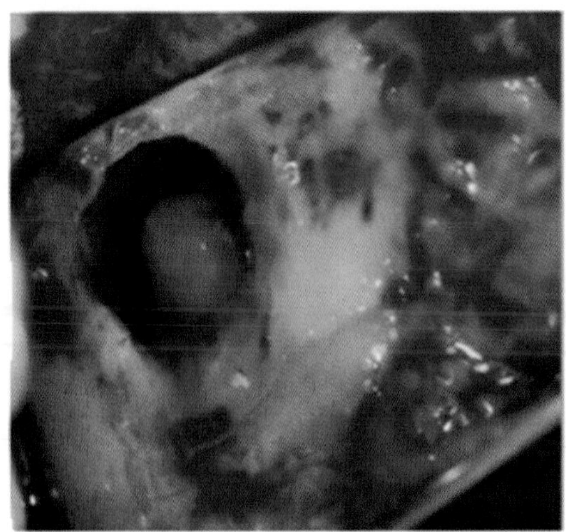

Figure 9.30 After ostectomy and apical curettage, the apical 3 to 4 mm of the root should be "suspended in space" to facilitate root-end resection. (Image courtesy of Dr. Kathleen McNally.)

initially be used [2]. For more precise cuts around the root ends, smaller round burs should be used [3]. The goal for exposure of the apical 3 or 4 mm of the root is to isolate the root end so as to have it appear suspended in space. This allows adequate access for apical curettage and root-end resection (Figure 9.30).

If the cortical bone is intact and there is no apical lesion, the removal of bone must be more exact. By recording the length of the root from radiographs, the site of the ostectomy can be calculated or measured. A preoperative CBCT is useful in demonstrating where and how much bone should be removed.

The osteotomy begins approximately 3 mm coronal to the estimated length of the apex of the root. The bur is used to shave away the cortical bone using slight pressure, and with the aid of the microscope the subtle difference in color between bone and the tooth root can be appreciated. Once the root is identified, the surgeon proceeds to remove bone from around the apical 3 or 4 mm of the root, including bone on the mesial and distal surfaces of the root, so the root appears suspended in space. Bone on the lingual or palatal side of the root does not need to be removed. The cuts should be deep enough to allow a straight fissure bur or an all-purpose bur to pass through to the lingual or palatal surface of the root, allowing root-end resection. If locating the root end becomes difficult, a piece of disinfected gutta-percha may be placed on the bone and a radiograph may be exposed to orient the surgeon to which direction to proceed in order to locate the root [3].

When a periapical lesion is present, and the cortical bone is intact over the lesion, the remaining bone may be quite thin. The bone may be sounded or penetrated by a sharp instrument to locate the lesion. This thin cortical bone may be scraped away with a curette or a periosteal elevator, exposing the lesion and root. From this point, the bone may be dissected from around the root end with the surgical high-speed handpiece to expose the apical 3 or 4 mm of the root and curette the lesion out of the bony crypt. The goal is to have the apical 3 or 4 mm of the root suspended in space to facilitate the root-end resection.

If the periapical lesion has resorbed the cortical bone, the lesion is easily located. However, some additional bone may need to be removed to allow adequate access to the lesion for curettage and to expose enough of the root in the apical area to perform root-end resection. In general, if the lesion extends more than 3 mm beyond the margin of cortical bone, it becomes difficult to curette the lesion out of the bony crypt, so additional bone may need to be removed to facilitate complete removal of the apical pathosis.

Piezoelectric devices are available for ostectomy procedures. These devices allow removal of cortical bone to create a window into bone and then replacing the piece of cortical bone back into its original place when the procedure is completed. More studies are needed; however, it appears to be a promising technique to go along with the other uses of ultrasonics in endodontic microsurgery [31].

Curettage

Curettage of the periapical lesion is an important step during surgery. Removal of a longstanding lesion enhances healing and may be the only way to resolve apical pathosis, particularly if the lesion is a true cyst. Any tissue curetted out of the lesion should be submitted for histologic examination by an oral pathologist. In infected cases, there may be a purulent exudate that can be drained during the curettage of the periapical tissues. In many instances, periapical tissues contain the remnants of extruded endodontic filling materials that may have provoked a foreign-body reaction [3]. From a purely operational perspective, the removal of this granulomatous tissue improves hemostasis and enhances visibility in the surgical field. Although not all of the tissues present in the periapical lesion must be removed to achieve a favorable outcome [32], the more tissue removed, the better hemostasis and visibility will be.

Microsurgical techniques support small ostectomy sites, the opening must be large enough to allow instrumentation so tissues can be adequately curetted from the bony crypt. This can require enlarging the opening in bone to provide access. An alternative is to first do the root-end resection, and then curette the lesion out of bone.

Curettes and periodontal scalers are typically used to curette the periapical tissues from bone. Curettes should initially be used by cleaving the soft tissue away from the walls of the bony crypt using the concave surface of the curette against osseous wall. After the tissues comprising the lesion have been separated from bone, the convex surface of the curette is used to scoop the detached soft tissue away from the bony wall and out of the lesion [3]. Tissue forceps can be used to grasp the periapical lesion to enhance removal from the bony crypt. Removing the lesion in one piece is ideal, because this reduces the amount of bleeding in the area and enhances the accuracy of the histopathological examination. Small soft tissue pieces removed in segments tend to increase bleeding and give a fragmented picture when the tissue is prepared and stained for microscopic examination.

The periapical inflamed tissue may be painful when it is being removed. It has been demonstrated that periapical lesions have innervation that accounts for this pain during curettage [33]. This scenario requires subsequent local anesthetic to be injected into the periapical lesion to provide anesthesia in this area.

Once the bulk of the periapical lesion has been removed from the bone and placed in 10% formalin solution, an ultrasonic scaler may be used to remove the small tissue tags left in the bony crypt. This removes the remaining soft tissue that is attached to the root and the bony walls that surrounded the lesion. This step reduces bleeding and enhances hemorrhage control and visualization of the surgical field. Control of bleeding, in turn, facilitates root-end resection and root-end preparation (Figure 9.31).

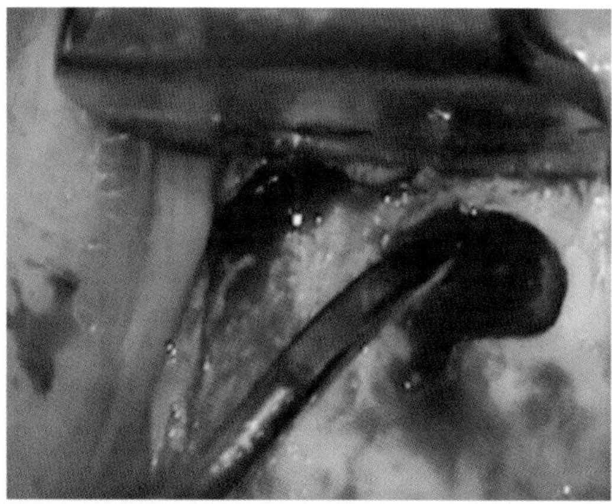

Figure 9.31 Ultrasonic scaler used after curettage of the periapical lesion to remove the remaining small tissue tags left behind in the bony crypt. (Image courtesy of Dr. Dean Whiting.)

Biopsy and microscopic histopathological examination

It is a surgical principle that tissue that warrants removal warrants histological examination to confirm the actual microscopic diagnosis. Whereas most periapical lesions are the result of inflammatory processes arising from infection of the root canal system, in some instances the periapical lesion, when examined histologically has an etiology of nonendodontic origin. Cyst and dental granulomas account for more than 90% of periapical radiolucencies [34–37]. Other noninflammatory conditions such as keratocystic odontogenic tumors (odontogenic keratocysts) [38], central giant cell granulomas [39], metastatic lesions [40, 41], ameloblastomas [44], central odontogenic fibromas [45], nasopalatine duct cysts [46–48], traumatic bone cysts (simple bone cysts) [49, 50], non-Hodgkin's lymphomas [51, 52], and chronic lymphoblastic leukemia [53] have all been reported in the literature. To rule out these uncommon but potentially serious diseases, every periapical lesion that is removed during root-end surgery should be sent for histopathological examination by an oral maxillofacial pathologist.

Root-end resection

Root-end resection involves removing 3 to 3.6 mm of the apical end of the root. The resection should be at a right angle to the long axis of the root. In some instances a slight 10- to 20-degree bevel of the root-end resection is necessary. By resecting 3 mm of the root end, most of the lateral and accessory canals will be resected, as well as the isthmuses that are found running between two canals in roots with multiple canals [54, 55]. In the case of the mesiobuccal root of the maxillary first molar, Degerness and Bowles [56] found that a 3.6-mm resection would adequately expose the isthmus between the mesiobuccal 1 canal and the mesiobuccal 2 canal, as well as placing the resection at a level where there was adequate thickness of dentin to resist vertical root fractures.

Historically, before the use of microscopes, the root end was resected at a 45-degree angle to the long axis of the root to facilitate visualizing the root end and to make the root-end preparation easier. With the magnification and illumination provided by the dental operating microscope, the root can be resected at right angles to the long axis of the root.

As Gilheany and colleagues [57] demonstrated, with a flat 0-degree bevel provided by a root-end resection that is at 90 degrees to the long axis of the root, the apical preparation does not have to be as deep to ensure a good apical seal, and there will be less leakage through cut dentinal tubules. A 45-degree bevel or a 30-degree bevel cuts through more dentinal tubules in the apical portion of the root than does a 0-degree bevel. Because more dentinal tubules are cut with a steeper bevel, more tubules will leak bacteria and bacterial toxins into the

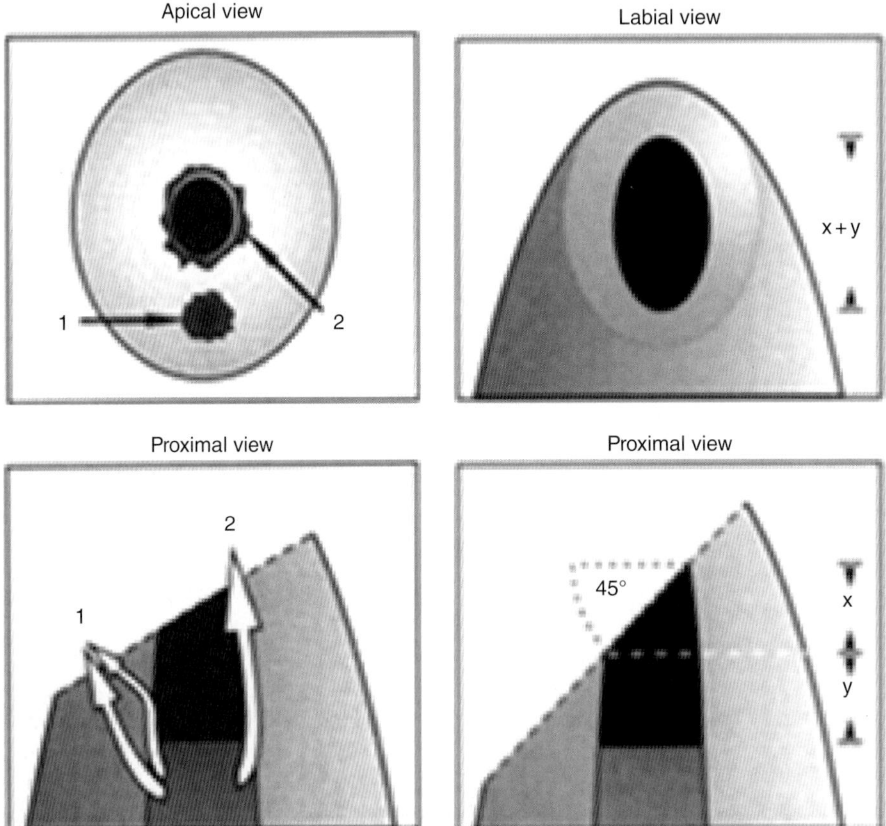

Figure 9.32 The angle of the root-end resection can affect leakage from the canal and around the root-end filling. Leakage occurs from the canal through dentinal tubules that are cut, as illustrated in the panels on the left. Leakage can occur around the root-end filling with a more-severe bevel, as the root-end filling is not deep enough on the facial surface to seal the canal. (From Gilheany PA, Figdor D, Tyas MJ. Apical dentin permeability and microleakage associated with root end resection and retrograde filling. *J Endod* 1994;20(1):22–26.)

periapical tissues, initiating a periapical inflammatory response. A 45-degree bevel requires the root-end preparation to be 2.5 mm in depth, and a 30-degree bevel requires the root-end preparation to be 2.1 mm in depth to prevent apical leakage [57]. With a flat 0-degree bevel, the depth of the root-end preparation of 1.0 mm in depth will prevent apical leakage [57] (Figure 9.32).

The root-end resection can be made with a #56 or #57 straight fissure bur or with a multipurpose bur (Dentsply Maillefer, Ballaigues, Switzerland) in a surgical high-speed handpiece. The multipurpose bur has been found to provide a smoother surface on the resected root end [58]. There are basically two methods for resecting the root end. One is to visualize where the resected point is on the root (3–3.6 mm) and then begin the resection slightly apical to that point so that if adjustments are needed with the bevel, this may be refined without sacrificing too much of the root. With this method, the surgeon must account for the width of the bur to ensure the bur width is not added to the depth of the resection (Figure 9.33).

The second method is to picture the point where the ideal resection should be, and reduce the root length to that point by gradually shaving down the root end. With either method, care should be exercised to ensure that the resection is close to right angles to the long axis of the root in both a buccolingual (palatal) direction and a mesiodistal direction. In some cases, to preserve root length, the resection may be less than 3 mm. In other cases it may be necessary to have a bevel of 10 degrees or more to visualize the root end for the root-end preparation and fill.

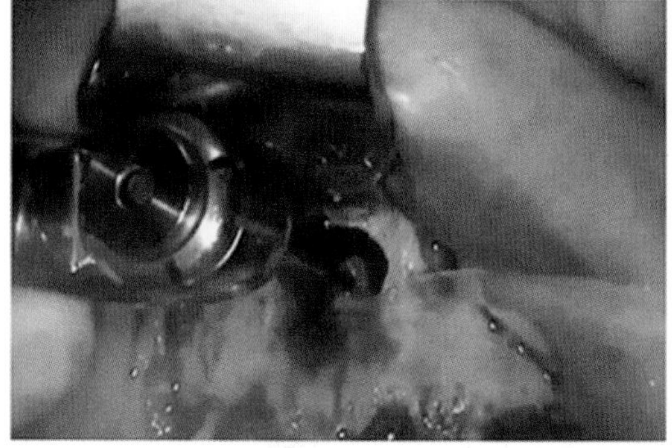

Figure 9.33 Surgical handpiece with straight fissure bur resecting apical 3 mm of the root at right angles to the long axis of the root. (Image courtesy of Dr. Dean Whiting.)

The endodontic microsurgeon should avoid placing a reverse bevel on the root end. A reverse bevel makes it extremely difficult to visualize the root end through the microscope, reducing the visualization required for root-end preparation and subsequent root-end fill. In some instances when trying to observe the site for the root-end resection through the microscope, the head of the handpiece blocks the view of the bur. It is essential that the bur be visualized while making the resection. To overcome this problem, the patient can be repositioned, or the handpiece can be rotated slightly while still keeping the bur in the proper orientation to the root end. If the granulomatous tissue is curetted from the periapical area, and the osseous tissue has been carefully removed from around the root end, the root-end resection is made easier, and the proper bevel of the root end is produced.

After the root-end resection is completed, the microscope can be slightly repositioned in order to view the root face created by the root-end resection. This may also be accomplished, at times, by having the patient slightly move their head, allowing the cut root face to be visible through the microscope.

The root-end resection may be better visualized by using methylene blue dye and then rinsing it away. The methylene blue dye will leave a blue stain on soft tissue such as the periodontal ligament. The stained periodontal ligament should resemble a target, where the outer circle of the periodontal ligament is the outside of the target, and the debris or unprepared canal and gutta-percha forms the inner portion of the target. The methylene blue will also stain any vertical fractures or cracks that may be present. Close microscopic visualization of the cut root face, in conjunction with the methylene blue staining, shows if the resection is smooth and flat and confirms that all of the root has been resected. Any discrepancies in the root-end resection can be corrected at this time.

Impregnated epinephrine pellets may now be placed into the bony crypt to allow time for them to help achieve hemostasis before it is time to place a root-end filling (Figures 9.34 and 9.35).

Root-end preparation

The root-end preparation is accomplished with ultrasonic surgical tips in the ultrasonic handpiece

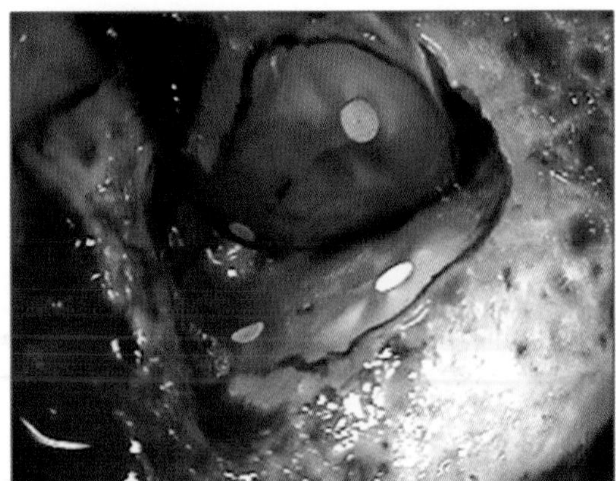

Figure 9.34 Methylene blue dye is used to stain the periodontal ligament to confirm that the entire root-end has been resected. It can also be used to verify the existence other canals, an isthmus, or cracks. (Image courtesy of Dr. Stephen Niemczyk)

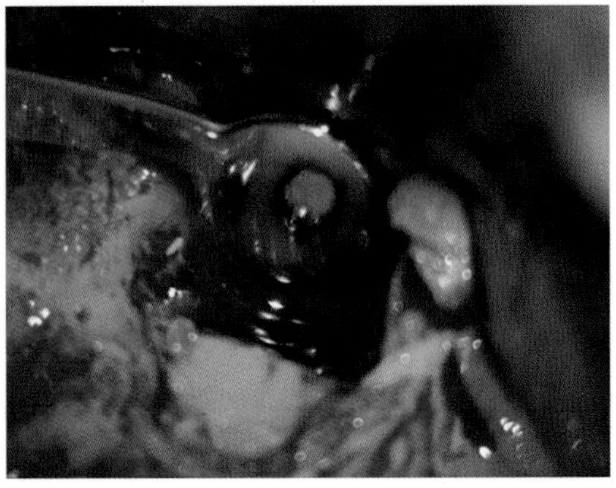

Figure 9.35 Methylene blue dye will stain remaining debris around the root canal filling, indicating leakage.

(Figures 9.36–9.38). The setting must be low enough to decrease the chances of creating cracks or causing the tip to break. Irrigation is necessary to ensure dissipation of heat and to prevent tissue damage.

The root-end preparation should be a class I preparation 3 mm in depth, centered in the canal, and in the long axis of the root. All canals in the root, as well as the isthmus areas between the canals, should be prepared. The instrument should be allowed to do the cutting without using heavy hand pressure. The ultrasonic tip is allowed to vibrate, permitting the gutta-percha to flow out of the canal. The preparation should be as small as possible while adequately cleaning the canal space. Enough dentin should remain to leave the walls of the canal thick enough to resist fracture. Special attention should be paid to the buccal wall of the canal, because gutta-percha often remains on this portion of the canal. When all the gutta-percha is removed, a microplugger is used to tamp down the gutta-percha to create a flat surface against which the root-end filling may be condensed.

Ultrasonic tips are available in various angles to facilitate preparing different roots in different areas of the mouth. In some instances, an empty or poorly obturated canal requires a deeper root-end preparation and root-end fill. Acteon North America (Mount Laurel, NJ, USA) manufactures Satelec ultrasonic tips, which are 6 mm and 9 mm in length.

To ensure the root-end preparation is in the long axis of the root, an ultrasonic tip can be used to place a groove on the cortical bone; the groove lines up with the long axis of the root to allow easy visualization through the microscope while doing the root-end preparation (Figure 9.39). When the root-end preparation is complete, the root-end can be conditioned and acid etched with 50% solution of citric acid. This removes the smear layer from the root-end resection, opens dentinal tubules to allow attachment of Sharpey's fibers to the resected dentin during healing, and improves healing and reattachment [59].

Hemostatic agents and hemostasis

Salem and El Deeb [60] determined that the average amount of blood loss during root-end surgery was 9.5 mL. This is not a great amount of blood loss in comparison to other surgeries in the oral cavity; blood loss can be greater if the procedure is longer. However, even a small amount of bleeding in the surgical area during endodontic microsurgery can complicate techniques, making the surgery more difficult and negatively affecting the outcomes.

Hemostasis

Proper hemostasis gives the microsurgeon control of the surgical field by enhancing visualization through the microscope and ensuring the field is free of excessive moisture, which can effect root-end filling materials. Hemostasis begins with the review of the medical history to identify conditions and medications that can cause

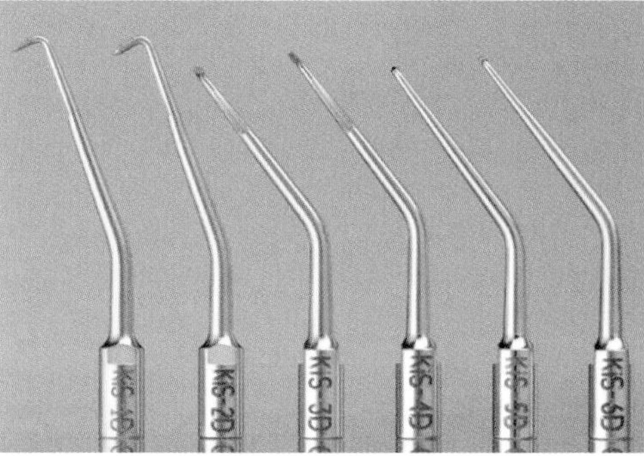
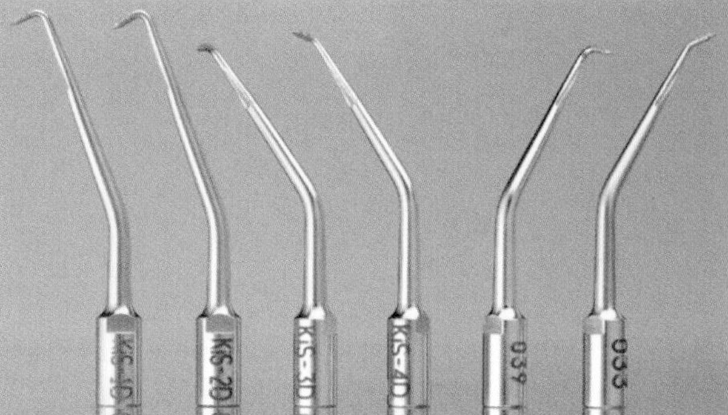

Figure 9.36 The KiS microsurgical ultrasonic tips are coated with zirconium nitride for a more-active cutting surface. They come in different sizes and angles to work on any roots in the mouth.

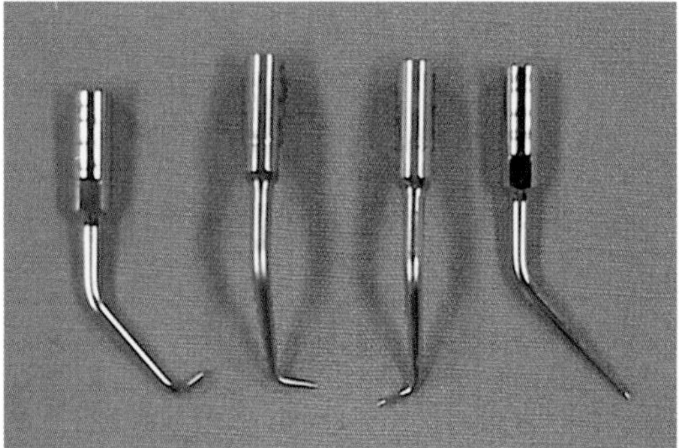

Figure 9.37 Stainless steel ultrasonic tips with varying angles. (Images courtesy of Dr. Scott McClanahan)

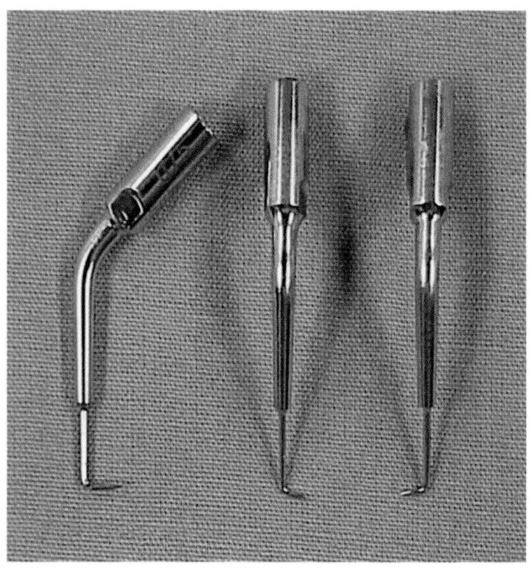

Figure 9.38 Smaller "Slim Jim" tips for preparing narrow canals and isthmuses. (Image courtesy of Dr. Scott McClanahan)

increased bleeding during endodontic microsurgery, as noted earlier in the chapter.

The next phase of hemostasis involves using local anesthetics with vasoconstrictors, as discussed earlier in the chapter. The debridement of vascular granulomatous tissue present in periapical lesions greatly reduces bleeding that otherwise would arise from these tissues.

The third phase of hemostasis is accomplished with local hemostatic agents. These agents are important in providing the amount of hemostasis needed when attempting to complete root-end preparation and root-end filling.

The mechanism of hemostasis after an injury or cutting of a blood vessel has three stages [61]. The first stage is contraction of the severed vessel, which will limit blood flow. The second stage is formation of a platelet plug when circulating platelets come in contact with the collagen in the wall of the injured blood vessel. This causes the platelets to swell and become tacky and attract more platelets by means of chemoattraction. The third stage of the mechanism is the activation of clotting factors and initiation of the clotting cascade, which ultimately converts prothrombin into thrombin, which, in turn, converts fibrinogen into fibrin fibers, forming a clot that contains platelets, blood cells, and plasma [61, 62].

Hemostatic agents

Controlling bleeding after incisions are made and the tissue is reflected during endodontic microsurgery will rely on local hemostatic agents to produce adequate hemostasis allowing minute manipulations required

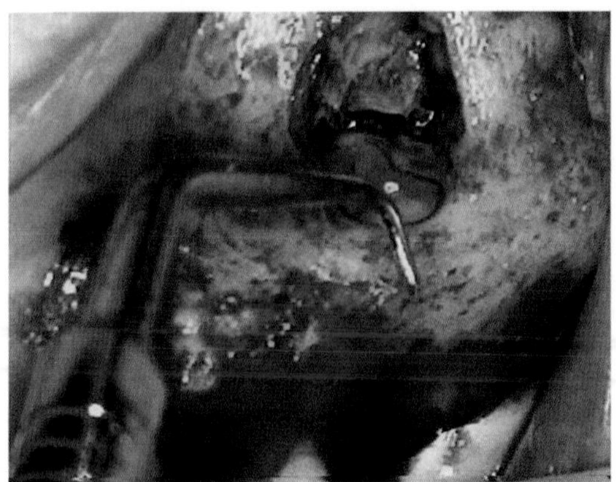

Figure 9.39 A groove can be placed in bone with the ultrasonic tip to correspond to the long axis of the root. This groove can be a reference point to follow to keep the root-end preparation in the long axis of the root. (Image courtesy of Dr. Stephen Niemczyk.)

during microsurgery. A number of local hemostatic agents are available to achieve local hemostasis in endodontic microsurgery.

Bone wax provides a tamponade effect by occluding vessels in bone. Bone wax should not be used in endodontic microsurgery as a foreign body reaction will ensue if the bone wax is not completely removed.

Ferric sulfate (15.5%–20%) causes coagulation of proteinaceous material. Ferric sulfate provides good local hemostasis; however, it produces a dark reddish-brown color in the surgical field, which hampers visualization. Most of the coagulation produced should be removed to improve access and visualization of the surgical site. It has a very low pH [62]. It must only be placed in the bony crypt, and it must be carefully and completely removed. Otherwise, it can delay healing and give rise to a foreign-body reaction [63, 64]. Cut-Trol (Kisco, Witchita, KS) is a very concentrated solution of ferric sulfate, and its high acidity makes it caustic to bony tissues, and it should be avoided, despite its good hemostatic properties.

Aluminum chloride has been used in various products, including Hemodette (DUX Dental, Oxnard, CA), which is a 20% buffered aluminum chloride gel. It is blue, providing better visibility for placement and removal. Aluminum chloride acts by hemagglutination and will cause necrosis, so it must be removed completely when the procedure is finished, and the area must be thoroughly irrigated with normal saline [21].

Collagen-based products include Avitene (Medline Industries, Inc., Mundelein, IL) and CollaPlug, CollaTape, and CollaCote (Zimmer Dental, Carlsbad, CA). Collagen-based products cause platelet adhesion, aggregation, and a release reaction that also activates factor XII. They may also have a mechanical tamponade effect and cause a release of serotonin [62]. Avitene is a fluffy white material that is difficult to apply when wet, and it is very sticky. It will adhere to instruments, gloves, and areas of bone where it is not needed, but it is effective and biocompatible [61].

Gelfoam (Pharmacia and Upjohn Company, Kalamazoo, MI) is a gelatin-based sponge-type material that stimulates the clotting cascade. It may initially cause inflammation in a wound, but studies suggest that with time there is no effect [61, 62].

Oxygenated regenerated cellulose products include Surgicel (Ethicon, Johnson & Johnson, Somerset County, NJ), and Oxycel (Oxycel, Worthington, UK). These are made by oxygenation of regenerated alpha cellulose products. The product becomes sticky and then physically occludes vessels; it does not enhance the clotting cascade by the adhesion and aggregation of platelets as do the collagen local hemostatic agents [62]. Bony healing may be impaired by these products, and the manufacturer does not recommend leaving them in a bony defect [61].

Thrombogen (ZymoGenetics, Inc., Seattle, WA) and like products are topical thrombin-containing materials. The thrombin acts to initiate the intrinsic and extrinsic pathways. It is somewhat difficult to handle and place [61, 62].

Calcium sulfate has been used as a local hemostatic agent. It acts by a mechanical tamponade effect that plugs blood vessels. It is placed into the bony crypt, and then the outer layer is removed to allow visualization and manipulation of the root end. It may be left in the bony defect because it will not cause an increase in the inflammatory response. It is also relatively inexpensive [61, 62].

Epinephrine pellets (Racellets, Pascal Co., Bellevue, WA) are racemic epinephrine–impregnated pellets that cause vasoconstriction by affecting the α-adrenergic receptors on the smooth muscle in the walls of small arterioles and precapillary sphincters. The amount of racemic epinephrine in the pellets can vary; however, because they are used topically there is little systemic absorption [61]. Epinephrine pellets (Racelett pellets) or CollaCote strips impregnated with epinephrine produce a dry field for root-end surgery due to efficient hemostasis, and studies indicate there are no cardiovascular effects or increase in heart rate or blood pressure [65, 66]. In a patient with significant cardiovascular disease, caution should be exercised when using epinephrine pellets. If there is concern about cotton fibers from epinephrine pellets being left behind after the pellets are removed, racemic epinephrine may be placed on nonstick (Teflon) pads (3M Nexcare, St. Paul, MN) and used for hemostasis in place of the epinephrine pellets in the surgical area.

It is critical to count the number of epinephrine pellets that are inserted into the bony lesion, to ensure all the pellets are removed at the end of the procedure. In cases of large periapical defects, a CollaPlug (Zimmer Dental, Carlsbad, CA) can be placed before the epinephrine pellets to fill in the defect, rather than placing too many epinephrine pellets, which can subject the patient to more systemic epinephrine than desirable.

The endodontic microsurgeon should be aware of the "epi clock." In this condition, the initial vasoconstriction produced by epinephrine in local anesthetic is lost over time, and a rebound phenomenon causes a vasodilation effect. This phenomenon is termed *reactive hyperemia rebound* [61], and it causes increased hemorrhage in the area. Once this occurs, it is difficult to regain hemostasis. In patients who have no contraindications to an increased amount of epinephrine and local anesthetic, a block may be given with local anesthetic containing 1:50,000 epinephrine. This will, after a few minutes, restore some of the vasoconstriction previously obtained. Again, caution must be exercised, and aspiration, as always, must verify that the anesthetic solution is not being deposited into a vessel.

Besides racemic epinephrine pellets, other local hemostatic agents that have few undesirable properties are calcium sulfate and Avitene.

For small "bleeders" in bone, burnishing the bone and applying pressure to the site of the bleeding is often enough to stop the seepage of blood.

In summary, the strategy for hemostasis involves the first phases of hemostasis, medical history, and local anesthetics with a vasoconstrictor. The next step is thorough curettage of the periapical lesion and use of ultrasonics, if needed, to remove tags of granulation tissue. Epinephrine pellets are the suggested material for a local hemostatic agent. In most cases, a few epinephrine pellets can be placed into the bleeding crypt with some pressure to achieve hemostasis. Ideally, the epinephrine pellets should be applied before the root-end preparation to allow time for hemostasis to occur before placing the root-end filling.

Stopping arterial bleeding

During any surgical procedure, one should be prepared to tie off a bleeding artery that may have been severed. This technique is termed a *stick tie*, and it can prevent an emergency bleeding problem. If significant bleeding ensues or if blood squirts from an artery, direct pressure should be applied over the vessel. If this is not successful in stopping the arterial bleeding, the surgical assistant should again apply pressure. A stick tie is performed by clamping the artery with hemostats. The artery is then tied off with 2–0 or 4–0 suture, which is preferably a resorbable suture.

The stick-tie procedure is performed by passing a needle proximal to where the hemostat has clamped the vessel. The needle is passed deep to the vessel, and then the suture is tied with just one throw. The assistant releases the pressure on the vessel, and the hemostat that is clamping the vessel is released. If the arterial bleeding has stopped, then the suture knot is secured with a second and third throw. If bleeding has not stopped after the first throw and release of pressure and the hemostat, then the surgical assistant again applies pressure to the vessel, and the vessel tissue is clamped to close off the artery. The needle and suture are passed deeper and more proximal to tie off the artery. Check again by releasing pressure. This can be repeated until the bleeding has been stopped [67].

Root-End Filling Materials and Placement of Root-End Filling Materials

Endodontic materials are described in detail in the chapter covering materials used in the practice of endodontics and will not be described here. Various materials have been used over the years as a root-end filling material. Many of these materials have been replaced by materials that are more biocompatible and provide a better seal. The requirements of an ideal root-end filling material are listed in Box 9.3 [68–72].

In the past, many materials have been used for root-end fillings, including amalgam, cold-burnished

Box 9.3 Requirements for an ideal root-end filling material

The requirements for an ideal root-end filling material were compiled by Chong and Pitt Ford [69] from other articles [70–73]. The ideal root-end filling material should

- Adhere or bond to tooth tissue and seal the root-end three dimensionally
- Not promote, and preferably inhibit, the growth of pathogenic microorganisms
- Be dimensionally stable and unaffected by moisture in either the set or unset state
- Be well tolerated by periradicular tissues with no inflammatory reactions
- Stimulate the regeneration of a normal periodontium
- Be nontoxic both locally and systemically
- Not corrode or be electrochemically active
- Not stain the tooth or the periradicular tissues
- Be easily distinguishable on radiographs
- Have a long shelf life
- Be easy to handle

gutta-percha, Cavit (3M), zinc oxide eugenol (ZOE), glass ionomer cement, resin-bonding agents, intermediate restorative material (IRM), and super ethoxybenzoic acid (Super EBA). Newer the choices are mineral trioxide aggregate (MTA) and the newer bioceramics materials.

Amalgam fell out of favor as a root-end filling material due to poor sealing ability, corrosion, dimensional changes, amalgam tattoos, poor biocompatibility, cytotoxicity, and poor outcomes [68, 70, 73]. To fill the void left with the abandonment of amalgam as a root-end filling material, several materials were developed, most notably Super EBA [70]. MTA and the newer bioceramics have largely replaced Super EBA and IRM as the root-end filling materials in greatest use.

The best choices today for a root-end filling material, and ones that satisfy many of the requirements for an ideal root-end filling material include MTA, the newer bioceramics, and occasionally IRM or Super EBA. On rare occasions a composite resin–glass ionomer might be indicated.

Intermediate restorative material

IRM (LD Caulk Company, Milford, DE, USA) is a polymer-resin reinforced zinc oxide eugenol material [74]. IRM demonstrated good healing outcomes when compared to amalgam as a root-end filling material [70]. In two clinical trials IRM has been demonstrated to have a high success rate and comparable to MTA [75, 76].

IRM is easy to mix and place. A thick mix can be prepared and then rolled out in a long, thin rope. An instrument is used to cut off a small portion and carry it to the root-end preparation. The IRM is condensed into the preparation using micro condensers. The excess is removed flush with the edge of the root-end preparation [2].

Super ethoxybenzoic acid

Super EBA (Harry J. Bosworth Co., Skokie, IL, USA) is a modified ZOE cement. The powder component contains 60% zinc oxide, 34% alumina, and 6% natural resin [2]. The liquid contains 62.5% ortho-ethoxy benzoic acid and 37.5% eugenol. Oynick and Oynick [77] confirmed collagen fibers growing on Super EBA. It has a short setting time, seals well, is well tolerated by tissues, and is dimensionally stable. Successful outcomes with Super EBA and microsurgical techniques have been reported in several studies [70, 78–81].

Super EBA is more difficult to mix than IRM. When enough powder has been incorporated into the mix, the shine is lost. The mix is then rolled out in a long, thin rope. An instrument is used to cut off a small portion and carry it to the dried root-end preparation. It is then condensed into the preparation using micro condensers [2]. The excess Super EBA is removed from the margins of the root-end preparation before it sets. Once the Super EBA begins to set, there should be no more manipulation of the material until it completely sets. The set Super EBA can now be trimmed and polished with a 30 fluted composite resin finishing bur. Citric acid (50%) can be applied to the root end for one minute [59].

Mineral Trioxide Aggregate

MTA is considered the gold standard against which other materials are compared because it satisfies many of the requirements for an ideal root-end filling material. The composition of MTA is described in the chapter on endodontic materials and the references for this chapter [74]. Desirable properties include good sealing ability [82–88], biocompatibility [89, 90], low solubility [91], high pH [91, 92], calcium release [91], antibacterial activity [93], and acceptable radiopacity. Cementoblasts can deposit cementum on MTA [94], which is an obvious benefit to healing in the periapical area.

The main drawbacks of MTA are its long setting time of 4 hours and its difficult handling properties. With experience, the clinician can overcome the less-desirable handling properties. MTA is marketed as ProRoot MTA (Dentsply Tulsa Dental Specialties, Tulsa, OK, USA). Once mixed, MTA can be carried to the preparation by different methods.

The first method is the utilization of the Lee MTA Forming Block (G. Hartzell & Son, Concord, CA, USA). The Lee block is a four-sided block with grooves of varying lengths which can be filled with MTA. The MTA mix is carried to the Lee block with the mixing spatula and spread across the surface and into the grooves. A sterile 2 × 2 gauge or a gloved finger is used to wipe off the excess MTA, leaving MTA in the grooves. A half Hollenbeck carver or similar instrument removes the MTA from the groove in the block. The MTA is in the form of a cylinder and is carried to the root-end preparation. With the Lee Block, the powder-to-liquid ratio in the MTA mix is important. If the mix is too wet, it will slump, and there will not be a well-formed cylinder of MTA to place into the root-end preparation. If the mix is too dry, it will crumble when the clinician attempts to take it out of the groove in the Lee block, or it will fall off of the instrument before reaching the root-end preparation. The mix can be manipulated to the desired consistency by absorbing water from the mix with a cotton roll or by adding additional water (Figures 9.40 and 9.41).

The second method employs a carrier to take the MTA to the root-end preparation. Several MTA carriers are on the market, including the Retrofill Amalgam Carrier (Miltex, York, PA, USA), the Messing Root Canal Gun (Miltex, York, PA), the Dovgan MTA Carrier (Quality Aspirators, Duncanville, TX), and the MAP System (Produits Dentaires, Vevey, Switzerland) [95].

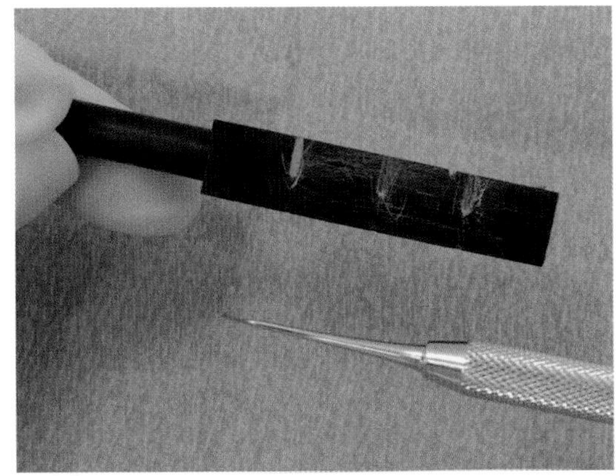

Figure 9.40 MTA cylinder formed in the Lee block and placed on an instrument to carry it to the root-end preparation.

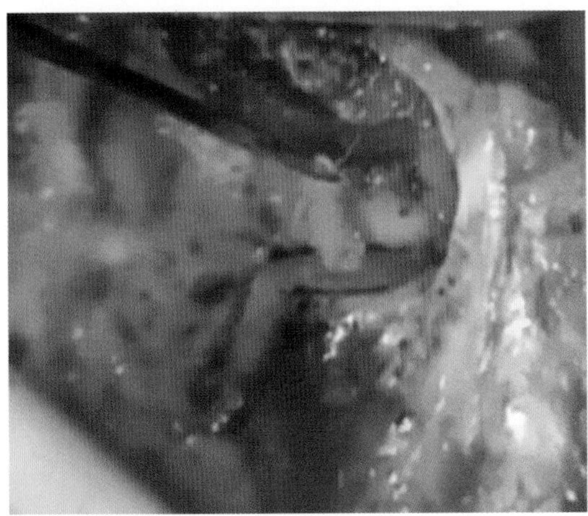

Figure 9.41 MTA that was formed in the Lee block being placed into a root-end preparation. (Image courtesy of Dr. Dean Whiting.)

The Messing Gun and the Retrofill Amalgam Carrier are older instruments and were not specifically designed to carry MTA to the root-end preparation. The Dovgan MTA carrier is a syringe device that comes in three different tip diameters. The diameters are 1.6 mm, 0.99 mm, and 0.8 mm [68]. The MTA is loaded into the tip and carried to the root-end preparation, where it is deposited.

The MAP System has a syringe with a ringed handle and a Teflon plunger that pushes the MTA forward and

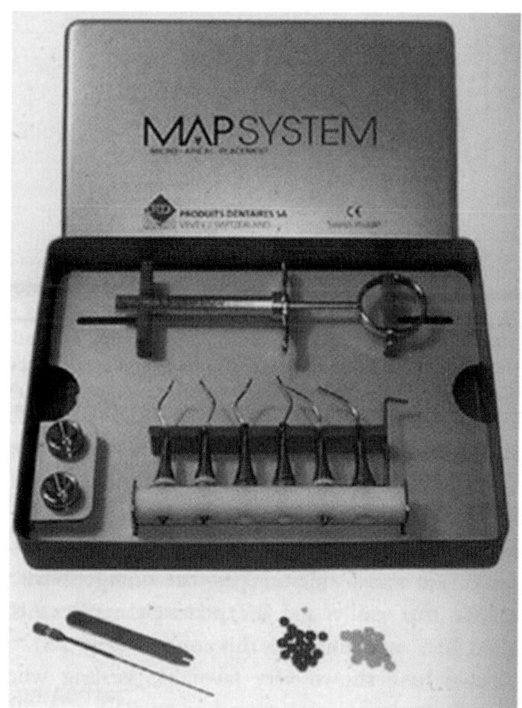

Figure 9.42 MAP System (PD, Vevey, Switzerland) comes with syringe tips of different diameters and angles for placement of MTA.

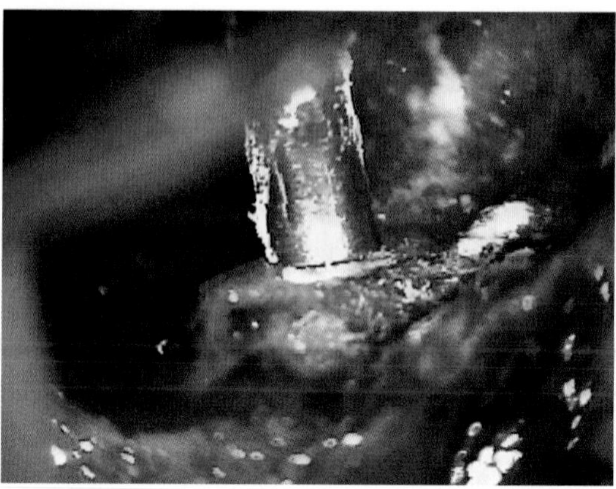

Figure 9.43 MTA being placed with the MAP System into a root-end preparation. (Image courtesy of Dr. Stephen Niemczyk.)

out of the tip. The system has six tips with two different diameters and three different tip curvatures. The tip is loaded with MTA and carried to the root-end preparation. The handle should not be twisted relative to the tip, because that twists the Teflon plunger and distorts it, preventing it from reaching the tip, and it will need to be replaced. Nickel–titanium tips are also available for the MAP System (Figures 9.42 and 9.43). The carrier tips must be thoroughly cleaned before the MTA sets inside. Once the MTA sets inside the tip, it cannot be removed and the tip must be discarded.

The ProRoot MTA manual carrier (Dentsply Tulsa Dental Specialties, Tulsa, OK) comes with a plastic sleeve that can be cut to the appropriate length. The carrier resembles a plugger. The sleeve is placed over the end of the Manual Carrier and resembles an amalgam carrier. MTA is loaded into the sleeve on the end of the carrier and then inserted into the root-end preparation. The first load is difficult to express out of the carrier because the sleeve is very stiff initially. As the plastic sleeve is stretched with repeated loads, it becomes easier to place the MTA into the root-end preparation (Figure 9.44).

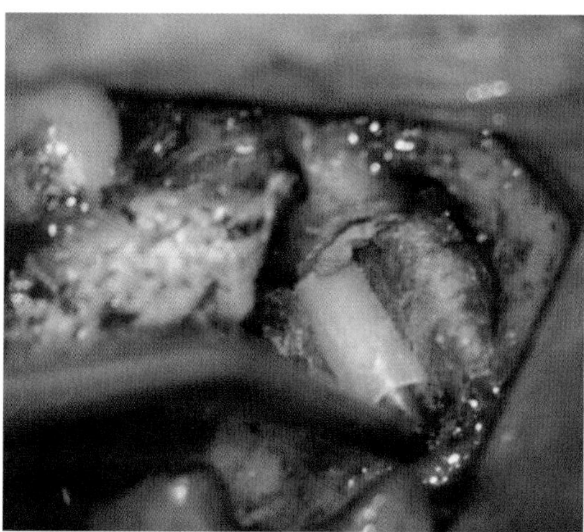

Figure 9.44 ProRoot MTA (Tulsa Dentsply, Tulsa, OK, USA) being placed into a root-end preparation with the ProRoot MTA Manual Carrier. (Image courtesy of Dr. Brandon Seto.)

Once the MTA is placed into the root-end preparation, it is condensed. MTA does not condense like amalgam or other dental materials [68]. A microplugger that has been prefitted is used to compact the MTA. The MTA must be manipulated into place and not condensed with hard pressure to avoid having the MTA move up the sides of the root-end preparation. Once the preparation is slightly overfilled, the MTA can be carved back to the margins of the root-end preparation by first using a carver and then a microbrush. Care should be taken that a divot is not left in the MTA. If the root-end preparation is deeper than 3 mm, the MTA can be condensed by placing a microplugger over the MTA and placing the noncutting side of an ultrasonic tip on the microplugger. The ultrasonic tip is then activated, moving the MTA to the depth of the preparation [68, 69]. MTA can be made to set up to a degree, so that it will not wash out, by blowing a gentle stream of air across the MTA with the Stropko irrigator tip.

Newer bioceramic root-end filling materials

Bioceramic materials have been developed with properties that overcome the shortcomings of MTA, including difficult handling and long setting time. Bioceramic materials have calcium silicates as the major ingredient. They are very biocompatible [96–101], have better handling properties [99], are antimicrobial [102], have shorter setting times, have cementogenic [101] and osteogenic properties [101], and have acceptable radiopacity and sealing ability [103, 104].

EndoSequence Root Repair Material (Brasseler USA, Savannah, GA, USA), Biodentine (Septodont, Saint Maurdes Fossés, France), and BioAggreate Root Repair Material (Innovative BioCeramix, Vancouver, BC, Canada) are some of the newer bioceramic root-end filling materials and are described in detail in the chapter on endodontic materials (Figure 9.45). One study evaluated the outcome of root-end surgeries that used EndoSequence Root Repair Material. At one year, the overall success rate was 92% [124].

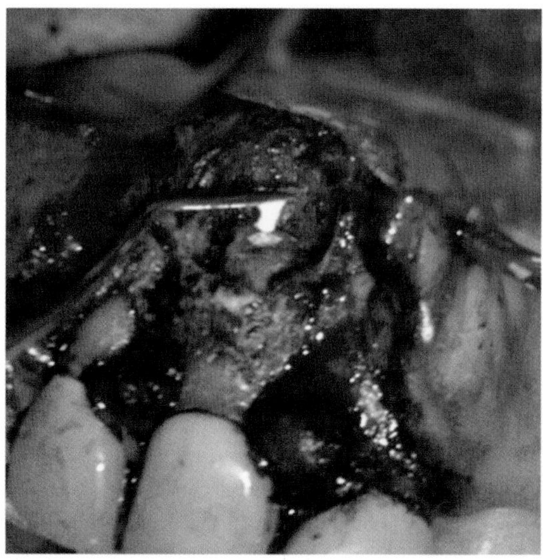

Figure 9.45 EndoSequence Root Repair Material (Brasseler USA, Savanah, GA, USA) being placed into a root-end preparation. (Image courtesy of Dr. Joao Barbizam.)

Bioceramic root-end filling materials are biocompatible, have shorter setting times, and have better handling characteristics. Bioceramics are very promising, but more long-term outcome studies are needed.

After the placement of the root-end filling is complete, the epi-pellets may be removed and counted to be sure that all have been removed. If another material was used to aid with hemostasis, that material should also be removed. The bony crypt may now be rinsed with sterile saline. The root-end filling material should be protected with a broad instrument to ensure that any unset root-end filling material is not washed out of the root-end preparation.

Flap closure and suturing techniques

After the root-end procedure is completed, the reflected tissue is ready to be re-approximated and closed with sutures. The mucoperiosteal flap should be repositioned and held in place with pressure for up to five minutes. Because the mucoperiosteal flap tends to retract during the procedure, it often needs to be stretched so that it can be positioned to its original position and then held in place. Once the flap is repositioned and will stay in that position, suturing may begin. Depending on circumstances, different sutures and types of sutures are needed to provide wound closure. Circumstances that dictate the size and type of suture materials are location of the incision, the thickness of the flap, and the suturing technique to be used [1].

Needles

The choice of needle is an important criterion for the surgical procedure as different needles have different characteristics. The chord length is the straight-line distance from the tip of a curved needle to the swage of the needle where it is attached to the suture material. The needle length is the distance measured along the needle from point to the swaged end. The radius of the needle is the distance from the center of the circle of a curved needle to the body of the needle [1]. Needles come in different shapes for penetration of tissue. These needle shapes include taper points, conventional cutting, reverse cutting, and taper cutting tips.

A needle with a shorter chord length is better for microsurgical techniques. For closure of most endodontic microsurgical flaps, a 3/8 circle needle is the most appropriate. The triangular cross-shaped reverse cutting needles are generally preferred for endodontic microsurgery. A needle length of 16 to 20 mm is needed to suture a buccal flap with a sulcular incision, including triangular and rectangular flaps. For closing horizontal incisions in submarginal incisions or papilla base incisions, a length of 8 mm or shorter is best [1]. Needles of other lengths may be required for certain situations.

Suture

The 4–0 silk sutures have been replaced by monofilament 5–0, 6–0, and 7–0 suture sizes. Silk sutures wick bacteria and quickly become contaminated in the oral environment; whereas the monofilament sutures are not as easily contaminated by oral bacteria. Contaminated suture leads to more inflammation at the suture site [105, 106].

Sutures are also classified as absorbable and nonabsorbable. Absorbable sutures include catgut, polyglycolic acid, and glycolide and e-caprolactone materials. Nonabsorbable sutures include silk, braded polyester, nylon, polyviolene, and polypropylene.

Suturing should start in the unattached reflected flap and go to the attached unreflected tissue. A surgeon's knot is used to close the incision. The surgeon's knot lies flat on the tissue and is locked, which keeps it from unraveling. A surgeon's knot is a modified square knot with two overhand knots that are completed in an opposite direction. The first knot is a double overhand knot, the second can be a single knot [1]. A second single knot can be added, if needed. The knot should lie on tissue, and not in the incision line.

In the case of papilla base incisions, using a smaller 7–0 suture, a single overhand knot is used first because the tightness of a first overhand double throw will cut through the tissue. This first single overhand knot is then followed with a double overhand knot in the papilla base incision closure.

When suturing with the aid of the microscope, it is useful to gather the extra suture material in the opposite hand, to ensure the surgeon has control of the extra suture, preventing it from hanging down into the surgical field. The surgical assistant should keep the free end of the suture away from the needle end. This allows the microsurgeon to stay focused through the microscope and maintain efficiency.

Single interrupted suture

The most elemental suturing technique to close wounds in endodontic microsurgery is the single interrupted suture. This is ideal for closing the vertical releasing incisions. It starts in the unattached reflected tissue and then continues into the attached tissue. A surgeon's knot is then tied off of the incision line.

This type of suture can also be used to suture the reflected papilla portion of an intrasulcular incision; it is used with 7–0 suture to close the horizontal portion of the papilla base incision. To close the papilla base incision, the papilla is divided into thirds horizontally. An interrupted suture is placed at the junction of each of the thirds using 7–0 suture. Then, if a gap exists in the middle third of the papilla, it can be closed with another interrupted suture in the middle third of the papilla.

The submarginal flap can be closed with interrupted sutures along the scalloped horizontal incision by suturing the points of the scalloped margin first, and then closing any gaps that exist in the areas between the points. It is important to check for gaps by placing a finger on either side of the incision and gently trying to separate the wound edges. If needed, more interrupted sutures may be placed. Mucoperiosteal flaps tend to shrink away from the incision line, and this is especially pronounced where there are two soft tissue edges to the incision. This is the case in the submarginal incision. Because of this shrinkage, it is important to stretch the and reposition the flap before suturing and to make sure that the sutures hold the reapproximated incision margins together so that healing can occur by primary intention

Modified vertical mattress suture

The modified vertical mattress suture is indicated when reattaching the free papilla of an intrasulcular flap, or when both the facial and palatal or lingual papillae have been reflected. The initial penetration of the needle is in the apical third of the interdental papilla on the facial side. The needle then goes through to the apical third of the lingual or palatal papilla. The needle is reinserted on the lingual or palatal papilla coronal to where it emerged and will be in the middle one third of the papilla. The needle is passed through the interdental space until the reflected side of the facial papilla is encountered, and then the needle is inserted and comes out coronal to the initial point of penetration on the facial papilla. The suture forms a bracket, and the two ends of the suture can be tightened so that the papilla lies in its original position. A surgeon's knot is then tied. In relation to the interdental papilla and the tooth structure, the insertion points of the needle are low-low (base of the papilla in the apical one third) and then high-high (more coronal in the middle one third of the papilla).

Sling suture

In cases when it is not possible to engage tissue on the lingual or palatal side of the tooth, a regular sling suture can be employed. After passing the needle through the mesial facial papilla and through the embrasure, the suture is brought around the lingual or palatal aspect of the tooth without engaging the tissue. On the distal aspect of the lingual or palatal side, the needle and suture is passed through to the distal embrasure to penetrate the distal facial papilla on the reflected side. It is then passed back through the distal facial papilla and back through the distal embrasure to the lingual or palatal side and brought around the lingual or palatal side near the gingival tissues to the mesial lingual or palatal side. The needle and suture is then passed through the mesial embrasure to the underside of the mesial facial papilla, to pierce the papilla. A surgeon's knot is then tied. The surgeon has the choice of either penetrating tissue on the lingual or palatal side or using the undercuts on the crown structure on the lingual or palatal side near the gingiva. The later method may be used, providing there is enough of an undercut to hold the suture below the height of contour on the lingual or palatal aspect of the tooth.

The sling suture, or modifications of it, is an excellent way to close intrasulcular incisions, especially around the tooth that was treated with a root-end resection, because it wraps around the tooth and holds the papilla in place on both the mesial and the distal side of the tooth.

A modification of the sling suture with elements of the vertical mattress suture is known as the *modified basket suture*. The initial needle insertions are low (apical) in all areas first, followed by high (coronal) insertions the last time through. Starting on the mesial facial side of the tooth to be included in the sling suture, the needle is inserted in the base of the interdental papilla and passed through the tissue and into the lingual or palatal papilla, much like an interrupted suture. The needle is then moved to the distal lingual or distal palatal side of the tooth and is inserted at the base of the papilla, through to the distal facial side of the tooth, entering the distal facial papilla on the reflected side of the flap and through to the facial side of the papilla. This should be at the apical third or base of the distal facial papilla. The needle is then reinserted coronally in the middle third of the distal facial papilla and passed through to the distal lingual or distal palatal papilla.

The needle should penetrate the distal lingual or distal palatal papilla and exit coronal to the previous needle insertion. From the distal lingual or distal palatal side, the needle is brought to the mesial lingual or mesial palatal side of the tooth, and the papilla is penetrated coronal to the previous site where the needle and suture penetrated the mesial lingual or mesial palatal papilla. The needle is then passed through the interdental tissues to the mesial facial papilla coronal to the first insertion point. The suture is secured with a surgeon's knot.

Figure-of-eight suture

A suture that is used after extraction and site preservation is an X, or a figure-of-eight suture, which holds a membrane in place in the socket. The suture begins at the mesial facial papilla of a socket to the distal lingual or distal palatal papilla of the socket, then is directed to the distal facial papilla of the socket. The suture completes the X over the socket by traversing to the mesial lingual or mesial palatal papilla. To complete the figure-of-eight, the suture goes from the mesial lingual or mesial palatal papilla to the mesial facial papilla, where a surgeon's knot is tied. Care must be taken to not catch the membrane with the needle and displace it out of the socket. The suture should hold the membrane in place.

Suture Removal

Sutures should be removed between 2 and 4 days after they are placed, because this allows sufficient reattachment of tissues and will not cause undue inflammation. In guided tissue-regenerative procedures, sutures may be needed for a longer period for membrane stabilization and to ensure the membrane is not exposed.

Postoperative Management and Instructions

The following procedures and instructions should be provided after suturing is completed. The tissue should again be held in place with firm finger pressure through a 2 × 2 moist gauze for 5 minutes to ensure good tissue readaptation. Postoperative vital signs should be taken to confirm stability of the patient. If needed, an angled radiograph or image can be exposed, if one was not previously taken.

Block anesthesia should be given with 0.5% (9 mg) bupivacaine with 1:200,000 epinephrine to provide long-acting anesthesia, so that the pain medications will have time to take effect. Oral and written postoperative instructions should be given to the patient. These should include postoperative expectations, the use of an ice pack, the gauze pack, oral hygiene instructions, and how to take the prescribed medications.

An ice pack should be provided to the patient, and should be applied before the patient leaves the office. The ice will constrict blood flow to the area, which reduces swelling and pain. It is applied by alternating 15 to 20 minutes on, and then 15 to 20 minutes off for the first 8 to 12 hours. Ice is applied alternately because continuous application of ice will cause vasodilation and increased blood flow to the area [107]. The patient may use bags of frozen vegetables, such as peas or corn, once the initial ice pack is no longer cold. The skin should be protected with a washcloth from the cold plastic. After 8 hours, the application of ice is discontinued

The patient should expect some swelling and possible ecchymosis in the first 48 hours; however, pain is usually well controlled with ibuprofen or other non-steroidal antiinflammatory drugs (NSAIDs). Narcotics and acetaminophen, such as codeine or hydrocodone with acetaminophen, should be prescribed in the event of more-severe pain. Instructions should be given to follow a flexible pain strategy of NSAIDs used alternately with acetaminophen for moderate pain, and narcotics (codeine or hydrocodone) with acetaminophen alternated with NSAIDs for more-severe pain.

In the event of bleeding, instructions are given to apply pressure with the extra gauze packs for 30 minutes or more. Alternatively, pressure can be applied with a tea bag for 30 minutes or more; tannic acid in the tea promotes hemostasis. In the event of uncontrolled bleeding, the patient should be seen immediately, because sutures and other measures may need to be employed to stop bleeding.

Generally, antibiotics are not required for surgeries. Exceptions are for existing swelling or in the case of guided tissue regeneration. If swelling occurs after the initial postoperative swelling, then antibiotics may be warranted, and incision and drainage may be required, or even reflection of the flap again for drainage. If antibiotics are required, the choices should be penicillin V, amoxicillin, or clindamycin.

Chlorhexidine gluconate, 0.12%, without alcohol, should be prescribed as a mouth rinse postoperatively. Patients should be instructed to carry out their normal oral hygiene regimen, being careful not to disturb the surgical area, and may use a soft wash cloth to clean the teeth in the area where the surgery was performed. After the first 24 hours, use of warm moist heat in the area may be permitted if there is little or no swelling.

Tsesis and colleagues [108] found that one day postoperatively, 76.4% of the patients were completely pain free, less than 4% had moderate pain, and 64.7% did not report any swelling. The preoperative symptoms significantly influenced the pain experience after surgery. Ideally, the patient should be contacted the evening of the surgery to confirm stability and assess pain level. Postoperative instructions can be reinforced, questions can be answered, and concern for the patient's well-being can be reinforced.

Surgical Wound Healing

Surgical wound healing in periapical surgery was investigated in classic research by Harrison and Jurosky [109–111]. Wound healing depends upon the type of tissue that is wounded and the type of wound or injury that the tissue receives [3, 112].

The tissues that are involved in the surgical wound include alveolar mucosa, palatal mucosa, marginal gingiva, attached keratinized gingiva, gingival fibers, periodontal ligament, periosteum, cementum, dentin, blood vessels, and cortical and cancellous bone.

Wound healing can occur either by primary or secondary intention. Primary-intention healing occurs when the wound edges are closely approximated and separated only by a thin clot. Regeneration is the end result of this mechanism, and wounded tissues are ultimately restored to their normal anatomy.

Secondary-intention healing occurs when the wound edges are not closely approximated, leading to an accumulation of granulation tissue between the wound edges. Repair is the end result of this mechanism, the wounded tissues do not preserve their normal anatomy, and scar tissue forms [112]. Intentional wounding during surgery initiates a series of vascular, cellular, and biochemical mechanisms leading to regeneration (primary-intention healing) or repair (secondary-intention healing) [112].

Healing was studied in an animal model in three distinct phases, which included the incisional wound, the dissectional wound, and the osseous excisional wound [109–111].

Incisional wound healing

The mechanisms of incisional wound healing can be described in four phases: clotting and inflammation, epithelial healing, connective tissue healing, and maturation and remodeling. Healing cannot be separated into distinct "phases" because considerable overlapping occurs and several phases can occur simultaneously [109]. Incisional wounds studied were vertical releasing incisions, intrasulcular horizontal incisions, and submarginal incisions. All incision lines healed similarly, but the submarginal incisions were less predictable.

Clotting occurs immediately in an incisional wound to stop bleeding, and it is followed by fibrin strands that run parallel to the wound. A surface coagulum forms over the wound. Inflammation due to tissue injury is imitated with inflammatory mediators and a cellular response. Initially, polymorphonuclear neutrophils (PMNs) respond, followed by macrophages [109].

Epithelial healing occurs in the incisional wound as epithelial cells elongate and migrate across the fibrin scaffolding. Once this occurs, an epithelial seal is formed. The seal forms a barrier that increases wound strength, prevents loss of fluids, and keeps the wound edges together. An epithelial seal was found to form within 2 days [109].

The connective tissue healing in the incisional wound begins when the epithelial seal is formed. This complex phase has fibroblast becoming the dominant cell. The fibroblasts secrete type I and type III collagen to form a connective tissue matrix. Angiogenesis and revascularization also occur in the connective tissue. There is a transition from granulomatous tissue to granulation tissue, signifying connective tissue healing [109].

As maturation and remodeling occurs, reorganization and realignment of collagen produces an organized pattern resembling a normal appearance [109]. This is usually evident by day 28.

Dissectional wound healing

The dissectional wound occurs with the elevation of the mucoperiosteal flap, and healing is similar for both triangular and submarginal flaps. Initially, the periosteum is lost, but it reforms by 14 days. The lamina propria of the attached gingiva shows little inflammation, whereas the lamina propria of the alveolar mucosa is usually highly inflamed on the first day after surgery. However, by the 14th day after surgery there is no inflammation. PMNs are the initial inflammatory cells to respond, followed by macrophages and fibroblasts. Angiogenesis and formation of type I collagen are noted on the 4th day after surgery. By the 28th day, the tissues in the dissectional wound are normal [110].

Excisional wound healing

The excisional wound is the wound produced in bone from the ostectomy. The osseous excisional wound fills with a disorganized coagulum and widely spaced fibrin strands. There is evidence of devitalized bone around the wound edges in cortical and cancellous bone for the first three days after surgery. Inflammatory cells and undifferentiated ectomesenchymal cells and fibroblast appear by day 3. Endosteal tissues proliferate from medullary spaces between trabeculae into the coagulum in the bony cavity on the fourth day. By the 14th day after surgery, 80% of the excisional wound is occupied by endosteal tissue and woven bone.

The woven bone is seen as appositional growth on the surface of cortical and cancellous devitalized bone around the excisional wound edges. A thick band of highly cellular tissue and dense fibrous connective tissue forming the periosteum is evident by the 14th day. This newly formed periosteum subsequently functions to repair the cortical plate destroyed in the excisional wound. By day 28, there is maturing of new trabecular bone arising from the endosteal side of the wound because these trabeculae had coalesced to occupy more of the osseous defect than endosteal tissue. Osteoid-like tissue is also deposited on the endosteal surfaces of the trabeculae. A fibrous periosteum forms with an architectural pattern similar to a mature periosteum, forming cortical bone over the newly formed trabeculae [111].

Clinical importance

Understanding the different aspects of wound healing will help the endodontic microsurgeon perform surgery. In the case of the incisional wound, clean incision lines that go completely to bone on the first pass will make reapproximation of the wound edges more predictable and lead to more-rapid epithelial healing. Compression of the flap both before and after suturing will prevent accumulation of a large surface coagulum or a collection of blood and fibrin between the replaced flap and the bone. Both of these can lead to delayed healing. Also, removing the surface coagulum of dried blood on the wound edges with a moistened cotton-tipped applicator will lead to better reapproximation of the wound edges. The loss of soft tissue attachment due to apical epithelial downgrowth can be prevented following intrasulcular incisions by maintaining the vitality of root-attached tissues. This can be accomplished by initiating flap reflection and elevation in the vertical incision rather than in the gingival sulcus against the marginal gingiva, by avoiding curettage or planing of the root surface, and by frequent irrigation of the root surface to prevent dehydration. Because an epithelial seal is formed by the second postoperative day, sutures can be removed as early as 2 or 3 days after the surgery [109]. The early removal of sutures reduces the risk of inflammation from bacteria wicking onto the sutures.

Outcomes

When evaluating microsurgical outcomes, only studies of modern microsurgical techniques and materials should be included. Studies have documented that the outcomes using newer endodontic microsurgery techniques tend to be significantly better than with the historical methods that were used in prior studies [76–78, 113–120]. After four years, very few changes in outcome are recorded [118]. The nonoperated roots of mandibular molars developed signs of apical pathosis in 8.1% of the cases [120]. Meta-analyses from different groups have concluded that successful outcomes with modern endodontic microsurgical techniques is in the 91% to 94% range [113–116].

Factors affecting the prognosis of root-end resection

Effect of type of filling material

In 1999, Rubinstein and Kim [78] reported initial healing of 96.8% of cases one year after performing root-end microsurgery with Super EBA root-end fills. In a follow-up study five to seven years after the one-year study, they reported 91.5% of the cases remained healed, but 8.5% of the cases showed apical breakdown [79].

Maddalone and Gagliani [80] in 2003, using modern endodontic microsurgical procedures with Super EBA as a root-end filling material, reported a 92.5% success rate of cases over three years. Chong and colleagues [75] in 2003 reported that a success rate for MTA was 84% at twelve months and 92% at twenty-four months, whereas filling with IRM only had a success rate of 76% at twelve months, and 87% at twenty-four months; however, the difference was not statistically significant.

Von Arx and colleagues [121] in 2010 compared the outcomes of MTA versus composite resin. MTA-treated teeth demonstrated a significantly higher rate of healing (91.3% of cases) compared with Retroplast-treated teeth (79.5%). In 2010 Tang and colleagues [122] did a systematic review to evaluate outcomes when MTA is used as a root-end filling material. From the five studies that met their criteria, they concluded that MTA as a root-end filling material is better than amalgam and gutta-percha and is similar to IRM.

Song and Kim 81] in 2012 did a prospective randomized controlled study of MTA and super EBA as root-end filling materials in endodontic microsurgery. The overall success rate was 94.3%, with a success rate of 95.6% for MTA and 93.1% for super EBA. There was no statistically significant difference between the groups.

Li and colleagues ([123] in a two-year retrospective study in 2014 evaluated the results of microsurgery with super EBA. The overall healing rate was 93.1%. Shinbori and colleagues [124] in 2015 did a retrospective study on the outcome of root-end surgery with EndoSequence BC Root Repair material used as a root-end filling material. At the one-year follow-up, the overall success rate was 92%. Rud and colleagues [125] reported a 97% success rate with an eight-year follow-up using a dentin-bonded composite resin (Retroplast). In a later study, they reported complete healing in 92% of cases using the same composite resin material [126].

Effect of preoperative pain

Von Arx and colleagues [127] in 2010 performed a meta-analysis of the factors that affect the prognosis of apical surgery with root-end filling. They cited a shortage of evidence-based information regarding healing determinants. They found the following factors were significantly associated with higher healed rates: patients without preoperative pain or signs, patients with good density of the root canal filling, and patients with no or a very small periapical lesion (less than 5 mm). They also [128] studied the influence of various predictors on healing outcome after one year. The only factor that reached statistical significance was the presence of pain at the initial presentation. Factors that nearly reached significance were lesion size, root-end filling material, and postoperative healing course.

Effect of prior surgery (resurgery)

Peterson and Gutmann [129] in 2001 did a systematic review of initial apical surgery versus apical resurgery. Most of the articles included were from the 1970s. This meant that the methods in most of the studies were not those used in endodontic microsurgery today. Although success rates were much higher for initial surgeries, the success and uncertain healing categories for resurgeries were close to success rates for initial surgeries.

In 2005 Gagliani and colleagues [130] showed that five years after surgery, 86% of the roots that received a first periapical surgery showed complete healing, and 59% of the roots receiving a resurgery (second periapical surgery) showed complete healing. They still recommended surgical retreatment of teeth previously treated with surgery as a valid alternative to extraction.

Song and colleagues [131] performed a retrospective clinical study on the outcomes of endodontic micro-resurgery. They found an overall success rate of 92.9%. The most common possible causes of failure were no root-end filling and incorrect root-end preparation. The use of microsurgical techniques and biocompatible materials such as MTA and super EBA resulted in a high clinical success rate, even in endodontic resurgery.

Effect of longer-term versus shorter-term recall

Song and colleagues [132] in 2014 compared the clinical outcomes of endodontic microsurgery at one year versus long-term follow-up. They found the overall success rate of cases with four or more years of follow-up was 87.8%, compared with 91.3% at one year of follow-up, which was not statistically significant. Song and colleagues [133] in 2012 found 93.3% of endodontic microsurgery cases that were considered healed in a prior five-year study remained healed after more than six years.

Effect of interproximal bone height

Von Arx and colleagues [133] performed a five-year longitudinal assessment of the prognosis of apical microsurgery. They found the healing rate at five years after apical microsurgery was eight percentage points poorer than when it was assessed at one year (from 83.8% to 75.9%). The prognosis was significantly affected by the interproximal bone levels around the treated tooth. If interproximal bone level was greater than 3 mm from the cementoenamel junction, it healed less often than if it was 3 mm or less. Cases with root-end fillings of ProRoot MTA healed more often than those filled with super EBA.

Effect of the size of the apical lesion

Wang and colleagues [135], as part of the Toronto outcome studies in 2004, reported an overall healed rate of 74%. The healed rate was significantly higher for teeth with small lesions (5 mm or less) and with preoperative root canal fillings that were inadequate in length, either long or short, rather than at an adequate length. Thus, preoperative lesion size and root canal filling length were significant predictors of outcomes for root-end surgery. Not all of the surgeries were completed with modern microsurgical techniques. The effect of lesion size on outcome was also observed in a later Toronto study [136].

Effect of age

Most studies show no effect of the patient's age on the outcome or root-end surgery; however, Barone and colleagues [136], as part of the Toronto outcome studies, found that age did affect endodontic surgical outcomes. Three significant outcome predictors were identified: age, preoperative root-filling length, and the size of the apical crypt. Patients older than 45 years healed 84% of the time, whereas those 45 years of age or younger healed 68% of the time. If the preoperative root canal filling was inadequate, healing was seen in 84% of the cases, whereas those with adequate preoperative filling length healed in 68% of the cases. If the surgical crypt was 10 mm or less, the healing rate was 80%, but if it greater than 10 mm, the healing rate was 53%.

Effect of the length of the access window into the bony crypt

Von Arx and colleagues [137] in 2007 did a prospective study to evaluate how the dimensions of the bone defect affect healing outcomes one year after apical surgery. The only parameter that was found to be significantly related to healing outcome was the length of the access window to the bony crypt.

Summary

In summary, most studies evaluating modern microsurgical techniques have found a healing rate of greater than 90%. A high success rate was observed when modern root-end fillings were placed. The high success rate for endodontic microsurgery makes it a viable treatment option for patients.

Guided tissue regeneration in endodontic surgery

Pecora and colleagues [138] listed the following indications for guided tissue regeneration applications in endodontic surgery:

- Through-and-through periapical lesion
- Large periapical lesion
- Endo-perio lesion
- Periapical lesion communicating with the alveolar crest
- Furcation involvement as a result of a perforation
- Root perforation with bone loss to alveolar crest

Rankow and Krasner [139] listed conditions encountered in endodontic surgery that could require the use of guided tissue regenerative procedures:

- Apical pathosis without communication to the alveolar crest
- Apical pathosis with communication to the alveolar crest (dehiscence, proximal bone loss, developmental grooves)
- Root or furcation bone loss due to perforation
- Cervical root resorption
- Oblique root fractures
- Ridge augmentation

The conditions that most often require guided tissue regeneration in endodontic surgery are apical–marginal bone defects where there is no bone over the root surface from apex to crestal bone; through-and-through defects where the lesion perforates both the facial cortical bone as well as the lingual or palatal cortical plate of bone; and furcation defects from perforations, some large bony defects, and ridge preservation. These conditions are encountered during endodontic surgical therapy, not as independent surgeries that fall within the scope of periodontal practice.

Guided tissue regeneration is based on the principle that specific cells contribute to the formation of specific tissues. It consists of placing barriers of different types to cover the bone and periodontal ligament, thus temporarily separating them from the gingival epithelium. Excluding the epithelium and the gingival connective tissue from the root surface during the postsurgical healing phase not only prevents epithelial migration into the wound but also favors repopulation of the area by cells from the periodontal ligament and the bone.

Guided bone regeneration employs the same principles of specific tissue exclusion as guided tissue regeneration uses. However, because the objective of guided bone regeneration is to regenerate a single tissue, namely bone, it is theoretically easier to accomplish than guided tissue regeneration, which strives to regenerate multiple tissues in a complex relationship.

Barriers, or membranes, used to exclude the faster-growing epithelium from the underlying connective tissue are classified as either resorbable or nonresorbable. Resorbable membranes do not require a second surgery to remove them; nonresorbable membranes do require a second surgery to remove them.

Resorbable membranes may be made from collagen, polylactic acid, polyglycolic acid, or calcium sulfate [138, 139]. Nonresorbable membranes that have been used include polytetrafluorethylene (PTFE or Gore-Tex) membranes [138, 139]. The amount of cross-linking in the membrane structure can affect how rapidly the membrane is turned over and resorbs.

Gortex membranes are no longer available, but the suture still can be purchased. dPTFE membranes (with and without titanium struts for reinforcement) have replaced the Gortex membranes in the marketplace.

Bone grafts

Bone or osseous grafts may be classified by their action on new bone formation. Grafts that act as a template or scaffold to assist in bone formation are classified as *osteoconductive grafts*. Grafts that act to stimulate or induce new bone formation are classified as *osteoinductive grafts*. Grafts that have cells that actually produce new bone are classified as *osteogenic grafts*.

Bone-grafting materials are further classified by their origin. *Autogenous grafts* are the patient's own bone from another site in their body. Autogenous bone is considered the gold standard. Autogenous bone uses osteoconduction, osteoinduction, and osteogenesis in the formation of new bone. Bone can be harvested from iliac crest or from intraoral sites.

Allografts are grafts from another member of the same species; in the case of humans, it is bone from another human. Allografts may be frozen bone, freeze-dried (lyophilized) bone (FDB), demineralized freeze-dried bone (DFDBA), or irradiated bone. It may be ordered as cortical or cancellous bone. Allografts are osteoconductive and osteoinductive. Demineralization removes the mineral phase and exposes the underlying bone collagen and growth factors, particularly bone morphogenetic proteins (BMPs), which induce new bone formation. Combination allografts have recently entered the market place that combine mineralized (70%) and demineralized (30%) bone and have done well in a human ridge preservation study [140].

Xenografts are bone grafts from a different species. Currently, there are two available sources of xenografts used as bone substitutes in clinical practice: bovine bone and natural coral. Both provide products that are biocompatible and structurally similar to human bone. Xenografts are osteoconductive, and their advantage is that they are readily available and almost entirely free of the risk of disease transmission. Materials marketed in the United States are certified that they are derived from animals approved by the US Department of Agriculture (USDA) and should not carry disease.

Alloplasts are grafts from natural or synthetic bone substitutes. They are biocompatible space fillers. Most bone substitutes are osteoconductive, inert filling materials and integrate with new bone; histologically, they produce only limited periodontal regeneration. Included in alloplast graft materials are bioceramics, such as tricalcium phosphate and hydroxyapatite, bioactive glasses, polymers, and calcium sulfate (plaster of Paris).

Bone-grafting materials should only be ordered from a reputable licensed certified tissue bank [141].

Technique

With an apical–marginal defect, the membrane is trimmed so that it extends 2 to 3 mm beyond the margins of the bony defect. The membrane should be at least 2 to 3 mm from the cementoenamel junction [138], so there is no interference with epithelial reattachment. The membrane should be completely covered and not exposed to oral fluids, which would increase the risk of infection [138, 139]. The membrane should be stable and not move when the flap is reapproximated and sutured in place. Once the membrane is trimmed and hydrated in normal saline, it will adapt better because it will be more pliable. This can be accomplished while the bone-grafting material is being placed in the bony defect. Exposed root surfaces that will be contacted with the bone-grafting material should be etched with either 50% citric acid or tetracycline (100 mg/mL) for 3 minutes [138].

The bone-grafting material should be hydrated prior to placing it into the defect. The grafting material is then placed into the bony defect. The roots must be covered with the grafting material to provide space between the root surface and the membrane. It is important to provide this space so that the membrane does not rest upon the root surface, because, if it does, there will be no regeneration of periodontal ligament or bone. The bony defect should be very slightly overfilled (Figure 9.46).

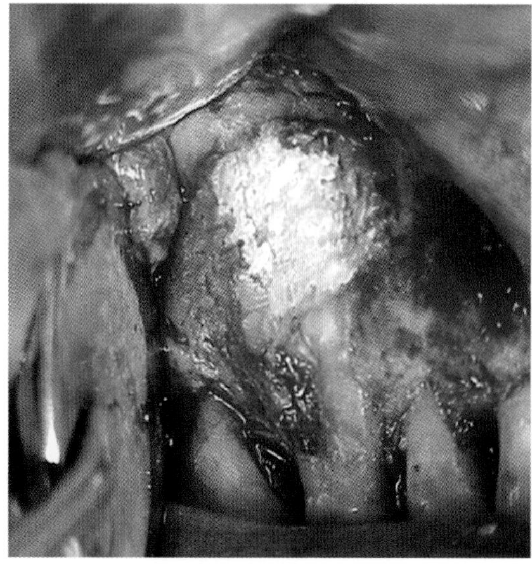

Figure 9.46 Bone-grafting material placed into large periapical defect and over root structure. (Image courtesy of Dr. Dwight Moss.)

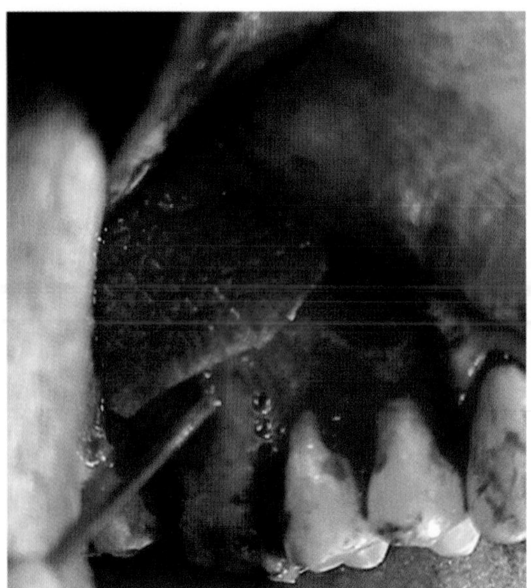

Figure 9.47 A resorbable membrane is placed over the bony defect, which has been filled with a bone-grafting material. The flap is replaced, held in place, and then sutured in place. (Image courtesy of Dr. Dwight Moss.)

The hydrated membrane is now placed over the graft material with the membrane edges covering the edges of the bony defect by at least 2 mm and not encroaching on the cementoenamel junction or the biological width [138, 139]. The membrane should be stable as the flap is repositioned and sutured, so that it will not move during suturing or the healing phase. This ensures that the membrane will be in place and exclude epithelium from areas where connective tissue needs to re-form (Figure 9.47).

Regeneration of through-and-through bony defects is similar to apical–marginal bone defects, except an additional membrane is required on the palatal or lingual aspect of the bony defect. Radiographic evidence or CBCT imaging may indicate a through-and-through lesion. The radiographic image will show a lesion within a lesion if there is a through-and-through lesion. The CBCT will show a loss of cortical bone or a break in the cortical bone on both sides of lesion. When a through-and-through defect is suspected from periapical radiographs or CBCT, after completion of the root-end resection, preparation, and fill, the palatal (or lingual) bone in the bony crypt should be sounded with a sharp instrument to determine the size of the perforation of the bone. This can also be confirmed by going through the perforation of the cortical plate and having the sharp instrument penetrate the palatal (or lingual) mucosa.

Once the size of the perforation is determined, a membrane can be trimmed to cover the opening in the palatal (or lingual) bone. The membrane should extend over the margins of the defect by at least 2 mm. Additionally, a membrane must be trimmed for the opening of the defect on the facial side. The exposed root surfaces should be etched with either citric acid or tetracycline solution. Both membranes are hydrated. The palatal (or lingual) opening in the cortical bone is covered with the membrane. The hydrated bone-grafting material is then placed into the defect and built up to the facial cortical plate. The membrane for the facial opening of the bony defect is placed after that, covering the lesion by at least 2 mm and resting on solid cortical bone. The flap is replaced and sutured back into place. Pecora and colleagues [142] found improved outcomes of root-end surgeries with the use of calcium sulfate for bone regeneration.

Calcium sulfate can be used as a bone-grafting material, as well as a membrane. It may also be used in combination with bone allograft material. If the two materials are mixed, the ratio is usually 80% bone grafting material and 20% calcium sulfate [139]. If calcium sulfate is used as both the bone-grafting material and the membrane, the procedure is similar to other grafting procedures. The exposed root surface is scaled and root planed, and all granulation tissue is removed from the bony crypt. The roots are etched with 50% citric acid, ethylenediamenetetraacetic acid (EDTA), or tetracycline solution. The bony defect is filled with calcium sulfate or a combination of calcium sulfate and bone. The material is then pressed into the defect with gauze. A second layer of pure calcium sulfate is then placed over the previous layer to very slightly overfill the defect. This second layer of calcium sulfate serves as a membrane. The flap is replaced and sutured in place.

It is best to not manipulate the flap too much because the calcium sulfate is somewhat brittle, and it could fracture and then move under the flap. The patient should also be instructed, during postoperative instructions, to not touch the flap with any pressure because this could also fracture the calcium sulfate.

The benefit of using guided tissue regeneration techniques in large periapical lesions is not fully decided because of conflicting evidence. Murashima and colleagues [143] found that calcium sulfate was effective in bone regeneration on large osseous defects and on through-and-through osseous defects. It was less effective in osseous defects communicating with the gingival sulcus. Tobon and colleagues [144] found the use of regenerative materials, such as nonbioresorbable membranes and resorbable hydroxyapatite improved the predictability of clinical, radiographic, and histological healing in cases of regenerative techniques following periapical surgery. Garret and colleagues [145], however, found that the use of a resorbable guided tissue regeneration membrane with a four-walled osseous defect confined to the apical region did not improve healing.

Ridge preservation

Ridge preservation or site preservation after an extraction can be a valuable service for a patient who has to lose a tooth. For the endodontist, this can occur after an exploratory surgery determines there is a vertical root fracture or when an endodontically treated tooth is deemed unsalvageablei during a root-end surgery. Tooth extraction will lead to loss of alveolar bone, which will affect prosthodontic restoration of either a fixed or removable partial denture or of a dental implant. The tooth should be extracted as atraumatically as possible to preserve cortical plates of bone. A membrane is then trimmed to cover the extraction site. The size of the membrane depends on the amount of bone lost prior to the extraction or as a result of the extraction. It may only need to cover the socket, if it has been a flapless extraction, or it might need to cover the socket, as well as the missing cortical plate of bone. It may be necessary to undermine the gingival attachments in order to get the membrane to lie down over the socket.

The bone-grafting material of choice is hydrated and placed in the socket. It is often better to place the bone graft in a tuberculin syringe with an end cut off, so it can be compacted tighter than other grafting sites are packed. Collagen products (CollaPlug, Zimmer Biomet, Warsaw, IN, USA) may be placed in the socket before the grafting material in some cases to occupy space and promote healing. The membrane is placed over the bone-grafting material and sutured in place to cover the grafting material. The suturing may need to cross the membrane in a figure-of-eight or X shape to hold the membrane in place.

As another option, calcium sulfate can be mixed with the grafting bone in an 80% bone and 20% calcium sulfate mix. The mixture is then placed into the socket. Calcium sulfate without the bone can then be placed as a membrane over the grafting material mix. The choice of grafting material—FDB, DFDBA, bovine bone, or synthetic graft material—depends on the preference of the patient and the surgeon, whether the surgeon wishes to have more rapid bone turnover or slower bone turnover, and the type of bone being regenerated.

Often during guided tissue regeneration procedures, a periosteal releasing incision is required to free the mucoperiosteal flap enough so that there can be adequate coverage of the membrane and bone graft. The procedure is to stretch the mucoperiosteal flap in an apical direction to put tension on the flap. The extent of the reflection and length of vertical releasing incisions should be noted. Only the periosteal tissue is incised. The alveolar mucosa is not incised, and great care must be taken to avoid cutting or perforating the entire mucoperiosteal flap. Once the periosteum is cut, the flap can be extended enough to cover the membrane and graft. This is a technically difficult procedure, but it is one that should be mastered to avoid exposing the membrane.

Extraction–Replantation

Extraction–replantation, intentional replantation, or replantation are all terms for treating a tooth that cannot be treated by other means. It is generally reserved for teeth where surgical access would be difficult, non-healing lesions, or patient limitations that prevent conventional root-end surgery. The procedure calls for atraumatic extraction of a tooth, and then submergence into Hank's balanced salt solution (HBSS) where root-end resection, root-end preparation, and root-end filling is completed. The tooth is then replanted back into the socket.

Kratchman [146] listed several indications for extraction–replantation procedures. They include difficult access, anatomic limitations, inaccessible perforations, patients' limitations, failure to heal, and chronic pain.

Teeth with *difficult access* include mandibular second molars because the apices of these roots are more lingual in the mandible. Thick buccal bone and the external oblique ridge also interfere with access. Access to the apices of this tooth is extremely challenging because locating and instrumenting through a deep tunnel in bone is very demanding.

Anatomic limitations include a mandibular premolar that is in very close proximity to the mental foramen and mandibular molars that are in very close proximity to the inferior alveolar canal [146].

Perforations in areas not accessible surgically include the proximal surface of tooth in the interdental area or in a furcation [146].

Patient management and limitations can prevent disabled patients from being able to undergo endodontic microsurgical procedures or to maintain the position required for the surgeon to use the microscope. Extraction–replantation is a much shorter procedure than endodontic microscopic root-end surgery [2, 146].

Failure to heal after endodontic therapy, nonsurgical retreatment, or surgical endodontic procedures is another reason for extraction–replantation. Any evidence of persistent disease, such as pain, sinus tract, swelling, or radiographic evidence that the lesion is not healing would be an indication for extraction–replantation if the tooth could not be treated by the more conventional methods [2, 146].

Persistent chronic pain can be an indication for extraction–replantation, if other treatment methods have been unsuccessful, and there is a good reason to believe that there is an endodontic cause that cannot be addressed in any other manner [146].

Contraindications for extraction–replantation include preexisting moderate to severe periodontal disease, curved or flared roots, nonrestorable teeth, and cases where there is missing interseptal bone [147].

It is important to explain the procedure to the patient and to present the risks and benefits of the procedure. The risk of fracture and resorption should be explained, as well as the understanding that if the procedure is not performed the tooth would probably have to be extracted.

Procedure

One of the critical steps in the extraction–replantation procedure is atraumatically extracting the tooth and avoiding damage to the cementum or fracturing the tooth. Evaluation of the root form of the tooth is important. Teeth with fused roots are generally good candidates, unless they have interseptal bone. Teeth with straight roots and a furcation where bone is present are good candidates. Teeth with wide and/or dilacerated roots are poor candidates for extraction–replantation because it is difficult to extract without fracturing them.

Extraction–replantation procedures have been refined to follow many of the principles in the dental traumatology literature for the avulsed tooth. Historically, extraction–replantation procedures had to be completed as rapidly as possible to avoid extended extraoral dry time, which would increase the chances of replacement resorption. Antibiotics are used to reduce the likelihood of inflammatory resorption in both management of the avulsed tooth and in extraction–replantation.

Before the extraction–replantation procedure, it is important to make sure the crown of the tooth is solid and restored, to reduce the susceptibility to fracture during extraction. The occlusal surface of the tooth should be relieved, so the tooth has little or no occlusal contact.

It is necessary to be organized before and during extraction–replantation procedures to limit extraoral time. Instruments and materials required for the procedure should be in order, and the HBSS should be placed in two emesis basins. If a stainless steel emesis basin is used, 2 × 2 gauze should be placed on the bottom of the basin to prevent reflection of light back through the microscope, which would be too bright for the surgeon's eyes. A sterilized rubber band is placed over the handle of the extraction forceps, ensuring the forceps beaks will stay closed once the tooth is extracted. This allows the tooth to be held in the forceps for the entire procedure while the tooth is out of the mouth [146].

The extraction should be a slow, deliberate procedure. The gingival attachment must be severed with a surgical blade. Elevators and periotomes should not be used to elevate against the root of the tooth. Likewise, the beaks of the forceps should be kept off of the cementum on the root above the cementoenamel junction. This increases the chance of fracture of the crown during extraction, but it decreases the chance of resorption developing later. It is important to be patient during the extraction, because expanding the cortical plates of bone is a slow and deliberate process. The procedure can take 20 to 30 minutes [146]. Once the tooth is extracted, it should immediately be transferred to one of the basins containing the HBSS. The root surface should never be touched.

If there is a cyst or granuloma attached to the root and it comes out with the tooth, the socket does not need to be curetted. Even if granulation tissue remains in the socket, nothing should be curetted from the socket. It will heal once the etiology is removed from the canal of the tooth [2]. The socket should be gently irrigated with HBSS or normal saline to keep the periodontal ligament cells moist and nourished.

Under the surgical operating microscope, the root-end procedures should be completed while keeping the tooth root moist with HBSS. If the extraction–replantation is to correct another problem, such as repairing a perforation, that procedure should be completed while the root surface is kept moist with the HBSS.

When the root-end procedure is completed, the tooth can be rinsed with HBSS from the "clean" basin. The tooth is then replanted back into its socket. Due to the root-end resection and the expansion of the cortical plates of bone, it is generally easy to replant the tooth. Once the tooth is back in the socket, the facial and lingual (or palatal) cortical plates of bone are compressed and the patient is asked to bite on a cotton roll or a wooden stick to insure the tooth is seated properly and stabilized [146]. Splinting is often not required because the tooth usually snaps into place. The tooth should be in minimal or no occlusion; however, slight occlusal function will speed healing. If splinting is required, it should be minimal, such as sutures crossed over the occlusal surface, or a periodontal pack [146]. If a splint is used, it should be flexible and removed within one week [148]. Borrowing from the dental traumatology literature, a flexible splint produces the best outcome [149]. To be consistent with dental traumatology guidelines [149], tetracycline, penicillin, or amoxicillin for one week should be prescribed to help prevent inflammatory resorption, although definitive human studies are lacking on their benefit. The patient should follow a soft dental diet for one to two weeks and should be instructed in home oral hygiene care to keep the area clean.

The most common reason for a poor outcome of extraction–replantation procedures is resorption, either replacement or inflammatory in nature. Other negative outcomes include periapical rarefaction due to periapical inflammation, chronic pain, or fracture of the crown or root [146].

Most failures occur during the first year [150]. Fortunately, there is a favorable outcome in most studies, although the success rates and techniques are varied. There have not been studies using the techniques recommended by Kratchman [146]. The success rate for extraction–replantation using older studies range from 80% to 95% [151–153]. These outcomes make extraction–replantation a viable option in carefully selected cases.

Root amputations and hemisection techniques in endodontics

Although the topic for root amputations and hemisections of molars are now less common due to the success of osteointegrated implants, there are still cases when these techniques are the best option for a patient. This is especially true in teeth with endodontic involvement.

Root amputation is the removal of one or more roots of a multirooted tooth. The involved root is separated at the junction of the root and the crown. In general, this procedure is performed in maxillary molars. *Hemisection* is the surgical division of a multirooted tooth. The defective or periodontally involved root and that part of the crown are then removed. *Bicuspidization* is the surgical division of a mandibular molar (as in a hemisection), but the crown and root of both halves of the tooth are retained.

Teeth requiring root resections, should have adequate endodontic treatment before the root resection. The root canal in the root to be resected should be filled with either amalgam or a composite resin to the level where the resection will be made. Gutta-percha does not provide an adequate seal in the resected root because it will be exposed to oral fluids. It is essential that there is a restorative plan for the proper coronal restoration of teeth undergoing respective procedures.

Indications [154–157] and contraindications [155–158] for root resection are listed in Box 9.4. Indications [154–156] and contraindications [154, 155] for bicuspidization are listed in Box 9.5.

Mandibular molars that require resective treatment should almost always only be treated by hemisection or bicuspidization, because a root amputation leaves an unfavorable leverage situation on the remaining root and will lead to fracture of the tooth [156].

Box 9.4 Indications and contraindications for root resection

Indications for root resection [154–157]

- There is a severe osseous defect around one root that is not amenable to traditional or regenerative therapy, but there is adequate bone support on the adjacent root or roots.
- There is grade II or III horizontal furcation involvement with minimal bone loss on roots to be retained.
- There is close root proximity to a root on an adjacent tooth.
- A root cannot be treated with restoration owing to severe caries, perforation, or resorption.
- There is a vertical root fracture.
- There is an endodontically untreatable root due to obstructed canal or separated instrument.
- A strategically important root (or roots) and crown can be preserved.

Contraindications to root resection [155–158]

- The tooth is not restorable or not strategic.
- There is unfavorable anatomy, such as fused roots or a tall root trunk.
- There is excessive mobility that did not improve after initial therapy.
- There is a poor crown-to-root ratio on the remaining root(s).
- The adjacent teeth mesial and distal to the affected tooth have large restorations that might warrant a three-unit fixed bridge.
- Nonsurgical root canal therapy cannot be completed on the remaining root(s).
- There are patient risk factors such as poor plaque control, or the patient is a smoker.
- An implant or a three-unit bridge is a better option for the patient.

Box 9.5 Indications and contraindications for bicuspidization

Indications for bicuspidization [154–157]

- There is a furcation perforation.
- There is a furcation defect from periodontal disease.
- There is a fracture into the furcation.

Contraindications for bicuspidization [154, 155]

The mesial or the distal segment is not restorable or has a poor periodontal prognosis.
Root canal treatment cannot be completed on either half of the tooth.
The roots are fused or the furcation is too far apical.

The type of flap that should be reflected depends on how difficult it will be to section and remove the root to be resected, how much access is needed, and how much bone loss is present. Often, bone has to be removed in order to deliver the resected root. This requires more access than an envelope flap would allow.

Root amputations

Amputation of a root of a maxillary molar may be accomplished by one of two techniques. If a new crown is to be placed, a vertical root amputation can be used. This has the advantage of having a crown placed that will more closely match the support from the remaining roots, and it will have a more favorable contour for cleansing. The vertical root amputation can require less removal of bone if the resected root can be removed by forceps. This procedure has also been called a *trisection* [157] (Figure 9.48). A second technique used for root amputations is a horizontal resection, where the root is resected at the furcation level apical to the crown. This technique is employed when the coronal restoration will be left in place. Buccal and palatal mucoperiosteal

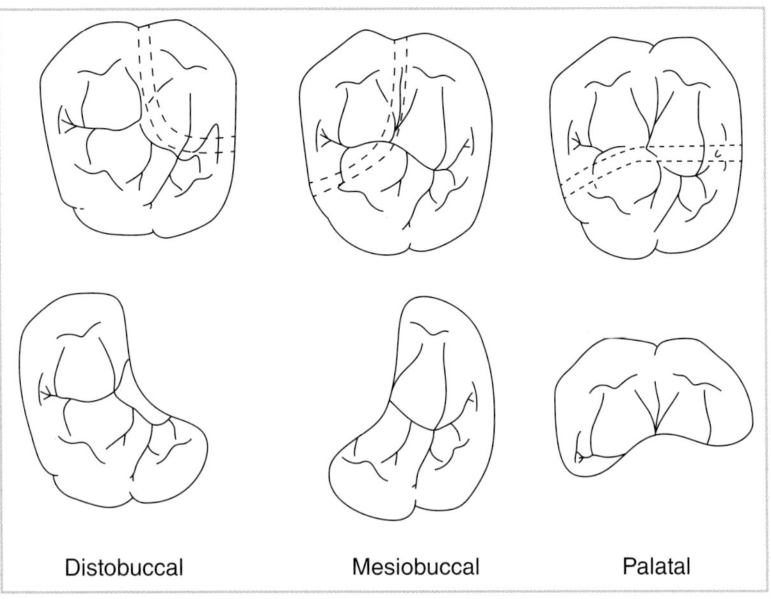

Figure 9.48 The occlusal view of crown shapes after vertical root amputations. The crown shape will resemble the remaining root structure after root amputation of the other root. (Adapted from Newell DH, Morgano SM, Baima RF. Fixed prosthodontics with periodontally compromised dentitions. In: Malone WFP, Koch DL, editors. *Tylman's theory and practice of fixed prosthodontics*. 8th ed. St Louis: Ishiyaky EuroAmerica;1989 pp 80–1.) [158]

flaps are reflected, which provides access to the involved tooth and the osseous structures as well [157].

Vertical Root Amputation

In vertical root amputation, a buccal and palatal mucoperiosteal flap is elevated to improve access to the involved tooth and osseous structures [157]. A silver point or stainless steel wire can be threaded through the furcation area, if possible, to outline the affected root to be resected. If not, marker cuts can be placed at the furcation entrances and extended coronally. A rubber dam is placed, and coronal cuts are made to connect the silver point furcation exits. Most of the root-amputation procedure should be accomplished with rubber dam isolation to prevent debris from contaminating the wound site. The cuts with a surgical-length fissure bur, or an Endo Z bur, are made more on the portion of the tooth to be removed and are gradually moved toward the furcation. The cuts are on the portion of the crown over the root to be removed. From the occlusal view, the cut will resemble a C shape extending from the buccal furcation to the interproximal furcation [157, 158].

Once the bur cuts into the furcation, the root is separated from the rest of the tooth. Care must be taken when approaching the furcation. A non–end-cutting bur, such as an Endo Z bur (Dentsply International, York, PA), may be used to avoid cutting too deep. The root can now be removed with a periosteal elevator or extraction forceps [157].

The tooth is contoured and refined to ensure that there is not a spur left in the furcation area from the incomplete resection of the root in the furcation area. This should be confirmed with a radiograph. The bone should be recontoured so the bony contours match the tooth contours, which allows reattachment of the supracrestal attachment apparatus and 3 mm of biologic width [157]. The reflected flaps are then sutured into place, and postoperative instructions are given, along with any prescription for pain control. It is important to have a definite restorative commitment to place a crown to match the root structure left after the vertical root amputation, before attempting a vertical root amputation.

Horizontal Root Amputation

A full-thickness flap should be elevated on both the facial and palatal surfaces to provide access to the root. All visible granulomatous tissue is removed from the area. Some cortical bone might need to be removed to facilitate root delivery. A silver point or stainless steel wire can be threaded through the furcation area, if possible, to outline the affected root to be resected. If not, marker cuts can be placed at the furcation entrances and extended coronally. Threading of a silver point or a stainless steel wire through the furcation entrances is not possible in teeth with normal periodontal support.

A tapered or straight small fissure bur is used to separate the root in the furcal area with copious sterile saline irrigation. A horizontal cut is made from the proximal side of the root to the furcation, apical to the crown. As the cut approaches the furcation, especially in the palatal areas, a non–end-cutting bur, such as an Endo Z bur, can be used to avoid unwanted cuts in bone or other roots. The root is delivered with elevators.

Sometimes additional bone needs to be removed in order to extract the root. Ensure there are no furcal overhangs or spurs and that proper crown shape is achieved [154, 156, 157]. This should be verified radiographically (Figure 9.49). There should be no sharp edges, and all surfaces should be rounded and shaped to enhance cleansing. This is very important for oral hygiene and final prosthodontic restoration. The flaps are repositioned and sutured to provide closure.

Hemisection

Hemisection involves sectioning and removing either the mesial or the distal root of a mandibular molar. In most cases, a buccal and a lingual flap should be elevated. The lingual flap can be an envelope flap. The buccal flap in some instances can be an envelope flap; however, a triangular or rectangular flap will be required if the root cannot be extracted with forceps.

The two buccal grooves and the lingual groove on the crown do not conform to the underlying root

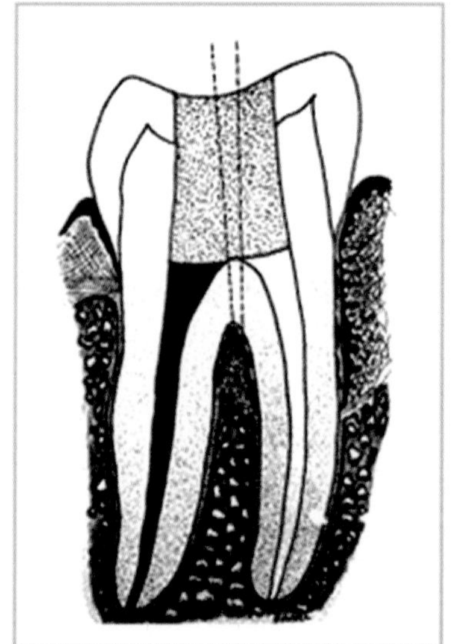

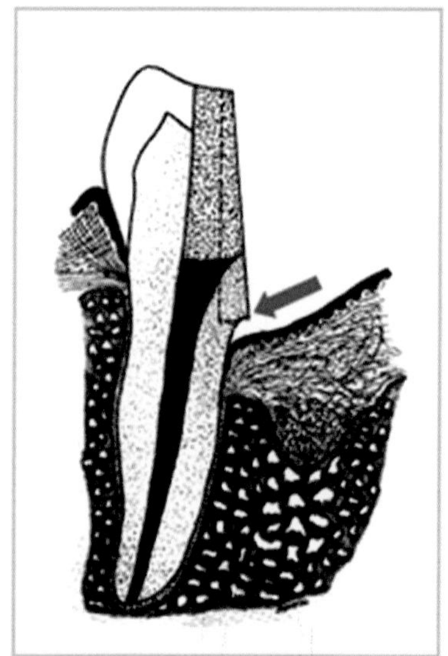

Tylman's

Figure 9.49 Hemisection of a mandibular molar. The arrow on the right diagram is pointing to a spur left after resection in the furcation. It is important to remove this overhang in all root resections, because it can be a site for plaque accumulation and makes it difficult for the patient to clean the area.

structure; therefore, a silver point or stainless steel wire is placed through the furcation from the lingual to the buccal side, which indicates correct vertical cut positions. Extend the vertical cuts apically through the furcation, cheating toward the root to be extracted. An orientation radiograph may be required before complete hemisection. After separation, the silver point may be withdrawn occlusally. Forceps can be used to deliver the root. It the root cannot be easily removed, the buccal cortical bone is removed to facilitate extraction of the root. Once the root is removed, the edges of the resection are smoothed, and overhangs or a spur at the furcation is removed. If bone had to be removed to extract the root, the bony edges are rounded and smoothed.

Bicuspidization

The technique for bicuspidization is very similar to the technique used for hemisection of a tooth, but neither root is removed. They are merely separated through the furcation. It requires skill because neither root can be encroached upon, as they both will receive crowns. Hence, enough tooth structure needs to remain. Indications are more limited for bicuspidization.

The outcome for resection of roots depends upon how the tooth is used, how it will be loaded, and the maintenance of periodontal health around the tooth. A more negative outcome can be expected if a tooth with a resected root is expected to serve as an abutment. Outcome studies show a wide percentage of successful outcomes for teeth with resected roots.

Blomlof and colleagues [159] found that at ten years, 68% of root-resected molars and 77% of root-filled single-rooted teeth remained in the mouth. Root resection appears to have a similar prognosis to single rooted teeth that are equally susceptible to periodontitis. Langer and colleagues [160] found that 38% of molar root resections failed during a ten-year period (2:1 ratio of mandibular-to-maxillary failures). Basten and collegues [161] found that the prognosis for root-resected molars may be better than previously thought, because this retrospective study showed 49 root-resected molars had a 92% survival rate over 12 years. Fugazzoto [162] found that root-resected molars showed a 96.8% success rate for up to 15 years of follow-up, and implants yielded a success rate of 97% in up to 13 years of follow-up. These therapies are not interchangeable and must be carefully considered in treatment-planning decisions. In selected cases, the success of root resections is high enough to justify the procedure.

Surgical repair of resorptive lesions or perforations

Management of resorptive defects is covered in the chapter on resorption. Repair of external resorptive defects or external repair of root perforations requires reflecting a mucoperiosteal flap to gain access to the defect. Often an envelope flap is sufficient to access defects in the cervical area of a root. Defects located more apically on the root require a triangular or rectangular flap design to achieve adequate reflection of the flap and proper access to the defect.

MTA or newer bioceramics work well, if the perforation is below crestal bone and does not communicate with the oral cavity. In areas where the defect is exposed to oral fluids and there is a risk of the restorative material washing out, a composite resin or glass ionomer would be the appropriate restorative material.

Management of Complications

Kim [2] lists surgical sequelae and complications after root-end surgery. Surgical sequelae are part of the normal surgical procedure and postoperative course. Included in postoperative sequelae are pain, hemorrhage, swelling, and ecchymosis. Complications from root-end surgery include maxillary sinus infringement and perforation, lacerations, paresthesia, and serious infection [2].

Pain occurs after any surgical procedure, but after endodontic microsurgery it is only mild to moderate in most cases. Pain can be managed in most cases by administering long-acting local anesthetics such as bupivacaine and using a flexible pain strategy of ibuprofen, acetaminophen, and narcotic medications, depending on the severity of pain.

Hemorrhage is a rare problem and can usually be prevented by good suturing technique and pressure with a 2 × 2 gauze moistened with saline after the flap has been sutured in place. Ice packs also decrease bleeding when held in place with some pressure. Postoperative instructions will allay the patient's fears about slight oozing of blood versus heavy bleeding.

Swelling is common after root-end surgery. The patient should be informed that swelling is very likely, and that it may be worse the day after surgery. Ecchymosis is caused by the extravasation and breakdown of blood in the subcutaneous tissues. This discoloration in the face or neck areas is more likely to occur in fair-skinned patients and the elderly, but it can occur in any patient [2]. It also may occur in patients on anticoagulant or aspirin therapy. It is not a serious problem, except esthetically for the patient, and it will resolve in a few days.

Paresthesia after surgery occurs most often when the inferior alveolar nerve is involved due to impingement, incorrect handling, laceration, severance, or chemical injury. Fortunately, unless the nerve is completely cut and not reapproximated or severely burned with a chemical, the paresthesia will be transitory and should return within 4 weeks [2]. The surgeon should chart the extent of the paresthesia and record it in the patient's record. In the event of a completely severed nerve, the patient should be referred to a oral maxillofacial surgeon.

It is fairly common to have a *perforation of the maxillary sinus* when performing root-end surgery in the maxillary posterior teeth because the sinus lies close to roots of the maxillary molars and premolars, especially the mesial buccal root of the second molar, the palatal root of the first molar, and the distal buccal root of the second molar [163].

Oberli and colleagues [164] found that perforation of the Schneiderian membrane of the maxillary sinus during root-end surgery occurred in 9.6% of the root-end surgeries. Exposure of the membrane without rupture occurred in 12% of the cases. It was found that the distance between the apex or the periapical lesion and the sinus floor did not predict a possible sinus membrane rupture. However, if the radiograph showed a distinct distance between the lesion and the sinus floor, there was an 82.5% probability that oral antral communication would not occur. Friedman and Horowitz [165] found in a review of 472 such procedures that the occurrence of sinus perforations was 10.4% (23% in molars, 13% in second premolars, and 2% in first premolars). This low incidence, coupled with no recorded sinusitis, favors this treatment before extraction, but it demands meticulous surgical technique and appropriate postoperative care.

Sinus perforation occurs in many cases of root-end surgery involving maxillary posterior teeth. Radiographs and CBCT imaging can give the surgeon an idea of the proximity of the root apex to the maxillary sinus. Perforation of the sinus is a very manageable condition, and the endodontic microsurgeon should be equipped to handle this complication.

Confirmation of a sinus perforation can be verified visually under the microscope or by squeezing the patient's nose and having the patient blow out. Air bubbles will be visible coming from the perforation if the sinus floor has been perforated. Preventing the introduction of debris from tooth fragments or root-end filling materials into the maxillary sinus should a perforation occur is the first consideration. In larger perforations, a suture should be placed through a CollaPlug, leaving two long ends of the suture on either side of the CollaPlug. Attention must be paid to the condition of the CollaPlug, because as it absorbs more moisture and blood, it will decrease in size and become less rigid and could tear or disintegrate easily. Although it is not a problem if the CollaPlug disintegrates and falls into the maxillary sinus, because it will be resorbed, it would be better to remove the CollaPlug if it becomes too small or not structurally sound so as to prevent debris from entering the maxillary sinus. The CollaPlug can be easily removed when the root-end surgery is completed and before closing the flap.

Tataryn and colleagues [166] in an animal study found that sinus perforations during root-end surgery showed that defects, regardless of their size, tended to repair with limited bony covering and fibrous scar. Resorbable collagen membranes did not improve osseous repair. Because sinus perforations that occur during root-end surgery are closed off from the oral cavity once the flap is closed, there is no communication between the maxillary sinus and the oral cavity. This is unlike when a sinus perforation occurs during an extraction and there is an open socket that provides an opening into the oral cavity and creates an oral antral fistula. According to Watzek and colleagues [167], antral perforations that occur during root-end surgery constitute no risk to the maxillary sinus, even if a transantral approach was used.

After closing and suturing the mucoperiosteal flap in cases where there has been a sinus perforation, the patient should be given postoperative instructions that inform them that they may experience some evidence of bleeding from nasal discharges, but no frank bleeding will be noted. The patient is instructed not to blow their nose and to elevate the head at night [2]. Lin and colleaguges [168] recommended antihistamines, nasal drops such as 0.5% phenylephrine (Neo-Synephrine), and antibiotics if signs of a maxillary sinus infection are seen. The AAA management of sinus exposure calls for *a*ntihistamines, *a*nalgesics, and *a*ntibiotics. Waiting to see if any signs or symptoms of maxillary rhinosinusitis develop before prescribing any of these medications is also a very plausible option.

Lacerations can accidently occur during surgery. If they require closure, they may be sutured. *Cracks* around the corners of the mouth can occur due to the stretching of tissues. These can be prevented, or certainly lessened, if a thin layer of petroleum jelly is applied to these areas preoperatively [2].

Postoperative infection can occur with any surgery. Swelling into fascial spaces should be closely monitored, and appropriate therapy should be rendered, including incision and drainage and drain placement, antibiotics, and other supportive care. Appropriate referral should be made to an oral maxillofacial surgeon or a hospital emergency department in cases of the most serious and highest risk fascial space infections, including those that can obstruct an airway, spread to the cavernous sinus, or progress into cervical spaces.

Conclusions

Endodontic microsurgery has provided patients and endodontists with the possibility of very good outcomes. Patients may retain their natural teeth due to the skill of the endodontic microsurgeon and the precise instrumentation afforded by microsurgical techniques. Endodontic microsurgical procedures offer the patient a valuable option.

Endodontic microsurgeons must become proficient in the various microsurgical techniques through training and experience in order to provide their patients the very best care available. Continued advancements in technology will make outcomes even more predicable for our patients.

Disclaimer

The views expressed in this chapter are those of the authors and do not necessarily reflect the official policy or position of the Department of the Navy, Department of the Army, Department of Defense, or the US government.

References

1 Merino EM. *Magnifying the surgical field with an operation microscope: Endodontic microsurgery*. London: Quintessence Publishing, 2009. pp. 5–32.
2 Kim S. *Color atlas of microsurgery in endodontics*. Philadelphia: WB Saunders; 2001.
3 Gutmann JL, Harrison JW. *Surgical endodontics*. Boston: Blackwell Scientific Publications; 1991.
4 McDonald NJ, Torabinejad M. Endodontic surgery. In: Walton RE, Torabinejad M, editors. *Principles and practice of endodontics*. Philadelphia: WB Saunders; 2002. pp. 424–444.
5 Morrow SG, Rubenstein RA. Endodontic surgery. *Endodontics*. 5th ed. Hamilton, Ontario: BC Decker; 2002. pp. 669–745.
6 Little JW, Falace DA, Miller CS, Rhodus NL. Acquired bleeding and hypercoagulable disorders. In: Little JW, Falace DA, Miller CS, Rhodus NL, editors. *Dental management of the medically compromised patient*. 8th ed. St. Louis: Elsevier Mosby; 2013. p;. 409–36.
7 Little JW, Falace DA, Miller CS, Rhodus NL. Congenital bleeding and hypercoagulable disorders. In: Little JW, Falace DA, Miller CS, Rhodus NL, editors. *Dental management of the medically compromised patient*. 8th ed. St. Louis: Mosby Elsevier; 2013. p. 437–58.
8 Beirne OR. Evidence to continue oral anticoagulant therapy for ambulatory oral surgery. *J Oral Maxillofac Surg* 2005; 63: 540–545.
9 Karsli ED, Erdogan O, Esen E, Acarturk E. Comparison of the effects of warfarin and heparin on bleeding caused by dental extraction: a clinical study. *J Oral Maxillofac Surg* 2011; 69: 2500–2507.
10 Krishnan B, Shenoy NA, Alexander M. Exodontia and antiplatelet therapy. *J Oral Maxillofac Surg* 2008; 66: 2063–2066.
11 Napenas JJ, Oost FC, DeGroot A, Loven B, Hong CH, Brennan MT, et al. Review of postoperative bleeding risk in dental patients on antiplatelet therapy. *Oral Surg Oral Med Oral Pathol Oral Radiol* 2013; 115: 491–499.
12 Bajkin BV, Popovic SL, Selakovic SD. Randomized, prospective trial comparing bridging therapy using low-molecular-weight heparin with maintenance of oral anticoagulation during extraction of teeth. *J Oral Maxillofac Surg* 2009; 67: 990–995.

13 Ang-Lee MK, Moss J, Yuan CS. Herbal Medicines and perioperative care. *J Am Med Assoc* 2001; 286: 208–216.

14 Cohan RP, Jacobsen PL. Herbal supplements: considerations in dental practice. *J Calif Dent Assoc* 2000; 28: 600–610.

15 Drugs.com. Medications for herbal supplementation. http://www.drugs.com/condition/herbal-supplementation.html.

16 MedlinePlus. Herbal medicine. https://www.nlm.nih.gov/medlineplus/herbalmedicine.html.

17 University of Maryland Medical Center. Herbal medicine. http://umm.edu/health/medical/altmed/treatment/herbal-medicine.

18 Little JW, Falace DA, Miller CS, Rhodus NL. Drugs used in complementary and alternative medicine of potential importance in dentistry. In: Little JW, Falace DA, Miller CS, Rhodus NL, editors. *Dental management of the medically compromised patient*. St Louis: Elsevier Mosby; 2013. pp. 624–630.

19 Buckley JA, Ciarcio SE, McMullen JA. Efficacy of epinephrine concentration in local anesthesia during periodontal surgery. *J Periodontol* 1984; 55: 653–657.

20 Malamed SF. Clinical action of specific agents. In: Malamed SF, editor. *Handbook of local anesthesia*. St. Louis: Mosby; 1997. pp. 49–75.

21 Niemczyk SP. Essential of endodontic microsurgery. *Dent Clin North Am* 2010; 54: 375–399.

22 Rubinstein R. The anatomy of the surgical operating microscope and operating positions. *Dent Clin North Am* 1997; 41: 391–414.

23 Grandi C, Pacifici L. The ratio in choosing access flap for surgical endodontics: a review. *Oral Implantol* 2009; 2(1): 37–52.

24 Johnson BR, Fayad MI, Witherspoon DE. Periradicular surgery. In: Hargreave KM, Cohen S, editors. *Cohen's pathways of the pulp*. 10th ed. St. Louis: Mosby Elsevier; 2011. pp. 720–776.

25 Morrmann W, Ciancio SG. Blood supply of human gingiva following periodontal surgery. A fluorescein angiographic study. *J Periodontol* 1977; 48: 681–692.

26 Velvart P, Peters CI. Soft tissue management in endodontic surgery. *J Endod* 2005; 31: 4–16.

27 Kramper BJ, Kaminski EJ, Osetek EM, Heuer MA. A comparative study of the wound healing of three types of flap design used in periapical surgery. *J Endod* 1984; 10: 17–25.

28 Velvart P. Papilla base incision: a new approach to recession-free healing of the interdental papilla after endodontic surgery. *Int Endod J* 2002; 35: 453–460.

29 Velvart P, Ebner-Zimmermann U, Ebner JP. Comparison of papilla healing following sulcular full-thickness flap and papilla base flap in endodontic surgery. *Int Endod J* 2003; 36: 653–659.

30 Velvart P, Ebner-Zimmermann U, Ebner JP. Comparison of long-term papilla healing following sulcular full thickness flap and papilla base flap in endodontic surgery. *Int Endod J* 2004; 37: 687–693.

31 Abella F, de Ribot J, Doria G, Duran-Sindreu F, Roig M. Applications of piezoelectric surgery in endodontic surgery: a literature review. *J Endod* 2014; 40: 325–332.

32 Lin LM, Gaengler P, Langeland K. Periradicular curettage. *Int Endod J* 1996; 29: 220–227.

33 Lin L, Langeland K. Innervation of the inflammatory periapical lesions. *Oral Surg* 1981; 51: 535–543.

34 Bhaskar SN. Periapical lesions: types, incidence and clinical features. *Oral Surg* 1966; 21: 657–671.

35 Lalonde ER, Luebke RG. The frequency and distribution of periapical cysts and granulomas: an evaluation of 800 specimens. *Oral Surg* 1968; 25: 861–868.

36 Spatafore CM, Griffin JA, Keyes GG, Wearden S, Skidmore AE. Periapical biopsy report: an analysis over a 10-year period *J Endod* 1990; 16: 239–241.

37 Nair PNR, Pajorola G, Schroeder HE. Types and incidence of human periapical lesions obtained with extracted teeth. *Oral Surg* 1996; 81(1): 93–102.

38 Garlock JA, Pringle GA, Hicks ML. The odontogenic keratocyst: a potential endodontic misdiagnosis. *Oral Surg* 1998; 85: 452–456.

39 Lombardi T, Bischof M, Nedir R, Vergain D, Galgano C, Samson J, et al. Periapical central giant cell granuloma misdiagnosed as odontogenic cyst. *Int Endod J* 2006; 39: 510–515.

40 Grimm M, Henopp T, Hoefert S, Schaefer F, Kluba S, Krimmel M, et al. Multiple osteolytic lesions of intraosseous adenoid cystic carcinoma in the mandible mimicking apical periodontitis. *Int Endod J* 2012; 45: 1156–1164.

41 Fujihara H, Chikazu D, Saijo H, Suenaga H, Mori Y, Iino M, et al. Metastasis of hepatocellular carcinoma into the mandible with radiographic findings mimicking a radicular cyst: a case report. *J Endod* 2010; 36: 1593–1596.

42 Bueno MR, De Carvalhosa AA, Castro PH, Pereira KC, Borges FT, Estrela C. Mesenchymal chondrosarcoma mimicking apical periodontitis. *J Endod* 2008; 34: 1415–1419.

43 Svirsky JA, Epstein RA. Small cell carcinoma of the lung metastatic to the wall of a radicular cyst *J Endod* 1994; 20(10): 512–514.

44 Faitaroni LA, Bueno MR, De Carvalhosa AA, Ale KAB, Estrela C. Ameloblastoma suggesting large apical periodontitis. *J Endod* 2008; 34(2): 216–219.

45 Huey MW, Bramwell JD, Hutter JW, Kratochvil FJ. Central odontogenic fibroma mimicking a lesion of endodontic origin. *J Endod* 1995; 21(12): 625–627.

46 Moss HD, Hellstein JW, Johnson JD. Endodontic considerations of the nasopalatine duct region. *J Endod* 2000; 26(2): 107–110.

47 Suter VG, Buttner M, Altermatt HJ, Reichart PA, Bornstein MM. Expansive nasopalatine duct cysts with nasal

involvement mimicking apical lesions of endodontic origin: a report of two cases. *J Endod* 2011; 37: 1320–1326.

48 Faitaroni LA, Bueno MR, Carvalhosa AA, Mendonca EF, Estrela C. Differential diagnosis of apical periodontitis and nasopalatine duct cyst. *J Endod* 2011; 37: 403–410.

49 Rodrigues CD, Estrela C. Traumatic bone cyst suggestive of large apical periodontitis. *J Endod* 2008; 34(4): 484–489.

50 Fregnani ER, de Moraes Ramos FM, Nadalin MR, Silva-Sousa YT, da Cruz Perez DE. Simple bone cyst: Possible misdiagnosis in periapical pathology. *Gen Dent* 2007; 55: 129–131.

51 Jessri M, Abdul Majeed AA, Matias MA, Farah CS. A case of primary diffuse large B-cell non-Hodgkin's lymphoma misdiagnosed as chronic periapical periodontitis. *Aust Dent J* 2013; 58: 250–255.

52 Mendonca EF, Sousa TO, Estrela C. Non-Hodgkin lymphoma in the periapical region of a mandibular canine. *J Endod* 2013; 39: 839–842.

53 Morgan LA. Infiltrate of chronic lymphocytic leukemia appearing as a periapical radiolucent lesion. *J Endod* 1995; 21(9): 475–478.

54 DeDeus QD. Frequency, location and direction of the lateral, secondary, and accessory canals. *J Endod* 1975; 1: 361–366.

55 Weller RN, Niemczyk SP, Kim S. Incidence and position of the canal isthmus. Part I. Mesiobuccal root of the maxillary first molar *J Endod* 1995; 21(7): 380–383.

56 Degerness R, Bowles W. Anatomic determination of the mesiobuccal root resection level in maxillary molars. *J Endod* 2008; 34(10): 1182–1186.

57 Gilheany PA, Figdor D, Tyas MJ. Apical dentin permeability and microleakage associated with root end resection and retrograde filling. *J Endod* 1994; 20(1): 22–26.

58 Morgan LA, Marshall JG. The topography of root ends resected with fissure burs and refined with two types of finishing burs. *Oral Surg* 1998; 85: 585–591.

59 Craig KR, Harrison JW. Wound healing following demineralization of resected root ends in periradicular surgery. *J Endod* 1993; 19(7): 339–347.

60 Selim HA, El Deeb ME, Messer HH. Blood loss during endodontic surgery. *Endod Dent Traumatol* 1987; 3: 33–36.

61 Kim S, Rethnam S. Hemostasis in endodontic microsurgery. *Dent Clin North Am* 1997; 41(3): 499–511.

62 Witherspoon DE, Gutmann JL. Haemostasis in periradicular surgery. *Int Endod J* 1996; 29: 135–149.

63 Lemon RR, Steele PJ, Jeansonne BG. Ferric sulfate hemostasis: effect on osseous wound healing. I. Left in situ for maximum exposure. *J Endod* 1993; 19: 170–173.

64 Jeansonne BG, Boggs WS, Lemon RR. Ferric sulfate hemostasis: effect on osseous wound healing. II. With curettage and irrigation. *J Endod* 1993; 19: 174–176.

65 Vickers FJ, Baumgartner JC, Marshall G. Hemostatic efficacy and cardiovascular effects of agents used during endodontic surgery. *J Endod* 2002; 28: 322–332.

66 Vy CH, Baumgartner JC, Marshall JG. Cardiovascular effects and efficacy of a hemostatic agent in periradicular surgery. *J Endod* 2004; 30: 379–383.

67 Edgerton M. *Art of surgical technique*: Baltimore: Williams & Wilkins; 1988.

68 Chong BS, Pitt Ford TR. Root-end filling materials: rationale and tissue response. *Endod Topics* 2005; 11(July): 114–130.

69 Chong BS. A surgical alternative. In: *Managing endodontic failure in practice*. London: Quintessence Publishing; 2004. pp. 123–147.

70 Dorn SO, Gartner AH. Retrograde filling materials: a retrospective success-failure study of amalgam, EBA and IRM. *J Endod* 1990; 16: 391–394.

71 Gartner AH, Dorn SO. Advances in endodontic surgery. *Dent Clin North Am* 1992; 36: 357–378.

72 Kim S, Pecora G, Rubinstein RA, Dorcher-Kim J. Retrofilling materials and techniques. *Color atlas of microsurgery in endodontics*. Philadelphia: WB Saunders; 2001. pp. 115–124.

73 Frank AL, Glick DH, Patterson SS, Weine FS. Long-term evaluation of surgically placed amalgam fillings. *J Endod* 1992; 18: 391–398.

74 Johnson JD. Root canal filling materials. In: Ingle JI BL, Baumgartner JC, editors. *Ingle's endodontics*. Hamilton: BC Decker; 2008. pp. 1019–1052.

75 Chong BS, Pitt Ford TR, Hudson MB. A prospective clinical study of mineral trioxide aggregate and IRM when used as root-end filling materials in endodontic surgery. *Int Endod J*. 2003; 36: 520–526.

76 Lindeboom JAH, Frenken JWFH, Kroon FHM, van den Akker HP. A comparative prospective randomized clinical study of MTA and IRM as root-end filling materials in single-rooted teeth in endodontic surgery. *Oral Surg Oral Med Oral Pathol Oral Radiol Endod*. 2005; 100: 495–500.

77 Oynick J, Oynick T. A study of a new material for retrograde fillings. *J Endod* 1978; 4: 203–206.

78 Rubinstein RA, Kim S. Short-term observation of the results of endodontic surgery with the use of a surgical operation microscope and super-EBA as root-end filling material. *J Endod* 1999; 25: 43–48.

79 Rubinstein RA, Kim S. Long-term follow-up of cases considered healed one year after apical microsurgery. *J Endod* 2002; 28: 378–383.

80 Maddalone M, Gagliani M. Periapical endodontic surgery: a 3-year follow-up study. *Int Endod J* 2003; 36: 193–198.

81 Song M, Kim E. A prospective randomized controlled study of mineral trioxide aggregate and super ethoxy-benzoic acid as root-end filling materials in endodontic microsurgery. *J Endod* 2012; 38: 875–879.

82 Torabinejad M, Watson TF, Pitt Ford TR. Sealing ability of a mineral trioxide aggregate when used as a root-end filling material. *J Endod* 1993; 19: 591–595.

83 Torabinejad M, Hong CU, Pitt Ford TR. Physical properties of a new root end filling material. *J Endod* 1995; 21: 349–353.
84 Torabinejad M, Higa RK, Mckendry DJ, Pitt Ford TR. Dye leakage of four root end filling materials: effects of blood contamination. *J Endod* 1994; 20(4): 159–163.
85 Torabinejad M, Rastegar AF, Kettering JD, Pitt Ford TR. Bacterial leakage of mineral trioxide aggregate as a root end filling material. *J Endod* 1995; 21(3): 109–112.
86 Xavier CB, Weismann R, de Oliveira MG, Demarco FF, Pozza DH. Root-end filling materials: apical microleakage and marginal adaptation *J Endod* 2005; 31(7): 539–542.
87 Tang HM, Torabinejad M, Kettering JD. Leakage evaluation of root end filling materials using endotoxin. *J Endod* 2002; 28(1): 5–7.
88 Torabinejad M, Smith PW, Kettering JD, Pitt Ford TR. Comparative investigation of marginal adaptation of mineral trioxide aggregate and other commonly used root-end filling materials. *J Endod* 1995; 21(6): 295–299.
89 Torabinejad M, Hong CU, Pitt Ford TR, Kettering JD. Cytotoxicity of four root end filling materials *J Endod* 1995; 21: 489–492.
90 Sarkar NK, Caicedo R, Ritwik P, Moiseyeva R, Kawashima I. Physiochemical basis of the biologic properties of mineral trioxide aggregate. *J Endod* 2005; 31(2): 97–100.
91 Fridland M, Rosado R, Eng C. MTA solubility: a long term study. *J Endod* 2005; 31(5): 376–379.
92 Durarte MAH, Demarchi ACCO, Yamashita JC, Kuga MC, Fraga SC. pH and calcium ion release of 2 root-filling materials *Oral Surg Oral Med Oral Pathol Oral Radiol Endod* 2003; 95: 245–247.
93 Eldeniz AU, Hadimli JJ, Ataoglu H, Orstavik D. Antibacterial effect of selected root-end filling materials. *J Endod* 2006; 32(4): 345–349.
94 Thompson TS, Berry JE, Somerman MJ, Kirkwood KL. Cementoblasts maintain expression of osteocalcin in the presence of mineral trioxide aggregate. *J Endod* 2003; 29: 407–412.
95 Stropko JJ, Doyon G, Gutmann JL. Root-end management: resection, cavity preparation, and material placement. *Endod Topics* 2005; 11(July): 131–151.
96 Mukhtar-Fayyad D. Cytocompatibility of new bioceramic-based materials on human fibroblast cells (MRC-5). *Oral Surg Oral Med Oral Pathol Oral Radiol Endod* 2011; 112(6): e137–142.
97 Yan P, Yuan Z, Jiang H, Peng B, Bian Z. Effect of bioaggregate on differentiation of human periodontal ligament fibroblasts. *Int Endod J* 2010; 43: 1116–1121.
98 Yuan Z, Peng B, Jiang H, Bian Z, Yan P. Effect of bioaggregate on mineral-associated gene expression in osteoblast cells *J Endod* 2010; 36: 1145–1148.
99 Damas BA, Wheater MA, Bringas JS, Hoen MM. Cytotoxicity comparison of mineral trioxide aggregates and EndoSequence bioceramic root repair materials. *J Endod* 2011; 37: 372–375.
100 Al Anezi AZ, Jiang J, Safavi KE, Spangberg LS, Zhu Q. Cytotoxicity evaluation of EndoSequence Root Repair Material *Oral Surg Oral Med Oral Pathol Oral Radiol Endod* 2010; 109e: 122–125.
101 Chen I, Karabucak B, Wang C, Wang HG, Koyama E, Kohli MR, et al. Healing after root-end microsurgery by using mineral trioxide aggregate and a new calcium silicate–based biorceramic materials as root-end filling materials in dogs. *J Endod* 2015; 41: 389–399.
102 Zhang J, Pappen FG, Haapassalo M. Dentin enhances the antibacterial effect of mineral trioxide aggregate and bioaggregate. *J Endod* 2019; 35: 221–224.
103 Leal F, De-Deus G, Brandao C, Luna AS, Fidel SR, Souza EM. Comparison of the root-end seal provided by bioceramic repair cements and white MTA. *Int Endod J* 2011; 44: 661–668.
104 Nair U, Ghattas S, Saber M, Natera M, Walker C, Pileggi R. A comparative evaluation of the sealing ability of 2 root-end filling materials: an *in vitro* leakage study using *Enterococcus faecalis. Oral Surg Oral Med Oral Pathol Oral Radiol Endod* 2011; 112: e74–77.
105 Selvig KA, Biagiotti GR, Leknes KN, Wikesjo ME. Oral tissue reactions to suture materials. *Int J Periodont Rest Dent* 1998; 18: 475–487.
106 Leknes KN, Roynstrand IT, Selvig KA. Human gingival tissue reactions to silk and expanded polytetrafluoroethylene sutures. *J Periodontol* 2005; 76: 34–42.
107 Gutmann JL. Surgical endodontics: post-surgical care. *Endod Topics* 2005; 11(July): 196–205.
108 Tsesis I, Fuss Z, Lin S, Tilinger G, Peled M. Analysis of postoperative symptoms following surgical endodontic treatment. *Quintessence Int* 2003; 34: 756–760.
109 Harrison JW, Jurosky KA. Wound healing in the tissues of the periodontium following periradicular surgery. I. The incisional wound. *J Endod* 1991; 17: 425–435.
110 Harrison JW, Jurosky KA. Wound healing in the tissues of the periodontium following periradicular surgery. II. The dissectional wound. *J Endod* 1991; 17: 544–552.
111 Harrison JW, Jurosky KA. Wound healing in the tissues of the periodontium following periradicular surgery. III The osseous excisional wound. *J Endod* 1992; 18: 76–81.
112 Harrison JW. Healing of surgical wounds in oral mucoperiosteal tissues. *J Endod* 1991; 17: 401–408.
113 Tsesis I, Rosen E, Schwartz-Arad D, Fuss Z. Retrospective evaluation of surgical endodontic treatment: traditional versus modern technique *J Endod* 2006; 32: 412–416.
114 Tsesis I, Rosen E, Taschieri S, Telishevsky Strauss Y, Ceresoli V, Del Fabbro M. Outcomes of surgical endodontic treatment performed by a modern technique: An updated meta-analysis of the literature. *J Endod* 2013; 39: 332–339.
115 Setzer FC, Shah SB, Kohli MR, Karabucak B, Kim S. Outcome of endodontic surgery: a meta-analysis of the literature-part 1: comparison of traditional root-end

surgery and endodontic microsurgery. *J Endod* 2010; 36: 1757–1765.

116 Setzer FC, Kohli MR, Shah SB, Karabucak B, Kim S. Outcome of endodontic surgery: a meta-analysis of the literature: part 2: comparison of endodontic microsurgical techniques with and without the use of higher magnification. *J Endod* 2012; 38: 1–10.

117 Tsesis I, Faivishevsky V, Kfir A, Rosen E. Outcome of surgical endodontic treatment performed by a modern technique: a meta-analysis of literature. *J Endod* 2009; 35: 1505–1511.

118 Rud J, Andreasen JO, Moller Jensen JE. A follow-up study of 1000 cases treated by endodontic surgery. *Int J Oral Surg* 1972; 1: 215–228.

119 Friedman S. The prognosis and expected outcome of apical surgery. *Endod Topics* 2005; 11: 219–262.

120 Kraus RD, von Arx T, Gfeller D, Ducommun J, Jensen SS. Assessment of the nonoperated root after apical surgery of the other root in mandibular molars: A 5-year follow-up study. *J Endod* 2015; 41: 442–446.

121 von Arx T, Hanni S, Jensen SS. Clinical results with two different methods of root-end preparation and filling in apical surgery: mineral trioxide aggregate and adhesive resin composite. *J Endod* 2010; 36: 1122–1129.

122 Tang Y, Li X, Yin S. Outcomes of MTA as root-end filling in endodontic surgery: a systematic review. *Quintessence Int* 2010; 41: 557–566.

123 Li H, Zhai F, Zhang R, Hou B. Evaluation of microsurgery with Super EBA as root-end filling material for treating post-treatment endodontic disease: a 2-year retrospective study. *J Endod* 2014; 40: 345–350.

124 Shinbori N, Grama AM, Patel Y, Woodmansey K, He J. Clinical outcome of endodontic microsurgery that uses EndoSequence BC root repair material as the root-end filling material. *J Endod* 2015; 4: 607–612.

125 Rud J, Rud V, Munksgaard ED. Long-term evaluation of retrograde root fillings with dentin-bonded resin composite. *J Endod* 1996; 22: 90–93.

126 Rud J, Rud V, Munksgaard ED. Effect of root canal contents on healing of teeth with dentin-bonded resin composite retrograde seal. *J Endod* 1997; 23: 535–541.

127 von Arx T, Penarrocha M, Jensen S. Prognostic factors in apical surgery with root-end filling: a meta-analysis. *J Endod* 2010; 36: 957–973.

128 Von Arx T, Jensen SS, Hanni S. Clinical and radiographic assessment of various predictors for healing outcome 1 year after periapical surgery. *J Endod* 2007; 33: 123–128.

129 Peterson J, Gutmann JL. The outcome of endodontic resurgery: a systematic review. *Int Endod J* 2001; 34: 169–175.

130 Gagliani MM, Gorni FG, Strohmenger L. Periapical re-surgery versus periapical surgery: a 5-year longitudinal comparison. *Int Endod J* 2005; 38: 320–327.

131 Song M, Shin SJ, Kim E. Outcomes of endodontic micro-resurgery: A prospective clinical study. *J Endod* 2011; 37: 316–320.

132 Song M, Nam T, Shin SJ, Kim E. Comparison of clinical outcomes of endodontic microsurgery: 1 year versus long-term follow-up. *J Endod* 2014; 40: 490–494.

133 Song M, Chung W, Lee SJ, Kim E. Long-term outcome of the cases classified as successes based on short-term follow-up in endodontic microsurgery *J Endod* 2012; 38: 1192–1196.

134 Von Arx T, Jensen SS, Hanni S, Friedman S. Five-year longitudinal assessment of the prognosis of apical microsurgery. *J Endod* 2012; 38: 570–579.

135 Wang N, Knight K, Dao T, Friedman S. Treatment outcome in endodontics—the Toronto study. *Phases I and II: apical surgery. J Endod* 2004; (30): 751–761.

136 Barone C, Dao TT, Basrani BB, Wang N, Friedman S. Treatment outcome in endodontics—the Toronto study. Phases 3, 4, and 5: apical surgery. *J Endod* 2010; 36: 28–35.

137 von Arx T, Hänni S, Jensen SS. Correlation of bone defect dimensions with healing outcome one year after apical surgery. *J Endod* 2007; 33(9): 1044–1048.

138 Pecora G, Baek S-H, Rethnam S, Kim S. Barrier membrane techniques in endodontic microsurgery. *Dent Clin North Am* 1997; 41(3): 585–602.

139 Rankow HJ, Krasner PR. Endodontic applications of guided tissue regeneration in endodontic surgery. *J Endod* 1996; 22(1): 34–43.

140 Borg TD, Mealey BL. Histiologic healing following tooth extraction with ridge preservation using mineralized versus combined mineralized-demineralized freeze-dried bone allografts: a randomized controlled clinical trial. *J Periodontol.* 2015; 86: 348–355.

141 Holtzclaw D, Toscano N, Eisenlohr L, Callan D. The safety of bone allografts used in dentistry: a review. *J Am Dent Assoc* 2008; 139: 1192–1199.

142 Pecora G, DeLeonardis D, Ibrahim N, Bovi M, Cornelini R. The use of calcium sulphate in the surgical treatment of a "through and through" periradicular lesion. *Int Endod J* 2001; 34(3): 189–197.

143 Murashima Y, Yoshikawa G, Wadachi R, Sawada N, Suda H. Calcium sulphate as a bone substitute for various osseous defects in conjunction with apicectomy. *Int Endod J* 2002; 35(9): 768–774.

144 Tobon SI, Arismendi JA, Marin ML, Mesa AL, Valencia JA. Comparison between a conventional technique and two bone regeneration techniques in periradicular surgery. *Int Endod J* 2002; 35: 635–641.

145 Garrett K, Kerr M, Hartwell G, O'Sullivan S, Mayer P. The effect of a bioresorbable matrix barrier in endodontic surgery on the rate of periapical healing: An in vivo study. *J Endod* 2002; 28: 503–506.

146 Kratchman S. Intentional replantation. *Dent Clin North Am* 1997; 41(3): 603–617.

147 Lindeberg RW, Girardi AF, Troxell JB. Intentional replantation: management in contraindicated cases. *Comp Cont Educ* 1986; 7: 248–258.

148 Nasjleti CE, Castelli WA, Caffesse RG. The effects of direct splinting times on replantation of teeth in monkeys. *Oral Surg* 1982; 53: 557–566.

149 Andersson L, Andreasen JO, Day P, Heithersay G, Trope M, Diangelis AJ, et al. International Association of Dental Traumatology guidelines for the management of traumatic dental injuries: 2. Avulsion of permanent teeth. *Dent Traumatol* 2012; 28: 88–96.

150 Koenig KH, Nguyen NT, Barkhorder RA. Intentional replantation: a report of 192 cases. *Gen Dent* 1988; 36: 327–331.

151 Bender IB, Rossman LE. Intentional replantation of endodontically treated teeth. *Oral Surg Oral Med Oral Pathol Oral Radiol* 1993; 76: 623–630.

152 Grossman LI. Intentional replantation of teeth: a clinical evaluation. *J Am Dent Assoc* 1966; 104: 633–636.

153 Kingsbury BC, Weisenbaught JM. Intentional replantation of mandibular molars and premolars. *J Am Dent Assoc* 1971 ;83: 1053–1057.

154 Torabinejad M, Johnson BR. Endodontic surgery. In: Torabinejad M, Walton RE, Fouad AF, editors. *Endodontics principles and practice*. 5th ed. St Louis: Elsevier Saunders; 2015. pp. 376–396.

155 Carranza FA, Takei HH. Treatment of furcation involvement and combined periodontal–endodontic therapy. In: Carranza FA, Newman MG, editors. *Clinical periodontology*. 8th ed. Philadelphia: WB Saunders; 1996. pp. 640–651.

156 Glickman GN, Hartwell GR. Endodontic surgery. In: Ingle JI BL, Baumgartner JC, editors. *Ingle's endodontics*. 6th ed. Hamilton: BC Decker; 2008. pp. 1233–1294.

157 Hempton T, Leone C. A review of root resective therapy as a treatment option for maxillary molars. *J Am Dent Assoc* 1997; 128: 449–455.

158 Newell DH, Morgano SM, Baima RF. Fixed prosthodontics with periodontally compromised dentitions. In: Malone WFP, Koth DL, editors. *Tylman's theory and practice of fixed prosthodontics*. 8th ed. St Louis: Ishiyaku EuroAmerica; 1989. pp 80–1

159 Blomlof L, Jansson L, Appelgren R, Ehnevid H, Lindskog S. Prognosis and mortality of root-resected molars. *Int J Perio Rest Dent* 1997; 17: 190–201.

160 Langer B, Stein SD, Wagenberg B. An evaluation of root resections. A ten-year study. *J Periodontol* 1981; 52: 719–722.

161 Basten CH, Ammons WF, Persson R. Long-term evaluation of root-resected molars: a retrospective study *Int J Perio and Rest Dent* 1996; 16: 206–219.

162 Fugazzotto PA. A comparison of the success of root resected molars and molar position implants in function in a private practice: results of up to 15-plus years. *J Periodontol* 2001; 72: 1113–1123.

163 Eberhardt JA, Torabinejad M. A computed tomographic study the distances between the maxillary sinus floor and the apices of the maxillary posterior teeth. *Oral Surg* 1992; 73: 345–346.

164 Oberli K, Bornstein MM, von Arx T. Periapical surgery and the maxillary sinus: radiographic parameters for clinical outcome. *Oral Surg Oral Med Oral Pathol Oral Radiol Endod* 2007; 103(6): 848–853.

165 Freedman A, Horowitz I. Complications after apicoectomy in maxillary premolar and molar teeth. *Int J Oral Maxillofac Surg* 1999; 28: 192–194.

166 Tataryn RW, Torabinejad M, Boyne PJ. Healing potential of osteotomies of the nasal sinus in the dog. *Oral Surg* 1997; 84: 196–202.

167 Watzek G, Bernhart T, Ulm C. Complications of sinus perforation and their management. *Dent Clin North Am* 1997; 41: 563–583.

168 Lin L, Chance K, Skovlin F, Skribner J, Langeland K. Oroantral communication in periapical surgery of maxillary posterior teeth. *J Endod* 1985; 11: 40–44.

Questions

1 A vertical releasing incision for an intrasulcular incision for a triangular or rectangular mucoperiosteal flap should meet the marginal gingiva at right angles and should be at the junction of the
A apical and middle third of the interdental papilla.
B middle and coronal third of the interdental papilla.
C attached gingiva and alveolar mucosa.
D coronal third of the interdental papilla and alveolar crest.

2 What is the ideal degree of angle for the root-end to be resected in a root-end surgery?
A 0
B 15
C 30
D 45

3 Which local hemostatic agent has the most desirable properties for control of bleeding during root-end surgery?
A Bone wax
B Surgicel
C Racemic epinephrine pellets
D Ferric sulfate

4 Which of the following is an advantage of a papilla base incision and flap design for root-end surgery?
A Incision is not technically difficult.
B The flap is easily reflected.
C The flap is easily sutured.
D It allows excellent healing of the papilla.

5 How far should the root-end resection be from the root apex?
A 3 mm or less for teeth with long roots
B 3 mm except for the mesiobuccal root of maxillary first molars
C 3.6 mm for curved roots
D 4 mm for canine teeth

6 For direct visualization through the dental operating microscope while performing root-end surgery on the mesiobuccal root of the right maxillary first molar, the patient should be positioned on their
A left side
B right side
C back, with head turned to the left side
D back, with head turned to the right side

7 What is needed postoperatively after a palatal flap has been sutured back into place?
A Warm saline rinses
B Ice chips against the palate
C A palatal stent
D A 2 × 2 gauze pack against the palate

8 Which is an indication for guided tissue regeneration after root-end surgery?
A Preoperative pain
B The presence of an isthmus
C A 2 × 3-mm periapical lesion
D A through-and-through defect

9 Tissue from a periapical lesion is
A sent for histopathological examination.
B left in place if hemostasis can be achieved.
C not innervated.
D usually a cyst.

10 Which of the following is an indication for the submarginal incision?
A On maxillary posterior teeth with porcelain–metal crowns
B On mandibular anterior teeth with porcelain–metal crowns
C On anterior teeth with 2 mm of keratinized attached gingiva
D On anterior teeth with 3 mm of keratinized attached gingiva

CHAPTER 10

Lasers

Mohammed Alshahrani[1], Brian Beebe[2], and Sami M. Chogle[1]
[1] *Boston University Henry M. Goldman School of Dental Medicine, Boston, Massachusetts, USA*
[2] *Private practice, Bozeman, Montana, USA*

Einstein was the first physicist who laid the foundation of postulated laser theories that concluded the formation of the special light in early 1960s [1]. In 1951 at the spring meeting of American Physical Society in Washington Town, Einstein's student came up with the acronym MASER, which stands for *m*icrowave *a*mplification by *s*timulated emission of *r*adiation. It was not long until another American physicist, Gordon Gould, in 1957 proposed the term laser, when it was used for the first time [2]. The 1960s saw what many have described as the beginning of the use of laser technology in dentistry and endodontics, with attention given to developing basic laser parameters as applied to dental hard and soft tissues [3]. The first report of the use of lasers in endodontics attempted to seal the apical foramen in vitro by means of a high power–infrared (CO_2) laser [4].

The word *laser* is an acronym for *l*ight *a*mplification by the *s*timulated *e*mission of *r*adiation. The laser beam implicates stimulated emission of radiation. It is monochromatic (single wave), collimated (low divergence), coherent (photons in phase) and intense [2]. The main difference between the laser and regular light is that laser has a spontaneous emission because it happens without any additional interference and results in the formation of individual waves from each atom versus in phase with one another (not coherent) polychromatic light.

The construction of a light source based on stimulated emission of radiation requires an important active medium, the source of atoms. The active medium can be a solid material, liquid, or gas. These active media are enclosed in a tube usually made of ceramics or glass. The laser beam is generated by flash lamp or electric current, which is applied to the medium. Once applied to the medium, the flash lamp or electric current transforms the atoms from the ground state to the exited state (population inversion). The mirrors at both ends of the laser medium direct the photon population back and forth through the medium, which stimulates more radiation emission from multiple excited electrons. Some of the produced photons are released through one of the mirrors at the end through the delivery device.

Based on the active medium, laser units are classified into different types, such as carbon dioxide (CO_2), erbium (Er), neodymium (Nd), argon, diode, and excimer. Classification can include other substances added to the medium, such as yttrium, aluminum, garnet (YAG) or yttrium, scandium, gallium, garnet (YSGG). Each kind of laser produces light of a specific wavelength. For example, CO_2, Er:YAG, Cr:YSGG, and Nd:YAG lasers emit an invisible laser beam within the infrared range. (Figure 10.1) Laser energy interacts with tissues in one of four ways: absorption by tissues, transmission through tissues, reflection from tissues, or scattering on tissue surfaces (Figure 10.2).

When the photon of laser is transmitted through the tissues without interaction, it results in no changes of the lased tissues. If the light is reflected from the tissues, there is almost no absorption of the energy, which results in no thermal effect. Scattering of the light in different directions allows a greater absorption of light energy and results in a thermal effect but to a lesser extent. However, when the light is absorbed, the whole light energy is converted to thermal energy.

The soft and hard tissues, due to the high water content of their structure, readily absorb CO_2 laser.

Current Therapy in Endodontics, First Edition. Edited by Priyanka Jain.
© 2016 John Wiley & Sons, Inc. Published 2016 by John Wiley & Sons, Inc.

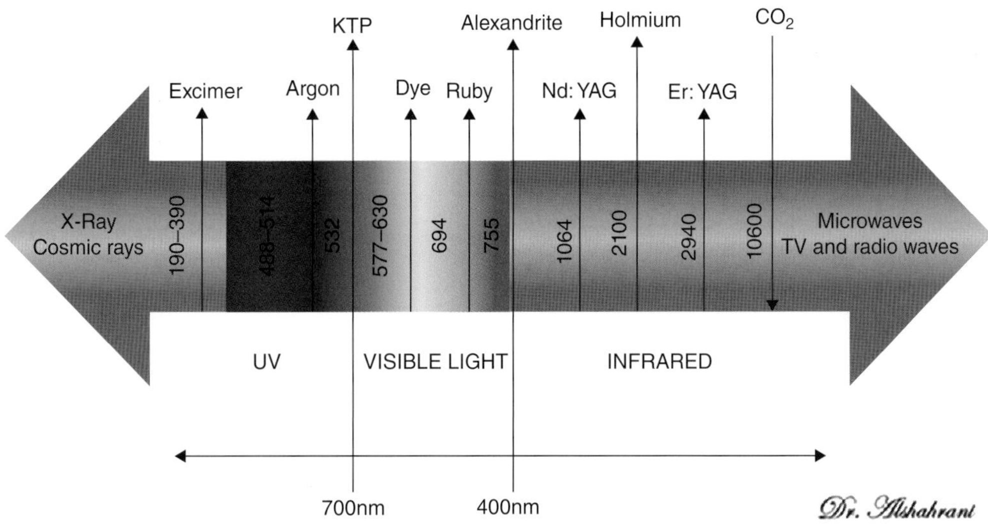

Figure 10.1 Wavelength of various types of lasers according to their emission.

However, the high thermal effect makes the CO_2 laser unsuitable for use in operative dentistry because it damages the dental pulp [5].

There have been marked evolutions in the use of lasers in endodontics. The development of new laser systems, optics, and fiber optics and better understanding of laser mechanism of action and new endodontic tips have made it possible to reconsider the laser application in the field of endodontics.

However, there are still concerns about laser use due to the lack of well-designed clinical studies, the limited number of endodontic tips, the selection of the appropriate wavelengths, and the energy used. Yet there is no consensus on the ideal energy settings for each specified procedure, which makes it difficult to standardize the procedure protocols. Another important obstacle is the high-priced laser machines, which limit their availability for dentists. The purpose of this chapter is to review the history and current concept of laser in endodontics as well as clinical applications of the laser with best available evidence.

History of lasers in endodontics

The first use of laser in endodontics was an attempt to investigate the effect of Nd:YAG lasers on dentin. The fiber optic was used to lase the dentin after preparing the root canal system. In this study, the effect of the laser ranged between melting the dentin to completely destroying the mounted specimen [6]. These severe effects resulted from the high wattage that was used: It melted and occluded the dentinal tubules. Occluding the dentinal tubule might be a beneficial effect of the laser to seal the root canal system. However, it generates a lot of heat (thermal damage), which is a concern during root canal treatment. This thermal effect damages not only the lased tooth but also the supporting tooth structures. Thus, laser use in endodontics was limited during that time.

Another attempt was made to investigate the feasibility of using lasers in cleaning and shaping of root canal systems [7]. There were no differences between the conventional method and the use of the laser to clean and shape the root canal system. In fact, the laser actually caused more mishaps than a conventional technique like ledges, where the fiberoptic came in touch with root canal walls, caused thermal damage, and weakened tooth structure (Figure 10.3). The treated area also had carbonization areas, which signified the high temperature increase during the procedure (Table 10.1) and (Figure 10.4).

In 1992, Bahcall's group did an in vivo study to determine the biological effect of Nd:YAG lasers on the periapical tissues [5]. Twelve teeth, which included 24 roots,

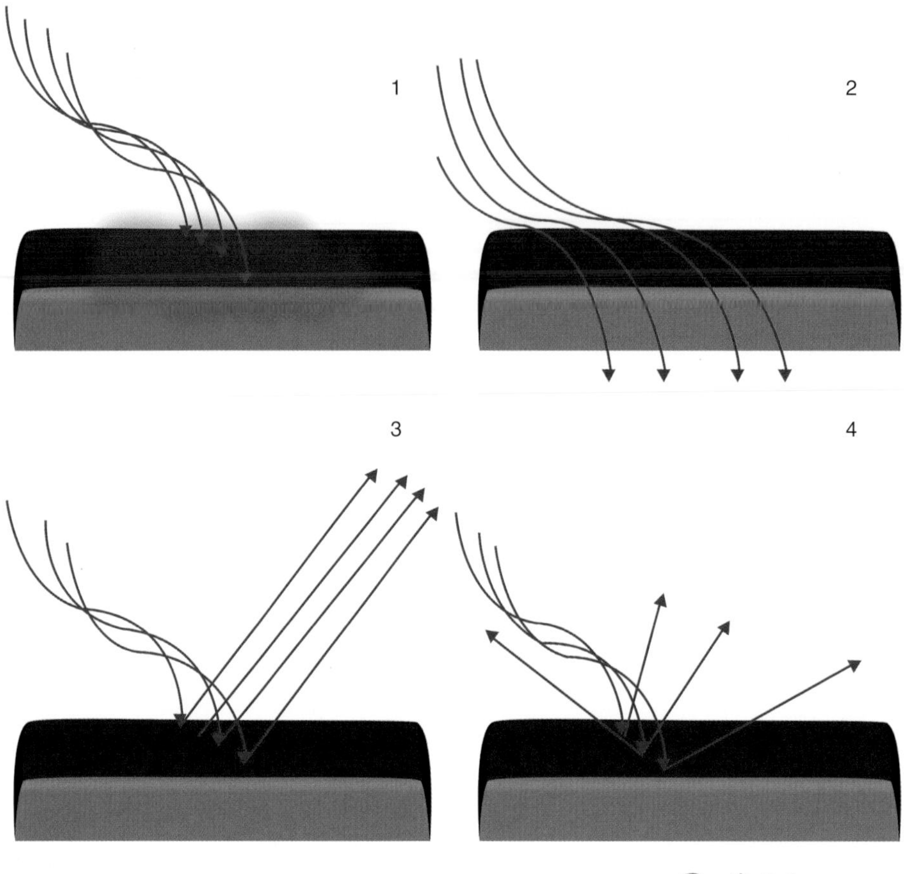

Figure 10.2 Laser energy interactions with tissues. 1, Absorption,. 2, Transmission. 3, Reflection. 4, Scatter.

in two mixed-breed dogs were included in this experiment. Half of the tooth specimens received the conventional root canal treatment and the second half received the laser treatment. The histological findings indicated a major bone remodeling and periodontal ligament necrosis. The latter led to ankylosis and replacement resorption. The laser in the in vivo settings appeared to be more efficient than in vitro settings. One explanation is the fact that laser energy is well absorbed by tissues due its high water content.

The concept of laser use in endodontics shifted from using the laser thermal effect to using lasers at subablative energy to create shock waves and shear forces that stream the irrigant throughout the root canal system.

The modern concept of laser in endodontics

The main etiology of apical periodontitis is the infected root canal system with microorganisms [8]. Mostly it involves a set of pathogenic species rather than single species, which are organized in mixed bacterial biofilms [9, 10]. Although complete eradication of microorganisms is not possible, the goal of endodontic treatment is the reduction of microorganism counts to a level where they do not cause disease. The complex root canal anatomy is another challenge that makes it difficult to clean and shape the root canal system completely [10].

During the cleaning and shaping process, a smear layer forms. It has an amorphous, irregular, and granular appearance when observed under the scanning

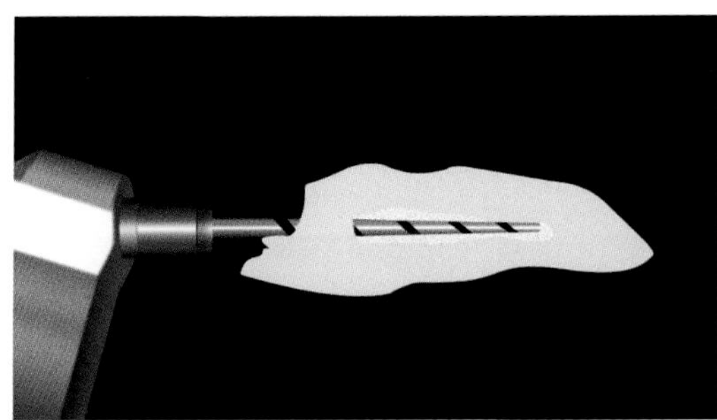

Figure 10.3 Laser tip used in cleaning and shaping of the root canal system. The figure shows the placement of the fiberoptic as close as possible to the working length, which creates a challenge during cleaning and shaping process.

Table 10.1 Effect of temperature on tissues.

Type of reaction	Temperature (°C)
Hyperemia	37–43
Decline of enzyme activity	43–50
Protein coagulation, protein damage	50–60
Collagen and cell membrane damage	70–80
Molecular destruction	80–100
Carbonization	100–140
Evaporation and desquamation	140–400
Cutting	500–800

electron microscope [11]. It consists of dentin, remnants of odontoblastic processes, pulpal tissues, and bacterial biofilms [12]. The smear layer affects the cleaning of the root canal system. (Box 10.1)

The development of new laser devices has allowed the use of less energy at subablative power, which reduced the undesirable effects of old laser techniques (Figure 10.5). Also, the tip designs that have been used were quite large and difficult to use within the root canal system. It requires an extremely large preparation that weakens the tooth structure. Thus, thinner endodontic tips have been developed, and these enable the clinician to place the tip close to working length while maintaining the integrity of the tooth structure. (Figure 10.6)

The goals of the newer systems and techniques are smaller fiberoptics, no thermal effects, antibacterial activity, safety, and low cost.

Laser uses in the field of dentistry, especially endodontics, were disappointing to a point where endodontists did not use lasers due to the side effects. The benefits of laser use have overcome its benefits. The possibility of using the energy of laser as a delivery system for irrigant solution was raised. Studies have shown that lasers at lower energy (subablative) produce no heat; rather, they induce bubbles to form, primary and secondary. Collapse of the bubbles creates turbulence that carries the irrigant solutions to the deepest points in the root canal system.

Clinical applications of lasers

Pulpal diagnosis

The pulpal diagnosis is a difficult assay due to a lot of factors. One of these factors is that the available pulpal testing methods do not assess the vitality of dental pulp. Testing rather reproduces the signs and symptoms of the diseased pulp, which depends on subjective and objective findings during the testing procedure. Thus any errors during diagnosis (false diagnosis) can result in accidental removal of the dental pulp. Studies have shown that there is no correlation between the histology of dental pulp and signs and symptoms. Laser Doppler flowmetry (LDF) is the only way to accurately assess the vitality of dental pulp by measuring the blood flow in the microvasculature system [13] .

Pulp capping

Pulp capping is the treatment of an exposed vital pulp by sealing the pulpal wound with a dental material such as calcium hydroxide (CaOH) or mineral trioxide aggregate (MTA) to facilitate the formation of reparative dentin and maintenance of a vital pulp. (AAE).

The pulp capping treatment is indicated when one of the following conditions occurs:

- The tooth has a deep carious lesion that is considered likely to result in pulp exposure during excavation.
- There is no history of subjective pretreatment symptoms.
- Pretreatment radiographs exclude periradicular pathosis.
- Mechanical exposure of a clinically vital and asymptomatic pulp occurs.
- Bleeding is controlled at the exposure site.
- Exposure permits the capping material to make direct contact with the vital pulp tissue.
- Exposure occurs when the tooth is under dental dam isolation.

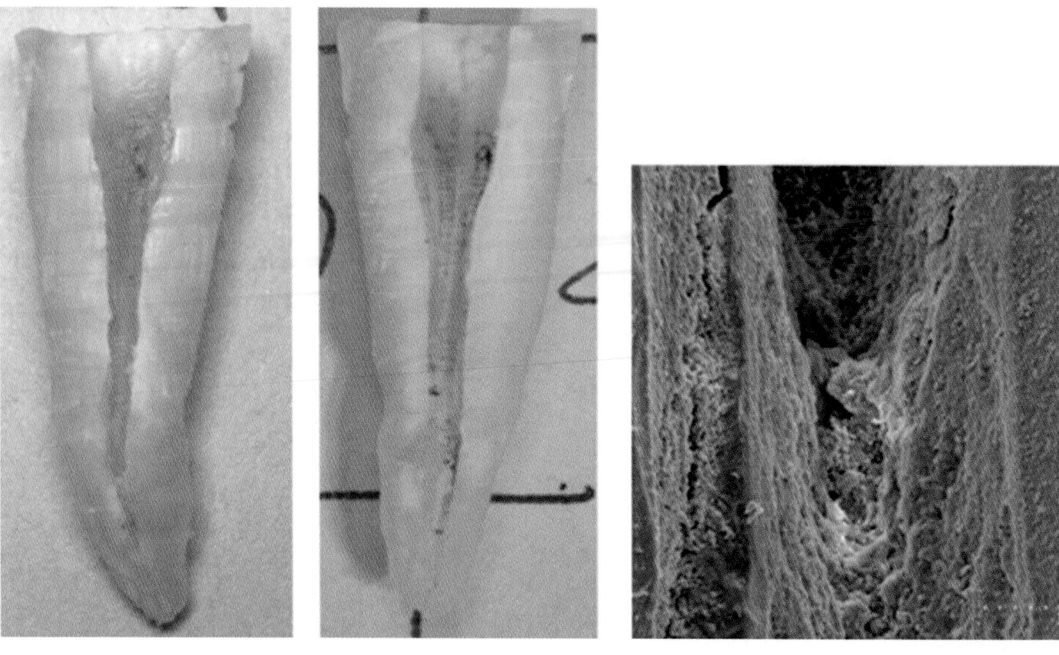

Figure 10.4 *Left* and *center,* Use of conventional erbium chromium YSGG laser caused thermal damage to tooth structure (carbonization). *Right,* Scanning electron microscope (SEM) image of thermal damage and ledging. (Images courtesy of Dr. Enrico DiVito.)

Box 10.1 Disadvantages of a smear layer

- Not a strict barrier against bacteria
- Interferes with sealing ability of the obturation material
- Acts as a substrate for unremoved bacteria
- Harbors microorganisms
- Interferes with cleaning action of irrigants
- Interferes with intracanal medicaments

Several attempts have been made to test the effect of various types of laser devices on dental pulp tissues. Melcer and colleagues used the ruby laser, and it caused damage to pulp tissues [14]. On the other hand, when CO_2 laser was used on exposed dental pulps of dogs, new mineralized dentin was produced without alteration at the cellular level.

When Jokic and colleagues used Nd:YAG and CO_2 lasers on dental pulps of dogs [15], coagulation necrosis, inflammation, hemorrhage, edema, and degeneration occurred in dental pulp. The energy level used in these studies was in a range between 3 and 60 W, which is considered high.

Moritz and colleagues used CO_2 laser in cases where direct pulp capping was indicated [16]. The energy level was 1 W for a 0.1-second exposure time. He applied the laser for one-second pulse intervals until the area was completely treated. Then it was followed by the application of CaOH. The control had no laser treatment; CaOH was directly placed over the exposure site. The symptoms and vitality testing were recorded before, 1 week after, and every month after for a period of one year. The results were 89% success rate versus 68% of the control.

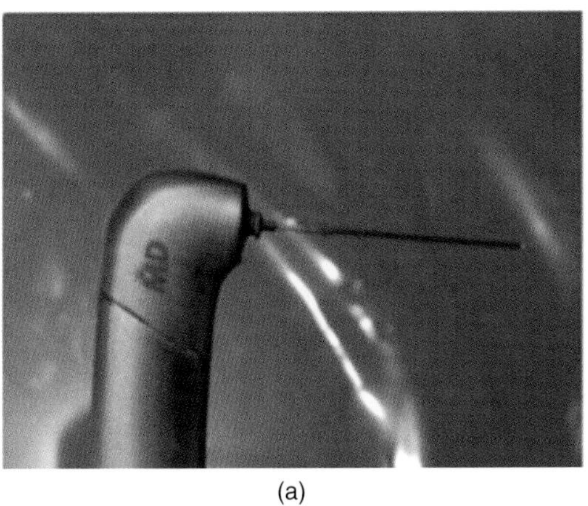

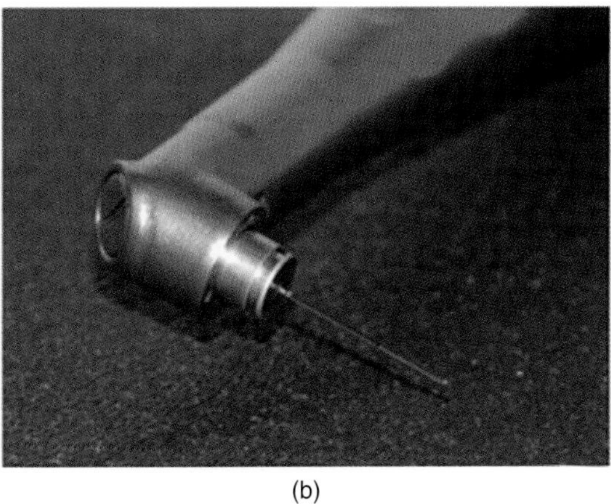

Figure 10.5 A, Conventional laser tip used on samples with thermal damage. B, A more recent modern tapered and stripped non-thermal photoacoustic PIPS laser tip. (Image courtesy of Dr. Enrico DiVito.)

The introduction of newer techniques using laser with reduced energy and a shorter period of lasing enabled clinicians to have better outcome of pulpal capping. The most recent studies reported an almost 90% success rate when the laser is used along with the capping material. Conventional pulpal capping resulted in a 60% success rate, which is significantly lower than when laser was used in pulp capping [17].

Laser and modified glass ionomer cement (GIC) were used in the direct pulp capping procedure to compare it with the modified GIC alone. The results with laser and modified GIC were a more-predictable response in the first 6 months than with the modified GIC alone. The survival rate of these teeth was recorded for a period of 54 months and was greater for laser and modified GIC than for modified GIC alone [18].

Laser technology is also used to treat dentin or root hypersensitivities by blocking the dentinal tubule to reduce fluid movement, which is responsible for pain sensation. When CO_2 laser is used at a low level of energy (less than 1 W), 10-Hz repletion rate, and an overall 10 seconds of exposure time, it did not elevate the intrapulpal temperature. The researchers consider these energy parameters to be a safe limit. Because it is different in clinical situations due to variable thicknesses of remaining dentin, it is recommended to use parameters lower than the safety limits [19].

Pulpotomy has been tested clinically on primary teeth. Interestingly out of the 68 laser-treated teeth, 66 were clinically successful with no signs and symptoms. Clinically and radiographically, the success rates were 97% and 94.1%, respectively [20].

Evidence-based current and future research

Since the introduction of LAI using the photon-initiated photoacoustic streaming (PIPS) technique and other newly designed endodontic fiberoptics, efforts have been made to investigate the efficiency of this technique. Peters's group made one of the earliest attempts. They tested the disinfection ability of sodium hypochlorite and the PIPS technique compared to ultrasonic and conventional irrigation. Interestingly, they found that LAI using the PIPS technique yielded more negative samples than ultrasonic and LAI [21]. The histological slices showed a significant reduction of bacterial biofilms, especially at apical cross sections (Figure 10.7).

The protocol used was activation of laser for a period of 30 seconds for one round only. It has been concluded that multiple activation rounds are needed to enhance the disinfection ability of the PIPS technique and to allow enough time for the active component of sodium hypochlorite to completely remove tissues and bacterial biofilms. Laser activation for 20 seconds is as effective as three rounds of ultrasonic activation [22]. Possible explanations could be the high absorbance of energy throughout the irrigant solution [23].

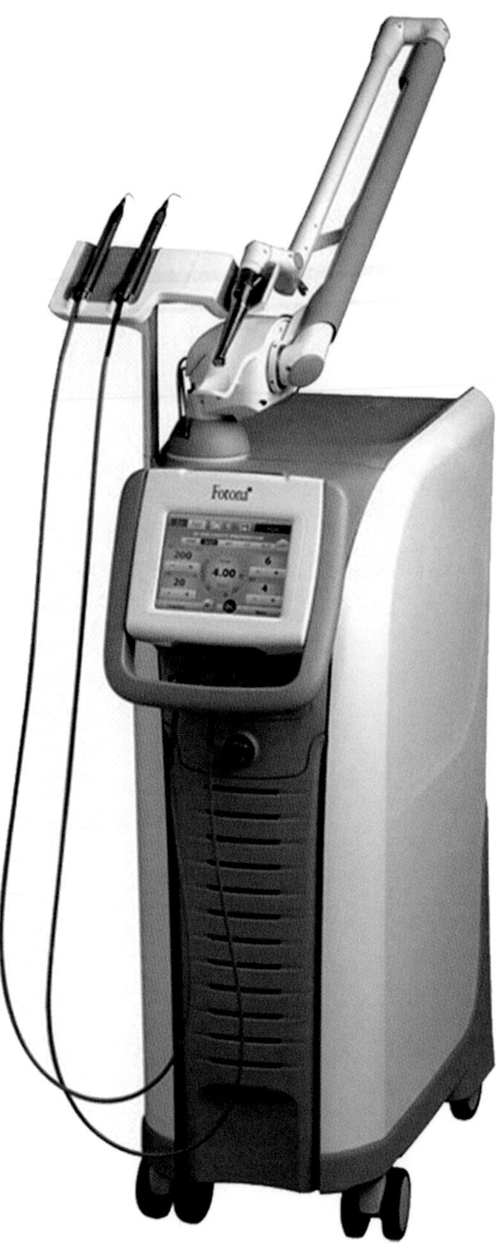

Figure 10.6 Er:YAG laser unit from Fotona.

On the other hand, when Pedulla and colleagues investigated the efficacy of the PIPS technique, they did not find any difference [24]. They inoculated the tooth specimens with *Enterococcus faecalis* and compared laser-activated irrigation with sodium hypochlorite and distilled water to needle irrigation with sodium hypochlorite. They did not find a significant difference between the PIPS technique and sodium hypochlorite and needle irrigation with sodium hypochlorite. This could be because they used a very short period of 30 seconds of activation time only.

Al Shahrani and colleagues in their study have attempted to investigate the effectiveness of LAI by PIPS using Er:YAG laser energy and sodium hypochlorite in decontaminating heavily colonized root canal systems in vitro compared to PIPS plus saline and needle irrigation [23]. Extracted single-rooted human teeth were cleaned and shaped to a minimally noninvasive preparation 25 0.08 taper. *E. faecalis* was used to inoculate the tooth specimens. Analysis of colony-forming units (CFU) showed that PIPS plus sodium hypochlorite was the most effective technique followed by sodium hypochlorite alone and PIPS and saline (Figure 10.8). Scanning electron microscopy showed clean and patent dentinal tubules compared to PIPS plus saline and sodium hypochlorite alone. Confocal laser microscopy confirmed the result of CFU count and standard error of the mean (SEM). (Figure 10.9)

The protocol of Alshahrani's study was different from what was previously described [22, 24, 25]. Al Shahrani's group used 90-second laser activation in three intervals of 30 seconds each, with a total amount of 21 mL of irrigant solution followed by 7 mL of irrigation with sodium hypochlorite for 60 seconds.

Arslan's group has done multiple studies to test the efficacy of the PIPS technique [25]. Their first study was to evaluate the efficacy of the PIPS technique in the removal of apically placed dentinal debris compared to ultrasonic, sonic, and conventional irrigation. They prepared their tooth specimen to size 40 and created an artificial groove at the apical area. After the treatment protocol, the amount of remaining dentinal debris was evaluated using stereomicroscope under 20× magnification. The result revealed that LAI using the PIPS technique was the most effective method for removing the smear layer, followed by sonic, ultrasonic, and conventional irrigation techniques. There was no significant difference between sonic and ultrasonic irrigation techniques. The protocol used during the experiment is activation of laser irrigation for 1 minute with a total amount of sodium hypochlorite of 6 mL. They concluded that the LAI using the PIPS technique

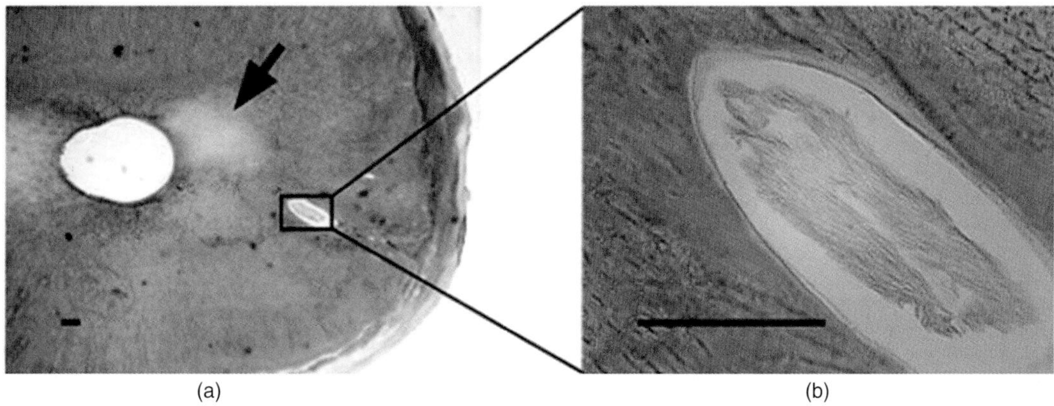

Figure 10.7 *A*, Cross section shows the main canal cleaned. Arrow points to area that is free of bacteria. *B*, A magnified lateral canal that had intact pulpal tissues. Scale bar is 100 μm in both images. (Images courtesy of Drs. Peters, Bardsley, Fong, Pandher, and Divito [21].)

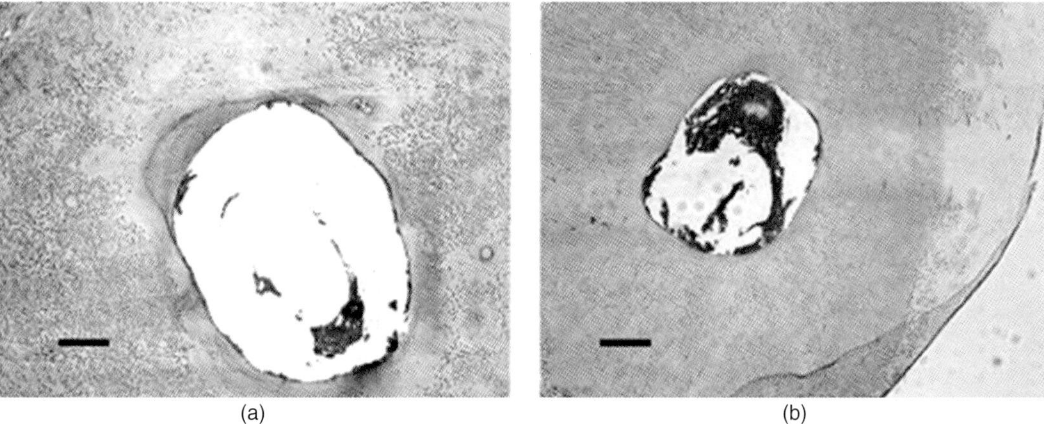

Figure 10.8 *A*, Cross section at 1-mm level shows remnant bacterial biofilms after PIPS and NaOCl use. *B*, Cross section at 1-mm level shows significantly more remnants of bacterial biofilms after ultrasonic and NaOCl use. Scale bar is 100 μm in both images. (Images courtesy of Drs. Peters, Bardsley, Fong, Pandher, and Divito [21].)

was the most effective protocol to remove the artificial debris from the apical third compared to passive ultrasonic and sonic irrigation techniques.

One of the unsatisfactory results of the irrigation procedure during root canal treatment is the accidental extrusion of the irrigant beyond the apex. It represents a concern during the cleaning and shaping process. It has been reported in the literature multiple times [26, 27]. In a survey by Kliere and colleagues on diplomates of the American Board of Endodontics, it has been shown that approximately 42% experienced sodium hypochlorite accident in their practice at least once, and 38% of the respondents experienced more than one accident [28]. It results in complications such as facial swelling, pain, and, to some extent, infection. The consequences also include treatment alteration and delay. The laser-activated irrigation creates shock waves; therefore, precautions should be taken when using such a technique to safely complete the treatment with minimal complications. Thus, the next step is to determine the safety of the PIPS technique.

The safety of laser-activated irrigation using PIPS at different power levels has been investigated by Arslan and colleagues [29]. In their study they used intact mandibular premolars with single straight canals. Tooth specimens were instrumented to F3 size ProTaper

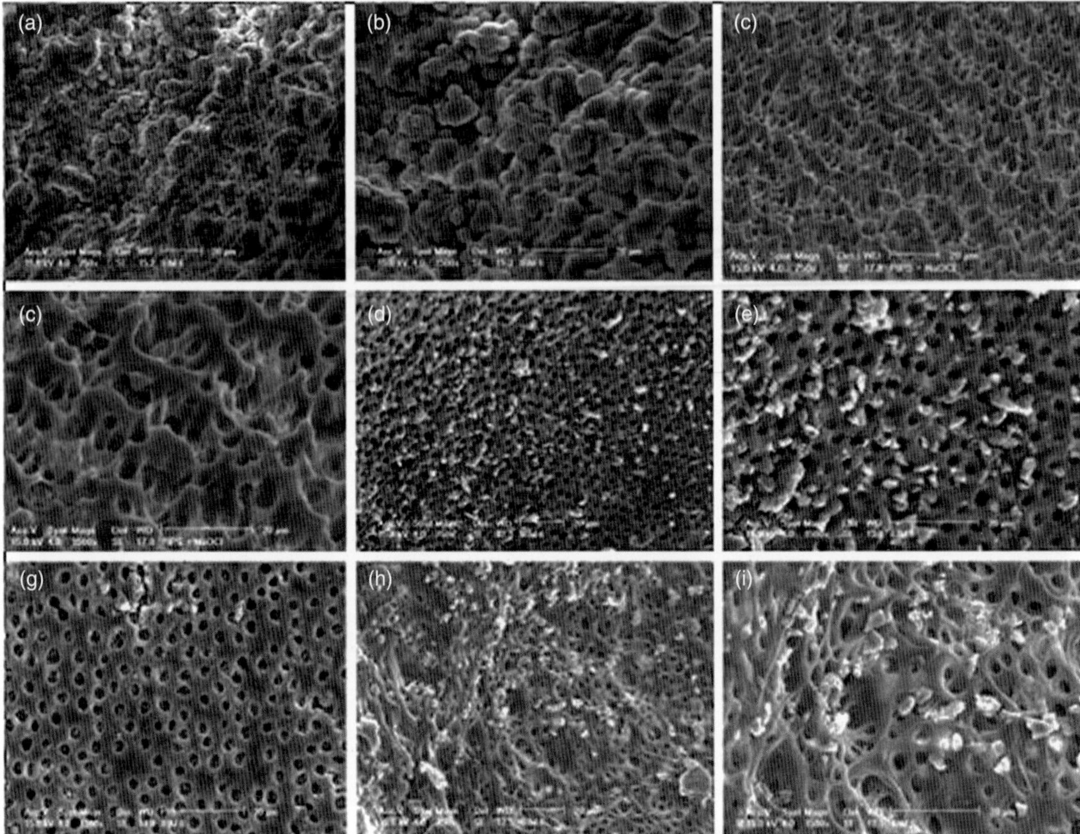

Figure 10.9 Scanning electron microscope analysis of root canal surface. *A* and *B*, Group I shows *E. faecalis* colonies attached to the root canal surface. *C* and *D*, Group II (PIPS + NaOCl) shows a clean root canal surface. *E* and *F*, Group III (PIPS + saline) shows colonies attached to the root canal surface. *G* to *I*, Group IV (irrigation with NaOCl) shows some colonies and the other image shows no colonies. (Image courtesy of Dr. Al Shahrani.)

(Dentsply, Ballaigues, Switzerland). The method used was a modification of Altundasar's group's, where they used flower arrangement foam to replicate the resistance of apical tissue (refer to Figure 1) [30]. To quantify the amount of extruded irrigant, the foam was weighed before and after. They did not find any significant difference among all techniques. LAI using PIPS at 0.3 W and 0.9 W did not result in more extrusion of irrigant than did the conventional technique. All groups had equal amounts of extrusion (Figure 2). One reason could be the close placement of the irrigation needle to working length as well as the continuous irrigation.

Treatment success depends on the complete removal of root canal contents, including pulpal tissues, dentinal debris, microorganisms (bacterial biofilms), and irritants [31]. The irrigant of choice in endodontics is sodium hypochlorite, as it is a broad-spectrum disinfectant. It exhibits bactericidal activity and, more importantly, tissue dissolution activity, which is something that other available irrigants used in endodontics do not have [32–37]. However, due to the complexity of the root canal anatomy, including lateral canals, isthmuses, anastomosis, and accessory canals, it is difficult to completely debride the root canal system [38]. Therefore, and irrigation-delivery system is mandatory to deliver the irrigation to the deepest parts of root canal systems to enhance the debridement of the root canals. LAI using PIPS is shown to be an effective technique in dissolving pulpal tissues [39]. (Figure 10.10)

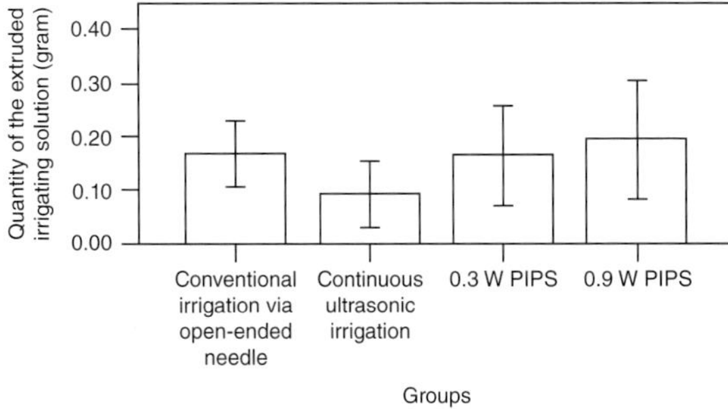

Figure 10.10 The amount of irrigant extrusion. There is no statistically significant difference. (Image courtesy of Arslan H, Capar ID, Saygili G, Gok T, Akcay M. Effect of photon-initiated photoacoustic streaming on removal of apically placed dentinal debris. *Int Endod J* 2014; 47(11): 1072–1077.)

Guneser and colleagues proposed an experiment to test the dissolving ability of sodium hypochlorite and PIPS and compared it with EndoActivator. They used bovine pulpal tissues extracted from central incisors. The bovine pulpal tissue was mixed with dentin shavings and placed in equal amounts in 1.5-mL Eppendorf tubes, and 1 mL of sodium hypochlorite was then added to the mixture. The experimental group was divided into four treatment groups: sodium hypochlorite plus PIPS, sodium hypochlorite plus Er:YAG with 300 μm fiberoptic using the R14 handpiece, sodium hypochlorite plus EndoActivator, and PIPS plus distilled water. Each group received the treatment. The Er:YAG laser group, PIPS plus sodium hypochlorite group, and sodium hypochlorite plus EndoActivator were activated for 5 minutes with a total amount of 1 mL of sodium hypochlorite. The result showed a superiority of the Er:YAG plus sodium hypochlorite in dissolving the tissues, followed by sodium hypochlorite plus PIPS and sodium hypochlorite plus EndoActivator. As is well known, dentin has a remarkable buffering effect against sodium hypochlorite [40]. Therefore, it reduces sodium hypochlorite's action by reducing its alkalinity. Thus, dentin shavings were used to simulate clinical situations. The Er:YAG laser with both endodontic optic fiber tip and PIPS tip dissolved the most tissue, and sonic activation using EndoActivator had no effect.

It has been shown in multiple studies that the efficacy of LAI using the PIPS technique is a promising adjunctive endodontic tool (Table 10.2). It resulted in better cleaning and decontamination of the root canal system. The unique design of the tip made of quartz and the implemented taper at the end allowed better delivery of the energy to the root canal system without the need to insert the tip close to the working length. It instead promotes minimally invasive preparations by placing the tip at the pulp chamber level (Figure 10.11).

Conclusions and future studies

Studies of LAI have shown the following:

- LAI used with sodium hypochlorite was an effective protocol in eradicating bacterial biofilm.
- LAI showed no thermal effect.
- LAI saves time.
- LAI promotes minimally invasive endodontics.

The current use of lasers in endodontics is to use the laser energy to enhance the sterility of root canal

Table 10.2 Comparison between modern lasers and old lasers.

Present-day laser-activated irrigation	Old lasers
Requires minimal preparation of the root canal system	Requires an extremely large preparation
Has no thermal effect	Has a thermal effect
Uses a subablative energy (less than 1W)	Uses a high energy (5–60W)
Tips are place at coronal pulpal chamber	Fiberoptics and metal files must be placed deep within (1 mm from working length)
Time saving	Takes longer
Laser-activated irrigation at subablative energy removes smear layer	Melts and carbonizes the root canal surface
Does not affect the tooth	Causes inflammation and edema of supporting tooth structure

Polyamide Sheath
Sheath stripped away 10mm approx
Laser Tip
Tapered Included a

(a)

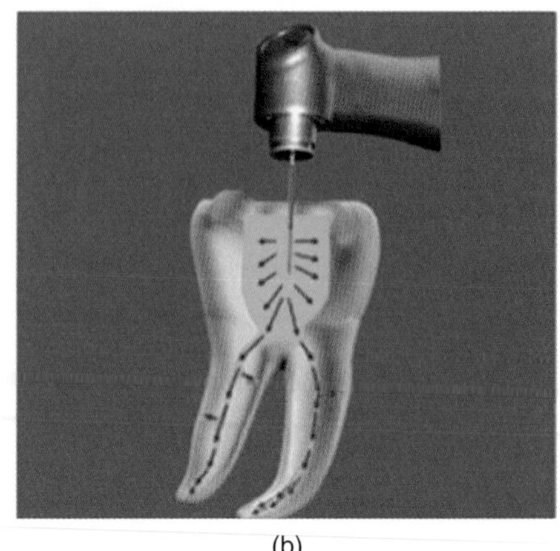

(b)

Figure 10.11 A close-up view of the PIPS tip and its composition, including the striped sheath that helps propagate the shock waves in the root canal system (a). The illustration shows how the PIPS is placed and how it delivers the shock waves (b).

systems. It has been used as an adjunctive tool to activate the irrigation solution. Although numerous studies showed the efficacy of LAI, there is still a need to investigate its safety in clinical settings followed by multicenter clinical outcome studies to evaluate the feasibility of LAI.

References

1 Gordon JP, Zeiger HJ, Townes CH. The maser—new type of microwave amplifier, frequency standard, and spectrometer. *Physical Review* 1955; 99(4): 1264–1274.

2 Schawlow AL, Townes CH. Infrared and optical masers. *Physical Review* 1958; 112(6): 1940–1949.

3 Mohammadi Z. Laser applications in endodontics: an update review. *Int Dent J* 2009 59(1): 35–46.

4 Weichman JA, Johnson FM. Laser use in endodontics: a preliminary investigation. *Oral Surg Oral Med Oral Pathol* 1971; 31(3): 416–420.

5 Bahcall J, Howard P, Miserendino L, Walia H. Preliminary investigation of the histological effects of laser endodontic treatment on the periradicular tissues in dogs. *J Endod* 1992; 18(2): 47–51.

6 Dederich DN, Zakariasen KL, Tulip J. Scanning electron microscopic analysis of canal wall dentin following neodymium-yttrium-aluminum-garnet laser irradiation. *J Endod* 1984; 10(9): 428–431.

7 Levy G. Cleaning and shaping the root canal with a Nd:YAG laser beam: a comparative study. *J Endod* 1992; 18(3): 123–127.

8 Kakehashi S, Stanley HR, Fitzgerald RJ. The effects of surgical exposures of dental pulps in germ-free and conventional laboratory rats. *Oral Surg Oral Med Oral Pathol* 1965; 20(3): 340–349.

9 Baumgartner JC. Microbiologic aspects of endodontic infections. *J Calif Dent Assoc* 2004; 32(6): 459–468.

10 Sakamoto M, Rôças IN, Siqueira JF Jr, Benno Y. Molecular analysis of bacteria in asymptomatic and symptomatic endodontic infections. *Oral Microbiol Immunol* 2006; 21(2): 112–122.

11 Sen BH, Wesselink PR, Turkun M. The smear layer: a phenomenon in root canal therapy. *Int Endod J* 1995; 28(3): 141–148.

12 Cameron JA. The use of ultrasound for the removal of the smear layer. The effect of sodium hypochlorite concentration; SEM study. *Aust Dent J* 1988; 33(3): 193–200.

13 Kimura Y, Wilder-Smith P, Matsumoto K. Lasers in endodontics: a review. *Int Endod J* 2000; 33(3): 173–185.

14 Melcer J, Chaumette MT, Zeboulon S, Melcer F, Hasson R, Merard R, Pinaudeau Y, Dejardin J, Weill R. Preliminary report on the effect of the CO_2 laser beam on the dental pulp of the *Macaca mulatta* primate and the Beagle dog. *J Endod* 1985; 11(1): 1–5.

15 Jukić S, Anić I, Koba K, Najzar-Fleger D, Matsumoto K. The effect of pulpotomy using CO_2 and Nd:YAG lasers on dental pulp tissue. *Int Endod J* 1997; 30(3): 175–180.

16 Moritz A, Schoop U, Goharkhay K, Sperr W. The CO_2 laser as an aid in direct pulp capping. *J Endod* 1998; 24(4): 248–251.

17 Olivi G, Genovese MD, Maturo P, Docimo R. Pulp capping: advantages of using laser technology. *Eur J Paediatr Dent* 2007; 8(2): 89–95.

18 Santucci PJ. Dycal versus Nd:YAG laser and Vitrebond for direct pulp capping in permanent teeth. *J Clin Laser Med Surg* 1999; 17(2): 69–75.

19 Fried D, Glena RE, Featherstone JD, Seka W. Permanent and transient changes in the reflectance of CO_2 laser-irradiated dental hard tissues at lambda = 9.3, 9.6, 10.3, and 10.6 microns and at fluences of 1-20 J/cm^2. *Lasers Surg Med* 1997; 20(1): 22–31.

20 Liu JF. Effects of Nd:YAG laser pulpotomy on human primary molars. *J Endod* 2006; 32(5): 404–407.

21 Peters OA, Bardsley S, Fong J, Pandher G, Divito E. Disinfection of root canals with photon-initiated photoacoustic streaming. *J Endod* 2011; 37(7): 1008–1012.

22 De Moor RJ, Meire M, Goharkhay K, Moritz A, Vanobbergen J. Efficacy of ultrasonic versus laser-activated irrigation to remove artificially placed dentin debris plugs. *J Endod* 2010; 36(9): 1580–1583.

23 Al Shahrani M, DiVito E, Hughes CV, Nathanson D, Huang GT. Enhanced removal of *Enterococcus faecalis* biofilms in the root canal using sodium hypochlorite plus photon-induced photoacoustic streaming: an *in vitro* study. *Photomed Laser Surg* 2014; 32(5): 260–266.

24 Pedullà E, Genovese C, Campagna E, Tempera G, Rapisarda E. Decontamination efficacy of photon-initiated photoacoustic streaming (PIPS) of irrigants using low-energy laser settings: an *ex vivo* study. *Int Endod J* 2012; 45(9): 865–870.

25 Arslan H, Capar ID, Saygili G, Gok T, Akcay M. Effect of photon-initiated photoacoustic streaming on removal of apically placed dentinal debris. *Int Endod J* 2014; 47(11): 1072–1077.

26 Behrents KT, Speer ML, Noujeim M. Sodium hypochlorite accident with evaluation by cone beam computed tomography. *Int Endod J* 2012; 45(5): 492–498.

27 Motta MV, Chaves-Mendonca MA, Stirton CG, Cardozo HF. Accidental injection with sodium hypochlorite: report of a case. *Int Endod J* 2009; 42(2): 175–182.

28 Kleier DJ, Averbach RE, Mehdipour O. The sodium hypochlorite accident: experience of diplomates of the American Board of Endodontics. *J Endod* 2008; 34(11): 1346–1350.

29 Arslan H1, Akcay M, Ertas H, Capar ID, Saygili G, Meşe M. Effect of PIPS technique at different power settings on irrigating solution extrusion. *Lasers Med Sci* 2015 Aug; 30(6): 1641–1645.

30 Altundasar E, Nagas E, Uyanik O, Serper A. Debris and irrigant extrusion potential of 2 rotary systems and irrigation needles. *Oral Surg Oral Med Oral Pathol Oral Radiol Endod* 2011; 112(4): e31–e35.

31 Siqueira JF Jr, Rocas IN. Clinical implications and microbiology of bacterial persistence after treatment procedures. *J Endod* 2008; 34(11): 1291–1301 e3.

32 Al-Jadaa A, Paqué F, Attin T, Zehnder M. Acoustic hypochlorite activation in simulated curved canals. *J Endod* 2009; 35(10): 1408–1411.

33 Cobankara FK, Ozkan HB, Terlemez A. Comparison of organic tissue dissolution capacities of sodium hypochlorite and chlorine dioxide. *J Endod* 2010; 36(2): 272–274.

34 Haapasalo M, Wang Z, Shen Y, Curtis A, Patel P, Khakpour M. Tissue dissolution by a novel multisonic ultracleaning system and sodium hypochlorite. *J Endod* 2014; 40(8): 1178–1181.

35 Rossi-Fedele G, Steier L, Dogramaci EJ, Canullo L, Steier G, de Figueiredo JA. Bovine pulp tissue dissolution ability of HealOzone, Aquatine Alpha Electrolyte) and sodium hypochlorite. *Aust Endod J* 2013; 39(2): 57–61.

36 Slutzky-Goldberg I, Hanut A, Matalon S, Baev V, Slutzky H. The effect of dentin on the pulp tissue dissolution capacity of sodium hypochlorite and calcium hydroxide. *J Endod* 2013; 39(8): 980–983.

37 Stojicic S, Zivkovic S, Qian W, Zhang H, Haapasalo M. Tissue dissolution by sodium hypochlorite: effect of concentration, temperature, agitation, and surfactant. *J Endod* 2010; 36(9): 1558–1562.

38 Peters LB, Wesselink PR. Periapical healing of endodontically treated teeth in one and two visits obturated in the presence or absence of detectable microorganisms. *Int Endod J* 2002; 35(8): 660–667.

39 Guneser MB, Arslan D, Usumez A. Tissue dissolution ability of sodium hypochlorite activated by photon-initiated photoacoustic streaming technique. *J Endod* 2015; 41(5): 729–732.

40 Wang JD, Hume WR. Diffusion of hydrogen ion and hydroxyl ion from various sources through dentine. *Int Endod J* 1988; 21(1): 17–26.

Questions

1 What was the major disadvantage of lasers in the initial studies in root canal cleaning?
A Thermal damage
B Apical extrusion
C Patient compliance
D Operator fatigue

2 The major shift in the use of lasers in endodontics has been from attempting to shape the root canal to cleansing the root canal.
A True
B False

3 All of the following are disadvantages of a smear layer left on root canal walls except
A It interferes with sealing ability of obturation material
B It acts as a substrate for unremoved bacteria.
C Smear layer harbors microorganisms.
D Smear layer interferes with intracanal medicaments.
E Smear layer is a strict barrier against bacteria.

4 Which was another disadvantage of the older laser tips?
A Color
B Length
C Size
D Metal

5 Laser Doppler flowmetry (LDF) may be useful in
A Controlling flow of irrigant in the canal
B Measuring pulp vitality
C Measuring the bacterial load in the canal
D Measuring pulp sensitivity

6 The energy level of the CO_2 laser influences the pulp-capping prognosis. What level of energy is more conducive to pulp survival and successful healing after pulpotomy?
A 60 W
B 30 W
C 3 W
D 1 W
E 0.1 W

7 In the Peters *et al.* study [21], which irrigation technique yielded the most negative culture samples?
A LAI alone
B LAI using PIPS
C Ultrasonics using PIPS
D Ultrasonics alone

8 Arslan and colleagues [25] demonstrated that LAI with PIPS was significantly better in what aspect of the endodontic procedure?
A Apical extrusion
B Canal disinfection
C Debris removal
D Tubule cleanliness

9 Where is the appropriate position to place the PIPS during the irrigation procedure?
A The apical third of each canal
B At full working length for complete disinfection
C At 1 to 2 mm into the orifice of each canal
D In the pulp chamber
E At the occlusal surface of the accessed tooth

10 What do the studies demonstrate so far in terms of apical extrusion with different irrigation technique?
A Ultrasonic activation is the best with minimal apical extrusion.
B Conventional irrigation demonstrates the most apical extrusion.
C Side-vented needles are significantly better than LAI.
D LAI with PIPS shows the least apical extrusion.
E No significant difference exists among the irrigation techniques for apical extrusion.

CHAPTER 11
Dental pulp regeneration

Sahng G. Kim
Columbia University College of Dental Medicine, New York, New York, USA

The dental pulp is a loose connective tissue consisting of a variety of cells such as odontoblasts, fibroblasts, endothelial cells, nerve cells, immune cells, and stem/progenitor cells, and an extracellular matrix including fibrillar proteins and ground substance [1]. Owing to its physiological and anatomical relationship with dentin, dental pulp functions as the pulp–dentin complex. The dental pulp is small in scale but has a highly complex structure that exerts multiple functions such as tooth development, mineralized tissue formation, nutrition supply to the surrounding mineralized tissues, immune response, and neurogenic/immunogenic inflammation as well as sensory function [1]. Research that endeavors to understand the underlying mechanisms of dental pulp regeneration is still in its early stage, but the laboratory and preclinical findings have been translated into successful clinical applications. In this chapter, the development and limitations of clinical dental pulp regeneration therapy, and cell-based and cell-free therapy for dental pulp regeneration, are reviewed and discussed.

History: early attempts to regenerate dental pulp

The first attempts to regenerate pulp tissue were found in case studies by Nygaard Ostby [2, 3]. In these studies, root canals were intentionally overinstrumented to evoke bleeding and then filled with gutta-percha and Kloroperka N-O paste short of the root apices to allow tissue ingrowth into the root canals. A 4% formaldehyde solution was used to disinfect the canals in necrotic cases. Histology showed mineral tissue deposition along the root canal walls and connective tissue formation in the root canal space. However, the ingrowth of fibrous connective tissue was not observed in most of the necrotic cases, although it was identified in the majority of vital cases [3].

To enhance root canal disinfection for pulp regeneration in immature nonvital teeth, Rule and Winter [4] introduced polyantibiotics consisting of neomycin sulfate, polymyxin B sulfate, bacitracin, and nystatin and absorbable iodoform into the root canals. They found continued root development and apical barrier formation in their nonvital cases. Nevins and colleagues [5, 6] reported revitalization and hard tissue formation in immature pulpless teeth in monkeys and humans when root canals were mechanically instrumented and collagen–calcium phosphate gels were used as a scaffold.

Clinical dental pulp regeneration

How did early research efforts evolve into a current treatment modality?

The early efforts to regenerate dental pulp in patients did not provide reliable clinical outcomes. However, the anecdotal or empirical evidence from early clinical trials was regarded as a useful groundwork to develop more sophisticated clinical protocols. The role of inducing bleeding into the root canal space, the methods of disinfection in nonvital teeth, and the possible need for scaffold materials were rediscovered in recent clinical studies.

There was a paucity of clinical studies that had attempted to achieve dental pulp regeneration until Iwaya and colleagues [7] reported a treatment of an immature necrotic mandibular second premolar with

Current Therapy in Endodontics, First Edition. Edited by Priyanka Jain.
© 2016 John Wiley & Sons, Inc. Published 2016 by John Wiley & Sons, Inc.

a sinus tract. The tooth had a developmental anomaly, dens evaginatus, and the fracture of the dental protuberance on the occlusal surface, which led to pulp necrosis and a chronic apical abscess. The root canal was mechanically instrumented, chemically irrigated using 5% sodium hypochlorite and 3% hydrogen peroxide, and medicated with two antibiotics (metronidazole and ciprofloxacin). At the fifth visit of root canal disinfection, vital tissue ingrowth was observed clinically in the root canal, and a calcium hydroxide/iodoform paste was applied to the tissue. The tooth was sealed with a glass ionomer and composite resin restorative material. Complete root apex closure and the thickening of root canal walls with the resolution of the periapical radiolucency were confirmed radiographically at a 30-month follow-up.

Banchs and Trope [8] demonstrated a similarly successful clinical case with a more-controlled clinical protocol, which has served as a basis for many current clinical pulp regeneration studies. An immature mandibular second premolar diagnosed with pulp necrosis and a chronic apical abscess was chemically disinfected with 5.25% sodium hypochlorite and 0.12% chlorhexidine in addition to intracanal medication with a triple antibiotic paste (ciprofloxacin, metronidazole, and minocycline). At the second visit, bleeding was evoked using an explorer for the formation of blood clots over which mineral trioxide aggregate and a temporary filling material were placed. At the third visit, the temporary filling material was replaced with a composite resin. At a 24-month follow-up, the tooth showed complete root formation with thickening of root canal walls, the resolution of the periapical radiolucency, and a positive response to a cold test.

Medicaments, materials and induced bleeding in pulp regeneration therapy

The previous clinical trials have provided useful information such as the use of the intracanal medicament for sufficient disinfection and the importance of induced bleeding [2–8]. The use of the triple antibiotic paste became the most common intracanal medicament for pulp regeneration [8]. The rationale of the use of this antibiotic paste was based on the in vitro studies by the Hoshino group [9, 10], which showed that the mixture of three antibiotics (ciprofloxacin, metronidazole, and minocycline) was effective in disinfection of both infected pulp and root canal dentin. An in vivo study by Windley and colleagues [11] in a dog model also demonstrated a significantly higher disinfection in teeth after an additional two weeks of the antibiotic dressing compared with teeth that had sodium hypochlorite irrigation alone.

As an alternative to the antibiotics for pulp regeneration, calcium hydroxide has been suggested. Chueh and colleagues [12] showed that root canal disinfection with a short-term (less than 3 months) and a long-term (more than 3 months) calcium hydroxide application was equally conducive to healing of apical pathosis with continued root development in immature necrotic teeth. An *in vitro* study by Ruparel and colleagues [13] showed that the combinations of antibiotics consisting of the triple antibiotics, the double antibiotics, and modified triple antibiotics, and amoxicillin–clavulanic acid (Augmentin) had a detrimental effect on the survival of stem cells of the apical papilla in concentrations higher than 1 mg/mL. The concentrations of commonly used antibiotic pastes for pulp regeneration are around 1000 mg/mL, suggesting the paste form of antibiotics can cause the death of the cells that would be recruited to the root canal space and contribute to the regeneration of vital tissues. On the other hand, calcium hydroxide did not demonstrate any harmful effect on the cells in all concentrations tested [13]. Therefore, calcium hydroxide or a low concentration of antibiotics (liquid form, 0.01–0.1 mg/mL) should be used as an antibacterial medicament in pulp regeneration.

When the triple antibiotic paste is placed in contact with the anterior teeth, discoloration can occur. Minocycline, which is one of the components of the triple antibiotic paste, is the main cause of tooth discoloration. Minocycline can penetrate the tooth through dentinal tubules, and it can integrate with the crystal structure of the tooth. Administration of minocycline is contraindicated in pregnant women who are in the third trimester or in children who are younger than 8 years of age, due to the induction of tooth discoloration, reduction of bone growth, and amelogenesis imperfecta.

Another material used for pulp regeneration therapy is calcium silicate–based cement such as mineral trioxide aggregate (MTA). The coronal space is usually filled with MTA after inducing bleeding with a file. MTA has a remarkable biocompatibility and sealing ability and is able to set in a moist environment such as the bleeding area of the tooth. It permits cell proliferation and cell attachment,

Box 11.1 Differences among treatment procedures for immature teeth

1. Apexification

a. Calcium hydroxide

- Requires a long time for treatment results
- Increased risk of tooth fracture

b. Mineral trioxide aggregate

- Root remains thin
- Neither strengthens the root nor promotes further development

2. Revascularization

- Promotes further root development
- Results in reinforcement of the dentinal walls by deposition of hard tissue
- Strengthens the root

which enhance the tissue healing process and may prevent the weakening of the dentin structure.

Induction of bleeding into root canals is considered a critical step for successful pulp regeneration. Lovelace and colleagues [14] reported that evoked bleeding could trigger a greater influx of stem cells into the root canal space based on the finding that significantly higher mesenchymal stem cells markers (CD73, CD105) were observed in the intracanal blood after bleeding was induced, compared with the concentration of those markers in systemic blood. Ding and colleagues [15], in their clinical study, showed that all cases of unfavorable clinical outcomes were related to a failure to evoke bleeding into the root canal space. Petrino and colleagues [16] suggested that anesthesia without a vasoconstrictor (3% mepivacaine) should be used to avoid the constriction of blood vessels, thereby allowing more bleeding to be induced into the root canals.

Current clinical protocols and American Association of Endodontists considerations or pulp regeneration

In January 2011, the American Dental Association adopted pulp-regeneration procedures as a new treatment modality. Since then, there have been numerous clinical case reports and series [17–27] and several outcome studies [28–33] with different clinical protocols. Clinical protocols vary in the use of mechanical instrumentation, type of irrigants, and intracanal medicaments, yet they all have led to successful outcomes (root maturation with or without return of vitality). An example of clinical pulp regeneration in an immature tooth is presented in Figure 11.1. A review by Kontakiotis and colleagues [34] showed that most of the studies did not use mechanical instrumentation and only used sodium hypochlorite as a chemical irrigant and antibiotics as the main intracanal medicament for pulp regeneration. The American Association of Endodontists has developed a recommended clinical protocol based on clinical and preclinical studies [35].

The American Association of Endodontists (AAE) suggests that regenerative endodontic treatment can be used for teeth of a compliant patient with necrotic pulp, an immature apex, and pulp space not needed for post and core. At the first appointment for regenerative endodontic treatment, risks and potential benefits should be explained to the patient in detail.

This protocol includes the case selection, the treatment procedures, and the follow-up methods. As was described previously by Andreasen and colleagues [36] and Kling and colleagues [37], the tooth selected for pulp regeneration should have an open apex with diameters bigger than 1.0 mm or 1.1 mm. As for the clinical recommendation, low concentrations of sodium hypochlorite and calcium hydroxide or low concentrations of triple antibiotics as an intracanal medicament should be used for chemical disinfection at the first appointment. The use of anesthesia without a vasoconstrictor [16], and ethylenediaminetetraacetic acid (EDTA) as a single irrigant to promote the release of growth factors from dentin by chelating the inorganic components of root dentin , induced bleeding by overinstrumentation to recruit the stem/progenitor cells, a resorbable matrix as a barrier to aid cement placement, and a calcium silicate–based cement such as Biodentine to seal the coronal extension of the root canal space are recommended at the second appointment [35]. At the follow up visits, the resolution of clinical signs and symptoms, radiographic healing such as the absence of a periapical radiolucency and the increased root lengths and widths, and the return of a positive vitality response are assessed [35].

The limitations of current treatment protocols

There are several treatment options for a necrotic or infected immature permanent tooth. Traditionally, apexification has been recommended for treating an immature tooth that has an open apex. Apexification is a procedure that promotes the formation of an apical barrier to prevent the extrusion of filling materials. Materials such as calcium hydroxide and MTA, which induce the formation of a calcified apical barrier, are used for apexification. MTA has been proposed as a material to create an apical barrier that prevents the extrusion of obturation materials.

The goal of pulp regeneration therapy is to restore the functional integrity of the dental pulp and dentin [38–40]. The dental pulp and dentin, originated from the neural crest-derived mesenchyme, work as a functional unit called the pulp–dentin complex due to their physiological and anatomical relationships [41–43]. Pulp regeneration therapy can offer biological and clinical benefits to patients. From a biological perspective, the neurovascular system can be reconstituted along with tubular dentin and odontoblast layers. This functional structure of the pulp–dentin complex may restore the immune response to the pulp that will function as the first line of defense against microbial invasion during the infection [41, 44]. From a clinical perspective, pulp regeneration therapy meets our general goal in endodontic treatment, which is to cure and prevent apical periodontitis. In addition, mineralized tissue deposition along the root canal walls in necrotic teeth with immature root apices can make a tooth more resistant to fracture. Differences among treatment procedures for immature teeth were highlighted in Box 11.1.

Several clinical studies showed successful clinical outcomes when the current treatment protocols were used (Table 11.1). Histological observation, however, showed bone-like and cementum-like tissues without odontoblasts and regenerated dentin. Becerra and colleagues [45] showed successful root maturation and complete resolution of a periapial radiolucency

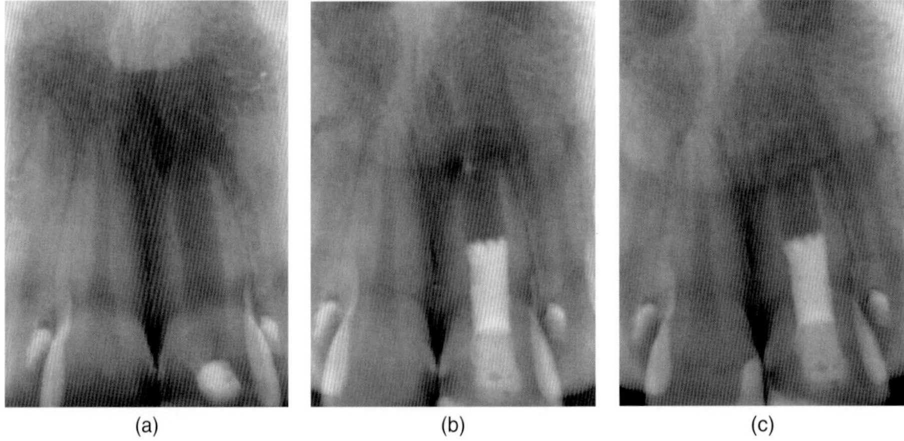

Figure 11.1 Clinical pulp regeneration therapy. A, Preoperative radiograph shows an immature necrotic maxillary left central incisor with a periapical radiolucency. B, Postoperative radiograph. Sodium hypochlorite and ciprofloxacin were used to disinfect the canal. Bleeding was evoked and the tooth was sealed with a mineral trioxide aggregate and bonded resin. C, Seven-month recall radiograph. The resolution of the periapical radiolucency and apical closure were observed. (Image courtesy of Dr. Victoria Tountas.)

Table 11.1 Clinical protocols and success rates of pulp regeneration outcome studies.

Study	Type of study	Initial irrigation	Medication	Final irrigation	Success rate (healed and healing)
Jeeruphan *et al.* [28]	Retrospective	2.5% NaOCl	Triple antibiotic paste	2.5% NaOCl	100%(20/20)
Nagy *et al.* [29]	Prospective	2.6% NaOCl	Double antibiotic paste	2.6% NaOCl and saline	85% (17/20)
Kahler *et al.* [30]	Prospective	1% NaOCl	Triple antibiotic paste	1% NaOCl	90.3%
Nagata *et al.* [31]	Prospective	6% NaOCl and 2% chlorhexidine	Triple antibiotic paste Calcium hydroxide and chlorhexidine gel	17% EDTA and saline	95.6% (22/23)
Alobaid *et al.* [32]	Retrospective	Varying concentrations of NaOCl, chlorhexidine, and/or EDTA	Triple antibiotic paste or double antibiotic paste and/or calcium hydroxide	Unknown	79% (15/19)
Saoud *et al.* [33]	Prospective	2.5% NaOCl	Triple antibiotic paste	Saline	100% (20/20)

in an immature necrotic mandibular second premolar with chronic apical abscess two years after pulp regeneration therapy. The histological assessment of the tooth extracted for the orthodontic reason revealed the formation of periodontal ligament-like tissue and bone-like or cementum-like tissue in the root canal space [45]. Another histological observation by Lei and colleagues [46] also showed islands of bone-like tissue and deposition of cementum-like tissue along the root canal wall with fibrous connective tissue similar to periodontal ligament ten months after pulp regeneration therapy in an immature necrotic second premolar. This finding was in accordance with the observations of animal studies using current treatment protocols. A dog study by Wang and colleagues [47] showed the deposition of cementum onto dentin and bone-like and periodontal ligament–like tissues in the root canal space in immature necrotic teeth with apical periodontitis. Another dog study by Gomes-Filho and colleagues [48] showed newly formed vital tissues in the necrotic teeth that consisted of cementum-like and bone-like tissues and fibrous connective tissue attached to cementum-like tissues. No significant differences in histological outcomes were found among three experimental groups with different protocols including use of blood clots with or without platelet-rich plasma protein gels and/or bone marrow aspirate gels.

Current clinical protocols have only allowed ectopic tissue formation in the root canal. The ectopic tissues such as cementum, bone, and periodontal ligament in the root canal have a functional quality inferior to the normal pulp–dentin complex with respect to immune defenses and regeneration after infection or injury. From a biological perspective, tissue-engineering strategies should be considered for dental pulp regeneration.

Dental pulp tissue engineering

Tissue engineering: cell-based versus cell-free strategies

Stem/progenitor cells are the centerpiece of tissue engineering, along with other essential components that involve biomaterial scaffolds and signaling molecules. After tooth development, some mesenchymal cells in the dental pulp maintain their properties as stem cells and reside in a specialized microenvironment called a *stem cell niche*. The stem cell niche plays a critical role in regulating the balance between self-renewal and differentiation of stem cells by asymmetric/symmetric divisions. Mesenchymal stem cells (MSCs) in the niche function as reservoirs of cells to initiate tissue regeneration during infection and/or injury from trauma and/or disease.

Stem cells of the apical papilla (SCAPs), bone marrow mesenchymal stem cells, dental pulp stem cells (DPSCs), periodontal ligament stem cells, and inflamed periapical progenitor cells are MSCs that may contribute to the regeneration of the pulp–dentin complex. SCAPs are capable of differentiating into odontoblast-like cells forming root dentin, and DPSCs have the ability to differentiate into odontoblast-like cells and form dentin/pulp-like tissues. Even when the pulp becomes

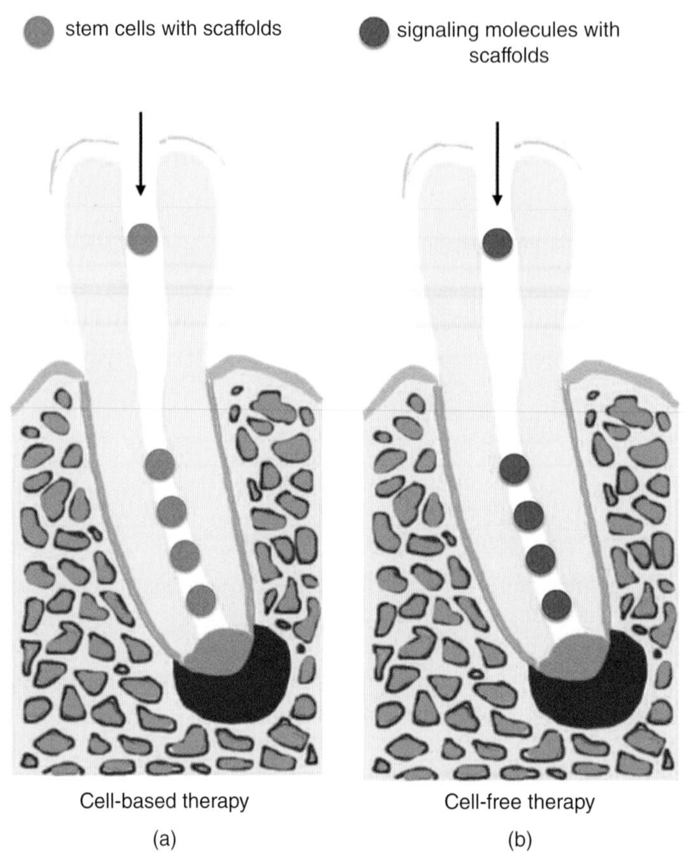

Figure 11.2 Tissue-engineering strategies. *A*, Cell-based therapy using the delivery of stem cells into the defect site. A gel-type scaffold can carry stem cells into the root canal space. Stem cells participate in tissue formation by differentiating into the resident cells. This strategy has been widely used in animal studies. *B*, Cell-free therapy using the delivery of signaling molecules into the defect site. A gel-type scaffold can carry signaling molecules into the root canal space. The signaling molecules can modulate cellular events of endogenous cells and enhance tissue formation. This strategy has fewer translational barriers.

necrotic, SCAPs can survive perhaps due to collateral circulation from the periapical area.

Current tissue-engineering strategies for dental pulp regeneration use the regenerative potentials of the mesenchymal stem/progenitor cells. Two therapeutic strategies have been proposed (Figure 11.2). One is cell-based therapy: isolation and ex vivo expansion of MSCs from different tissue sources and their transplantation into the pulp space. This strategy has been widely used in animal studies. The other is cell-free (cell-homing) therapy: delivery of signaling molecules into the pulp space to control the cellular activities including migration, attachment, proliferation, and differentiation of endogenous MSCs. This strategy has fewer barriers to clinical translation.

Previous work in animal models

Some preclinical studies have attempted to regenerate the pulp–dentin complex using cell-based therapy. Cordeiro and colleaguges [49] demonstrated engineered pulp-like tissues in tooth slices when the tooth slices were seeded with two cell populations, including stem cells from human deciduous teeth and human dermal microvascular endothelial cells, and were implanted into subcutaneous tissues of immunodeficient mice. Huang and colleagues [50] also showed de novo dentin and pulp-like tissues in root fragments when the fragments that contained synthetic scaffolds and tooth-derived stem cells were implanted into the dorsum of severe combined immunodeficiency mice. Iohara and colleagues [51] first showed orthotopic dentin–pulp regeneration when CD105^{+} side population cells, which were a highly angiogenic and neurogenic subpopulation of stem cells with a cell migratory factor or stromal derived factor-1, were transplanted in pulpectomized teeth of dogs. The cell-free strategy was applied in a study by Kim and colleagues [52], where collagen gels with a cocktail of growth factors such as basic fibroblast growth factors, vascular endothelial growth factors, platelet-derived growth factors, nerve growth factors, and bone morphogenetic protein-7 were introduced in emptied root canals of human teeth and transplanted into the dorsum of mice. Pulp-like connective tissues with vasculatures and nerves as well as dentin-like structures were observed after three-week subcutaneous transplantation.

Factors affecting pulp regeneration therapy

To achieve successful results of the treatment procedure, a thorough understanding of the case is very important. The first important consideration is the disinfection of the canal. Researchers suggest that regenerative endodontic treatment will be successful if it is possible to create an environment similar to that for the avulsed tooth. Therefore, if the canals are effectively disinfected and the coronal access is properly sealed, regenerative endodontic treatment should be successful as in an avulsed tooth.

The second consideration is the apex diameter. A tooth with an open apex permits the migration of mesenchymal stem cells into the root canal space, thus allowing the host cell homing to form new tissue in the root canal space. An apical opening of 1.1 mm in diameter or larger is desirable, although the regeneration of the pulp–dentin complex can be achieved in a tooth with a smaller apical opening when biological cues are used in the root canal to promote cell homing.

The third factor is the patient's age. Regeneration might not be as robust in older patients as in young patients because the regeneration potential of patients' endogenous MSCs can decrease with age.

Clinical implications

In cell-based therapy, the ability to select the best subpopulation of stem cells to be transplanted can be considered a strong therapeutic benefit [53]. However, the therapy may suffer from other potential issues such as immunorejection, tumorigenesis, pathogen transmission from donor cells, high cost of manufacturing and commercializing stem cell products, and the special training required for cell manipulation during the transplantation [38]. Cell-free (cell-homing) therapy, on the other hand, may not have these obstacles to clinical translation because it uses a patient's endogenous cells to be mobilized and controlled by exogenous biological molecules. Indeed, a few commercial products approved by the U.S. Food and Drug Administration (FDA) [54, 55] have been used for periodontal regeneration therapy, and similar biological products are anticipated to be available for dental pulp regeneration in the near future.

Conclusions

Despite the high therapeutic promises of clinical dental pulp regeneration therapy, histological findings in clinical cases have thus far not demonstrated the restoration of the pulp–dentin complex. Two main tissue-engineering strategies, cell-based therapy and cell-free therapy, have been suggested to regenerate dentin pulp and dentin. Cell-based therapy has many translational obstacles resulting from safety and regulatory issues, although it has clear scientific merits such as the selection of the best stem cell subpopulation for pulp regeneration. Cell-free therapy can overcome major translational hurdles that cell-based therapy suffers from, with promising therapeutic potentials for the regeneration of dental pulp and dentin.

References

1 Okiji T. Pulp as a connective tissue. In: Hargreaves KM, Goodis EG, Tay FR, editors. *Seltzer and Bender's Dental Pulp*, 2nd edition. Quintessence Publishing; 2012. pp. 67–90.

2 The role of the blood clot in endodontic therapy. An experimental histologic study. *Acta Odontol Scand* 1961; 19: 324–353.

3 Nygaard-Ostby B, Hjortdal O. Tissue formation in the root canal following pulp removal. *Scand J Dent Res* 1971; 79: 333–349.

4 Rule DC, Winter GB. Root growth and apical repair subsequent to pulpal necrosis in children. *Br Dent J* 1966; 120: 586–590.

5 Nevins A, Finkelstein F, Borden B, Laporta R. Revitalization of pulpless open apex teeth in rhesus monkeys using collagen–calcium phosphate gel. *J Endod* 1976; 2: 159–165.

6 Nevins A, Wrobel W, Valachovic R, Finkelstein F. Hard tissue induction into pulpless open-apex teeth using collagen–calcium phosphate gel. *J Endod* 1977; 3: 431–433.

7 Iwaya SI, Ikawa M, Kubota M. Revascularization of an immature permanent tooth with apical periodontitis and sinus tract. *Dent Traumatol* 2001; 17: 185–187.

8 Banchs F, Trope M. Revascularization of immature permanent teeth with apical periodontitis: new treatment protocol? *J Endod* 2004; 30: 196–200.

9 Hoshino E, Kurihara-Ando N, Sato I, Uematsu H, Sato M, Kota K, Iwaku M. In-vitro antibacterial susceptibility of bacteria taken from infected root dentine to a mixture of ciprofloxacin, metronidazole and minocycline. *Int Endod J* 1996; 29: 125–30.

10 Sato I, Ando-Kurihara N, Kota, Iwaku M, Hoshino E. Sterilization of infected root-canal dentine by topical application of a mixture of ciprofloxacin, metronidazole and minocycline in situ. *Int Endod J* 1996; 29: 118–24.

11 Windley W 3rd,, Teixeira F, Levin L, Sigurdsson A, Trope M. Disinfection of immature teeth with a triple antibiotic paste. *J Endod* 2005; 31: 439–443.

12 Chueh LH, Ho YC, Kuo TC, Lai WH, Chen YH, Chiang CP. Regenerative endodontic treatment for necrotic immature permanent teeth. *J Endod* 2009; 35: 160–164.

13 Ruparel NB, Teixeira FB, Ferraz CC, Diogenes A. Direct effect of intracanal medicaments on survival of stem cells of the apical papilla. *J Endod* 2012; 38: 1372–1375.

14 Lovelace TW, Henry MA, Hargreaves KM, Diogenes A. Evaluation of the delivery of mesenchymal stem cells into the root canal space of necrotic immature teeth after clinical regenerative endodontic procedure. *J Endod* 2011; 37: 133–138.

15 Ding RY, Cheung GS, Chen J, Yin XZ, Wang QQ, Zhang CF. Pulp revascularization of immature teeth with apical periodontitis: a clinical study. *J Endod* 2009: 35: 745–749.

16 Petrino JA, Boda KK, Shambarger S, Bowles WR, McClanahan SB. Challenges in regenerative endodontics: a case series. *J Endod* 2010; 36: 536–541.

17 Jung IY, Kim ES, Lee CY, Lee SJ. Continued development of the root separated from the main root. *J Endod* 2011; 37: 711–714.

18 Torabinejad M, Turman M. Revitalization of tooth with necrotic pulp and open apex by using platelet-rich plasma: a case report. *J Endod* 2011; 37: 265–268.

19 Chen MY, Chen KL, Chen CA, Tayebaty F, Rosenberg PA, Lin LM. Responses of immature permanent teeth with infected necrotic pulp tissue and apical periodontitis/abscess to revascularization procedures. *Int Endod J* 2012; 45: 294–305.

20 Jadhav G, Shah N, Logani A. Revascularization with and without platelet-rich plasma in nonvital, immature, anterior teeth: a pilot clinical study. *J Endod* 2012; 38: 1581–1587.

21 Lenzi R, Trope M. Revitalization procedures in two traumatized incisors with different biological outcomes. *J Endod* 2012; 38: 411–414.

22 Torabinejad M, Faras H. A clinical and histological report of a tooth with an open apex treated with regenerative endodontics using platelet-rich plasma. *J Endod* 2012; 38: 864–868.

23 Narayana P, Hartwell GR, Wallace R, Nair UP. Endodontic clinical management of a dens invaginatus case by using a unique treatment approach: a case report. *J Endod* 2012; 38: 1145 –1148.

24 Paryani K, Kim SG. Regenerative endodontic treatment of permanent teeth after completion of root development: a report of 2 cases. *J Endod* 2013; 39: 929–934.

25 Martin G, Ricucci D, Gibbs JL, Lin LM. Histological findings of revascularized/revitalized immature permanent molar with apical periodontitis using platelet-rich plasma. *J Endod* 2013; 39: 138–144.

26 Shimizu E, Ricucci D, Albert J, Alobaid AS, Gibbs JL, Huang GT, Lin LM. Clinical, radiographic, and histological observation of a human immature permanent tooth with chronic apical abscess after revitalization treatment. *J Endod* 2013; 39: 1078–1083.

27 Keswani D, Pandey RK. Revascularization of an immature tooth with a necrotic pulp using platelet-rich fibrin: a case report. *Int Endod J* 2013; 46: 1096–1104.

28 Jeeruphan T, Jantarat J, Yanpiset K, Suwannapan L, Khewsawai P, Hargreaves KM. Mahidol study 1: comparison of radiographic and survival outcomes of immature teeth treated with either regenerative endodontic or apexification methods: a retrospective study. *J Endod* 2012; 38:1330–1336.

29 Nagy MM, Tawfik HE, Hashem AA, Abu-Seida AM. Regenerative potential of immature permanent teeth with necrotic pulps after different regenerative protocols. *J Endod* 2014; 40:192–198.

30 Kahler B, Mistry S, Moule A, Ringsmuth AK, Case P, Thomson A, Holcombe T. Revascularization outcomes: a prospective analysis of 16 consecutive cases. *J Endod* 2014; 40: 333–338.

31 Nagata JY, Gomes BP, Rocha Lima TF, Murakami LS, de Faria DE, Campos GR, et al. Traumatized immature teeth treated with 2 protocols of pulp revascularization. *J Endod* 2014; 40: 606–612.

32 Alobaid AS, Cortes LM, Lo J, Nguyen TT, Albert J, Abu-Melha AS, et al. Radiographic and clinical outcomes of the treatment of immature permanent teeth by revascularization or apexification: a pilot retrospective cohort study. *J Endod* 2014; 40: 1063–1070.

33 Saoud TM, Zaazou A, Nabil A, Moussa S, Lin LM, Gibbs JL. Clinical and radiographic outcomes of traumatized immature permanent necrotic teeth after revascularization/revitalization therapy. *J Endod* 2014; 40: 1946–1952.

34 Kontakiotis EG, Filippatos CG, Tzanetakis GN, Agrafioti A. Regenerative endodontic therapy: a data analysis of clinical protocols. *J Endod* 2015; 41: 146–154.

35 American Association of Endodontists. AAE Clinical Considerations for a Regenerative Procedure, Revised 4-12-15

http://www.aae.org/uploadedfiles/publications_and_research/research/currentregenerativeendodontic considerations.pdf (accessed 1 July 2015)

36 Andreasen JO, Paulsen HU, Yu Z, Bayer T, Schwartz O. A long-term study of 370 autotransplanted premolars. Part II. Tooth survival and pulp healing subsequent to transplantation. *Eur J Orthod* 1990; 12: 14–24.

37 Kling M, Cvek M, Mejare I. Rate and predictability of pulp revascularization in therapeutically reimplanted permanent incisors. *Endod Dent Traumatol* 1986; 2: 83–89.

38 Mao JJ, Kim SG, Zhou J, Ye L, Cho S, Suzuki T, et al. Regenerative endodontics: barriers and strategies for clinical translation. *Dent Clin North Am* 2012; 56: 639–649.

39 Hargreaves KM, Giesler T, Henry M, Wang Y. Regeneration potential of the young permanent tooth: what does the future hold? *J Endod* 2008; 34: S51–S56.

40 Nakashima M, Akamine A. The application of tissue engineering to regeneration of pulp and dentin in endodontics. *J Endod* 2005; 31: 711–718.

41 Pashley DH. Dynamics of the pulpo-dentin complex. *Crit Rev Oral Biol Med* 1996; 7: 104–133.

42 Mjör IA, Sveen OB, Heyerass KJ. Pulp–dentin biology in restorative dentistry. Part 1: normal structure and physiology. *Quintessence Int 200*; 32: 427–446.

43 Byers MR, Närhi MV. Dental injury models: experimental tools for understanding neuroinflammatory interactions and polymodal nociceptor functions. *Crit Rev Oral Biol Med* 1999; 10: 4–39.

44 Hahn CL, Liewehr FR. Innate immune responses of the dental pulp to caries. *J Endod* 2007; 33: 643–651.

45 Becerra P, Ricucci D, Loghin S, Gibbs JL, Lin LM. Histologic study of a human immature permanent premolar with chronic apical abscess after revascularization/revitalization. *J Endod* 2014; 40: 133–139.

46 Lei L, Chen Y, Zhou R, Huang X, Cai Z. Histologic and immunohistochemical findings of a human immature permanent tooth with apical periodontitis after regenerative endodontic treatment. *J Endod* 2015; 41: 1172–1179.

47 Wang X, Thibodeau B, Trope M, Lin LM, Huang GT. Histologic characterization of regenerated tissues in canal space after the revitalization/revascularization procedure of immature dog teeth with apical periodontitis. *J Endod* 2010; 36: 56–63.

48 Gomes-Filho JE, Duarte PC, Ervolino E, Mogami Bomfim SR, Xavier Abimussi CJ, Mota da Silva Santos L, et al. Histologic characterization of engineered tissues in the canal space of closed-apex teeth with apical periodontitis. *J Endod* 2013; 39: 1549–1556.

49 Cordeiro MM, Dong Z, Kaneko T, Zhang Z, Miyazawa M, Shi S, et al. Dental pulp tissue engineering with stem cells from exfoliated deciduous teeth. *J Endod* 2008; 34: 962–969.

50 Huang GT, Yamaza T, Shea LD, Djouad F, Kuhn NZ, Tuan RS, Shi S. Stem/progenitor cell-mediated de novo regeneration of dental pulp with newly deposited continuous layer of dentin in an *in vivo* model. *Tissue Eng Part A* 2010; 16: 605–615.

51 Iohara K, Imabayashi K, Ishizaka R, Watanabe A, Nabekura J, Ito M, et al. Complete pulp regeneration after pulpectomy by transplantation of $CD105^+$ stem cells with stromal cell-derived factor–1. *Tissue Eng Part A* 2011; 17: 1911–1920.

52 Kim JY, Xin X, Moioli EK, Chung J, Lee CH, Chen M, et al. Regeneration of dental-pulp-like tissue by chemotaxis-induced cell homing. *Tissue Eng Part A* 2010; 16: 3023–3031.

53 Iohara K, Zheng L, Ito M, Ishizaka R, Nakamura H, Into T, et al. Regeneration of dental pulp after pulpotomy by transplantation of $CD31^-$/$CD146^-$ side population cells from a canine tooth. *Regen Med* 2009; 4: 377–385.

54 Pellegrini G, Seol YJ, Gruber R, Giannobile WV. Pre-clinical models for oral and periodontal reconstructive therapies. *J Dent Res* 2009; 88: 1065–1076.

55 White AP, Vaccaro AR, Hall JA, Whang PG, Friel BC, McKee MD. Clinical applications of BMP-7/OP-1 in fractures, nonunions and spinal fusion. *Int Orthop* 2007; 31: 735–741.

Questions

1 Which of the following statements is most likely true about the histological outcome of regenerative endodontic treatment?

- A Odontoblast-like cells were found along the predentin layer after regenerative endodontic treatment of immature necrotic teeth in most animal studies.
- B Cementum-like tissues were identified in root canals after the revitalization procedure of immature dog teeth with apical periodontitis.
- C Periodontal ligament–like tissues were not observed in root canals after the revascularization procedure of immature dog teeth with apical periodontitis.
- D Bone-like tissues were not found in the intracanal space after pulp revascularization procedure of immature dog teeth with apical periodontitis.

2 Which of the following statements is most likely true about the intracanal medicaments used in regenerative endodontic treatment?

- A Triple antibiotic pastes at the concentration of 1000 mg/mL did not decrease the survival of stem cells of the apical papilla.
- B Double antibiotic pastes at the concentration of 1000 mg/mL did not decrease the survival of stem cells of the apical papilla.
- C Calcium hydroxide at the concentration of 1 mg/mL increased the survival of stem cells of the apical papilla.
- D Calcium hydroxide at the concentration of 100 mg/mL decreased the survival of stem cells of the apical papilla.

3 Which of the following statements is most likely true?
- A Pulp regeneration therapy can prevent and cure apical periodontitis.
- B Reconstitution of neurovascular structure in pulp tissue is vital to natural immune defense.
- C Functional odontoblasts will function as the first line of defense against microorganisms.
- D All of the above

4 Which of the following statements is most likely true?
- A Cell-based therapy has been widely used in animal studies.
- B Cell-based therapy uses delivery of signaling molecules into the pulp space to control the cellular activities.
- C Cell-free therapy has more translational barriers.
- D Cell-free therapy suffers from immunorejection, tumorigenesis, and pathogen transmission of donor cells.

5 Which of the following statements in most likely false?
- A The goal of pulp regeneration therapy is to restore the functional integrity of the dental pulp and dentin.
- B Mineralized deposition along the root canal walls after pulp regeneration therapy may provide a tooth with fracture resistance.
- C The success rates of clinical pulp regeneration therapy ranged from 79% to 100% based on the clinical outcome studies.
- D The ectopic tissues such as cementum, bone, and periodontal ligament in the root canal have a functional quality superior to the normal pulp–dentin complex with respect to immune defenses.

CHAPTER 12

Teledentistry

Mansi Jain
Inderprastha Dental College and Hospital, Uttar Pradesh, India

Technological innovations in the medical field have been extensive in recent years. Just as communication technology and use of electronic information has developed over the years, terms to describe health care services at a distance, such as *telehealth* and *telemedicine,* have also evolved. Telemedicine may be defined as "the combined use of telecommunications and computer technologies to improve the efficiency and effectiveness of health care services by liberating caregivers from traditional constraints of space and time and empowering consumers to make informed choices in a competitive marketplace" [1].

Dental care, being constantly transformed by these latest innovations, in a synergistic combination with telecommunications technology and the Internet, has yielded a relatively new and exciting field that has immense potential called *teledentistry* [1]. *Tele* comes from Greek and means "distance." [2]. Teledentistry as defined by Cook is "the practice of using video-conferencing technologies to diagnose and to provide advice about the treatment over a distance." It is a combination of telecommunications and dentistry, involving the exchange of clinical information and images over remote distances for dental consultation and treatment planning [3].

Due to the enormous growth of technological capabilities, teledentistry possesses the potential to fundamentally change the current practice and the face of the oral health care [4]. It has the ability to improve access and delivery to oral healthcare, improve the delivery of oral healthcare, and lower its costs. It also has the potential to eliminate the disparities in oral healthcare between rural and urban communities.

This chapter reviews this current concept and how it is used in today's practice, especially its benefits in the field of endodontics. The words *telehealth, teleconsultation,* and *e-health* are used synonymously with *teledentistry* in the chapter. Ethical and legal issues related with this type of practice are also discussed in brief.

Historical background and origins

Radiology was one of the earliest medical specialties to use telecommunication: In 1959, Albert Jutra used communication cable to transmit videotaped telefluoroscopy examinations between two hospitals in Montreal, five miles apart [5]. In its simplest form, telehealth has been around for decades. The beginning of telemedicine can be traced back to 1924, when physicians started consulting patients in remote areas using telephones and radios as the means of communication. In 1989, the Westinghouse Electronics Systems Group in Baltimore conducted a conference focused on drafting a blueprint for dental informatics, combining computer and information science, engineering, and technology in all areas of oral health [6].

The U.S. Army's total dental access (TDA) project is seen as being at the frontier of teledentistry. Started in 1994, this project initially used a traditional plain old telephone system (POTS) with two different communication methods: real time and store and forward. It concluded that teledentistry reduced total patient care cost, improved dental care to distant and rural areas, and provided beneficial information regarding deeper analyses. [1, 7]

In 1995, Rocca and colleagues conducted a pilot study in Haiti to connect a general dentist to a dental specialist in Washington, D.C., via a satellite system. Two years later, integrated services digital network (ISDN)–based teledentistry was tested in Germany, Belgium, and

Current Therapy in Endodontics, First Edition. Edited by Priyanka Jain.
© 2016 John Wiley & Sons, Inc. Published 2016 by John Wiley & Sons, Inc.

Italy. Studies have also been conducted in Scotland, Japan, England, and Taiwan to examine ISDN-based teledentistry. Since then, the era of teledentistry has been expanding worldwide, and teledentistry is gaining ground in developing countries. [7]

Forms of teledentistry

Teleconsultation with specialists, through electronic health records, telecommunications technology, digital imaging, and Internet, can take place by several methods. Two common methods are real-time consultation and the store-and-forward method (Figure 12.1 and Figure 12.2) [8].

Real-time consultation involves using video conferencing, which transfers the information immediately. The dentist and patient at different locations can see, hear, and communicate with each other using advanced telecommunication technology.

The store-and-forward method involves the exchange of clinical information and images collected and stored in a local database for review by a specialist at a later stage. In this method, the patient is not present during the consultation. This stored information is then forwarded for treatment planning via established networks and the Internet. The treatment is provided in a far timelier, targeted, and cost-effective manner [9].

Remote monitoring may be home based or hospital based, where patients are monitored at a distance. A near-real-time consultation has also been mentioned in the literature; it makes use of a low resolution, low-frame-rate product like a jittery television [10].

Scope of teledentistry

Teledentistry improves access to oral health care, improve the delivery of oral healthcare, and lower its costs. It also has the potential to eliminate the disparities in oral healthcare between rural and urban communities. It is the fastest way to bridge the rural-urban health divide and also can help to bring specialized healthcare to the remotest corners of the world [11]. Interprofessional communications will improve dentistry's integration into the larger healthcare delivery system. The use of specialist consultations and continuity of care will provide aspects of decision support and facilitate a sharing of the contextual knowledge of the patient among dentists [12] (Box 12.1).

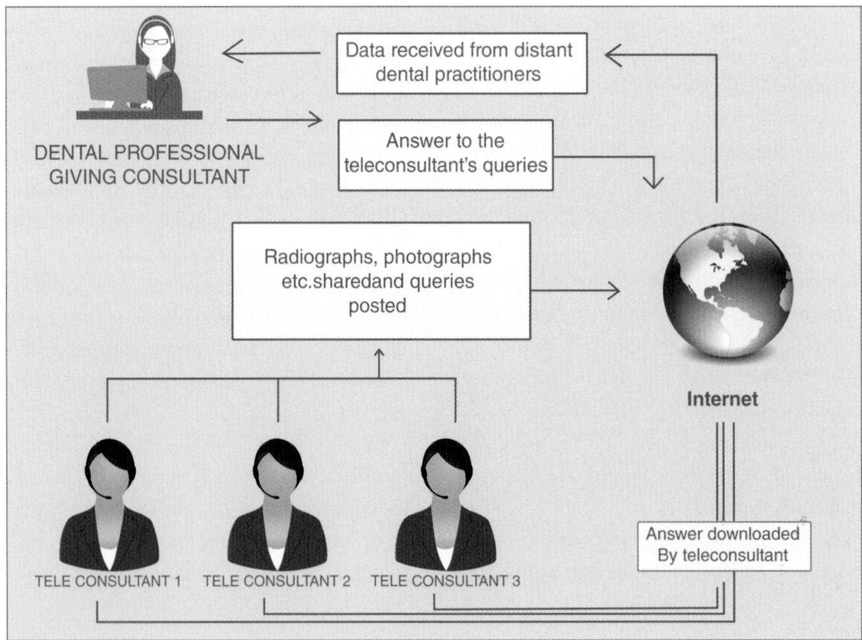

Figure 12.1 Store and forward method.

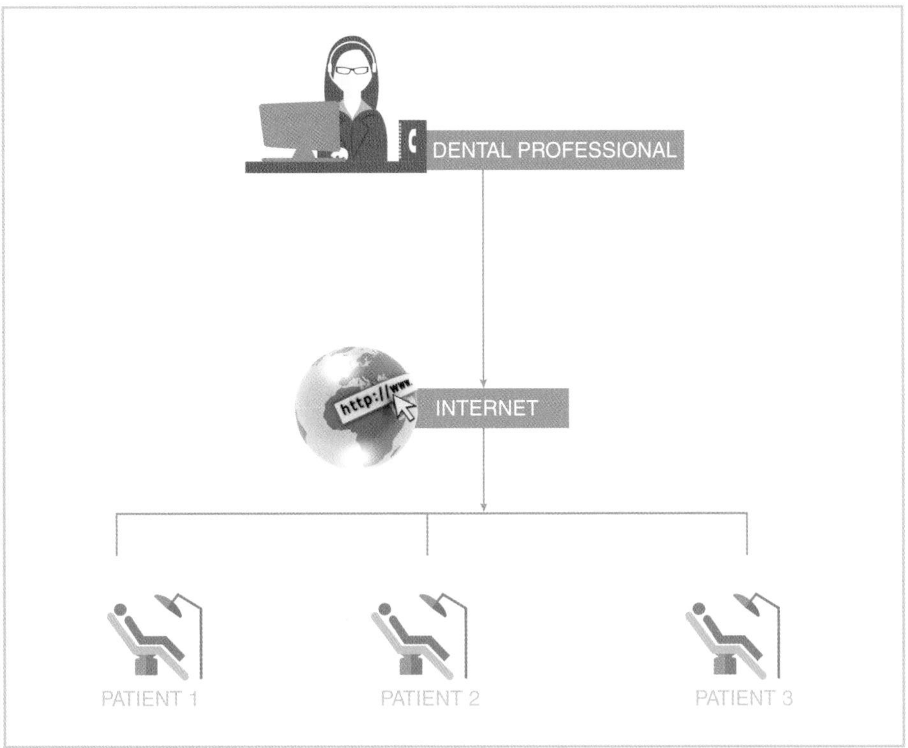

Figure 12.2 Real-time consultation.

Tele education is gaining popularity to supplement traditional teaching methods in dental education and provide new opportunities for dental students and dentists [13]. Formal online education can be divided into two main categories: Web-based self-instruction and interactive video- conferencing. The web-based self-instruction educational system contains information that has been developed and stored before the user accesses the program. The advantage of this is that the user can control the pace of learning and can review the material as many times as he or she wishes. The limitations have been noted in areas of satisfaction (lack of face to face communication with peers and instructors) and accuracy (lack of face to face patient examination) [13].

Interactive videoconferencing (conducted via POTS, satellite, ISDN, Internet or Intranet explained later in the chapter) includes both, a live interactive videoconference (with at least one camera set-up where the patient's information is transmitted or at both locations) and supportive information (such as patient's medical history and radiographs) that can be sent before or at the same time as the videoconference (with or without the patient present). The advantage of this educational style is that the user (typically the patient's health care provider) can receive immediate feedback. Dental chat rooms are available through numerous dental organizations and study clubs, as well as through individual practitioners who exchange information on a variety of topics [13].

Technological requirements

A typical system consists of a computer with substantial hard drive memory, adequate RAM, and a speedy processor; an intraoral video camera and a digital camera for the capture of pictures; a modem; and an Internet connection. A fax machine, a scanner, and a printer are also required in some cases [9]. To enable live videoconferencing, a widely available standalone IP/ISDN videoconferencing solution may be used, or a PCI codec board may be installed into the system. If a live group session

Box 12.1 Advantages and Disadvantages of Teledentistry

Advantages

Reduces the cost of service and improves quality of care
Decreases peer isolation and increases specialist support and education
Diagnosis is done and treatment plan is developed without seeing the patient
Improved diagnostic services and integration of dentistry into a better healthcare delivery system
Better communication with insurance industry with respect to requirements

Disadvantages

A back-up communication system and technical support group are required
Proper Internet connection is mandatory for video conferencing
Privacy and security are important issues
Chance of misdiagnosis, due to technical problems occurring during data transfer, is higher; this can lead to a malpractice claim
Reimbursement of services provided through this means of care is limited

is desired, a multipoint control unit that bridges three or more parties is required. The codec must be able to accommodate audio and visual functions [14].

There is not a recommended list of equipment, hardware or software, for designing a teledental model. Factors taken into consideration while determining selection of technology and equipment for designing a teledental model may include budget, information technology infrastructure, networks, telecommunication services, data security, real-time video conferencing versus store-and-forward communication, and comfort with technology. For most dental applications, store-and-forward technology provides excellent results without excessive costs for equipment or connectivity.

Another important aspect of designing or choosing the model is the teledental application and imaging software. Components to consider when choosing such an application are dental records storage, dental billing, and appointment scheduling. Dental records storage allows the collection of data critical in the clinical management of patients, including patient charts and histories. Dental billing may be a factor in choice of software. The billing and revenue component of management software allows the management of patients' financial records. Appointment scheduling permits the management of appointments, and scheduling can be a part of the management software. The software is designed to track patients from the moment they are entered into the system and also keeps track of missed, rescheduled, and canceled appointments.

Modes of transferring information

POTS (plain old telephone system)

POTS is still commonly used in teledentistry because of its low maintenance and technical support costs. The real-time method transfers the information immediately, whereas the store-and-forward method allows data to be stored in a local database to be forwarded as needed. POTS works through the telephone company with low-speed and sometimes unreliable connection. Information exchange is also possible with the help of fax machine [15].

ISDN (integrated services digital network)

ISDN provides a higher speed, and information can travel in both directions simultaneously, which increases accessibility and reliability in teledentistry. But building an international ISDN network is too expensive and impractical [16]. The World Wide Web is popular tool for easy access of information [15].

Web-based teledentistry

Unlike ISDN, Web-based teledentistry does not require a special network, and hence it is more cost-effective. However, there are no rules on the Internet: there is no licensure and no verification, and there is little accountability. A Web-based network poses privacy and security concerns because of hackers and crackers. An ISDN network, on the other hand, is connected from one point to another with no network sharing. Live interactive videoconferencing can also be conducted via satellite.

Several programs on computerized dental services currently in use are [17]. Some are

- Fluoride probe
- Electromyography: the Procera system
- Digital dental radiology
- Electronic patient record system
- Intraoral camera and computer imaging

Networked programs link hospitals and clinics with outlying clinics and community health centers in rural or suburban areas by dedicated high-speed lines or the Internet. Point-to-point connections using private networks are used by hospitals and clinics that deliver services directly at ambulatory care sites.

Primary or specialty care to home connections involves connecting primary care providers, specialists, and home health nurses with patients using single-line phone video systems for interactive clinical consultations. Home-to-center monitoring links are used for patient monitoring, home care, and related services that provide care to patients in the home, using normal phone lines and Internet.

With the help of an EPR (electronic patient record) system, it is now possible to make or get cumulative data (a longitudinal record) of the patient from different dental clinics, which aids in diagnosis and in proper management of the patient. Data storage does not require much space, and there is less risk of damaging or losing data. Data retrieval also becomes easy and quick, and information is more legible [18].

The universal dental diagnostic coding system (SNODENT, Systematized Nomenclature of Dentistry) consists of diagnostic terms and terms describing symptoms, clinical signs and findings, radiographic observations, and related test findings. It can provide a basis for designing digital record forms for artificial intelligence to further assist the dental care provider in making more-accurate diagnostic decisions [19].

Dental-Consults is a Web-based teledentistry consultation system developed for use by dentists. The referring dentist logs into the secure Web server, fills in the patient's details, specific reasons for consultation, chief complaints, and provisional diagnosis information, and uploads intraoral images and dental radiographs. The specialist reviews the consult and suggests a diagnosis and treatment plan within five working days after receipt of the complete patient case. Further discussion, if required, is possible [20].

The Dental-Consults teledentistry system uses secure sockets layer (SSL) to encrypt the information that flows between the Web browser and the server receiving the referral. When the lock or solid key is visible, the browser has established a secure encrypted connection with the server, meaning it is safe to send sensitive data. Confidentiality comes with SSL during the transmission of a patient's information [6, 20–25].

Teledentistry in endodontics

Periapical lesions are the most common pathology faced by dentists. Any faults in differential diagnosis and prognosis of treatment of periapical lesions can cause complications, problems, and a waste of time and money. However, these lesions are not always treated by specialists. In this regard, modern technology systems help in seeking timely expert advice and formulating a treatment plan. With the use of teledentistry methods, diagnosis of periapical lesions can be adequately assessed, and a necessary plan can be devised for proper endodontic management of the lesions. The method includes digital information for each of tooth of interest. Distant consultants, specialist in endodontics, are informed via their mobile phones about the received request, after which they download the digital images and accompanying anamnestic data. They establish the diagnosis and suggest a treatment, then post this information on an online server, which informs the consultation-requester dentist about the received response [14]. Baker and colleagues (2000) demonstrated no statistically significant difference in the assessment of periapical lesions between the images viewed locally and those transmitted via a videoconferencing between systems and viewed on a monitor screen [26].

Concerns in the use of teledentistry

Legal issues

Largely still untested by law and with significant variation among countries, issues such as accountability, jurisdiction, liability, privacy, consent, and malpractice are crucial to consider when attempting to use this mode of communication. The medicolegal issue arises mainly owing to lack of any well-defined standards. Currently, there is no method to ensure safety, quality, efficiency, or effectiveness of information and its exchange. The most significant barrier to a nationwide teledentistry practice even in developed countries is the traditional system of state-by-state licensing [27]. In 2000, 20 states in the United States enforced strict licensure laws requiring teledentistry practitioners to obtain full licenses to practice across states [28].

Confidentiality

Patients should be made aware that their information is to be transmitted electronically and the possibility exists that the information may be intercepted, despite maximum efforts to maintain security. The form should contain the name of both the referring and consulting practitioners to ensure adequate coverage for malpractice, and the consulting doctor should acquire a copy of the informed consent before any form of patient contact is established.

Liability

Teledentistry raises concerns about liability. There is no law to clarify the role of the teleconsulting dentist and his or her liability [14]. The payment of the health care professional who provides teleconsultation has been a major issue in recent years. The National Rural Health Association has recommended reimbursement of care provided by teleconsultants, eliminating separate billing for telemedicine, increasing reimbursement for the originating telemedicine sites, and providing reimbursement for store-and-forward procedures [29].

In the United States, Medicare, federally qualified health centers, Medicaid, and California Children's Services are some of the payers for telemedicine reimbursement. Private insurances such as Blue Cross of California are also available for such care [30]. However, none of these programs that reimburse telemedical consultations have included teledental consultations as yet. Hence, payment remains a big question.

Future prospects

Healthcare is being changed dramatically by the use of computers and telecommunications. Teledentistry has not yet become an integral part of mainstream oral health care. In the near future, teledentistry will be just another way to access oral health care, especially for isolated populations who may have difficulty accessing the oral health care system due to distance, inability to travel, or lack of oral health care providers in their area.

Although Internet-based dentistry has taken precedence over other ways of communication, potential shortcomings still exist, such as necessity for proper training, an instant response, message misunderstanding, privacy concerns, and the possibility of overlooking or neglecting the messages. It is important that practitioners choosing to include this form of delivery of care educate themselves as to the legal, technological, and ethical issues associated with teledentistry. They must take the initiative to become up to date and comfortable with the technology they are using. The instructors in teledentistry education courses need to be well versed in computer knowledge.

Future advances in technology will enable teledentistry to be used in many more ways, such as clinical decision support, quality and safety assessment, consumer home use, medication e-prescribing, and simulation training. In spite of some issues that need to be resolved, the potential of teledentistry is tremendous in developing countries, and this potential needs to be explored.

References

1 Kuszler PC. Telemedicine and integrated health care delivery: compounding malpractice liability. *Am J Law Med* 1999; 25: 297–326.

2 Sanjeev M., Sushant GK. Teledentistry: a new trend in oral health. *Int J Clin Cases Invest* 2011; 2(6): 49–53.

3 Cook J. ISDN videoconferencing in postgraduate dental education and orthodontic diagnosis. Learning Technology in Medical Education Conference 1997 (CTI Medicine). 1997: 111–116.

4 Kopycka-Kedzierawski DT, Billings RJ. Teledentistry in inner-city child-care centers. *J TelemedTelecare* 2006; 12: 176–181.

5 Subramanyamvenkata R. Telepathology: virtually a reality. *J Oral Maxillofac Pathol* 2002; 1(1): 1–15.

6 Chen JW, Hobdell MH, Dunn K, Johnson KA, Zhang J. Teledentistry and its use in dental education. *J Am Dent Assoc* 2003; 134(3): 342–346.

7 Rocca MA, Kudryk VL, Pajak JC, Morris T. The evolution of a teledentistry system within the Department of Defense. *Proc AMIA Symp*1999: 921–924.

8 Baheti MJ, Bagrecha SD, Toshniwal NG, Misal A. Teledentistry: a need of the era. *Int J Dent Med Res* 2014; 1(2): 80–91.
9 Bhambal A, Saxena S, Balsaraf SV. Teledentistry: potentials unexplored. *J Int Oral Health* 2010; 2(3): 1–6.
10 Jain A, Bhaskar DJ, Gupta D, Agali C, Gupta V, Karim B. Teledentistry: upcoming trend in dentistry. *J Adv Med Dent Sci Res* 2013;1(2):112–115.
11 Bagchi S. Telemedicine in rural India. *PLoS Med* 2006; 3: 297–299.
12 Kirshner M. The role of information technology and informatics research in the dentist–patient relationship. *Adv Dent Res* 2003; 17: 77–81.
13 Liu SC. Information technology in family dentistry. *Hong Kong Dent J* 2006;3: 61–66.
14 Chang SW, Plotkin DR, Mulligan R, Polido JC, Mah JK, Meara JG. Teledentistry in rural California: a USC Initiative. *J Calif Dent Assoc* 2003; 31: 601–608.
15 Bauer JC,Brown WT.The digital transformation of oral health care. Teledentistry and electronic commerce. *J Am Dent Assoc* 2001; 132(2): 204–209.
16 Yoshinaga L. The use of teledentistry for remote learning applications. *Pract Proced Aesthet Dent* 2001; 13(4): 327–328.
17 Liu, SC-Y. Information technology in family dentistry. *Hong Kong Dent J* 2006; 3: 61–66.
18 Schleyer TK, Dasari VR. Computer-based oral health records on the World Wide Web. *Quintessence Int July* 1999; 30: 451–460.
19 Rose LF, Mealey BL. *Periodontics: medicine, surgery and implants*. 1st edition. St. Louis: Elsevier Mosby; 2004. pp. 163–171.
20 Clark GT. Teledentistry: what is it now and what will it be tomorrow? *J Calif Dental Assoc* 2000; 28: 121–127.
21 Teledentistry: e consultations. Dentistry Magazine Article Feb 9, 2002.
22 Alipour L, Rocca V, Kudryk, Morris T. A teledentistry consultation system and continuing dental education via Internet. *J Med Internet Res* 1999; 1 (suppl1): e110.
23 Sood SP, Bhatia JS. Development of telemedicine technology in India: "Sanjeevani"—an integrated telemedicine application. *J Postgrad Med* 2005; 51(4); 308–311.
24 Birnbach JM. The future of teledentistry. *J Calif Dent Assoc* 2000; 28: 141–143.
25 Stephens CD, Cook J. Attitudes of UK consultants to teledentistry as a means of providing orthodontic advice to dental practitioners and their patients. *J Orthod* 2002; 29(2): 137–142.
26 Baker WP 3rd,, Loushine RJ, West LA, Kudryk LV, Zadinsky JR. Interpretation of artificial and *in vivo* periapical bone lesions comparing conventional viewing versus a video conferencing system. *J Endod* 2000; 26(1): 39–41.
27 Sfikas M. Teledentistry: legal and regulatory issues explored. *J Am Dent Assoc*1997; 128: 1716–1718.
28 Golder DT, Brennan KA. Practicing dentistry in the age of telemedicine. *J Am Dent Assoc* 2000; 131: 734–744.
29 Hughes M, Bell M, Larson D, *Weens J*. Telehealth reimbursement. National Rural Health Association Policy Brief May 2010.
30 Telemedicine Reimbursement Handbook. California Telemedicine and eHealth Center. Sacramento, California; 2006.

Questions

1 Teledentistry is a synergistic combination with
A Telecommunication and Internet
B Teleradiology and telemedicine
C Telemedicine and consultation
D Internet and health records

2 Who was the first to define teledentistry?
A US Army
B Albert Jutra
C Cook
D Westinghouse Electronics System Group

3 The method in which dentist and patient can see, hear, and communicate with use of videoconference is called
A Remote monitoring method
B Store and forward method
C Near real-time consultation
D Real-time consultation

4 Which of the following is *not* true?
A Teledentistry reduces the cost of services and improves quality of care.
B Privacy and security is not an issue.
C Diagnosis and treatment planning can be done without seeing the patient.
D None of the above

5 Cook defined teledentistry as
A a. The practice of using videoconferencing technologies to diagnose and to provide advice about the treatment over a distance.
B b. A practice to eliminate disparities in oral health between rural and urban communities.
C c. The exchange of clinical information and images over remote distances.
D d. The combined use of telecommunication and computer technologies to improve health care services.

6 The US Army's Total Dental Access project used which of the following methods?
A ISDN
B Network programs
C Electronic patient record system
D POTS

7 ISDN stands for
A Integrated services dental network
B Integrated services digital network
C Integrated solar dental network
D Integrated solar digital network

8 Which of the following are the benefits of using teledentistry?
A Expansion of healthcare services to remote or rural areas
B Decrease in peer isolation and increase in specialist support
C Improved diagnostic services
D All the above

9 The exchange of clinical information and images that is collected and stored to be reviewed by a specialist later is called
A Remote-monitoring method
B Near real-time consultation
C Store-and-forward method
D Real-time consultation

10 Which of the following is a concern in teledentistry?
A Confidentiality
B Liability
C Legal issues
D All of the above

Quiz answers

Answers

Chapter 1

1 b
2 a
3 a
4 a
5 b
6 b
7 a
8 a
9 a
10 e

Chapter 2

1 a
2 e
3 a
4 c
5 d
6 a

Chapter 3

1 c
2 e
3 a
4 c
5 a
6 d
7 d
8 a
9 b
10 b

Chapter 4

1 b
2 d
3 d
4 c
5 a
6 b
7 c

Chapter 5

1 b
2 d
3 d
4 d
5 d
6 a
7 a
8 d
9 b

Chapter 6

1 c
2 b
3 c
4 b
5 d
6 b
7 e
8 a
9 b
10 c

Current Therapy in Endodontics, First Edition. Edited by Priyanka Jain.
© 2016 John Wiley & Sons, Inc. Published 2016 by John Wiley & Sons, Inc.

Chapter 7

1 a
2 a
3 c
4 b
5 a
6 c
7 d
8 a
9 e
10 d

Chapter 8

1 d
2 c
3 a
4 d
5 c
6 c
7 d
8 a
9 d
10 d

Chapter 9

1 a
2 a
3 c
4 d
5 b
6 a
7 c
8 d
9 a
10 d

Chapter 10

1 a
2 a
3 e
4 c
5 b
6 d
7 b
8 c
9 d
10 e

Chapter 11

1 b
2 c
3 d
4 a
5 d

Chapter 12

1 a
2 c
3 d
4 b
5 a
6 d
7 b
8 d
9 c
10 d

Index

Current Therapy in Endodontics, First Edition. Edited by Priyanka Jain.

© 2016 John Wiley & Sons, Inc. Published 2016 by John Wiley & Sons, Inc.

U

V

W

X

Z

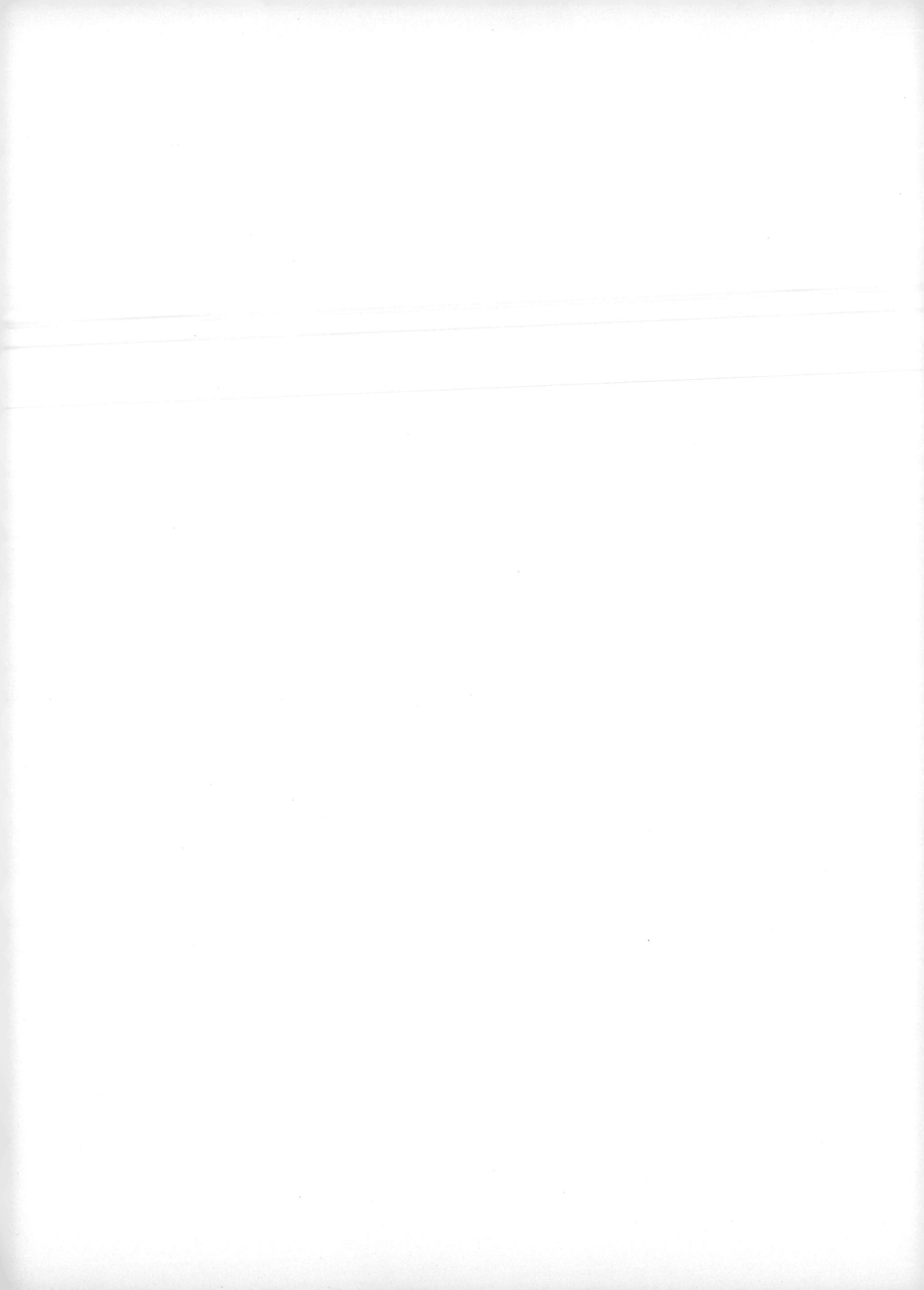